Natural Products for Cancer Prevention and Therapy

Natural Products for Cancer Prevention and Therapy

Special Issue Editors

Anupam Bishayee
Mukerrem Betul Yerer-Aycan

MDPI • Basel • Beijing • Wuhan • Barcelona • Belgrade

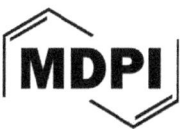

MDPI

Special Issue Editors

Anupam Bishayee
Larkin University
Miami, Florida, USA

Mukerrem Betul Yerer-Aycan
Erciyes University
Kayseri, Turkey

Editorial Office
MDPI
St. Alban-Anlage 66
Basel, Switzerland

This is a reprint of articles from the Special Issue published online in the open access journal *Nutrients* (ISSN 2072-6643) from 2017 to 2018 (available at: https://www.mdpi.com/journal/nutrients/special_issues/natural_products_cancer_prevention_therapy)

For citation purposes, cite each article independently as indicated on the article page online and as indicated below:

LastName, A.A.; LastName, B.B.; LastName, C.C. Article Title. *Journal Name* **Year**, *Article Number*, Page Range.

ISBN 978-3-03897-310-2 (Pbk)
ISBN 978-3-03897-311-9 (PDF)

Contents

About the Special Issue Editors

Anupam Bishayee's primary research interest during the last two decades encompasses natural products in health and disease, with special emphasis on cancer prevention and therapy. Dr. Bishayee's laboratory has been investigating the chemopreventive and therapeutic effects of various medicinal plants, natural products, dietary and synthetic agents using various pre-clinical models of cancer, and underlying cellular and molecular mechanisms of action. Dr. Bishayee has published more than 160 peer-reviewed original research papers and review articles, mostly in high-impact journals; 15 book chapters; and around 70 abstracts, as well as delivering more than 30 invited presentations at various national and international scientific meetings. Dr. Bishayee is serving as the editor-in-chief of the *Journal of Natural Products* in Cancer Prevention and Therapy, as well as being the editorial board member and reviewer of more than 60 reputed journals. Dr. Bishayee guest edited several Special Issues on natural products and cancer for high-impact journals.

Mukerrem Betul Yerer-Aycan is the head of the Pharmaceutical Sciences Division and Department of Pharmacology in Erciyes University, Faculty of Pharmacy, Kayseri Turkey. Dr. Yerer-Aycan served as the associate dean of the Faculty of Pharmacy for eight years. She is a pharmacist, and graduated from Hacettepe University, Ankara, Turkey. She has nearly 20 years of experience in the research and discovery of medications aimed to treat cancer and neurological disorders. Her laboratory is mainly focused on the cellular and molecular mechanisms of cell survival. She has several national and international grants and has been a member of various scientific societies. Notably, she has authored more than 30 manuscripts, as well as book chapters, and has served on the editorial board of several journals. She has presented as an invited speaker around 20 times at several national/international meetings and has been a guest editor for the journal Nutrients for a theme issue on natural products for cancer prevention and therapy.

Preface to "Natural Products for Cancer Prevention and Therapy"

Natural products represent an important source for the discovery and development of drugs for cancer prevention and therapy. Approximately 80% of all drugs approved by the United States Food and Drug Administration during the last three decades for cancer therapy are either natural products, per se, or are based on, or mimic, natural products. With the introduction and refinement of new technologies, including genetic tools for the production of secondary plant metabolites, combinatorial synthesis, and high-throughput assays, it is likely that novel compounds from natural sources, including medicinal plants and marine organisms, will be identified and developed as cancer preventive and anticancer drugs, with an acceptable toxicity. In this Special Issue book, contributions from eminent cancer researchers around the world present recent advances on our knowledge of natural products in cancer prevention and therapy.

This Special Issue book contains contributions from researchers working in the field of natural products in cancer prevention and therapy. We are working in the field of natural products and cancer. Several years ago, according to our experiences, we decided to organize an international conference series regarding the use of natural products for cancer prevention and treatment. Our aim was to gather researchers working in this field from all around the world, as many natural products are being used traditionally, and are also being prescribed as alternative medicines by physicians. Our first meeting was held in Istanbul between 31 August and 2 September 2015, along with the contributions of our invited speakers and the participants working in this field. With the success of our first meeting, we then organized our second meeting in Kayseri, between 8 and 11 November 2017. The abstracts of all of the presentations at our meeting were published in Proceedings, and the report of the meeting was published in Nutrients. Subsequently, we edited the Special Issue with the same topic, to include several full-length papers based on the presentations at the meeting, as well as on contributions from other scientists. We are indebted to those who have contributed to our Special Issue with their manuscripts, the reviewers, and the MDPI publishing group. We hope our Special Issue book will be considered a valuable source of new information on natural products in the cancer research field.

Anupam Bishayee and Mukerrem Betul Yerer-Aycan

Special Issue Editors

Conference Report

Report on Second International Conference on Natural Products for Cancer Prevention and Therapy Held in Kayseri, Turkey, 8–11 November 2017

Mükerrem Betül Yerer [1],* and Anupam Bishayee [2],*

[1] Department of Pharmacology, Faculty of Pharmacy, University of Erciyes, Kayseri 38039, Turkey
[2] Department of Pharmaceutical Sciences, College of Pharmacy, Larkin University, Miami, FL 33169, USA
* Correspondence: eczbetul@yahoo.com (M.B.Y.); abishayee@ularkin.org or abishayee@gmail.com (A.B.);
Tel.: +90-542-5322161 (M.B.Y.); +1-305-760-7511 (A.B.)

Received: 8 December 2017; Accepted: 21 December 2017; Published: 23 December 2017

1. Preface

Scientific experts from eight countries gathered to share their views and experience on the latest research on natural products for cancer prevention and therapy. The traditionally used herbal medicines, medicinal plants, plant extracts, fractions, and phytochemicals for cancer prevention and therapy were discussed throughout the meeting. The scientific program comprised of 12 plenary lectures, 23 oral presentations, and 72 posters, providing an opportunity for more than 130 natural product scientists to present their research in three days. Abstracts for plenary talks, oral presentations, and posters were published as proceedings of the meeting in the special issue of Proceedings, Volume 1 and Issue 10 (http://www.mdpi.com/2504-3900/1/10). The aim of this biannual meeting was to foster discussion and disseminate the results of the research on natural products that are used for cancer prevention and therapy. During the meeting, the scientific committee members of the meeting who attended the conference had been selected as judges to evaluate all of the oral and poster presentations and the three best oral and poster presentation awards have been granted to the young scientists. The participants were able to network and engage in discussion for potential collaboration to advance our knowledge on utility of natural products for prevention and treatment of cancer.

2. Summary of the Scientific Presentations

2.1. Plenary Lectures

The meeting was successfully focused on the natural products being investigated for their efficiency in several cancer types and for their potency in cancer prevention. Only the plenary lectures have been summarized here in this manuscript, and all of the other oral and poster presentations have been listed where the abstracts can be reached from http://www.mdpi.com/2504-3900/1/10.

2.1.1. Growth Factors Responsible from the Cancer Progress: Role of Natural Products

Mükerrem Betül Yerer

Growth factors are one of the main factors responsible from the uncontrolled cell progress in cancer. Up to date many scientists have focused on these factors either as the marker or as the targets in several cancer types. Yerer has presented a plenary lecture on the natural products targeting these factors (Nerve growth factor (NGF), epidermal growth factor (EGF), hepatocyte growth factors (HGF), fibroblast growth factors (FGF), vascular endothelial growth factors (VEGF), platelet derived growth factor (PDGF), and transforming growth factor (TGF-β) (http://www.mdpi.com/2504-3900/1/10/979) [1].

2.1.2. Natural Products for Cancer Prevention and Therapy: Progress, Pitfalls and Promise

Anupam Bishayee

The presentation of Bishayee highlighted studies on cancer preventive and therapeutic attributes of various naturally occurring agents and underlying mechanisms of action, with special emphasis on results reported from our laboratory. Current limitations, challenges, and future directions of research for successful cancer drug development based on natural products will also be discussed (http://www.mdpi.com/2504-3900/1/10/982) [2].

2.1.3. Novel Anticancer Capacities of Saffron

Amr Amin

Amr Amin has presented a plenary lecture on the anticancer effects of the saffron's main active ingredient "safranal" against HCC using in vitro, in silico, and network analyses. In their studies, in addition to the unique and differential cell cycle arrest, safranal showed pro-apoptotic effect through activation of both intrinsic and extrinsic initiator caspases implicating ER stress-mediated apoptosis (http://www.mdpi.com/2504-3900/1/10/834) [3].

2.1.4. Cardiac Glycosides as Novel Modulators of Cancer Cell Survival

Marc Diederich

This plenary lecture focused on Cardiac Glycosides (GCs) can be considered as pharmacological agents, allowing for cancer cells to switch from one cell death modality to another. All the findings encourage to further explore a potential for CGs in general as cancer cell death modulators alone or in combination with other targeted treatments (http://www.mdpi.com/2504-3900/1/10/972) [4].

2.1.5. Ins and Outs of Flavonoids in Cancer Prevention vs. Cancer Therapy: A Lesson from Quercetin in Leukemia

Gian Luigi Russo, Maria Russo, Carmela Spagnuolo, Idolo Tedesco, Stefania Moccia

Russo et al. has critically reviewed the clinical and pre-clinical studies on the concept that polyphenols, being antioxidant compounds, can fight cancer. They suggest that a clear distinction must be done between the use of polyphenols, such as flavonoids, in cancer treatment versus cancer prevention, starting from adequate and specifically selected cellular models. As an example, he has present data on the potential application of quercetin against chronic lymphocytic leukemia (CLL) (http://www.mdpi.com/2504-3900/1/10/977) [5].

2.1.6. Anticancer Potential of Flavones

Randolph RJ Arroo, Didem Şöhretoğlu, Demetrios A Spandidos, Vasilis P Androutsopoulos

Flavones are abundantly present in common fruits and vegetables, many of which have been associated with cancer prevention. Taking into account that no flavonoid based drugs are clinically used in cancer therapy, Randolph has focused on the flavones—which constitute a subgroup of the flavonoids—show some structural analogy with estrogen, and are known to interact with human estrogen receptors, either as agonist or as antagonist. Thus, whereas epidemiological and pre-clinical data seem to indicate a high potential for flavonoids, from the point of view of the pharmaceutical industry and drug developers, they are considered poor candidates (http://www.mdpi.com/2504-3900/1/10/975) [6].

2.1.7. Resveratrol in Cancer Prevention and Treatment: Focusing on Molecular Targets and Mechanism of Action

Adriano Borriello

The relevance of these mechanisms and their translation in clinical therapy has been discussed in Borelli's plenary lecture. Resveratrol and its mechanism of action has been emphasized by her in cancer cells and in experimental models of senescence, inflammation, obesity, and metabolic diseases. Its molecular targets act at different levels: (1) specific molecular pathways (like p53, NF-kappaB, PKC, PI3K, MDM2, LATS1, STK3 and several others); (2) epigenetic control of gene transcription through sirtuin activation; (3) cell division cycle and differentiation; (4) apoptosis and autophagy; and, (5) cellular redox homeostasis (http://www.mdpi.com/2504-3900/1/10/976) [7].

2.1.8. Cynaropicrin: A Promising Natural Agent with Antitumor and Antiviral Activities

Mahmoud F. Elsebai, Jukka Hakkola, Mohamed Mehiri, Juana Diez

Human infection with HCV is currently recognized as the leading cause of hepatocellular carcinoma (HCC), which demands liver transplantation, which was estimated to result in ~10,000 deaths in the US only in the year 2011. Elsebai has presented a plenary lecture on cynaropicrin as a potential agent for treatment and prevention of HCC by indirect way through inhibition of HCV and in a direct way evidenced by the many antitumor activities in literature (http://www.mdpi.com/2504-3900/1/10/974) [8].

2.1.9. Relationship between Structure of Phenolics and Anticancer Activity

Müberra Koşar

Many phenolic compounds have been investigated for their potential use as cancer chemopreventive agents. Phenolic compounds consist of one or more hydroxyl substitution on the aromatic ring system. Koşar has emphasized that Cinnamic acid esters, such as caffeic acid phenethyl and benzyl esters, display selective antiproliferative activity against some types of cancer cells. Flavonoids consist of a large group of polyphenolic compounds having a benzo-γ-pyrone structure, and are ubiquitously present in plants. This structure can be responsible from the anticancer acitvities of these compounds (http://www.mdpi.com/2504-3900/1/10/978) [9].

2.1.10. Pristimerin is a Promising Natural Product against Breast Cancer In Vitro and In Vivo through Apoptosis and the Blockage of Autophagic Flux

Buse Cevatemre, Konstantinos Dimas, Bruno Botta and Engin Ulukaya

Ulukaya has given a lecture on the pristimerin's cytotoxic potential on particularly cancer stem cells (CSCs) should be much more important due to the CSCs' recent role in recurrence of cancer. He has presented their studies on Pristimerin that has been shown to suppress the proliferation of various cancer cell lines at relatively lower concentrations, of which, the IC50 values are around 0.5–4 μM (http://www.mdpi.com/2504-3900/1/10/973) [10].

2.1.11. Can Curcumin Be Employed to Promote the Integration of Oncology and Natural Products?

Mutlu Demiray and Fatemeh Bahadori

Curcumin is multi-targeted molecule with pleotropic nature, which inhibits NF-κB and related proteins promoting effectiveness of tyrosine kinase inhibitors (TKIs). Demiray has presented their clinical studies with curcumin on adenoid cystic carcinoma where they have treated patients for 72 months by oral curcumin and eight months by i.v curcumin. Disease control rate was 89.3% (15/17), and no any grade III-IV toxicities was observed related to curcumin reflecting the clinical use of curcumin on adenoid cystic carcinoma patients (http://www.mdpi.com/2504-3900/1/10/980) [11].

2.1.12. Therapeutic Potential of Black Pepper Compound for BRaf Resistant Melanoma

Neel M. Fofaria, Sharavan Ramachandran, and Sanjay K. Srivastava

Srivastava's presentation mainly focused on the combination of BRAF inhibitors with Mcl-1 inhibitor such as piperlongumine may have therapeutic advantage to melanoma patients with acquired resistance to BRAF inhibitors alone or in combination with MEK1/2 inhibitors (http://www.mdpi.com/2504-3900/1/10/981) [12].

2.2. Oral and Poster Presentations

Oral Presentations		
Title	Authors	Link
Effect of Pomegranate Extract and Tangeretin on Specific Pathways in the Rat Breast Cancer Model Induced with DMBA [13].	H. Fatih Gul et al.	http://www.mdpi.com/2504-3900/1/10/983
Synergistic Cytotoxic Effects of Resveratrol in Combination with Ceramide Metabolizing Enzymes in Ph + Acute Lymphoblastic Leukemia [14].	Osman Oğuz et al.	http://www.mdpi.com/2504-3900/1/10/984
Characterization of cycloartane-type sapogenol derivatives for prostate cancer chemoprevention [15].	Bilge Debelec-Butuner et al.	http://www.mdpi.com/2504-3900/1/10/985
Epibrassinolide treatment caused autophagy or apoptosis decision in a time-dependent manner through ER stress in colon cancer cells [16].	Pınar Obakan-Yerlikaya et al.	http://www.mdpi.com/2504-3900/1/10/986
Determination of Silymarin molecule activity in colon cancer by AgNOR technique [17].	Merve Alpay et al.	http://www.mdpi.com/2504-3900/1/10/987
The cytotoxic effect of *Lysimachia savranii* on the neuroblastoma cells [18].	Gonca Dönmez et al.	http://www.mdpi.com/2504-3900/1/10/988
Autocrine Growth Hormone-triggered curcumin resistance abolished by NF-κB signaling pathway dependent on inflammatory cytokines and active polyamine catabolic machinery in MCF-7, MDA-MB-453 and MDA-MB-231 breast cancer cells [19].	Ajda Çoker Gürkan et al.	http://www.mdpi.com/2504-3900/1/10/989
The effect of *Lysimachia savranii* on the migration of the breast cancer cells [20].	Işıl Aydemir et al.	http://www.mdpi.com/2504-3900/1/10/990
Investigation of cytotoxic effect of *Origanum minutiflorum* on cancer cells [21].	Oktay Özkan et al.	http://www.mdpi.com/2504-3900/1/10/991
Celastrol modulates lipid synthesis via PI3K/Akt/mTOR signaling axis to finalize cell death response in prostate cancer cells [22].	Elif Damla Arisan et al.	http://www.mdpi.com/2504-3900/1/10/992

Oral Presentations		
Title	**Authors**	**Link**
Investigation of the Effect of Paclitaxel and Pycnogenol on Mitochondrial Dynamics in Breast Cancer Therapy [23].	Suna Saygılı et al.	http://www.mdpi.com/2504-3900/1/10/993
Effects of curcumin on lipid peroxidation and antioxidant enzymes in kidney, liver, brain and testis of mice bearing Ehrlich Solid Tumor [24].	Mustafa Nisari et al.	http://www.mdpi.com/2504-3900/1/10/994
Curcumin enhances the efficacy of 5-FU in Colo205 cell lines [25].	Ebru Öztürk et al.	http://www.mdpi.com/2504-3900/1/10/995
Effect of a New Sapogenol Derivative (AG-07) on Cell Death via Necrosis [26].	Yalcin Erzurumlu et al.	http://www.mdpi.com/2504-3900/1/10/996
Cytotoxic and Antiinflammatory Activity Guided Studies on *Plantago holosteum* Scop [27].	Yasin Genc et al.	http://www.mdpi.com/2504-3900/1/10/997
Continuously monitoring the cytotoxicity of API-1, α-chaconine and α-solanine on human lung carcinoma A549 [28].	Ebru Öztürk et al.	http://www.mdpi.com/2504-3900/1/10/998
The effects of α-chaconine on ER-α positive endometrium cancer cells [29].	Ayşe Kübra Karaboğa Arslan et al.	http://www.mdpi.com/2504-3900/1/10/999
Investigation of apoptotic effect of sinapic acid in Hep3B and HepG2 human hepatocellular carcinoma cells [30].	Canan Eroğlu et al.	http://www.mdpi.com/2504-3900/1/10/1000
Cytotoxic and Antioxidant Activity of four *Cousinia* Species of Stenocephalae Bunge. Section [31].	Leyla Paşayeva et al.	http://www.mdpi.com/2504-3900/1/10/1001
Apoptotic effect of Ginnalin A on MDA-MB-231 and MCF7 human breast cancer cell lines [32].	Ebru Avcı et al.	http://www.mdpi.com/2504-3900/1/10/1002
Cytotoxic effects of coumarin compounds imperatorin and osthole, alone and in combination with 5-fluorouracil in colon carcinoma cells [33].	Ayşe Eken et al.	http://www.mdpi.com/2504-3900/1/10/1003
Screening of some Apiaceae and Asteraceae plants for their cytotoxic potential [34].	Perihan Gürbüz et al.	http://www.mdpi.com/2504-3900/1/10/1004
Cyclodextrine Based Nanogels and Phase Solubility Studies of Flurbiprofen as a Chemopreventive Agent [35].	Ayşe Nur Oktay et al.	http://www.mdpi.com/2504-3900/1/10/1005
Poster Presentations		
Effect of a synthesized compound against cancerous cell line and synthesis of copper ion incorporated 1-(3,4-diaminophenyl) ethanone-based hybrid nanoflowers [36].	Burcu Somtürk Yılmaz et al.	http://www.mdpi.com/2504-3900/1/10/1006
Development of effective anticancer drug candidates against breast and colon cancers [37].	Senem Akkoç et al.	http://www.mdpi.com/2504-3900/1/10/1007

Poster Presentations		
Title	**Authors**	**Link**
Synthesis of copper ion incorporated aminoguanidine derivatives-based hybrid nanoflowers [38].	Sevtap Çağlar Yavuz et al.	http://www.mdpi.com/2504-3900/1/10/1008
Evaluation of anti-proliferative and cytotoxic properties of chlorogenic acid against breast cancer cell lines by real time monitoring [39].	Onur Bender et al.	http://www.mdpi.com/2504-3900/1/10/1009
Investigation of Apoptotic Effects of Usnic Acid on Hepatocellular Carcinoma [40].	Beste Yurdacan et al.	http://www.mdpi.com/2504-3900/1/10/1010
In vitro Cytotoxic Effect Evaluation of *Dioscorea communis* (L.) Caddick & Wilkin Rhizome and Stem Extracts on Hepatocellular Carcinoma Cells [41].	Ünal Egeli et al.	http://www.mdpi.com/2504-3900/1/10/1011
The Effect of Herbal Medicine on Neuroblastoma Cell Line in Culture [42].	Büşra Şen et al.	http://www.mdpi.com/2504-3900/1/10/1012
The foods containing miR-193b may inhibit the growth of breast cancer cells [43].	Dilek Asci Celik et al.	http://www.mdpi.com/2504-3900/1/10/1013
Is the dietary miR-193b a novel cell cycle arresting source for breast carcinoma? [44].	Nilgun Gurbuz et al.	http://www.mdpi.com/2504-3900/1/10/1014
The effects of Wortmannin and EGCG and combined treatments on MDA-MB-231 breast cancer cell lines via inactivation of PI3K signaling pathway [45].	Elgin Turkoz Uluer et al.	http://www.mdpi.com/2504-3900/1/10/1015
The effects of Paclitaxel and Metformin and combined treatments on TLR signaling pathway on MDA-MB-231 breast cancer cell lines [46].	Melike Ozgul et al.	http://www.mdpi.com/2504-3900/1/10/1016
Inhibition of telomerase activity by cucurbitacin I in colon cancer cell line, LS174T [47].	Emir Tosun et al.	http://www.mdpi.com/2504-3900/1/10/1017
Effect of cucurbitacin I on proliferation and migration in colorectal cancer cell line, LS174T [48].	Emir Tosun et al.	http://www.mdpi.com/2504-3900/1/10/1018
In vitro anticancer and cytotoxic activities of some plant extracts on HeLa and Vero cell lines [49].	Fulya Tugba Artun et al.	http://www.mdpi.com/2504-3900/1/10/1019
Anticancer Effects of Oleocanthal and *Pinus Pinaster* on Breast Cancer Cell in Culture [50].	Mahmud Özkut et al.	http://www.mdpi.com/2504-3900/1/10/1020
Antiproliferative and Apoptotic Effects of the Medicinal Plants on Breast Cancer Cell Lines [51].	Pınar Kılıçaslan Sönmez et al.	http://www.mdpi.com/2504-3900/1/10/1021
The role of trophoblastic stem cells conditioned media on JAR cell culture [52].	Hilal Kabadayı et al.	http://www.mdpi.com/2504-3900/1/10/1022
The effect of pycnogenol and paclitaxel on DNA damage in human breast cancer cell line [53].	Hülya Birinci et al.	http://www.mdpi.com/2504-3900/1/10/1023

Poster Presentations		
Title	**Authors**	**Link**
Investigation of the effects of paclitaxel and pycnogenol on inflammatory response (PTX3, BDNF, IGF2R) in human breast cancer cell line [54].	Hülya Birinci et al.	http://www.mdpi.com/2504-3900/1/10/1024
Is There Any Protective Effect of Pomegranate and Tangeretin on the DMBA-Induced Rat Breast Cancer Model? [55].	H. Fatih Gul et al.	http://www.mdpi.com/2504-3900/1/10/1025
The neurotoxic effects of *Origanum minutiflorum* [56].	İsmail Sari et al.	http://www.mdpi.com/2504-3900/1/10/1026
The Cytotoxic and Apoptotic Effects of Usnic Acid on Prostate Cancer versus Normal Cells [57].	Işıl Ezgi Eryılmaz et al.	http://www.mdpi.com/2504-3900/1/10/1027
Antiproliferative Effect of Methanolic Extract of *Linum arboretum* on A549 Cells [58].	Ozgur Vatan et al.	http://www.mdpi.com/2504-3900/1/10/1028
Investigation of *in vitro* Cytotoxic Effects of *Montivipera xanthina* on Healthy and Cancer Human Lung Cell Lines [59].	Huzeyfe Huriyet et al.	http://www.mdpi.com/2504-3900/1/10/1029
Development and Characterization of Paclitaxel-loaded PLGA Nanoparticles and Evaluation of Cytotoxicity on MCF-7 cell line by MTT Assay [60].	Merve Çelik Tekeli et al.	http://www.mdpi.com/2504-3900/1/10/1030
Effects of Fulvic Acid on Different Cancer Cell Lines [61].	S. Kerem Aydin et al.	http://www.mdpi.com/2504-3900/1/10/1031
Antioxidant, antibacterial and antiproliferative activities of Turkish rhubarb (*Rheum palmatum* L.) leaf extracts [62].	Mehmet Berköz et al.	http://www.mdpi.com/2504-3900/1/10/1032
The Effect of Herbal Medicine on Colon Cancer Cells in Culture [63].	Pelin Toros et al.	http://www.mdpi.com/2504-3900/1/10/1033
The Effect of Herbal Medicine on Prostate Cancer Cells in Culture [64].	Pelin Toro et al.	http://www.mdpi.com/2504-3900/1/10/1034
Determination of Antioxidant Capacity, Phenolic Acid Composition and Antiproliferative Effect Associated with Phenylalanine Ammonia Lyase (PAL) Activity in Some Plants Naturally Growing under Salt Stress [65].	Seda Şirin et al.	http://www.mdpi.com/2504-3900/1/10/1035
Development and Characterization of Paclitaxel-loaded PLGA Nanoparticles and Cytotoxicity Assessment by MTT assay on A549 cell line [66].	Sedaf Ünal et al.	http://www.mdpi.com/2504-3900/1/10/1036
Evaluation of in vitro anti-proliferative activity of St. John's wort (*Hypericum perforatum* Linn.) plant extract on cervix adenocarcinoma [67].	Rana Kavurmacı et al.	http://www.mdpi.com/2504-3900/1/10/1037
The cytotoxic effect of *Annona muricata* leaf extract on triple negative breast cancer cell line [68].	Rana Kavurmacı et al.	http://www.mdpi.com/2504-3900/1/10/1038

Poster Presentations		
Title	**Authors**	**Link**
Cytotoxic activity of *Achillea coarctata* Poir. Extract [69].	Sevil Albayrak et al.	http://www.mdpi.com/2504-3900/1/10/1039
Cytotoxic activity of Endemic *Astragalus argaeus* Boiss. from Turkey [70].	Sevil Albayrak et al.	http://www.mdpi.com/2504-3900/1/10/1040
Lactic Acid Bacteria Mediated Apoptosis Induction: Natural way of colon cancer cells' inhibition [71].	Şebnem Kurhan et al.	http://www.mdpi.com/2504-3900/1/10/1041
Synthesized a new organic compound's cytotoxic activity quantum mechanics calculations and docking studies [72].	Senem Akkoç et al.	http://www.mdpi.com/2504-3900/1/10/1042
Anticancer Activity of *Centaurea babylonica* L. [73].	Elif Dündar et al.	http://www.mdpi.com/2504-3900/1/10/1043
Cytotoxic Effects of Functional Foods *Momordica charantia* L. and *Lycium barbarum* L. Extracts on Prostate Cancer Cells [74].	Guzide Satir Basaran et al.	http://www.mdpi.com/2504-3900/1/10/1044
Cytotoxic Effects of Kynurenic acid and Quinaldic acid in Hepatocellular Carcinoma (HepG2) cell line [75].	Pınar Atalay Dündar et al.	http://www.mdpi.com/2504-3900/1/10/1045
The Effects of Benzoxasol Derivate Compounds in Breast Cancer Cells [76].	Funda Kosova et al.	http://www.mdpi.com/2504-3900/1/10/1046
Potential Cytotoxic Activity of *Psephellus pyrrhoblepharus* Extracts [77].	Pelin Taştan et al.	http://www.mdpi.com/2504-3900/1/10/1047
Screening of *Onosma* species for Cytotoxic Activity [78].	Özge Güzel et al.	http://www.mdpi.com/2504-3900/1/10/1048
Apoptotic Effects of *Mount Bulgar Viper (Montivipera bulgardaghica)* PLA2 and SVMPs Venom Peptide fractions on HeLa and A549 Cancer Cells [79].	Yalcin Erzurumlu et al.	http://www.mdpi.com/2504-3900/1/10/1049
Turkish Propolis Extract Increases Apoptosis via Induction of Mitochondrial Membrane Potential Loss in MCF-7 Cells [80].	Sema Misir et al.	http://www.mdpi.com/2504-3900/1/10/1050
The Effect of Gilaburu (*Viburnum opulus*) Juice on Ehrlich Ascites Tumor (EAT) Cell Culture [81].	Özge Al et al.	http://www.mdpi.com/2504-3900/1/10/1051
Synthesis and characterizations of folate-conjugated PLGA-PEG nanoparticles loaded with dual agents [82].	Yüksel Öğünç et al.	http://www.mdpi.com/2504-3900/1/10/1052
Selective cytotoxic activity of *Scutellaria* species [83].	Zeynep Dogan et al.	http://www.mdpi.com/2504-3900/1/10/1053
The Antiproliferative Effect of Alpha Tocopherol in F98 Cell Culture [84].	Remzi Soner Cengiz et al.	http://www.mdpi.com/2504-3900/1/10/1054
Analysis of the Cytotoxic Effects of *Eryngium billardieri* Delar. Extracts on MCF7 Cell Line [85].	Leyla Paşayeva et al.	http://www.mdpi.com/2504-3900/1/10/1055
Cytotoxic Effects of *Alchemilla mollis* (Buser) Rothm. Extracts on MCF 7 cell line [86].	Selen İlgün et al.	http://www.mdpi.com/2504-3900/1/10/1056

Poster Presentations		
Title	**Authors**	**Link**
Comparative Evaluation of the cytotoxic effects of stem and flower extracts of *Rhaponticoides iconiensis* (Hub.-Mor.) M.V.Agab. & Greuter [87].	Eren Demirpolat et al.	http://www.mdpi.com/2504-3900/1/10/1057
Goji berry fruit extract suppresses cell proliferation of breast cancer cells by inhibiting EGFR/ERK signaling [88].	Hatice Bekci et al.	http://www.mdpi.com/2504-3900/1/10/1058
Biologically transformed Propolis Exhibits Cytotoxic Effect on A375 Malignant Melanoma Cells in vitro [89].	Hikmet Memmedov et al.	http://www.mdpi.com/2504-3900/1/10/1059
Rheum ribes extract increase the expression level of miR-200 family in human colorectal cancer cells [90].	Ilknur Cinar et al.	http://www.mdpi.com/2504-3900/1/10/1060
Potential effects of *Liquidambar orientalis* Mill. against HT-29 and HCT-116 cell lines [91].	Sumeyra Cetinkaya et al.	http://www.mdpi.com/2504-3900/1/10/1061
The Effect of Tocopherol-α On the Cell Viability in Caco-2 Cell Line [92].	Ayşenur Gök et al.	http://www.mdpi.com/2504-3900/1/10/1062
In vitro Antioxidant and Anticancer Activities of Some Local Plants from Bolu Province of Turkey [93].	Kadriye Nur Kasapoğlu et al.	http://www.mdpi.com/2504-3900/1/10/1063
Survey of the apoptotic effect of Ginnalin A on Hep3B human hepatocellular carcinoma cell line [94].	Pınar Özden et al.	http://www.mdpi.com/2504-3900/1/10/1064
Ameliorative effects of Carvacrol on Cyclophosphamide-induced testis damage and oxidative stress [95].	Mustafa Cengiz et al.	http://www.mdpi.com/2504-3900/1/10/1066
Synthesis of Anthocyanin-rich Red Cabbage Nanoflowers and Their Antimicrobial and Cytotoxic Properties [96].	Suheyl Furkan Konca et al.	http://www.mdpi.com/2504-3900/1/10/1067
Cytotoxic potentials of some Asteraceae plants from Turkey on HeLa cell line [97].	Kübra Uzun et al.	http://www.mdpi.com/2504-3900/1/10/1068
The Role of Lidocaine in the Dunning Model Rat Prostate Cancer Cells: Cell Kinetics and Motility [98].	Esma Purut et al.	http://www.mdpi.com/2504-3900/1/10/1069
Pelargonium endlicherianum Fenzl. Root extract suppresses cell proliferation of prostate cancer cells [99].	Selda Eren et al.	http://www.mdpi.com/2504-3900/1/10/1070
Assessment of antioxidant and cytotoxic activity of known antioxidants compared to neopterin [100].	Gözde Girgin et al.	http://www.mdpi.com/2504-3900/1/10/1071
Comparison of radical scavenging and cytotoxic activities of well-known non-enzymatic antioxidants [101].	Suna Sabuncuoğlu et al.	http://www.mdpi.com/2504-3900/1/10/1072
A Study on the Synthesis and Anticancer Activities of Novel 6-Methoxy Flavonyl Piperazine Derivatives [102].	Meltem Ceylan-Ünlüsoy et al.	http://www.mdpi.com/2504-3900/1/10/1073

Poster Presentations		
Title	**Authors**	**Link**
Effect of Paclitaxel Loaded Chitosan Nanoparticles and Quantum Dots on Breast Cancer [103].	Gülen Melike Demir et al.	http://www.mdpi.com/2504-3900/1/10/1074
Turkish Medicinal Plants Used in Cancer Treatment and Evaluation of Plant Usage in the Oncology Clinic of the İstanbul University Faculty of Medicine [104].	Büşra Teke et al.	http://www.mdpi.com/2504-3900/1/10/1075
Is Acteosid Effects on Colon Cancer Stem Cells Via Inflamation and/or Apoptosis? [105].	Fatma Firat et al.	http://www.mdpi.com/2504-3900/1/10/1076
Analysis of the Cytotoxic Effects of *Achillea millefolium* L. Extracts on MCF7 Cell Line [106].	Esra Köngül et al.	http://www.mdpi.com/2504-3900/1/10/1077

3. Author Affiliations

- Abdurrahim Kocyigit, Department of Medical Biochemistry, Faculty of Medicine, Bezmialem Vakif University, Sarıyer, Turkey
- Ademi Fahri Pirhan, Department of Biology, Faculty of Science, Ege University, Izmir, Turkey
- Adnan Ayhanci, Biology Department, Art and Science Faculty, Eskişehir Osmangazi University, Eskişehir, Turkey
- Adriana Borriello, Department of Biochemistry, Biophysics and General Pathology, University of Campania "L. Vanvitelli", Naples, Italy
- Ahmet Baysar, Department of Chemical Engineering, Inonu University, Malatya, Turkey
- Ahmet Cumaoglu, Department of Biochemistry, Faculty of Pharmacy, Erciyes University, Kayseri, Turkey
- Ahmet Savran, Department of Arts and Sciences, Faculty of Medicine, Niğde Ömer Halisdemir University, Niğde, Turkey
- Ajda Çoker-Gürkan, Department of Molecular Biology and Genetics, Istanbul Kultur University, Atakoy Campus, Istanbul, Turkey
- Ali Karagoz, Department of Molecular Biology and Genetics, Faculty of Science, Istanbul University, Istanbul, Turkey
- Amr Amin, Biology Department, UAE University, Abu Dhabi, United Arab Emirates
- Anupam Bishayee, Department of Pharmaceutical Sciences, College of Pharmacy, Larkin University, Miami, FL, USA
- Arzu Atalay, Biotechnology Institute, Ankara University, Ankara, Turkey
- Asuman Bozkir, Department of Pharmaceutical Technology, Faculty of Pharmacy, Ankara University, Ankara, Turkey
- Ayhan Altıntaş, Department of Pharmacognosy, Faculty of Pharmacy, Anadolu University, Eskişehir, Turkey
- Aynur Işık, Department of Molecular Biology and Genetics, Faculty of Science, Gazi University, Ankara, Turkey
- Ayse Baldemir, Department of Pharmaceutical botany, Faculty of Pharmacy, Erciyes University, Kayseri, Turkey
- Ayse Nalbantsoy, Department of Bioengineering, Faculty of Engineering, Ege University, Izmir, Turkey
- Aysun Adan, Molecular Biology and Genetics, Faculty of Life and Natural Sciences, Abdullah Gul University, Kayseri, Turkey

- Aysun Ökçesiz, Department of Pharmaceutical Toxicology, Faculty of Pharmacy, Erciyes University, Kayseri, Turkey
- Ayşe Eken, Department of Pharmaceutical Toxicology, Faculty of Pharmacy, Erciyes University, Kayseri, Turkey
- Ayşe Kübra Karaboğa Arslan, Department of Pharmacology, Faculty of Pharmacy, Erciyes University, Kayseri, Turkey
- Ayşe Nur Oktay, Department of Pharmaceutical Technology, Faculty of Pharmacy, Gazi University, Ankara, Turkey
- Ayşe Zeynep Ünal, Toxicology Department, Faculty of Pharmacy, Hacettepe University, Ankara, Turkey
- Ayşenur Gök, Ankara University, Faculty of Veterinary Medicine, Ankara, Turkey
- Basseem Radwan, Department of Pharmacology, Faculty of Pharmacy, Erciyes University, Kayseri, Turkey
- Bayram Goçmen, Zoology Section, Department of Biology, Faculty of Science, Ege University, Izmir, Turkey
- Belma Aslım, Gazi University, Faculty of Science, Department of Biology, Teknikokullar, Ankara, Turkey
- Benjamin-Florian Hempel, Institut für Chemie, Technische Universitat Berlin, Strasse des 17. Juni 124, Berlin, Germany
- Beraat Özçelik, Department of Food Engineering, Faculty of Chemical and Metallurgical Enginerring, Istanbul Technical University, Turkey
- Berrin Tunca, Medical Biology Department, Faculty of Medicine, Uludag University, Bursa, Turkey
- Beste Yurdacan, Medical Biology Department, Faculty of Medicine, Uludag University, Gorukle, Bursa, Turkey
- Bijen Kıvçak, Deparment of Pharmacognosy, Faculty of Pharmacy, Ege University, İzmir, Turkey
- Bilge Debelec-Butuner, Department of Pharmaceutical Biotechnology, Faculty of Pharmacy, Ege University, Izmir, Turkey
- Bruno Botta, Dipartimento di Chimica e Tecnologie del Farmaco, Sapienza University of Roma, piazzale Aldo Moro 5, Roma, Italy
- Burak Durmaz, Department of Medical Biochemistry, Ege University, Turkey
- Burcu Somtürk Yılmaz, Department of Chemistry, Faculty of Sciences, Erciyes University, Kayseri, Turkey
- Burçin Türkmenoğlu, Department of Chemistry, Faculty of Sciences, Erciyes University, Kayseri, Turkey
- Buse Cevatemre, Department of Biology, Faculty of Arts and Sciences, Uludag University, Bursa, Turkey
- Büşra Şen, Department of Histology and Embryology, Faculty of Medicine, Celal Bayar University, Manisa, Turkey
- Büşra Teke, Faculty of Pharmacy, İstanbul University, Istanbul, Turkey
- Canan Eroğlu, Department of Medical Biology, Meram Faculty of Medicine, Necmettin Erbakan University, Konya, Turkey
- Canan Türkoğlu, Department of Biology, Faculty of Art and Life Sciences, Manisa Celal Bayar University, Manisa, Turkey
- Carmela Spagnuolo, Institute of Food Sciences, National Research Council, Avellino, Italy
- Çiğdem Yücel, Erciyes University Faculty of Pharmacy Department of Pharmaceutical Technology
- Damla Akogullari, Faculty of Medicine, Department of Histology & Embryology, Manisa Celal Bayar University, Manisa, Turkey

- Daniel Petras, Institut für Chemie, Technische Universitat Berlin, Strasse des 17. Juni 124, Berlin, Germany
- Demetrios A. Spandidos, Department of Toxicology, Medical School, University of Crete, Crete GR, Greece
- Didar Tasdemir, Department of Analytical Chemistry, Faculty of Pharmacy, Erciyes University, Kayseri, Turkey
- Didem Şöhretoğlu, Faculty of Pharmacy, Hacettepe Unıversıty, Ankara, Turkey
- Dilek Asci Celik, Department of Medical Biology, School of Medicine, Suleyman Demirel University, Isparta, Turkey
- Dilek Ceylan, Genome and Stem Cell Center, University of Erciyes, Kayseri, Turkey
- Ebru Avcı, Department of Medical Biology, Meram Faculty of Medicine, Necmettin Erbakan University, Konya, Turkey
- Ebru Öztürk, Department of Pharmacology, Faculty of Pharmacy, Erciyes University, Kayseri, Turkey
- Efe Kurtdede, Ankara, Turkey
- Elgin Turkoz Uluer, Department of Histology & Embryology, Faculty of Medicine, Manisa Celal Bayar University, Manisa, Turkey
- Elif Damla Arısan, Department of Molecular Biology and Genetics, Istanbul Kultur University, Atakoy Campus, Istanbul, Turkey
- Elif Dündar, Department of Pharmaceutical Botany, Graduate School of Health Sciences, Anadolu University, Eskişehir, Turkey
- Emin Sarıpınar, Department of Chemistry, Faculty of Sciences, Erciyes University, Kayseri, Turkey
- Emine Akalın Uruşak, Faculty of Pharmacy, İstanbul University, Istanbul, Turkey
- Emir Tosun, Department of Chemical Engineering, Inonu University, Malatya, Turkey
- Engin Ulukaya, Department of Clinical Biochemistry, Faculty of Medicine, Istinye University, Istanbul, Turkey
- Ercan Kurar, Department of Medical Biology, Meram Faculty of Medicine, Necmettin Erbakan University, Konya, Turkey
- Ercüment Ölmez, Faculty of Medicine, Department of Pharmacology, Celal Bayar University, Manisa, Turkey
- Erdal Bedir, Department of Bioengineering, Faculty of Engineering, Izmir Institute of Technology, Izmir, Turkey
- Erem Bilensoy, Hacettepe University Faculty of Pharmacy Department of Pharmaceutical Technology
- Eren Demirpolat, Department of Pharmacology, Faculty of Pharmacy, Erciyes University, Kayseri, Turkey
- Erkan Yilmaz, Biotechnology Institute, Ankara University, Ankara, Turkey
- Eser Yıldırım Sözmen, Department of Medical Biochemistry, Ege University, Turkey
- Esma Purut, Department of Biology, Faculty of Science, University of Istanbul, Istanbul, Turkey
- Esra Köngül, Department of Pharmacognosy, Faculty of Pharmacy, Erciyes University, Kayseri, Turkey
- Esra Küpeli Akkol, Department of Pharmaceutical Technology, Faculty of Pharmacy, Gazi University, Ankara, Turkey
- Evren Demircan, Department of Food Engineering, Faculty of Chemical and Metallurgical Enginerring, Istanbul Technical University, Turkey
- Ezgi Balkan, Department of Medical Biochemistry, Faculty of Medicine, Bezmialem Vakif University, Turkey
- Fatemeh Bahadori, Department of Pharmaceutical Biotechnology, Faculty of Pharmacy, Bezmialem Vakif University, Istanbul, Turkey

- Fatih Çöllü, Biology, Faculty of Science and Literature, Manisa Celal Bayar University, Manisa, Turkey
- Fatma Esin Kırık, Department of Medicinal Microbiology, Faculty of Medicine, Niğde Ömer Halisdemir University, Niğde, Turkey
- Fatma Firat, Department of Histology and Embryology, Faculty of Medicine, Manisa Celal Bayar University, Manisa, Turkey
- Feyzan Özdal Kurt, Department of Biology, Faculty of Art and Life Sciences, Manisa Celal Bayar University, Manisa, Turkey
- Fulya Tugba Artun, Institute of Science, Istanbul University, Istanbul, Turkey
- Funda Karbancıoğlu-Güler, Department of Food Engineering, Faculty of Chemical and Metallurgical Enginerring, Istanbul Technical University, Sarıyer, Turkey
- Funda Kosova, Faculty of Health Science, Celal Bayar University, Manisa, Turkey
- Funda Nuray Yalçın, Pharmacognosy Dept., Faculty of Pharmacy, Hacettepe University, Ankara, Turkey
- Gamze Güney Eskiler, Medical Biology Department, Faculty of Medicine, Sakarya University, Sakarya, Turkey
- Gian Luigi Russo Russo, Institute of Food Sciences, National Research Council, Avellino, Italy
- Gonca Dönmez, Department of Medicinal Biology, Faculty of Medicine, Niğde Ömer Halisdemir University, Niğde, Turkey
- Gorkem Kısmalı, Ankara, Turkey
- Gökçe Şeker Karatoprak, Erciyes University Faculty of Pharmacy Department of Pharmacognosy
- Gözde Girgin, Toxicology Department, Faculty of Pharmacy, Hacettepe University, Ankara, Turkey
- Gul Ozcan, Department of Biology, Faculty of Science, Istanbul University, Istanbul, Turkey
- Gulay Melikoglu, Department of Pharmacognosy, Faculty of Pharmacy, Istanbul University, Istanbul, Turkey
- Guzide Satır Basaran, Department of Biochemistry, Faculty of Pharmacy, Erciyes University, Kayseri, Turkey
- Gülen Melike Demir, Department of Pharmaceutical Technology, Faculty of Pharmacy, Gazi University, Ankara, Turkey
- Güliz Armagan, Department of Biochemistry, Faculty of Pharmacy, Ege University, İzmir, Turkey
- Gülşah Albayrak, Department of Histology and Embryology, Faculty of Medicine, Celal Bayar University, Manisa, Turkey
- Gülşah Çeçener, Medical Biology Department, Faculty of Medicine, Uludag University, Gorukle, Bursa, Turkey
- Gülşen Akalın Çiftçi, Department of Biochemistry, Faculty of Pharmacy, Anadolu University, Eskişehir, Turkey
- H. Fatih Gul, Department of Medical Biochemistry, Faculty of Medicine, Firat University, Elazig, Turkey
- H. Gul Dursun, Medical Biology Department, Meram Medical Faculty, Necmettin Erbakan University, Konya, Turkey
- H. Seda Vatansever, Department of Histology and Embryology, Faculty of Medicine, Manisa Celal Bayar University, Manisa, Turkey
- Hakkı Taştan, Department of Biology, Faculty of Science, Gazi University, Ankara, Turkey
- Harun Ülger, School of Medicine, Department of Anatomy, Erciyes University, Kayseri, Turkey
- Hasibe Vural, Department of Medical Biology, Meram Faculty of Medicine, Necmettin Erbakan University, Konya, Turkey
- Hatice Bekci, Department of Food Engineering, Engineering Faculty, Erciyes University, Kayseri, Turkey

- Kemal Sami Korkmaz, Department of Bioengineering, Faculty of Engineering, Ege University, Izmir, Turkey
- Konstantinos Dimas, Department of Pharmacology, Faculty of Medicine, University of Thessaly, Larissa, Greece
- Kübra Uzun, Pharmacognosy Dept., Faculty of Pharmacy, Erciyes University, Kayseri, Turkey
- Latife Merve Oktay, Faculty of Medicine Department of Medical Biology, Ege University, Turkey
- Leyla Paşayeva, Department of Pharmacognosy, Faculty of Pharmacy, Erciyes University, Kayseri, Turkey
- Mahmoud F. Elsebai, Pharmacognosy Department, Faculty of Pharmacy, Mansoura University, Mansoura, Egypt
- Mahmud Özkut, Department of Histology & Embryology, Faculty of Medicine, Manisa Celal Bayar University, Manisa, Turkey
- Marc Diederich, College of Pharmacy, Seoul National University, Seoul, Korea
- Maria usso, Institute of Food Sciences, National Research Council, Avellino, Italy
- Mehmet Berköz, Department of Pharmaceutical Biotechnology, Faculty of Pharmacy, Yuzuncu Yıl University, Van, Turkey
- Mehmet İbrahim Tuğlu, Department of Histology and Embryology, Faculty of Medicine, Manisa Celal Bayar University, Manisa, Turkey
- Mehmet Zülfü Yildiz, Zoology Section, Department of Biology, Faculty of Arts and Science, Adıyaman University, Adıyaman, Turkey
- Mehtap Nisari, Department of Anatomy, Faculty of Medicine, Erciyes University, Kayseri, Turkey
- Melike Ozgul, Department of Histology & Embryology, Faculty of Medicine, Manisa Celal Bayar University, Manisa, Turkey
- Meltem Ceylan-Ünlüsoy, Department of Pharmaceutical Chemistry, Faculty of Pharmacy, Ankara University, Ankara, Turkey
- Mert Burak Ozturk, Department of Bioengineering, Faculty of Engineering, Ege University, Izmir, Turkey
- Mert Ilhan, Department of Pharmaceutical Technology, Faculty of Pharmacy, Biruni University, İstanbul, Turkey
- Merve Alpay, Department of Biochemistry, Faculty of Medicine, Duzce University, Düzce, Turkey
- Merve Çelik Tekeli, Erciyes University Faculty of Pharmacy Department of Pharmaceutical Technology
- Merve Çelik, Department of Molecular Biology and Genetics, Faculty of Science and Letters, Istanbul Kultur University, Istanbul, Turkey
- Merve Karaman, Department of Biology, Balikesir University, Balikesir, Turkey
- Merve Uğur, Department of Molecular Biology and Genetics, Faculty of Science and Letters, Istanbul Kultur University, Istanbul, Turkey
- Metin Yıldırım, Department of Biochemistry, Faculty of Pharmacy, Mersin University, Mersin, Turkey
- Mirosław Krośniak, Department of Food Chemistry and Nutrition, Medical College, Jagiellonian University, Krakow, Poland
- Mohamed Mehiri, Nice, France
- Mustafa Cengiz, Department of Mathematics and Science Education, Education Faculty, Siirt University, Siirt, Turkey
- Mustafa Nisari, Department of Nutrition and Dietetics, Faculty of Health Sciences, University of Nuh Naci Yazgan, Kayseri, Turkey
- Mustafa Öztatlıcı, Department of Histology and Embryology, Faculty of Medicine, Manisa Celal Bayar University, Manisa, Turkey

- Mutlu Demiray, Department of Medical Oncology, KTO Karatay University, Konya, Turkey
- Müberra Koşar, Faculty of Pharmacy, Department of Pharmacognosy, Eastern Mediterranean University, Gazimağusa, North Cyprus via Mersin 10, Turkey
- Mükerrem Betül Yerer, Department of Pharmacology, Faculty of Pharmacy, Erciyes University, Kayseri, Turkey
- Müzeyyen Demirel, Department of Pharmaceutical Technology, Faculty of Pharmacy, Anadolu University, Tepebaşı, Turkey
- N. Nalan İmamoğlu, Department of Basic Sciences, Faculty of Pharmacy, Erciyes University, Kayseri, Turkey
- Nalan Özdemir, Department of Chemistry, Faculty of Sciences, Erciyes University, Talas Street, Kayseri, Turkey
- Narçın Palavan-Ünsal, Department of Molecular Biology and Genetics, Istanbul Kultur University, Atakoy Campus, Istanbul, Turkey
- Nazım Bozan, Department of Otorhinolaryngology, Faculty of Medicine, Yuzuncu Yil University, Van, Turkey
- Necip Ilhan, Department of Medical Biochemistry, Faculty of Medicine, Firat University, Elazig, Turkey
- Neel M. Fofaria, Department of Biomedical Sciences and Department of Immunotherapeutics and Biotechnology, Texas Tech University Health Sciences Center, Lubbock, USA
- Neriman İnanç, Department of Nutrition and Dietetics, Faculty of Health Sciences, University of Nuh Naci Yazgan, Kayseri, Turkey
- Nevin Çelebi, Department of Pharmaceutical Technology, Faculty of Pharmacy, Gazi University, Ankara, Turkey
- Nevin Ilhan, Department of Medical Biochemistry, Faculty of Medicine, Firat University, Elazığ, Turkey
- Nilgun Gurbuz, Department of Medical Biology, School of Medicine, Suleyman Demirel University, Isparta, Turkey
- Nilufer Cinkilic, Department of Biology, Science and Art Faculty, Uludag University, Bursa, Turkey
- Nur Selvi, Faculty of Medicine Department of Medical Biology, Ege University, Turkey
- Nurcan Silahtarlıoğlu, Graduate School Natural Applied Science, Erciyes University, Kayseri, Turkey
- Nurhayat Sutlupinar, Department of Pharmacognosy, Faculty of Pharmacy, Istanbul University, Istanbul, Turkey
- O. Faruk Kirlangic, Department of Molecular Biology and Genetic, Balikesir University, Balikesir, Turkey
- Oguzhan Tatar, Department of Medical Biochemistry, Faculty of Medicine, Firat University, Elazig, Turkey
- Oktay Özkan, Department of Medicinal Pharmacology, Faculty of Medicine, Niğde Ömer Halisdemir University, Niğde, Turkey
- Onur Bender, Biotechnology Institute, Ankara University, Ankara, Turkey
- Onur Kaya, Graduate School Natural Applied Science, Erciyes University, Kayseri, Turkey
- Oruc Allahverdiyev, Department of Pharmacology, Faculty of Pharmacy, Yuzuncu Yıl University, Van, Turkey
- Osman Oğuz, Molecular Biology and Genetics, Faculty of Life and Natural Sciences, Abdullah Gul University, Kayseri, Turkey
- Osman Tugay, Department of Biology Program of Botany, Faculty of Sciences, Selcuk University, Konya, Turkey

- Osman Üstün, Department of Pharmacognosy, Faculty of Pharmacy, Gazi University, Ankara, Turkey
- Oya Bozdağ-Dündar, Department of Pharmaceutical Chemistry, Faculty of Pharmacy, Ankara University, Ankara, Turkey
- Ozer Yılmaz, Department of Biology, Science and Art Faculty, Uludag University, Bursa, Turkey
- Ozgun Teksoy, Biology Department, Art and Science Faculty, Eskişehir Osmangazi University, Eskişehir, Turkey
- Ozgur Tag, Cancer Biology Laboratory, Department of Chemistry, Graduate School of Natural and Applied Sciences, Ege University, Izmir, Turkey
- Ozgur Vatan, Department of Biology, Science and Art Faculty, Uludag University, Bursa, Turkey
- Ömer Taş, Department of Pharmacognosy, Faculty of Pharmacy, Erciyes University, Kayseri, Turkey
- Özge Al, School of Medicine, Department of Anatomy, Erciyes University, Kayseri, Turkey
- Özge Güzel, Department of Bioengineering, Faculty of Engineering, Izmir Institute of Technology, Izmir, Turkey
- Özge Rencüzoğulları, Atakoy Campus, Department of Molecular Biology and Genetics, Istanbul Kultur University, Istanbul, Turkey
- Özlem Temiz-Arpacı, Department of Pharmaceutical Chemistry, Faculty of Pharmacy, Ankara University, Ankara, Turkey
- Pelin Taştan, Deparment of Pharmacognosy, Faculty of Pharmacy, Ege University, İzmir, Turkey
- Pelin Toros, Department of Histology & Embryology, Faculty of Medicine, Manisa Celal Bayar University, Manisa, Turkey
- Perihan Gürbüz, Pharmacognosy Dept., Faculty of Pharmacy, Erciyes University, Kayseri, Turkey
- Petek Ballar, Faculty of Pharmacy, Department of Biochemistry, Ege University, Izmir, Turkey
- Pınar Atalay Dündar, Department of Basic Sciences, Faculty of Pharmacy, Erciyes University, Kayseri, Turkey
- Pınar İkiz, Pharmacognosy Dept., Faculty of Pharmacy, Hacettepe University, Ankara, Turkey
- Pınar K. Sönmez, Department of Histology & Embryology, Faculty of Medicine, Manisa Celal Bayar University, Manisa, Turkey
- Pınar Kılıçaslan Sönmez, Department of Histology and Embryology, Faculty of Medicine, Celal Bayar University, Manisa, Turkey
- Pınar Obakan-Yerlikaya, Department of Molecular Biology and Genetics, Istanbul Kultur University, Atakoy Campus, Istanbul, Turkey
- Pınar Özden, Department of Medical Biology, Meram Faculty of Medicine, Necmettin Erbakan University, Konya, Turkey
- Pinar K. Sönmez, Department of Histology & Embryology, Faculty of Medicine, Manisa Celal Bayar University, Manisa, Turkey
- Rana Kavurmacı, Department of Advanced Technology, Ahi Evran University, Kırşehir, Turkey
- Randolph R. J. Arroo, Leicester School of Pharmacy, De Montfort University, The Gateway, Leicester LE1 9BH, UK
- Recep Eröz, Department of Genetics, Faculty of Medicine, Duzce University, Düzce, Turkey
- Remzi Soner Cengiz, Faculty of Veterinary Medicine, Turkey
- Remziye Kendirci, Department of Histology and Embryology, School of Medicine, Manisa Celal Bayar University, Manisa, Turkey
- Renata Francik, Department of Bioorganic Chemistry, Medical College, Jagiellonian University, Krakow, Poland
- Roderich D. Süssmuth, Institut für Chemie, Technische Universitat Berlin, Strasse des 17. Juni 124, Berlin, Germany

- Rojen Geylan, Department of Pharmacognosy, Faculty of Pharmacy, Erciyes University, Turkey
- Ruziye Daşkın, Botany Dept., Faculty of Science and Letters, Uludağ University, Bursa, Turkey
- S. Kerem Aydin, Sirri Yircali Anatolian High School, Balikesir, Turkey
- Sanjay K. Srivastava, Department of Biomedical Sciences and Department of Immunotherapeutics and Biotechnology, Texas Tech University Health Sciences Center, Lubbock, USA
- Seda Duman, Department of Bioengineering, Faculty of Engineering, Izmir Institute of Technology, Izmir, Turkey
- Seda Şirin, Gazi University, Faculty of Science, Department of Biology, Teknikokullar, Ankara, Turkey
- Sedat Ünal, Erciyes University Faculty of Pharmacy Department of Pharmaceutical Technology
- Seher Dalgic, Sirri Yircali Anatolian High School, Balikesir, Turkey
- Seher Yılmaz, School of Medicine, Department of Anatomy, Bozok University, Yozgat, Turkey
- Selda Eren, Faculty of Pharmacy, Erciyes University, Kayseri, Turkey
- Selen İlgün, Faculty of Pharmacy, Department of Pharmaceutical Botany, Erciyes University, Kayseri, Turkey
- Selim Demir, Department of Nutrition and Dietetics, Faculty of Health Sciences, Karadeniz Technical University, Trabzon, Turkey
- Sema Misir, Department of Biochemistry, Faculty of Pharmacy, Cumhuriyet University, Sivas, Turkey
- Senem Akkoç, Department of Chemistry, Faculty of Sciences, Erciyes University, Kayseri, Turkey
- Serap Yalcin, Department of Molecular Biology and Genetics, Ahi Evran University, Kırşehir, Turkey
- Serap Yalın, Department of Biochemistry, Faculty of Pharmacy, Mersin University, Mersin, Turkey
- Sevil Albayrak, Biology Department, Science Faculty, Erciyes University, Kayseri, Turkey
- Sevinç İnan, Department of Histology and Embryology, Faculty of Medicine, Celal Bayar University, Manisa, Turkey
- Sevtap Çağlar Yavuz, Department of Chemistry, Faculty of Sciences, Erciyes University, Kayseri, Turkey
- Seyhan Altun, Department of Biology, Faculty of Science, University of Istanbul, Istanbul, Turkey
- Sezin Anil, Department of Pharmacognosy, Faculty of Pharmacy, Istanbul University, Istanbul, Turkey
- Sharavan Ramachandran, Department of Biomedical Sciences and Department of Immunotherapeutics and Biotechnology, Texas Tech University Health Sciences Center, Lubbock, USA
- Sibel Gunes, Biology Department, Art and Science Faculty, Eskişehir Osmangazi University, Eskişehir, Turkey
- Sibel İlbasmiş Tamer, Department of Pharmaceutical Technology, Faculty of Pharmacy, Gazi University, Ankara, Turkey
- Sinem Yılmaz, Faculty of Pharmacy, Department of Biochemistry, Ege University, Izmir, Turkey
- Solmaz Susam, Department of Medical Biochemistry, Faculty of Medicine, Firat University, Elazig, Turkey
- Stefania Moccia, Institute of Food Sciences, National Research Council, Avellino, Italy
- Suheyl Furkan Konca, Department of Pharmaceutical Biotechnology, Faculty of Pharmacy, Erciyes University, Kayseri, Turkey
- Sukran Kultur, Department of Pharmaceutical Botany, Faculty of Pharmacy, Istanbul University, Istanbul, Turkey
- Sumeyra Cetinkaya, Medical Biology Department, Meram Medical Faculty, Necmettin Erbakan University, Konya, Turkey

- Suna Sabuncuoğlu, Toxicology Department, Faculty of Pharmacy, Hacettepe University, Ankara, Turkey
- Suna Sayğılı, Department of Histology and Embryology, Faculty of Medicine, Celal Bayar University, Manisa, Turkey
- Şamil Öztürk, Department of Histology & Embryology, Faculty of Medicine, Manisa Celal Bayar University, Manisa, Turkey
- Şebnem Kurhan, Novel Food Technologies Development, Application and Research Center, Abant İzzet Baysal University, Bolu, Turkey
- Taner Dağcı, Department of Physiology, Faculty of Medicine, Ege University, İzmir, Turkey
- Terken Baydar, Toxicology Department, Faculty of Pharmacy, Hacettepe University, Ankara, Turkey
- Tevhide Sel, Ankara Unıversıty, Faculty of Veterinary Medicine, Turkey
- Tolga Cavas, Medical Biology Department, Faculty of Medicine, Uludag University, Bursa, Turkey
- Tolga Ertekin, School of Medicine, Department of Anatomy, Kocatepe University, Afyon, Turkey
- Tuna Onal, Department of Histology & Embryology, Faculty of Medicine, Manisa Celal Bayar University, Manisa, Turkey
- U. Sebnem Harput, Department of Pharmacognosy, Faculty of Pharmacy, Hacettepe University, Ankara, Turkey
- Ünal Egeli, Medical Biology Department, Faculty of Medicine, Uludag University, Bursa, Turkey
- Varol Sahinturk, Vocational School of Health Services, Eskişehir Osmangazi University, Eskişehir, Turkey
- Vasilis P. Androutsopoulos, Department of Toxicology, Medical School, University of Crete, Crete GR, Greece
- Veysel Kayser, Faculty of Pharmacy, The University of Sydney, Sydney, Australia
- Vildan Betül Yenigun, Department of Medical Biochemistry, Faculty of Medicine, Bezmialem Vakif University, Turkey
- Yalcin Erzurumlu, Faculty of Pharmacy, Department of Biochemistry, Ege University, Izmir, Turkey
- Yasemin Tekin, Biology Department, Art and Science Faculty, Eskişehir Osmangazi University, Eskişehir, Turkey
- Yasin Genc, Department of Pharmacognosy, Faculty of Pharmacy, Hacettepe University, Ankara, Turkey
- Yeşim Aktaş, Erciyes University Faculty of Pharmacy Department of Pharmaceutical Technology
- Yuksel Aliyazicioglu, Medicinal Plants, Traditional Medicine Practice and Research Center, Gumushane University, Gumushane, Turkey
- Yüksel Öğünç, Department of Biochemistry, Faculty of Pharmacy, Anadolu University, Eskişehir, Turkey
- Zerrin Seller, Department of Biochemistry, Faculty of Pharmacy, Anadolu University, Eskişehir, Turkey
- Zeynep Dogan, Department of Pharmacognosy, Faculty of Pharmacy, Hacettepe University, Ankara, Turkey

Acknowledgments: The authors are indebted to Erciyes University Rectorate and Erciyes University Faculty of Pharmacy and Larkin University, College of Pharmacy for their valuable contributions to the organization and to the Research Foundation of Erciyes University (Project Number: TSS-2017-7720) for their financial support of this symposium. Also to the local organizing committee members (Perihan Gürbüz, Eren Demirpolat, Ahmet Cumaoğlu, Gökçe Şeker Karatoprak, Ayşe Kübra Karaboğa Aslan, Ebru Öztürk and Görkem Kısmalı) for their accomplished work.

Author Contributions: M.B.Y. wrote the manuscript and A.B. reviewed and edited the document.

Conflicts of Interest: There is not any conflict of interest to declare.

References

1. Yerer, M.B. Growth Factors Responsible from the Cancer Progress: Role of Natural Products. *Proceedings* **2017**, *1*, 979. [CrossRef]
2. Bishayee, A. Natural Products for Cancer Prevention and Therapy: Progress, Pitfalls and Promise. *Proceedings* **2017**, *1*, 982. [CrossRef]
3. Amin, A. Novel Anticancer Capacities of Saffron. *Proceedings* **2017**, *1*, 834. [CrossRef]
4. Diederich, M. Cardiac Glycosides as Novel Modulators of Cancer Cell Survival. *Proceedings* **2017**, *1*, 972. [CrossRef]
5. Russo, G.L.; Russo, M.; Spagnuolo, C.; Moccia, S. Ins and Outs of Flavonoids in Cancer Prevention vs. Cancer Therapy: A Lesson from Quercetin in Leukemia. *Proceedings* **2017**, *1*, 977. [CrossRef]
6. Arroo, R.R.J.; Şöhretoğlu, D.; Spandidos, D.A.; Androutsopoulos, V.P. Anticancer Potential of Flavones. *Proceedings* **2017**, *1*, 975. [CrossRef]
7. Borriello, A. Resveratrol in Cancer Prevention and Treatment: Focusing on Molecular Targets and Mechanism of Action. *Proceedings* **2017**, *1*, 976. [CrossRef]
8. Elsebai, M.F.; Hakkola, J.; Mehiri, M.; Diez, J. Cynaropicrin: A Promising Natural Agent with Antitumor and Antiviral Activities. *Proceedings* **2017**, *1*, 974. [CrossRef]
9. Koşar, M. Relationship between Structure of Phenolics and Anticancer Activity. *Proceedings* **2017**, *1*, 978. [CrossRef]
10. Cevatemre, B.; Dimas, K.; Botta, B.; Ulukaya, E. Pristimerin is a Promising Natural Product against Breast Cancer *in vitro* and *in vivo* through Apoptosis and the Blockage of Autophagic Flux. *Proceedings* **2017**, *1*, 973. [CrossRef]
11. Demiray, M.; Bahadori, F. Can Curcumin be Employed to Promote the Integration of Oncology and Natural Products? *Proceedings* **2017**, *1*, 980. [CrossRef]
12. Fofaria, N.M.; Ramachandran, S.; Srivastava, S.K. Therapeutic Potential of Black Pepper Compound for BRaf Resistant Melanoma. *Proceedings* **2017**, *1*, 981. [CrossRef]
13. Gul, H.F.; Ilhan, N.; Ilhan, N.; Ozercan, I.H. Effect of Pomegranate Extract and Tangeretin on Specific Pathways in the Rat Breast Cancer Model Induced with DMBA. *Proceedings* **2017**, *1*, 983. [CrossRef]
14. Oğuz, O.; Adan, A. Synergistic Cytotoxic Effects of Resveratrol in Combination with Ceramide Metabolizing Enzymes in Ph + Acute Lymphoblastic Leukemia. *Proceedings* **2017**, *1*, 984. [CrossRef]
15. Debelec-Butuner, B.; Ozturk, M.B.; Tag, O.; Akgun, I.H.; Bedir, E.; Korkmaz, K.S. Characterization of Cycloartane-Type Sapogenol Derivatives for Prostate Cancer Chemoprevention. *Proceedings* **2017**, *1*, 985. [CrossRef]
16. Obakan-Yerlikaya, P.; Adacan, K.; Arısan, E.D.; Çoker-Gürkan, A.; Palavan-Ünsal, N. Epibrassinolide Treatment Caused Autophagy or Apoptosis Decision in a Time-Dependent Manner through ER Stress in Colon Cancer Cells. *Proceedings* **2017**, *1*, 986. [CrossRef]
17. Alpay, M.; Eröz, R.; Kısmalı, G.; Kurtdede, E. Determination of Silymarin Molecule Activity in Colon Cancer by AgNOR Technique. *Proceedings* **2017**, *1*, 987. [CrossRef]
18. Dönmez, G.; Kırık, F.E.; Aydemir, I.; Sarı, İ.; Özkan, O.; Savran, A.; Tuğlu, M.İ. The Cytotoxic Effect of *Lysimachia savranii* on the Neuroblastoma Cells. *Proceedings* **2017**, *1*, 988. [CrossRef]
19. Gürkan, A.J.; Çelik, M.; Uğur, M.; Arisan, A.D.; Obakan Yerlikaya, P.; Palavan Ünsal, N. Autocrine Growth Hormone-Triggered Curcumin Resistance Abolished by NF-κB Signaling Pathway Dependent on Inflammatory Cytokines and Active Polyamine Catabolic Machinery in MCF-7, MDA-MB-453 and MDA-MB-231 Breast Cancer Cells. *Proceedings* **2017**, *1*, 989. [CrossRef]
20. Aydemir, I.; Sari, İ.; Dönmez, G.; Kırık, F.E.; Özkan, O.; Savran, A.; Tuğlu, M.İ. The Effect of *Lysimachia Savranii* on the Migration of the Breast Cancer Cells. *Proceedings* **2017**, *1*, 990. [CrossRef]
21. Özkan, O.; Aydemir, I.; Sarı, İ.; Dönmez, G.; Kırık, F.E.; Savran, A.; Tuğlu, M.İ. Investigation of Cytotoxic Effect of *Origanum Minutiflorum* on Cancer Cells. *Proceedings* **2017**, *1*, 991. [CrossRef]
22. Arisan, E.D.; Rencüzoğulları, Ö.; Çoker-Gürkan, A.; Obakan-Yerlikaya, P.; Palavan-Ünsal, N. Celastrol Modulates Lipid Synthesis via PI3K/Akt/mTOR Signaling Axis to finalize Cell Death Response in Prostate Cancer Cells. *Proceedings* **2017**, *1*, 992. [CrossRef]
23. Sayğılı, S.; Birinci, H.; Şen, B.; Öztatlıcı, M.; İnan, S.; Özbilgin, K. Investigation of the Effect of Paclitaxel and Pycnogenol on Mitochondrial Dynamics in Breast Cancer Therapy. *Proceedings* **2017**, *1*, 993. [CrossRef]

24. Nisari, M.; Yılmaz, S.; Ertekin, T.; Ceylan, D.; İnanç, N.; Al, Ö.; Ülger, H. Effects of Curcumin on Lipid Peroxidation and Antioxidant Enzymes in Kidney, Liver, Brain and Testis of Mice Bearing Ehrlich Solid Tumor. *Proceedings* **2017**, *1*, 994. [CrossRef]

25. Öztürk, E.; Karaboğa Arslan, A.K.; Radwan, B.; Yerer, M.B. Curcumin Enhances the Efficacy of 5-FU in Colo205 Cell Lines. *Proceedings* **2017**, *1*, 995. [CrossRef]

26. Erzurumlu, Y.; Tag, O.; Yılmaz, S.; Ballar, P.; Bedir, E. Effect of a New Sapogenol Derivative (AG-07) on Cell Death via Necrosis. *Proceedings* **2017**, *1*, 996. [CrossRef]

27. Genc, Y.; Harput, U.S.; Saracoglu, I. Cytotoxic and Antiinflammatory Activity Guided Studies on *Plantago holosteum* Scop. *Proceedings* **2017**, *1*, 997. [CrossRef]

28. Öztürk, E.; Karaboğa Arslan, A.K.; Yerer, M.B. Continuously Monitoring the Cytotoxicity of API-1, α-Chaconine and α-Solanine on Human Lung Carcinoma A549. *Proceedings* **2017**, *1*, 998. [CrossRef]

29. Karaboğa Arslan, A.K.; Yerer, M.B. The Effects of α-Chaconine on ER-α Positive Endometrium Cancer Cells. *Proceedings* **2017**, *1*, 999. [CrossRef]

30. Eroğlu, C.; Kurar, E.; Avcı, E.; Vural, H. Investigation of Apoptotic Effect of Sinapic Acid in Hep3B and HepG2 Human Hepatocellular Carcinoma Cells. *Proceedings* **2017**, *1*, 1000. [CrossRef]

31. Paşayeva, L.; Üstün, O.; Demirpolat, E.; Karatoprak, G.Ş.; Tugay, O.; Koşar, M. Cytotoxic and Antioxidant Activity of Four *Cousinia* Species of Stenocephalae Bunge Section. *Proceedings* **2017**, *1*, 1001. [CrossRef]

32. Avcı, E.; Eroğlu, C.; Özden, P.; Vural, H.; Kurar, E. Apoptotic Effect of Ginnalin A on MDA-MB-231 and MCF7 Human Breast Cancer Cell Lines. *Proceedings* **2017**, *1*, 1002. [CrossRef]

33. Eken, A.; Karaboğa Arslan, A.K.; Öztürk, E.; Ökçesiz, A.; Yerer, M.B. Cytotoxic Effects of Coumarin Compounds Imperatorin and Osthole, Alone and in Combination with 5-Fluorouracil in Colon Carcinoma Cells. *Proceedings* **2017**, *1*, 1003. [CrossRef]

34. Gürbüz, P.; Uzun, K.; Öztürk, E.; Yerer, M.B. Screening of Some Apiaceae and Asteraceae Plants for Their Cytotoxic Potential. *Proceedings* **2017**, *1*, 1004. [CrossRef]

35. Oktay, A.N.; İlbasmiş Tamer, S.; Çelebi, N. Cyclodextrine Based Nanogels and Phase Solubility Studies of Flurbiprofen as a Chemopreventive Agent. *Proceedings* **2017**, *1*, 1005. [CrossRef]

36. Somtürk Yılmaz, B.; Akkoç, S.; Özdemir, N. Effect of a Synthesized Compound against Cancerous Cell Line and Synthesis of Copper Ion Incorporated 1-(3,4-Diaminophenyl) Ethanone-Based Hybrid Nanoflowers. *Proceedings* **2017**, *1*, 1006. [CrossRef]

37. Akkoç, S.; Özer, İ.; Kayser, V. Development of Effective Anticancer Drug Candidates against Breast and Colon Cancers. *Proceedings* **2017**, *1*, 1007. [CrossRef]

38. Çağlar Yavuz, S.; Somtürk Yılmaz, B.; Özdemir, N.; Sarıpınar, E. Synthesis of Copper Ion Incorporated Aminoguanidine Derivatives-Based Hybrid Nanoflowers. *Proceedings* **2017**, *1*, 1008. [CrossRef]

39. Bender, O.; Atalay, A. Evaluation of Anti-Proliferative and Cytotoxic Properties of Chlorogenic Acid against Breast Cancer Cell Lines by Real Time Monitoring. *Proceedings* **2017**, *1*, 1009. [CrossRef]

40. Yurdacan, B.; Egeli, Ü.; Güney Eskiler, G.; Eryılmaz, I.E.; Çeçener, G.; Tunca, B. Investigation of Apoptotic Effects of Usnic Acid on Hepatocellular Carcinoma. *Proceedings* **2017**, *1*, 1010. [CrossRef]

41. Egeli, Ü.; Yurdacan, B.; Huriyet, H.; Güney Eskiler, G.; Eryılmaz, I.E.; Cavas, T.; Çeçener, G.; Malyer, H.; Tunca, B. In Vitro Cytotoxic Effect Evaluation of *Dioscorea communis* (L.) Caddick & Wilkin Rhizome and Stem Extracts on Hepatocellular Carcinoma Cells. *Proceedings* **2017**, *1*, 1011. [CrossRef]

42. Şen, B.; Toros, P.; Sönmez, P.K.; Özkut, M.; Öztürk, Ş.; Çöllü, F.; Inan, S.; Tuğlu, İ. The Effect of Herbal Medicine on Neuroblastoma Cell Line in Culture. *Proceedings* **2017**, *1*, 1012. [CrossRef]

43. Celik, D.A.; Gurbuz, N. The Foods Containing miR-193b May Inhibit the Growth of Breast Cancer Cells. *Proceedings* **2017**, *1*, 1013. [CrossRef]

44. Gurbuz, N.; Celik, D.A. Is the Dietary miR-193b a Novel Cell Cycle Arresting Source for Breast Carcinoma? *Proceedings* **2017**, *1*, 1014. [CrossRef]

45. Turkoz Uluer, E.; Ozgul, M.; Onal, T.; Ozbilgin, K.; Inan, S. The Effects of Wortmannin and EGCG and Combined Treatments on MDA-MB-231 Breast Cancer Cell Lines via Inactivation of PI3K Signaling Pathway. *Proceedings* **2017**, *1*, 1015. [CrossRef]

46. Ozgul, M.; Turkoz Uluer, E.; Onal, H.; Akogullari, D.; Ozbilgin, K.; Inan, S. The Effects of Paclitaxel and Metformin and Combined Treatments on TLR Signaling Pathway on MDA-MB-231 Breast Cancer Cell Lines. *Proceedings* **2017**, *1*, 1016. [CrossRef]

47. Tosun, E.; Baysar, A. Inhibition of Telomerase Activity by Cucurbitacin I in Colon Cancer Cell Line, LS174T. *Proceedings* **2017**, *1*, 1017. [CrossRef]

48. Tosun, E.; Baysar, A. Effect of Cucurbitacin I on Proliferation and Migration in Colorectal Cancer Cell Line, LS174T. *Proceedings* **2017**, *1*, 1018. [CrossRef]

49. Artun, F.T.; Karagoz, A.; Ozcan, G.; Melikoglu, G.; Anil, S.; Kultur, S.; Sutlupinar, N. In Vitro Anticancer and Cytotoxic Activities of Some Plant Extracts on HeLa and Vero Cell Lines. *Proceedings* **2017**, *1*, 1019. [CrossRef]

50. Özkut, M.; Albayrak, G.; Kılıçaslan Sönmez, P.; Şen, B.; Toros, P.; Öztürk, Ş.; Çöllü, F.; İnan, S.; Tuğlu, M.İ. Anticancer Effects of Oleocanthal and Pinus Pinaster on Breast Cancer Cell in Culture. *Proceedings* **2017**, *1*, 1020. [CrossRef]

51. Kılıçaslan Sönmez, P.; Albayrak, G.; Özkut, M.; Şen, B.; Toros, P.; Öztürk, Ş.; Çöllü, F.; İnan, S.; Tuğlu, M.İ. Antiproliferative and Apoptotic Effects of the Medicinal Plants on Breast Cancer Cell Lines. *Proceedings* **2017**, *1*, 1021. [CrossRef]

52. Kabadayı, H.; Kendirci, R.; Vatansever, H.S. The Role of Trophoblastic Stem Cells Conditioned Media on JAR Cell Culture. *Proceedings* **2017**, *1*, 1022. [CrossRef]

53. Birinci, H.; Şen, B.; Sayğılı, S.; Ölmez, E.; Türköz Uluer, E.; Özbilgin, K. The Effect of Pycnogenol and Paclitaxel on DNA Damage in Human Breast Cancer Cell Line. *Proceedings* **2017**, *1*, 1023. [CrossRef]

54. Birinci, H.; Şen, B.; Sayğılı, S.; Ölmez, E.; İnan, S.; Özbilgin, K. Investigation of the Effects of Paclitaxel and Pycnogenol on Inflammatory Response (PTX3, BDNF, IGF2R) in Human Breast Cancer Cell Line. *Proceedings* **2017**, *1*, 1024. [CrossRef]

55. Gul, H.F.; Ilhan, N.; Susam, S.; Tatar, O.; Ilhan, N. Is There Any Protective Effect of Pomegranate and Tangeretin on the DMBA-Induced Rat Breast Cancer Model? *Proceedings* **2017**, *1*, 1025. [CrossRef]

56. Sari, İ.; Dönmez, G.; Kırık, F.E.; Aydemir, I.; Özkan, O.; Savran, A.; Vural, K.; Tuğlu, M.İ. The Neurotoxic Effects of *Origanum minutiflorum*. *Proceedings* **2017**, *1*, 1026. [CrossRef]

57. Eryılmaz, I.E.; Güney Eskiler, G.; Yurdacan, B.; Egeli, Ü.; Çeçener, G.; Tunca, B. The Cytotoxic and Apoptotic Effects of Usnic Acid on Prostate Cancer versus Normal Cells. *Proceedings* **2017**, *1*, 1027. [CrossRef]

58. Vatan, O.; Yılmaz, O.; Huriyet, H.; Cavas, T.; Cinkılıç, N. Antiproliferative Effect of Methanolic Extract of Linum arboreum on A549 Cells. *Proceedings* **2017**, *1*, 1028. [CrossRef]

59. Huriyet, H.; Cavas, T.; Vatan, O.; Cinkilic, N. Investigation of In Vitro Cytotoxic Effects of Montivipera xanthina on Healthy and Cancer Human Lung Cell Lines. *Proceedings* **2017**, *1*, 1029. [CrossRef]

60. Tekeli, M.Ç.; Yücel, Ç.; Ünal, S.; Şeker Karatoprak, G.; Aktaş, Y.; Bilensoy, E. Development and Characterization of Paclitaxel-loaded PLGA Nanoparticles and Evaluation of Cytotoxicity on MCF-7 cell line by MTT Assay. *Proceedings* **2017**, *1*, 1030. [CrossRef]

61. Aydin, S.K.; Dalgic, S.; Karaman, M.; Kirlangic, O.F.; Yildirim, H. Effects of Fulvic Acid on Different Cancer Cell Lines. *Proceedings* **2017**, *1*, 1031. [CrossRef]

62. Berköz, M.; Yıldırım, M.; Allahverdiyev, O.; Krośniak, M.; Francik, R.; Bozan, N.; Yalın, S. Antioxidant, Antibacterial and Antiproliferative Activities of Turkish Rhubarb (*Rheum palmatum* L.) leaf Extracts. *Proceedings* **2017**, *1*, 1032. [CrossRef]

63. Toros, P.; Şen, B.; Sönmez, P.K.; Özkut, M.; Öztürk, Ş.; Çöllü, F.; İnan, S.; Tuğlu, İ. The Effect of Herbal Medicine on Colon Cancer Cells in Culture. *Proceedings* **2017**, *1*, 1033. [CrossRef]

64. Toros, P.; Şen, B.; Sönmez, P.K.; Özkut, M.; Öztürk, Ş.; Çöllü, F.; İnan, S.; Tuğlu, S. The Effect of Herbal Medicine on Prostate Cancer Cells in Culture. *Proceedings* **2017**, *1*, 1034. [CrossRef]

65. Şirin, S.; Aslım, B. Determination of Antioxidant Capacity, Phenolic Acid Composition and Antiproliferative Effect Associated with Phenylalanine Ammonia Lyase (PAL) Activity in Some Plants Naturally Growing under Salt Stress. *Proceedings* **2017**, *1*, 1035. [CrossRef]

66. Ünal, S.; Yücel, Ç.; Çelik Tekeli, M.; Şeker Karatoprak, G.; Aktaş, Y.; Bilensoy, E. Development and Characterization of Paclitaxel-Loaded PLGA Nanoparticles and Cytotoxicity Assessment By MTT Assay on A549 Cell Line. *Proceedings* **2017**, *1*, 1036. [CrossRef]

67. Kavurmacı, R.; Yalcin, S. Evaluation of In Vitro Anti-Proliferative Activity of St. John's Wort (*Hypericum perforatum* Linn.) Plant Extract on Cervix Adenocarcinoma. *Proceedings* **2017**, *1*, 1037. [CrossRef]

68. Kavurmacı, R.; Yalcin, S. The Cytotoxic Effect of Annona muricata Leaf Extract on Triple Negative Breast Cancer Cell Line. *Proceedings* **2017**, *1*, 1038. [CrossRef]

69. Albayrak, S.; Silahtarlıoğlu, N. Cytotoxic Activity of *Achillea coarctata* Poir. Extract. *Proceedings* **2017**, *1*, 1039. [CrossRef]

70. Albayrak, S.; Kaya, O. Cytotoxic Activity of Endemic *Astragalus argaeus* Boiss. from Turkey. *Proceedings* **2017**, *1*, 1040. [CrossRef]

71. Kurhan, Ş.; Çakir, İ. Lactic Acid Bacteria Mediated Apoptosis Induction: Natural Way of Colon Cancer Cells' Inhibition. *Proceedings* **2017**, *1*, 1041. [CrossRef]

72. Akkoç, S.; Türkmenoğlu, B.; Çağlar Yavuz, S. Synthesized a New Organic Compound's Cytotoxic Activity Quantum Mechanics Calculations and Docking Studies. *Proceedings* **2017**, *1*, 1042. [CrossRef]

73. Dündar, E.; Akalın Çiftçi, G.; Altıntaş, A. Anticancer Activity of Centaurea babylonica L. *Proceedings* **2017**, *1*, 1043. [CrossRef]

74. Satir Basaran, G.; Bekci, H.; Baldemir, A.; İlgün, S.; Cumaoğlu, A. Cytotoxic Effects of Functional Foods *Momordica charantia* L. and *Lycium barbarum* L. Extracts on Prostate Cancer Cells. *Proceedings* **2017**, *1*, 1044. [CrossRef]

75. Atalay Dündar, P.; İmamoğlu, N.N. Cytotoxic Effects of Kynurenic Acid and Quinaldic Acid in Hepatocellular Carcinoma (HepG2) Cell Line. *Proceedings* **2017**, *1*, 1045. [CrossRef]

76. Kosova, F.; Temiz-Arpacı, Ö.; Ölmez, E.; Tuğlu, İ. The Effects of Benzoxasol Derivate Compounds in Breast Cancer Cells. *Proceedings* **2017**, *1*, 1046. [CrossRef]

77. Taştan, P.; Armagan, G.; Dağcı, T.; Kıvçak, B. Potential Cytotoxic Activity of Psephellus pyrrhoblepharus Extracts. *Proceedings* **2017**, *1*, 1047. [CrossRef]

78. Güzel, Ö.; Duman, S.; Yılmaz, S.; Pirhan, A.F.; Bedir, E. Screening of Onosma Species for Cytotoxic Activity. *Proceedings* **2017**, *1*, 1048. [CrossRef]

79. Erzurumlu, Y.; Petras, D.; Goçmen, B.; Hempel, B.F.; Heiss, P.; Yildiz, M.Z.; Süssmuth, R.D.; Nalbantsoy, A. Apoptotic Effects of Mount Bulgar Viper (*Montivipera bulgardaghica*) PLA2 and SVMPs Venom Peptide fractions on HeLa and A549 Cancer Cells. *Proceedings* **2017**, *1*, 1049. [CrossRef]

80. Misir, S.; Demir, S.; Turan, I.; Aliyazicioglu, Y. Turkish Propolis Extract Increases Apoptosis via Induction of Mitochondrial Membrane Potential Loss in MCF-7 Cells. *Proceedings* **2017**, *1*, 1050. [CrossRef]

81. Al, Ö.; Ülger, H.; Eetekin, T.; Nisari, M.; Susar, H.; Ceylan, D.; Şeker Karatoprak, G. The Effect of Gilaburu (*Viburnum opulus*) Juice on Ehrlich Ascites Tumor (EAT) Cell Culture. *Proceedings* **2017**, *1*, 1051. [CrossRef]

82. Öğünç, Y.; Demirel, M.; Seller, Z. Synthesis and Characterizations of Folate-Conjugated PLGA-PEG Nanoparticles Loaded with Dual Agents. *Proceedings* **2017**, *1*, 1052. [CrossRef]

83. Dogan, Z.; Saracoglu, I. Selective Cytotoxic Activity of Scutellaria Species. *Proceedings* **2017**, *1*, 1053. [CrossRef]

84. Cengiz, R.S.; Gök, A.; Kurtdede, E.; Kısmalı, G.; Sel, T. The Antiproliferative Effect of Alpha Tocopherol in F98 Cell Culture. *Proceedings* **2017**, *1*, 1054. [CrossRef]

85. Paşayeva, L.; Köngül, E.; Geylan, R.; Şeker Karatoprak, G.; Tugay, O. Analysis of the Cytotoxic Effects of Eryngium billardieri Delar. Extracts on MCF7 Cell Line. *Proceedings* **2017**, *1*, 1055. [CrossRef]

86. İlgün, S.; Şeker Karatoprak, G.; Koşar, M. Cytotoxic Effects of Alchemilla mollis (Buser) Rothm. Extracts on MCF 7 Cell Line. *Proceedings* **2017**, *1*, 1056. [CrossRef]

87. Demirpolat, E.; Paşayeva, L.; Tugay, O. Comparative Evaluation of the Cytotoxic Effects of Stem and Flower Extracts of *Rhaponticoides iconiensis* (Hub.-Mor.) M.V.Agab. & Greuter. *Proceedings* **2017**, *1*, 1057. [CrossRef]

88. Bekci, H.; Satır Basaran, G.; Baldemir, A.; Cumaoglu, A. Goji Berry Fruit Extract Suppresses Cell Proliferation of Breast Cancer Cells by Inhibiting EGFR/ERK Signalling. *Proceedings* **2017**, *1*, 1058. [CrossRef]

89. Memmedov, H.; Durmaz, B.; Merve Oktay, L.; Selvi, N.; Kalkan Yıldırım, H.; Yıldırım Sözmen, E. Biologically Transformed Propolis Exhibits Cytotoxic Effect on A375 Malignant Melanoma Cells In Vitro. *Proceedings* **2017**, *1*, 1059. [CrossRef]

90. Cinar, I.; Cetinkaya, S.; Dursun, H.G. Rheum ribes Extract Increase the Expression Level of miR-200 Family in Human Colorectal Cancer Cells. *Proceedings* **2017**, *1*, 1060. [CrossRef]

91. Cetinkaya, S.; Cinar, I.; Dursun, H.G. Potential Effects of *Liquidambar orientalis* Mill. Against HT-29 and HCT-116 Cell Lines. *Proceedings* **2017**, *1*, 1061. [CrossRef]

92. Gök, A.; Kurtdede, E.; Cengiz, R.S.; Kısmalı, G.; Sel, T. The Effect of Tocopherol-α on the Cell Viability in Caco-2 Cell Line. *Proceedings* **2017**, *1*, 1062. [CrossRef]

93. Kasapoğlu, K.N.; Kocyigit, A.; Yenigun, V.B.; Balkan, E.; Demircan, E.; Karbancıoğlu-Güler, F.; Özçelik, B. In Vitro Antioxidant and Anticancer Activities of Some Local Plants from Bolu Province of Turkey. *Proceedings* **2017**, *1*, 1063. [CrossRef]

94. Özden, P.; Avcı, E.; Vural, H. Survey of the Apoptotic Effect of Ginnalin A on Hep3b Human Hepatocellular Carcinoma Cell Line. *Proceedings* **2017**, *1*, 1064. [CrossRef]

95. Cengiz, M.; Teksoy, O.; Sahinturk, V.; Tekin, Y.; Gunes, S.; Ayhanci, A. Ameliorative Effects of Carvacrol on Cyclophosphamide-Induced Testis Damage and Oxidative Stress. *Proceedings* **2017**, *1*, 1066. [CrossRef]

96. Konca, S.F.; Tasdemir, D.; Aydogdu, G.; Yilmaz, E.; Bozkir, A.; Ocsoy, I. Synthesis of Anthocyanin-Rich Red cabbage Nanoflowers and Their Antimicrobial and Cytotoxic Properties. *Proceedings* **2017**, *1*, 1067. [CrossRef]

97. Uzun, K.; İkiz, P.; Daşkın, R.; Gürbüz, P.; Yalçın, F.N. Cytotoxic Potentials of Some Asteraceae Plants from Turkey on HeLa Cell Line. *Proceedings* **2017**, *1*, 1068. [CrossRef]

98. Purut, E.; Altun, S. The Role of Lidocaine in the Dunning Model Rat Prostate Cancer Cells: Cell Kinetics and Motility. *Proceedings* **2017**, *1*, 1069. [CrossRef]

99. Eren, S.; Bekci, H.; Satır Basaran, G.; Seker Karatoprak, G.; Cumaoglu, A. *Pelargonium endlicherianum* Fenzl. Root Extract Suppresses Cell Proliferation of Prostate Cancer Cells. *Proceedings* **2017**, *1*, 1070. [CrossRef]

100. Girgin, G.; Sabuncuoğlu, S.; Ünal, A.Z.; Baydar, T. Assessment of Antioxidant and Cytotoxic Activity of Known Antioxidants Compared to Neopterin. *Proceedings* **2017**, *1*, 1071. [CrossRef]

101. Sabuncuoğlu, S.; Ünal, A.Z.; Girgin, G. Comparison of Radical Scavenging and Cytotoxic Activities of Well-Known Non-Enzymatic Antioxidants. *Proceedings* **2017**, *1*, 1072. [CrossRef]

102. Ceylan-Ünlüsoy, M.; Bozdağ-Dündar, O. A Study on the Synthesis and Anticancer Activities of Novel 6-Methoxy Flavonyl Piperazine Derivatives. *Proceedings* **2017**, *1*, 1073. [CrossRef]

103. Demir, G.M.; Ilhan, M.; Küpeli Akkol, E.; Taştan, H.; Işık, A.; Tuncer Değim, İ. Effect of Paclitaxel Loaded Chitosan Nanoparticles and Quantum Dots on Breast Cancer. *Proceedings* **2017**, *1*, 1074. [CrossRef]

104. Teke, B.; Akalın Uruşak, E. Turkish Medicinal Plants Used in Cancer Treatment and Evaluation of Plant Usage in the Oncology Clinic of the İstanbul University Faculty of Medicine. *Proceedings* **2017**, *1*, 1075. [CrossRef]

105. Firat, F.; Türkoğlu, C.; Özdal Kurt, F.; Vatansever, H.S. Is Acteosid Effects On Colon Cancer Stem Cells via Inflamation and/or Apoptosis? *Proceedings* **2017**, *1*, 1076. [CrossRef]

106. Köngül, E.; Taş, Ö.; Paşayeva, L.; Şeker Karatoprak, G. Analysis of the Cytotoxic Effects of *Achillea millefolium* L. Extracts on MCF7 Cell Line. *Proceedings* **2017**, *1*, 1077. [CrossRef]

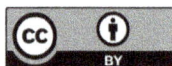

nutrients

MDPI

Article

Migration Rate Inhibition of Breast Cancer Cells Treated by Caffeic Acid and Caffeic Acid Phenethyl Ester: An In Vitro Comparison Study

Agata Kabała-Dzik [1,*], Anna Rzepecka-Stojko [2], Robert Kubina [1], Żaneta Jastrzębska-Stojko [3], Rafał Stojko [4], Robert Dariusz Wojtyczka [5] and Jerzy Stojko [6]

[1] Department of Pathology, School of Pharmacy with the Division of Laboratory Medicine in Sosnowiec, Medical University of Silesia in Katowice, Ostrogórska 30, 41-200 Sosnowiec, Poland; rkubina@sum.edu.pl

[2] Department of Pharmaceutical Chemistry, School of Pharmacy with the Division of Laboratory Medicine in Sosnowiec, Medical University of Silesia in Katowice, Jagiellońska 4, 41-200 Sosnowiec, Poland; annastojko@sum.edu.pl

[3] Department of Anesthesiology and Intensive Care, Prof. K. Gibiński University Clinical Center, Medical University of Silesia in Katowice, Ceglana 35, 40-514 Katowice, Poland; zak@czkstojko.pl

[4] Department of Women Health, School of Health Sciences, Medical University of Silesia in Katowice, Medyków 12, 40-752 Katowice, Poland; rstojko@sum.edu.pl

[5] Department and Institute of Microbiology and Virology, School of Pharmacy with the Division of Laboratory Medicine in Sosnowiec, Medical University of Silesia in Katowice, Jagiellońska 4, 41-200 Sosnowiec, Poland; rwojtyczka@sum.edu.pl

[6] Department of Toxicology and Bioanalysis, School of Pharmacy with the Division of Laboratory Medicine in Sosnowiec, Medical University of Silesia in Katowice, Jagiellońska 4, 41-200 Sosnowiec, Poland; jstojko@sum.edu.pl

* Correspondence: adzik@sum.edu.pl; Tel.: +48-32-364-13-54

Received: 19 September 2017; Accepted: 3 October 2017; Published: 19 October 2017

Abstract: One of the deadliest cancers among women is a breast cancer. Research has shown that two natural substances occurring in propolis, caffeic acid (CA) and caffeic acid phenethyl ester (CAPE), have significant anticancer effects. The purpose of our in vitro study was to compare cytotoxic activity and migration rate inhibition using CA and CAPE (doses of 50 and 100 μm) against triple-negative, MDA-MB-231 breast adenocarcinoma line cells, drawn from Caucasian women. Viability was measured by XTT-NR-SRB assay (Tetrazolium hydroxide-Neutral Red-Sulforhodamine B) for 24 h and 48 h periods. Cell migration for wound healing assay was taken for 0 h, 8 h, 16 h, and 24 h periods. CAPE displayed more than two times higher cytotoxicity against MDA-MB-231 cells. IC_{50} values for the XTT assay were as follows: CA for 24 h and 48 h were 150.94 μM and 108.42 μM, respectively, while CAPE was 68.82 μM for 24 h and 55.79 μM for 48 h. For the NR assay: CA was 135.85 μM at 24 h and 103.23 μM at 48 h, while CAPE was 64.04 μM at 24 h and 53.25 μM at 48 h. For the SRB assay: CA at 24 h was 139.80 μM and at 48 h 103.98 μM, while CAPE was 66.86 μM at 24 h and 47.73 μM at 48 h. Both agents suspended the migration rate; however, CAPE displayed better activity. Notably, for the 100 μM CAPE dose, motility of the tested breast carcinoma cells was halted.

Keywords: caffeic acid; CAPE; migration; wound healing; breast cancer; propolis

1. Introduction

Properly-fortified diets, especially those enriched with compounds such as polyphenols or phenolic acids, are found to counter the development of many diseases [1–3].

Propolis is one of many natural substances which are becoming increasingly popular for study by cancer research projects. Propolis is an amorphous, viscous substance, of a resin-like consistency, produced by honey bees (*Apis mellifera*) from collected plant pollen, which bees supplement with bee's wax or bee bread. The composition of propolis is extremely complex and varies depending on the locale, season, weather conditions, and plant species from which it is gathered [4–7].

Numerous scientific studies have shown that propolis has antiviral, antimicrobial, antifungal, and antiparasitic properties, as well as being known to have anti-inflammatory and antioxidant effects. Additionally, active, cardio-, and hepatoprotective effects have been measured using propolis. There are also research reports of propolis being used as a local anesthetic. Some authors report this compound has antitumor properties due to the antiproliferative, cytotoxic, and proapoptotic properties of propolis compounds. The high concentration of these substances in propolis determine its anti-inflammatory, anti-microbial, regenerative, immunomodulatory, hepatoprotective, antioxidative, and therefore antitumor activity [4–18].

There are hundreds of substances occurring in propolis. Two of these are caffeic acid (CA) and the caffeic acid phenethyl ester (CAPE). Some of their properties reported in research include: antioxidative, antibacterial, antiviral, anti-inflammatory, antiplatelet, antitumor, and antineoplastic effects [19–25].

In vitro research studies have clearly shown the cytotoxic properties of CAPE against: cells of pulmonary carcinoma, gastric carcinoma, colorectal carcinoma, malignant melanoma, hepatic carcinoma, pancreatic carcinoma, as well as cervical carcinoma [26–33].

Our earlier research showed that CA inhibits the viability and migration process of oral carcinoma SCC-25 cells and head and neck squamous carcinoma cells, while CAPE was directly reported as a growth inhibitor of breast cancer cells [34,35].

CAPE's antitumor activity was also reported. CAPE inhibits activity of cancer cells by using the significant nuclear transcription factor NF-κB. NF-κB inhibits apoptosis, induces proliferation, and intensifies angiogenesis. Evidence shows that NF-κB could be one of the most important factors in the process of oncogenesis and cancer progression. Moreover, it was shown that CAPE aggregates the Fas death-inducing receptors through a Fas-L-independent mechanism [36–38].

Research studies of breast cancer have shown CAPE is an inhibitor of FGF-2 (fibroblasts growth factor type 2), which is a factor of tumor growth. CAPE performance was evaluated positively, both for in vitro and in vivo research of MCF-7 and MDA-231 breast cancer cells. It is worth noting that CAPE did not affect healthy cells [23,39]. It was also shown that CAPE reduces expression of the mdr-1 gene, which causes increased sensitivity of tumor cells to chemotherapy. Also, after treatment with CAPE, the decreased vascular endothelial growth factor (VEGF) inhibited angiogenesis and tumor growth [40,41].

Breast cancer is one of the deadliest cancers among women. It is well known that genetic changes are conducive to the development of cancer. For instance, activation of oncogenes and alteration of tumor suppressor gene pathways leads to the development of tumor cells. Eventually, tumor cells lose complete control from highly regulated cell growth signals, leading to abnormal proliferation and avoiding apoptosis [42].

Breast cancer is a heterogeneous disease with many biological subtypes. One is triple negative breast cancer (TNBC). TNBC is much more aggressive than breast cancer of other molecular subtypes and known for its frequency of recurrence. As a result, the mortality rate of patients with TNBC is significantly higher than among patients with other types of breast cancer (estrogen receptor α and progesterone receptor positive) [43].

The treatment of a triple negative breast carcinoma depends on the severity of the disease. The choice of therapy is affected by the presence of metastases, the size of the primary tumor, and the result of detailed pathological tests, such as the degree of malignancy of the tumor, which determines the rate of division of tumor cells. Surgical methods, radiotherapy, and chemotherapy are used in the treatment of triple negative breast cancer. In the treatment of patients with TNBC, it is important to inhibit a formation of blood vessels providing nutrients to tumor tissues, the angiogenesis. However, the therapeutic options are very small here, but neither hormone therapy nor HER2 drugs works.

Therefore, the average survival time in this group is still less than in patients with other types of breast cancer. The biological characterization of the tumor cell is the method used to determine the type of tumor and to obtain valuable information on the factors influencing its growth. Triple negative breast cancer is diagnosed in patients under the age of 50. Factors that promote TNBC are: early menopause, obesity at menopausal age, and breast cancer in the family. The disease is characterized by an aggressive course, rapid tumor growth, and rapid onset of distal metastases (especially to the brain and lungs, and to a lesser extent bone and liver) and early relapse (within 1–3 years of diagnosis). A large number of patients with this type of cancer have a poor prognosis due to low remission during adjuvant therapy, and in the case of metastases a short survival time and high resistance to chemotherapy [44–48].

The response rate among patients with metastatic breast cancer is gradually decreasing, possibly due to the tumor's resistance to a wide range of cancer therapies [43,49–51]. Unfortunately, it must be mentioned that metastatic breast cancer's resistance to all forms of systemic treatments (hormonal, chemotherapy, and targeted) results in an estimated 90% or more of patients with metastatic disease developing tumors which will prove lethal [52].

The aims of decreasing toxicity levels of standard breast cancer treatment and increasing patients' survival chances have led researchers to test natural substances and their varying compounds. Such studies have yielded highly positive and encouraging results for breast cancer treatment. Taking into consideration the above facts, we compare in vitro effects of CAPE and CA (viability and migration) on MDA-MB-231 human breast cancer cells, which to the best of our knowledge is a new approach.

2. Materials and Methods

2.1. Cell Lines and Reagents

2.1.1. Breast Cancer Cell Line MDA-MB-231

In this research, the MDA-MB-231 line (human breast adenocarcinoma TNBC, No. 92020424 SIGMA from Sigma-Aldrich, Poznań, Poland) was used, as it is a model of human triple-negative breast cancer. The manufacturer's recommendations for preparations were all carefully followed. The MDA-MB-231 cells were cultured with Leibovitz's L-15 medium, with 10% of inactivated fetal bovine serum (FBS, Sigma-Aldrich, Poznań, Poland), and kept at 37 °C, without CO_2.

All cultured cells were supplemented with antibiotics of the following concentrations: penicillin—100 $U \cdot mL^{-1}$, streptomycin—100 $\mu g \cdot mL^{-1}$ and fungistatic amphotericin B with a concentration of 0.25 $\mu g \cdot mL^{-1}$. The medium was changed every 2–3 days, with the passage carried out with a confluence of 80% to 90%.

2.1.2. CA and CAPE

Both caffeic acid (CA, Sigma: C0625) and caffeic acid phenethyl ester (CAPE, Sigma: C8221) were purchased from Sigma-Aldrich, Poznań, Poland and were collected, stored, and used specifically according to the manufacturer's instructions.

2.2. Microscopic Evaluation of Carcinoma Cells Morphology. Hematoxylin and Eosin Staining Protocol

Initially, the MDA-MB-231 cells were inoculated into 2-chamber microscopic culture vessels (Lab-Tek, Waltham, MA, USA) at a count of 1000 cells/well. Depending on the time of the experiment, we added proper concentrations of the studied compounds to the media and left them for 24 and 48 h. This was followed by leaving the cultures for 24 h to obtain the cells' growth rate. They were then fixed for 12 h in 96% ethanol. The cells were then hydrated in the following series of dilutions: 99.6%, 96%, 90%, 80%, 70%, and 50% and stained with hematoxylin for 7 min (standard H&E staining protocol). Next, the plates were washed with PBS solution for approximately 30 min to blue up and were then incubated for 30 s with eosin. PBS solution was used again to wash the plates, and they were then dehydrated with ethanol of increasing concentrations of 50%, 70%, 80%, 90%, 96%, and 99.6%. Finally, the plates were immersed in the ethanol and xylene mixture (50:50) for 1 min and then in pure xylene. The plates were then mounted and analyzed under a microscope.

2.3. Cell Viability by Mitochondrial Activity, XTT Test Assay

Viable cells depend on an intact mitochondrial respiratory chain and an intact mitochondrial membrane. Activity of the measured compounds was determined using mitochondrial dehydrogenases from the viable cells. XTT (2,3-bis[2methoxy-4-nitro-5-sulfopheny]-2H-tetrazolium -5-carboxyanilide inner salt) is a tetrazolium salt that cleaves to formazan by the succinate dehydrogenase system, which belongs to the mitochondrial respiratory chain. This is significant, as it is only active in viable cells. Mitochondrial succinate dehydrogenase reduces yellow tetrazolium salt into a soluble orange formazan in the presence of an electron coupling reagent. The number of originating formazan is proportional to the amount of living cells [53]. We measured the enzyme activity at 480 nm, which is in line with the manufacturer's recommendation. The XTT assay was obtained from Xenometrix AG, Allschwil, Switzerland.

To measure cytotoxicity, the cells were inoculated on 96-well plates, at an amount of 10^4 cells/well. A fresh medium was added and left for 72 h to obtain the rate of cell growth. After the medium was decanted, separate culture mediums were added which contained 50 μM and 100 μM of either CA or CAPE, which had been prepared during a series of dilutions in the culture medium. A measure of 0.1 mL of medium with the defined concentrations of the substances was added to each well and left for 24 h/48 h in a CO_2 incubator at 37 °C. The test procedure was performed exactly in accordance with the instructions and protocol of the manufacturer.

2.4. Cytotoxicity by Lyzosomal Activity, NR Test Assay

Cell survival and viability can also be measured by using the ability of viable cells to incorporate and bind to neutral red (NR), which is best performed on adherent cells. Neutral red is a weak cationic dye that readily penetrates the cell membrane and accumulates intracellularly in lysosomes (lysosomal pH < cytoplasmic pH), where it binds to anionic sites of the lysosomal matrix. Lysosomal fragility and other effects, which gradually became irreversible, are caused by changes of the cell surface and the sensitivity of the lysosomal membrane. Such alterations, induced by the action of xenobiotics, result in decreased uptake and binding of NR. Therefore, it is possible to distinguish between viable, damaged, or dead cells [54]. The NR test was obtained from Xenometrix AG, Allschwil, Switzerland. We used CA and CAPE at concentrations of 50 μM and 100 μM, with 24 h and 48 h of incubation. The quantity of dye incorporated into cells was measured by spectrometry at 540 nm, which is directly proportional to the number of cells of the intact membrane. Test procedures were performed exactly following the instructions and protocol of the manufacturer.

2.5. Cell Proliferation by SRB Test Assay

Cell proliferation, measured as total protein synthesis, is a very sensitive toxicology marker. Sulforhodamine B (SRB, Acid Red 52) is an anionic dye that binds electrostatically to cellular proteins. SRB binds stoichiometrically to cellular proteins (when mild acidic conditions are guaranteed) and can then be extracted under basic conditions. The total amount of bound dye can be used as a proxy for cell mass, which is directly proportional to cell proliferation [55,56]. A fixed dye was solubilized and measured photometrically at OD 540 nm, with a reference filter of 690 nm. The OD values were correlated with total protein content and therefore with cell number. Concentrations of CA and CAPE of 50 μM and 100 μM were used to make the experiments for 24 h and 48 h of incubation. The SRB test was obtained from Xenometrix AG, Allschwil, Switzerland. Procedure of the test was performed exactly in accordance to the instructions and protocol of the manufacturer.

2.6. Migration—Cell Wound Closure Assay

Carcinoma cell migration is the result of variable biological processes, with a specific characteristic seen in their coordination. Wound-healing assays are standard and commonly used methods for investigation of cell migration. CA's and CAPE's ability to modify cell motility using the scratch wound healing assay was then analyzed [57,58]. This method was implemented to evaluate the migration activity rate of MDA-MB-231 cells exposed to CA and CAPE.

Briefly, the MDA-MB-231 cells (4×10^6 cells/well) were plated in 6-well plates for 48 h to a confluence of about 80%, then wounded by scratching with a p200 pipette tip. Thereafter, the debris was removed and we washed the cells once with 1 mL of the growth medium to assure the edges of the scratch were smoothed by washing. We took utmost care to make the wounds of the same dimensions, both for the experimental and control cells to minimize any possible variety resulting from a difference in scratch width.

The cells were then incubated with DMEM medium containing 0.5% FBS and treated with CA/CAPE doses of 50 μM and 100 μM, respectively. The control sample contained the cells and a standard medium without any active agents. The MDA-MB-231 cell migration was assessed by monolayer gap closure migration assay, embedded by free ImageJ software (version 1.50i, National Institute of Health, Bethesda, MD, USA), with a wound healing tool macro (Montpellier RIO Imaging, CNRS, Montpellier, France). The area of the initial wound was measured, followed by gap area measurements after 8 h, 16 h, and 24 h. The migration factor was presented as the gap area value over the initial scratch area.

2.7. Statistical Analysis

All results are expressed as means ± SD and were obtained from three separate experiments and performed in quadruplicates ($n = 12$). The results were performed with independent sample *t*-tests. The experimental means were compared to the means of untreated cells harvested in a parallel manner. Differences between 24 h/48 h and control samples were tested for significance using the one- and multiple-way Friedman ANOVA test. A *p*-value less than 0.05 was considered statistically significant.

3. Results

To obtain the quantitative assessment of breast cancer cells' viability, the XTT-NR-SRB (Tetrazolium hydroxide-Neutral Red-Sulforhodamine B) assay was used. IN a parallel fashion, the effects of selected times/concentrations of CA and CAPE on breast cancer cell motility and migration were evaluated. Figure 1 shows MDA-MB-231 carcinoma cells' morphology features as well as the impact of CA and CAPE on these cells. Examined cells were as phenotypical as the spindle shaped cells, with a visible hyperchromasia. Cell nuclei shapes were irregular. Small cells clustered around the large ones. The large, irregular nuclei contained several nucleoli in the nucleus. A pleomorphism of size and shape, as well as a coloration of nuclei, were visible. In the optical microscope, morphological characteristics of the apoptotic cells were visible, after the CA and CAPE treatment. Namely, we observed a cytoplasm density and changes in nuclear chromatin. The cytoplasmic shapes were changed. A fragmentation of a cytoplasm was visible. The cells were separated from each other.

For years, tetrazolium salts have been widely used as detection reagents in histochemical localization studies and cell biology assays. Like the MTT assay (reducing tetrazolium dye: 3-(4,5-dimethylthiazol-2-yl)-2,5-diphenyltetrazolium bromide to formazan), XTT measures cell viability based on the activity of enzymes in mitochondria of live cells, which reduces XTT and becomes inactive shortly after cell death. The data obtained in the experiment were normalized and presented as the percentage of control values (Figure 2).

When CA was used for treatment of MDA-MB-231, cell viability decreased as the dose increased, dropping from 93.1% for a dose of 10 μM, 89.8% for 25 μM, 77.9% for 50 μM, and a value of 66.4%

was reached with a dose of 100 µM after 24 h (Figure 2a,d). Simultaneously, when CAPE activity was compared to that of CA against MDA-MB-231 cells (Figure 2a,d), CAPE cell viability values for a dose of 10 µM were similar to CA (at 24 h, CA was 93.1%, while CAPE was 92.4%; after 48 h, CA was 92.4% and CAPE was 90.4%). The smallest doses of these two polyphenols had a similar cytotoxic effect on the examined cells. The effect increased in a dose-dependent manner for both agents. For CAPE, the values reached 68.4%, 51.9%, and 37.5% for respective doses of 25, 50, and 100 µM (Figure 2a,c), meaning that a stronger cytotoxic effect was achieved with CAPE at 24 h. After 48 h of incubation (Figure 2b), for both CAPE and CA, cell viability showed a dose-dependent effect and the values were as follows: for a 10 µM dose CAPE was 90.4% and CA 92.4%, for a dose of 25 µM CAPE was 53.5% and CA 79.5%, for 50 µM CAPE was 45.3% and CA 68.5%, and finally, for 100 µM CAPE was 31.6% and CA 55.5%.

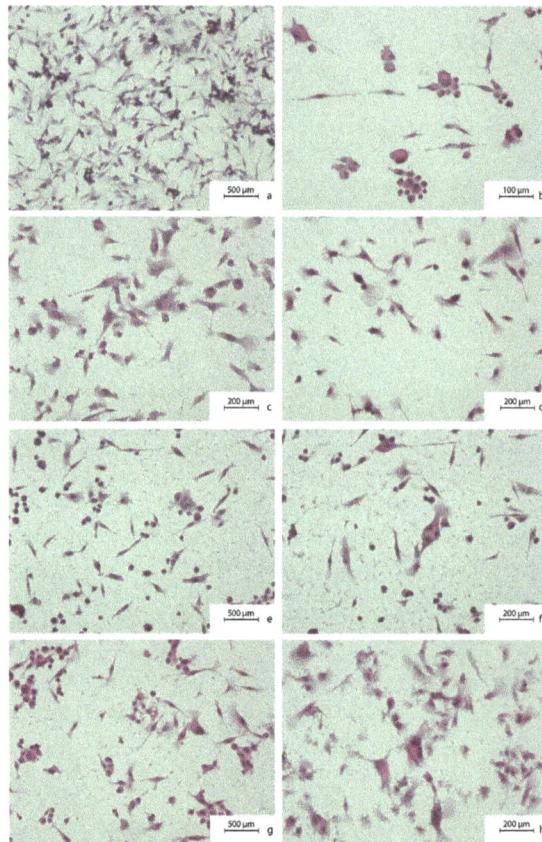

Figure 1. Cytomorphological view of MDA-MB-231 breast cancer cells without any treatment (**a–d**) as well as after 24 h of caffeic acid (CA) (**e,f**) and 24 h of caffeic acid phenethyl ester (CAPE) treatment (**g,h**), both with a 50 µM dose. To prepare the samples a hematoxylin and eosin staining was used. Exposition: optical magnification ×100 (**a,e,g**), ×400 (**c,d,f,h**), ×600 (**b**). Main features: (**a**) phenotypically as spindle-shaped cells (caudate, tadpole), hyperchromasia; (**b**) irregular nuclear shapes, small clusters of cells around the large ones; (**c**) large nuclei with irregular shape and several nucleoli in the nucleus; (**d**) pleomorphism of size, shape, and coloration of nuclei and whole cells; (**e**) karyopyknosis; (**f**) lower cell-cell contact; (**g**) karyopyknosis, cytoplasm density; (**h**) cytoplasm density and a shape change, cytoplasm fragmentation.

Comparing CAPE activity to that of CA, viability was again lower for CAPE at the same dosage after 48 h. This showed a dependent trend for the dose and time domain (smaller impact) for both examined substances (Figure 2c,d).

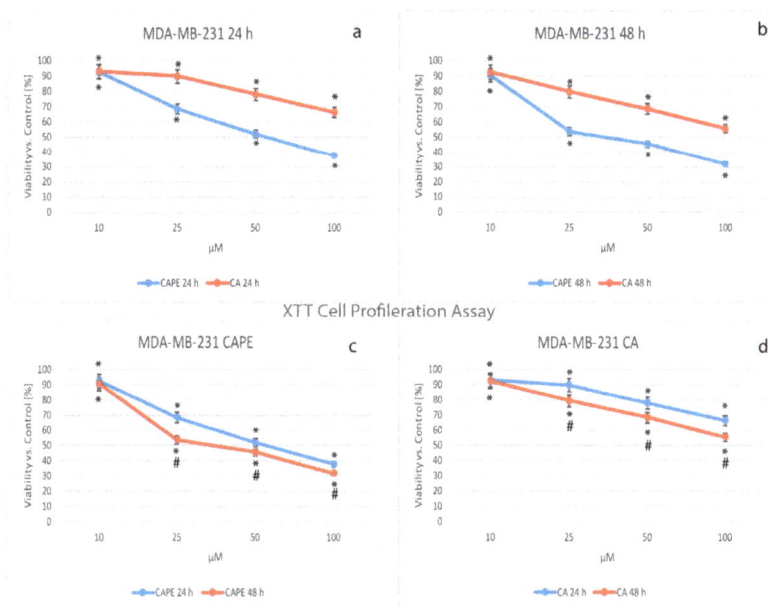

Figure 2. Cytotoxic effects of caffeic acid phenethyl ester (CAPE) and caffeic acid (CA) were both tested using concentrations of from 10 to 100 μM with 24 h and 48 h incubation times on the breast cancer cell line MDA-MB-231 using XTT (2,3-bis[2methoxy-4-nitro-5-sulfopheny]-2H-tetrazolium-5-carboxyanilide inner salt) Cell Proliferation Assay. Both polyphenols caused visible dose-dependent effects. Stronger activity was observed for CAPE than CA starting with a dose of 25 μM of each agent following 24 h (**a**) and 48 h (**b**) incubation times. A CAPE treatment of 48 h gave slightly stronger cytotoxic effect compared to 24 h (except a 10 μM dose) and was exclusively stronger for the 25 μM dose (**c**); however, succeeding dose increases of CAPE (50 and 100 μM) didn't yield symptomatic difference in viability, with both times reaching a low level. The experiment times (**c**,**d**) had only a small impact on cytotoxic activity. The results were presented as a mean and standard deviation of three independent experiments, with 12 wells each ($p < 0.05$; Friedman ANOVA test; *—significant difference vs. control, #—significant difference 48 h vs. 24 h).

The key component of the next viability test performed was the vital dye, neutral red (NR). Viable cells take up the dye by active transport and incorporate the dye into lysosomes, whereas non-viable cells do not take up the dye. The data obtained in the experiment were normalized and presented as % of viability over controls (Figure 3).

Using CA against MDA-MB-231 cells, the cell mortality increased in a dose-dependent manner. The viability values dropped from 93.26% for a dose of 10 μM, to 89.56% for 25 μM, 71.39% for 50 μM, and 64.54% with a dose of 100 μM of CA after 24 h (Figure 3a,d). Comparing CAPE's cytotoxic activity to that of CA against MDA-MB-231 cells (Figure 3a,b), cell viability values for a dose of 10 μM were similar: at 24 h CA was 93.26% and CAPE was 91.96%, while at 48 h CA was 91.08% and CAPE 90.36%. A dosage of 10 μM of both polyphenols had a similar cytotoxic effect on the examined cells (independent of time). Using CAPE against the examined cells, at 24 h the values reached 66.30%,

47.40%, and 35.12% for doses of 25, 50, and 100 μM, respectively (Figure 3a,c). The results sustain that CAPE achieved a stronger cytotoxic effect at 24 h.

For both substances, cell viability manifested a dose-dependent effect after 48 h of incubation (Figure 3b). The values were: at 10 μM CAPE was 90.36% and CA 91.08%, at 25 μM CAPE was 55.02% and CA 78.25%, for 50 μM CAPE was 41.38% and CA 65.80%, and finally, for 100 μM, CAPE was 29.46% and CA: 53.86%. Therefore, CAPE induces greater cell mortality than CA at the same dosage. Both CA and CAPE showed a dependent trend for the dose and time domain, but again a smaller impact (Figure 3c,d).

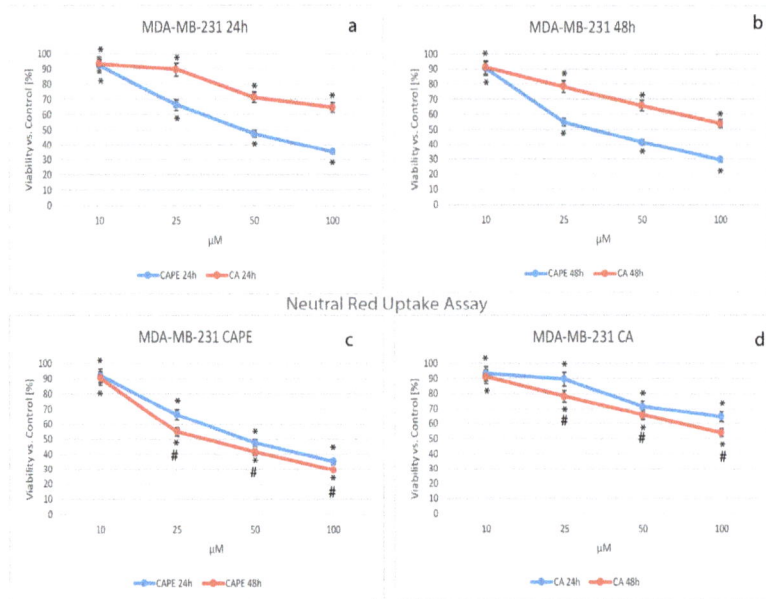

Figure 3. Cytotoxic effects of caffeic acid phenethyl ester (CAPE) and caffeic acid (CA) were tested using concentrations of from 10 to 100 μM with 24 h and 48 h incubation times on the breast cancer cell line MDA-MB-231 using neutral red (NR) Assay. Both polyphenols caused visible dose-dependent effects. A higher mortality factor was observed with CAPE than CA, starting from a dose of 25 μM of the tested compounds (**a,b**) for both 24 h and 48 h periods. In (**c**), using a dose of 10 μM of CAPE, the 48 h experiment did not produce any significant cytotoxic effects when compared to 24 h; nevertheless, a conspicuously stronger effect for 25 μM was observed. The succeeding dosage increases of CAPE (50 and 100 μM) displayed only a slight difference in viability factor, with both reaching a very low level. The cytotoxic activity of both substances showed no spectacular difference over time (**c,d**). The results were presented as mean and standard deviation of three independent experiments, with 12 wells each ($p < 0.05$; Friedman ANOVA test; *—significant difference vs. control, #—significant difference 48 h vs. 24 h).

The key component of the last cytotoxicity test performed was the dye, Sulforhodamine B (Acid Red 52). An increase or decrease in the number of cells causes an associated change in the amount of dye incorporated by the cells in the culture. This indicates the specific degree of cytotoxicity caused by the test material. Data received during the experiment were normalized and presented as % of viability over controls (Figure 4).

Testing CA against MDA-MB-231 cells, cell viability declined in a dose-dependent manner, falling after 24 h from 93.13% for a dose of 10 μM, to 92.78% for 25 μM, 67.46% for 50 μM, and to a value of 66.89% using a dose of 100 µM CA (Figure 4a,d). When CAPE cytotoxic activity was compared to CA against MDA-MB-231 cells (Figure 4a,b), cell viability values for a dose of 10 µM were again close to those of CA. At 24 h, CA was 93.19% and CAPE 92.21%, and at 48 h, CA was 91.99% while CAPE was 86.90% (where a slight difference was finally observed). At a dosage of 10 µM, both polyphenols had a similar cytotoxic effect on the examined cells, which was also observed in viability tests performed earlier for this study. The viability was dependent for the dose and time domain. For CAPE at 24 h, the values reached 68.85%, 50.05%, and 36.13% for doses of 25, 50, and 100 µM, respectively (Figure 4a,c). Again, CAPE's stronger cytotoxic effect than CA's was confirmed after 24 h.

After 48 h of incubation (Figure 4b) for both CAPE and CA, cell viability revealed a dose-dependent effect, with values as follows: for 10 µM CAPE was 86.90% and CA 91.99%, for 25 µM CAPE was 56.08% and CA 77.69%, for 50 µM CAPE was 37.80% and CA 64.22%, and finally, 100 µM CAPE reached 22.98% and CA 54.88%. Comparing CAPE to CA after 48 h, cell mortality was again higher for CAPE than CA at the same dosage. Dependent trends in the dose and time domain (greater impact than by XTT and NR) for both CA and CAPE were confirmed (Figure 4c,d).

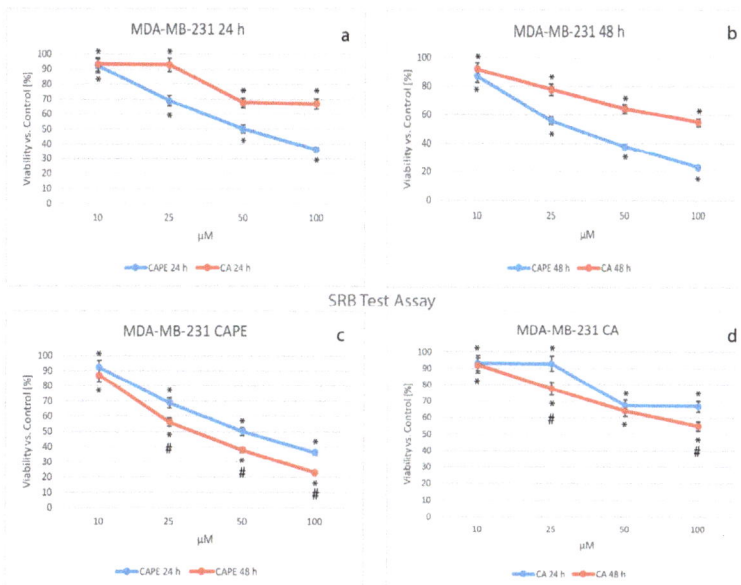

Figure 4. Viability results of the SRB (Sulforhodamine B) assay of caffeic acid phenethyl ester (CAPE) and caffeic acid (CA) at concentrations of from 10 to 100 µM for 24 h and 48 h incubation times on the breast cancer cell line MDA-MB-231. Like the XTT (2,3-bis[2methoxy-4-nitro-5-sulfopheny]-2H-tetrazolium-5-carboxyanilide inner salt) and NR (neutral red) tests, there was a visible dose-dependent effect for both polyphenols. Interestingly, for the 24 h experiment, CA (**a**) expressed 'two levels'—a first for 10 and 25 µM and a second (**d**), for 50 and 100 µM; this phenomenon could be explained by nonlinear absorbance; however, within a 48 h experiment it does not exist. Greater cancer cell mortality using CAPE rather than CA started again (just as with XTT and NR) from a dose of 25 µM of each tested compound for both 24 h (**a**) and 48 h (**b**) incubation times. After 48 h (**c**), CAPE treatment showed a stronger cytotoxic effect in comparison to the 24 h period (except the 10 µM dose). The experiment time had only slight impact on the cytotoxic activity of the tested compounds (**c**,**d**), which wasn't in opposition to the XTT and NR test assay. The results were presented as mean and standard deviation of three independent experiments 12 wells each ($p < 0.05$; Friedman ANOVA test; *—significant difference vs. control, #—significant difference 48 h vs. 24 h).

For both substances (CA and CAPE) used for the MDA-MB-231 breast cancer line, the half maximal inhibitory concentration (IC_{50}) was calculated by all three methods during the experiment. It is significant that the 50%-mortality of breast cancer cells (MDA-MB-231) were ca. twice as low for CAPE than CA for all methods. This showed that CAPE has a stronger cytotoxic effect on MDA-MB-231 cells than CA during 24 h and 48 h experiments. The IC_{50} results are shown in Table 1.

Table 1. IC_{50} (μM) values of caffeic acid (CA) and caffeic acid phenethyl ester (CAPE) in relation to breast cancer MDA-MB-231 for 24 h and 48 h, using different methods (XTT, NR, SRB, respectively: 2,3-bis[2methoxy-4-nitro-5-sulfopheny]-2H-tetrazolium-5-carboxyanilide inner salt, neutral red, Sulforhodamine B). All data demonstrated that lower doses of CAPE (ca. twice as low as CA) are needed to receive a similar mortality effect on MDA-MB-231 cells.

Method	Compound	Time of Incubation 24 h	Time of Incubation 48 h
XTT	CA	150.94	108.42
	CAPE	68.82	55.79
NR	CA	135.85	103.23
	CAPE	64.04	53.25
SRB	CA	139.80	103.98
	CAPE	66.86	47.73

Considering the cytotoxic effect of CA and CAPE (measured in this study by three methods), we clearly see that these two substances are active against MDA-MB-231 breast cancer cells, with CAPE displaying IC_{50} values more than twice as low as CA.

The next stage was an analysis of CA and CAPE's influence on migration of MDA-MB-231 cells. This was measured by wound healing, which is the complex, dynamic process of movement and replacement of missing cells. Observation of live cells' motility is an effective method to measure the rate of migration into the space created by the original wound. The desired situation is when the wound closes as little as possible, so the gap area value over the area of the original wound remains as great as possible, preferably for a prolonged period; this means the examined agent inhibits the migration of the carcinoma cells.

The results of the wound healing assay are presented in Figure 5. In the control group, cell migration was very dynamic, achieving a value of 16% after only 8 h. As seen, the wound's closure was practically complete, reaching a rate value of 1% after 16 h. There was no evidence of the wound after 24 h. Using a 50 μM dose of CA, the motility of the MDA-MB-231 cells was inhibited. The rate increased to 30% after 8 h, 11% after 16 h and 6% after 24 h. The wound closure was not complete following the CA treatment. Increasing the CA dose to 100 μM resulted in better closure rates and therefore promoted migration inhibition of the MDA-MB-231 cells. The wound area value was 49% in relation to the original scratch after 8 h. A value of 16% was achieved after 16 h, and, finally, 9% after 24 h. Inhibition of the cell migration showed a dose-dependent trend.

Using CAPE for wound healing resulted in deeper inhibition of cell migration when compared to CA. For a CAPE dose of 50 μM, the gap area factor was 66% for 8 h. The gap remained at 50% at 16 h and achieved a value of 28% after 24 h. Increasing the CAPE dose to 100 μM displayed better results, as was expected. CAPE stopped the MDA-MB-231 cells from migrating at 75%, after 8 h. The size of the gap remained stable, with a value of 72% after 16 h, to reach a minimal value of 68% after 24 h. CA and CAPE both inhibited migration of MDA-MB-231 cells in a dose-dependent manner. The CAPE treatment displayed better results, particularly for the 100 μM dose, where the motility of tested breast carcinoma cells was practically halted.

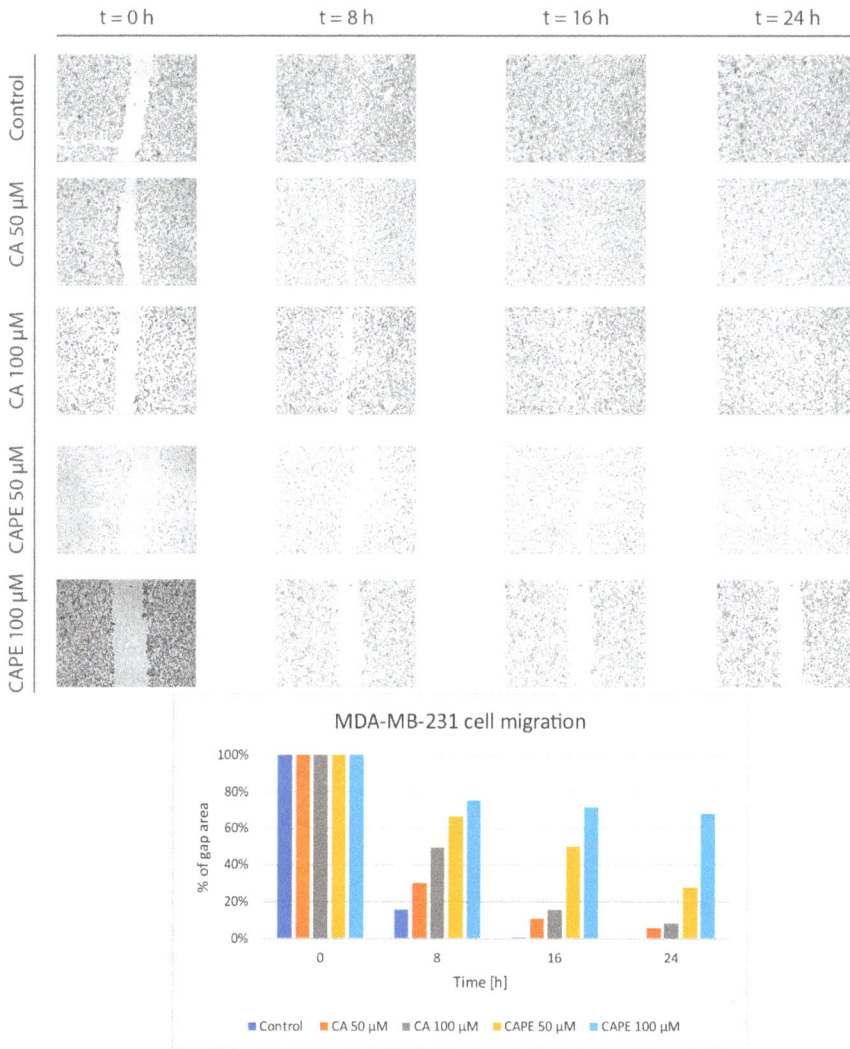

Figure 5. Caffeic acid (CA) and caffeic acid phenethyl ester (CAPE) at concentrations of 50 μM and 100 μM promote an inhibitory migration effect on MDA-MB-231 cells. There was a visible dose-dependent effect. The gap did not reach full closure for either agent. Comparison of these two substances shows CAPE has a greater influence on cell migration inhibition in MDA-MB-231 than CA. CAPE treatment with a dose of 100 μM demonstrated that the wound area basically remained unchanged over time. CAPE created a 'barrier' that was practically impassable and impenetrable by the MDA-MB-231 cells. The cell migration factor was performed by monolayer gap closure migration assay and embedded by free ImageJ software. The results are presented as the gap area in relation to the area value of the initial scratch, after 8 h, 16 h, and 24 h of observation.

4. Discussion

Research targeting finding new anticancer therapies is prompted by cancers' high mortality rate. Bioactive compounds have taken their place in the research arena as new, effective medicines [59,60].

Phytochemicals such as flavonoids, polyphenols, and phenolic acids are of great interest to scientists, due to their specific, active, anticancer effect on cancer cells [61,62].

Among patients diagnosed with breast cancer, complementary and targeted therapies using alternative natural substances are often employed. Between 63% to 80% of all breast cancer patients use at least one type of alternative medicine, while herbal or vitamin therapies are used by some 25% to 63% of the same patient group [63–67].

Simonetti et al. showed that CA is bioavailable and it may be correlated with the antioxidant potential of plasma, by intake of red wine [68].

The presence of the estrogen receptor is one of the priority classification factors of breast cancer cells [18,69]. For breast cancer, proliferation and survival of the cells is dependent on estrogen receptor signaling [22,70].

TNBC can be perfectly modeled using the MDA-MB-231 line because there are no estrogen receptors α and expression of estrogen receptor β is minimal [71,72]. It was initially classified as a basal line of breast cancer cells because of the lack of ER and PR expression, as well as HER2 amplification. At present, it is considered to belong to the claudin-low molecular subtype because the line displays a down-regulation of claudin-3 and claudinin-4, as well as low expression of the Ki-67 proliferative marker and an enrichment of markers associated with an epithelial-mesenchymal transition and an expression of traits associated with breast cancer stem cells (CSC), such as CD44+/CD24−/low phenotype. The cells of this line are distinguished by invasive phenotype [72]. In a bone metastasis researches, the MDA-MD-231 cell line was widely used [73]. Also, the MDA-MB-231 cell subclones have been isolated. They displayed easy bone, brain, and lung metastases, after intraventricular injection into a mice organism. It allowed for the identification of genes and pathways that are potential mediators of metastasis to the specific sites when using this cell line [69,74–77].

For this research, we used MDA-MB-231 cell line as a model of TNBC. Considering the above, this comparative study of CA and CAPE substances, which occur naturally in propolis, shows much promise for breast cancer research.

The estrogenic effect of CAPE was not fully investigated, however; its ability to bind estrogen receptors has been previously shown. CAPE modulates the estrogen receptor selectively and it is more likely related to the estrogen receptor β than α [22,69]. This may indicate that the estrogen-related compounds act better on estrogen-positive neoplastic cells [25,78].

Khoram et al. [79] showed that CAPE stimulated radiosensitivity in breast cancer cells. Clonogenicity was inhibited and radiation-induced DNA damage was maintained in two cell lines, particularly in T47D cells.

Chen et al. [28] and Lin et al. [80] observed that CAPE's anticancer activity was due to cell growth inhibition and a viability decline, both in a time and a dose-dependent manner. In another study, CAPE reduced the colony formation ability of PC-3 prostate cancer cells [26].

In an in vivo study, Wu et al. [27] showed CAPE's ability to reduce the volume of breast cancer tumors, respectively, by 40% and 60% for MDA-231 and MCF-7 xenografts. Interestingly, the lower dose of CAPE (10 μM) was more effective to inhibit the growth of MDA-231 xenografts than 50 μM for the MCF-7 xenografts.

In earlier research, we compared the in vitro cytotoxic activity of ethanol extract of propolis and CAPE against two cell lines, MDA-MB-231 and Hs578T, using MTT and lactate dehydrogenase (LDH) assays. IC_{50} values obtained for CAPE (both assays) were definitely lower than for ethanol extract of propolis [39].

Watabe et al. showed that CAPE inhibits nuclear factor NFκB. They also examined CAPE to confirm that death-inducing receptors clustered. They found that Fas death-inducing receptors were aggregated through a Fas-L independent mechanism in the MCF-7 cells. Consequently, it was shown that CAPE induced apoptosis. The aggregation of death receptors was executed through two pathways; FADD/caspase-8 and JNK/p38 [38].

Beauregard et al. tested CAPE and its 18 derivatives against breast cancer MCF-7 cells. Induction of caspase 3/7 resulted in apoptosis in five of eighteen CAPE-derivatives, which was even better than CAPE alone. Inhibition of NFκB was similar for all tested analogs and CAPE itself. They found that activation of the p53 pathway was realized by all CAPE derivatives [81].

Rosendahl et al. [82] tested caffeine and CA against breast cancer cells MCF-7, T47D, and MDA-MB-231. Their results showed that CA inhibited the proliferation of breast cancer cells, reducing the growth of breast cancer cells through modulating ER and IGFIR levels, thereby influencing downstream effectors and cell-cycle progression, but better CA activity in the MCF-7 cells (estrogen-positive) was observed. Their results displayed that CA suppressed the proliferation of breast cancer cells. They also tested an influence of coffee intake on a breast cancer disease. A higher coffee intake was correlated with a smaller invasion of primary tumors. On the other hand, it was reported by Wu [23] that CAPE inhibits MCF-7 and MDA-231 cells growth. In both cell lines, CAPE induced apoptosis and cell cycle arrest, and inhibited NF-κB as well as down-regulated the mdr-1 gene. VEGF formation was also suppressed by MDA-MB-231 cells. We can assume that activity of CA is closely related to the expression of estrogen, while CAPE acts independently of estrogen.

Our results showed that CAPE has a better cytotoxic effect than CA, which is in line with other research. However, our comparison of these two agents is novel, as it uses a triple cytotoxic assay.

Breast cancer metastasis is one of the primary reasons for its high mortality rate; therefore, migration and invasion research, as well as their mechanism, are part of the new era of breast cancer studies.

Wadhwa et al. used a free form of CAPE, as well as CAPE in a complex with gamma cyclodextrin (γCD) (equivalent doses), for cell viability studies of breast cancer lines MCF-7 and MDA-MB-231. They showed that CAPE displayed short-term toxicity, while CAPE-γCD complex caused permanent growth inhibition or apoptosis, which suggested that CAPE-γCD complex was characterized by a stronger effect. They also found that CAPE causes upregulation of p53 function by targeting mortalin-p53-interaction. The scratch and invasion studies on MCF-7 and MDA-MB-231 cells and their metastatic samples have shown that both CAPE-γCD complex and CAPE alone exhibit anti-migration activity [83].

Bonuccelli et al. showed that CAPE treatment significantly reduced wound closure (about 70% vs control) on breast cancer MCF-7 cells. In the 24 h period, CAPE acted as a natural mitochondrial OXPHOS inhibitor, which preventively targeted stem-like cancer cells. They also suggested that CAPE blocks formation of the mammosphere [84].

Recent research is being conducted to find a mechanism of the breast cancer cells migration.

Interesting results were proposed by Buchegger et al. [85]. They suggested potential mechanism of migration of MDA-MB-231 cells. They expressed Reprimo (RPRM) ectopically in MDA-MB-231 cells. RPRM is located at 2q23 and encodes a highly glycosylated protein that shows four bands (16, 21, 23, and 40 kDa) found predominantly in the cytoplasm. They found that RPRM overexpression suppressed migration and invasion of MDA-MB-231 cells. Another study on a mechanism of the migration was done by Bhat et al. [86]. Growth-regulated oncogene α (GROα) is a chemokine that plays a role not only in inflammation, but also in tumorigenesis. They found that MDA-MB-231 cells without GROα exhibited a significant migration decrease and invasion properties reduction. Liu et al. [87] showed that CD74 is involved in breast carcinoma metastasis. CD74 protein is the invariant chain of major histocompatibility complex (MHC) class II. Their results showed that this factor was highly expressed in MDA-MB-231 cells; furthermore, a downregulation of CD74 inhibited both migration and invasion of MDA-MB-231 cells. Wang et al. [88] reported that TBC1D3 oncogene promotes the migration of breast cancer cells, and its interaction with calmodulin enhances the effects of TBC1D3.

CAPE is known as a specific inhibitor of activation of nuclear transcription factor NF-κB in breast cancer cells [38,89]. Also, Wang et al. [90] found that an activation of NF-κB is required for the cell migration and TBC1D3-induced expression of OLR1, an oxidized low-density lipoprotein receptor 1, also known as lectin-like oxidized low-density lipoprotein (oxLDL) receptor-1. Our results showed a motility inhibition of human breast cancer cells by CAPE. It appears that CAPE addition inhibited the ability of the oncogene TBC1D3 to stimulate OLR1 expression in MDA-MB-231 cells. The tumor cells migration might be induced by TBC1D3, therefore an inhibition of NF-κB could result in the migration suppression thanks to CAPE addition.

CAPE influence on the migration of lung cancer A549 cells was tested by Shigeoka et al. They found that CAPE suppressed the motility promoted by TGF-beta-induced Akt phosphorylation [89].

Today, natural resources are being used more often. Also, a synthesis of analogues from natural remedies is proving to be an interesting source of substances that exhibit favorable activity for breast cancer treatment [90,91].

In earlier studies, we investigated the effect of CA on wound scratch on human squamous cell carcinoma cell line SCC-25. For ethanol treatment, approximately 5% of the wound was visible, while there was no closure if CA or a CA/ethanol mixture were used after 12 h. Total or nearly complete closure occurred after a treatment with 50 and 100 mmol/L of ethanol after 30 h, while with CA, a dose of 50 µM significantly inhibited migration of the cancer cells, leaving from 30% to 40% of wound closure after 30 h. The biggest gap (approx. 80%) was observed for pure CA treatment with a dose of 50 µM after 48 h [34].

We also compared the cytotoxic properties (by MTT) of CA and CAPE apoptosis induction and cell cycle arrest capabilities against MDA-MB-231 cells and found better activity of CAPE, with the same dosage and time of experiment [92].

Our novel comparative study confirms that CA and CAPE suspended migration rate of breast cancer MDA-MB-231 cells; however, much better results were obtained by the CAPE treatment.

5. Conclusions

In this limited in vitro study, we showed a comparison of CA and CAPE, two bioactive substances isolated from bee propolis. An XTT-NR-SRB assay and migration evaluation by wound healing assay were performed. We strongly believe, based on our results and other reports, that CA and CAPE can be used for chemoprevention. Nevertheless, more advanced studies are needed, particularly clinical trials. The mechanism of CA and CAPE's anticancer activity is becoming more well understood and documented; however, it remains a field in need of further investigation. Hopefully, this new approach of testing natural agents for breast cancer research will carefully explore the anti-cancer properties of all polyphenols. Our comparison of the effect of CA and CAPE on MDA-MB-231 cells clearly showed better results for CAPE-producing anticancer properties using the same dosages and experiment times.

Acknowledgments: This study was supported by a research grant from the Medical University of Silesia in Katowice, Poland, No. KNW 1-169/N/6/0.

Author Contributions: Agata Kabała-Dzik conceived the study idea, designed and performed the experiments, analyzed the data, and wrote the manuscript. Anna Rzepecka-Stojko carried out the experimental protocol; Robert Kubina performed the experiments and organized the data. Żaneta Jastrzębska-Stojko analyzed the data and made discussion research. Rafał Stojko consulted current treatments of breast cancer and analyzed the results; Robert Dariusz Wojtyczka organized the data and revised the manuscript. Jerzy Stojko contributed reagents and tools and critically revised the manuscript. All authors read and approved the final manuscript.

Conflicts of Interest: The authors declare no conflict of interest. The founding sponsor had no role in the design of the study; in the collection, analyses, or interpretation of data; in the writing of the manuscript, or in the decision to publish the results.

References

1. Rzepecka-Stojko, A.; Stojko, J.; Kurek-Gorecka, A.; Gorecki, M.; Kabala-Dzik, A.; Kubina, R.; Mozdzierz, A.; Buszman, E. Polyphenols from bee pollen: Structure, absorption, metabolism and biological activity. *Molecules* **2015**, *20*, 21732–21749. [CrossRef] [PubMed]

2. Rice-Evans, C.A.; Miller, N.J.; Paganga, G. Structure—Antioxidant activity relationships of flavonoids and phenolic acids. *Free Radic. Biol. Med.* **1996**, *20*, 933–956. [CrossRef]

3. Iriti, M. Editorial: Introduction to polyphenols, plant chemicals for human health. *Mini-Rev. Med. Chem.* **2011**, *11*, 1183–1185. [PubMed]

4. Castaldo, S.; Capasso, F. Propolis, an old remedy used in modern medicine. *Fitoterapia* **2002**, *73* (Suppl. 1), S1–S6. [CrossRef]

5. Popova, M.; Giannopoulou, E.; Skalicka-Wozniak, K.; Graikou, K.; Widelski, J.; Bankova, V.; Kalofonos, H.; Sivolapenko, G.; Gawel-Beben, K.; Antosiewicz, B.; et al. Characterization and biological evaluation of propolis from Poland. *Molecules* **2017**, *22*, 1159. [CrossRef] [PubMed]

6. Sforcin, J.M.; Bankova, V.; Kuropatnicki, A.K. Medical Benefits of Honeybee Products. *Evid. Based Complement. Altern. Med.* **2017**, *2017*, 2702106. [CrossRef] [PubMed]

7. Wojtyczka, R.D.; Dziedzic, A.; Idzik, D.; Kepa, M.; Kubina, R.; Kabala-Dzik, A.; Smolen-Dzirba, J.; Stojko, J.; Sajewicz, M.; Wasik, T.J. Susceptibility of Staphylococcus aureus clinical isolates to propolis extract alone or in combination with antimicrobial drugs. *Molecules* **2013**, *18*, 9623–9640. [CrossRef] [PubMed]

8. Dziedzic, A.; Kubina, R.; Wojtyczka, R.D.; Kabala-Dzik, A.; Tanasiewicz, M.; Morawiec, T. The antibacterial effect of ethanol extract of polish propolis on mutans streptococci and lactobacilli isolated from saliva. *Evid. Based Complement. Altern. Med.* **2013**, *2013*, 681891. [CrossRef] [PubMed]

9. Wang, P.; Liu, C.; Sanches, T.; Zhong, Y.; Liu, B.; Xiong, J.; Neamati, N.; Zhao, G. Design and synthesis of novel nitrogen-containing polyhydroxylated aromatics as HIV-1 integrase inhibitors from caffeic acid phenethyl ester. *Bioorg. Med. Chem. Lett.* **2009**, *19*, 4574–4578. [CrossRef] [PubMed]

10. Bufalo, M.C.; Bordon-Graciani, A.P.; Conti, B.J.; de Assis Golim, M.; Sforcin, J.M. The immunomodulatory effect of propolis on receptors expression, cytokine production and fungicidal activity of human monocytes. *J. Pharm. Pharmacol.* **2014**, *66*, 1497–1504. [CrossRef] [PubMed]

11. Jastrzebska-Stojko, Z.; Stojko, R.; Rzepecka-Stojko, A.; Kabala-Dzik, A.; Stojko, J. Biological activity of propolis-honey balm in the treatment of experimentally-evoked burn wounds. *Molecules* **2013**, *18*, 14397–14413. [CrossRef] [PubMed]

12. Kurek-Gorecka, A.; Rzepecka-Stojko, A.; Gorecki, M.; Stojko, J.; Sosada, M.; Swierczek-Zieba, G. Structure and antioxidant activity of polyphenols derived from propolis. *Molecules* **2013**, *19*, 78–101. [CrossRef] [PubMed]

13. Iriti, M.; Kubina, R.; Cochis, A.; Sorrentino, R.; Varoni, E.M.; Kabala-Dzik, A.; Azzimonti, B.; Dziedzic, A.; Rimondini, L.; Wojtyczka, R.D. Rutin, a quercetin glycoside, restores chemosensitivity in human breast cancer cells. *Phytother. Res.* **2017**, *31*, 1529–1539. [CrossRef] [PubMed]

14. Su, K.Y.; Hsieh, C.Y.; Chen, Y.W.; Chuang, C.T.; Chen, C.T.; Chen, Y.L. Taiwanese green propolis and propolin G protect the liver from the pathogenesis of fibrosis via eliminating TGF-beta-induced Smad2/3 phosphorylation. *J. Agric. Food Chem.* **2014**. [CrossRef] [PubMed]

15. Chen, Y.J.; Shiao, M.S.; Hsu, M.L.; Tsai, T.H.; Wang, S.Y. Effect of caffeic acid phenethyl ester, an antioxidant from propolis, on inducing apoptosis in human leukemic HL-60 cells. *J. Agric. Food Chem.* **2001**, *49*, 5615–5619. [CrossRef] [PubMed]

16. Kustiawan, P.M.; Puthong, S.; Arung, E.T.; Chanchao, C. In vitro cytotoxicity of Indonesian stingless bee products against human cancer cell lines. *Asian Pac. J. Trop Med.* **2014**, *4*, 549–556. [CrossRef] [PubMed]

17. Xuan, H.; Li, Z.; Yan, H.; Sang, Q.; Wang, K.; He, Q.; Wang, Y.; Hu, F. Antitumor activity of Chinese propolis in human breast cancer MCF-7 and MDA-MB-231 cells. *Evid. Based Complement. Altern. Med.* **2014**, *2014*, 280120. [CrossRef] [PubMed]

18. Kamiya, T.; Nishihara, H.; Hara, H.; Adachi, T. Ethanol extract of Brazilian red propolis induces apoptosis in human breast cancer MCF-7 cells through endoplasmic reticulum stress. *J. Agric. Food Chem.* **2012**, *60*, 11065–11070. [CrossRef] [PubMed]

19. Yildirim, O.; Yilmaz, A.; Oz, O.; Vatansever, H.; Cinel, L.; Aslan, G.; Tamer, L.; Adiguzel, U.; Arpaci, R.; Kanik, A.; et al. Effect of caffeic acid phenethyl ester on treatment of experimentally induced methicillin-resistant Staphylococcus epidermidis endophthalmitis in a rabbit model. *Cell Biochem. Funct.* **2007**, *25*, 693–700. [CrossRef] [PubMed]

20. Cho, M.S.; Park, W.S.; Jung, W.K.; Qian, Z.J.; Lee, D.S.; Choi, J.S.; Lee, D.Y.; Park, S.G.; Seo, S.K.; Kim, H.J.; et al. Caffeic acid phenethyl ester promotes anti-inflammatory effects by inhibiting MAPK and NF-kappaB signaling in activated HMC-1 human mast cells. *Pharm. Biol.* **2014**, *52*, 926–932. [CrossRef] [PubMed]

21. Altuntas, A.; Yilmaz, H.R.; Altuntas, A.; Uz, E.; Demir, M.; Gokcimen, A.; Aksu, O.; Bayram, D.S.; Sezer, M.T. Caffeic acid phenethyl ester protects against amphotericin B induced nephrotoxicity in rat model. *Biomed. Res. Int.* **2014**, *2014*, 702981. [CrossRef] [PubMed]

22. Zhou, K.; Li, X.; Du, Q.; Li, D.; Hu, M.; Yang, X.; Jiang, Q.; Li, Z. A CAPE analogue as novel antiplatelet agent efficiently inhibits collagen-induced platelet aggregation. *Pharmazie* **2014**, *69*, 615–620. [PubMed]

23. Wu, J.; Omene, C.; Karkoszka, J.; Bosland, M.; Eckard, J.; Klein, C.B.; Frenkel, K. Caffeic acid phenethyl ester (CAPE), derived from a honeybee product propolis, exhibits a diversity of anti-tumor effects in pre-clinical models of human breast cancer. *Cancer Lett.* **2011**, *308*, 43–53. [CrossRef] [PubMed]

24. Akyol, S.; Ozturk, G.; Ginis, Z.; Armutcu, F.; Yigitoglu, M.R.; Akyol, O. In vivo and in vitro antineoplastic actions of caffeic acid phenethyl ester (CAPE): Therapeutic perspectives. *Nutr. Cancer* **2013**, *65*, 515–526. [CrossRef] [PubMed]

25. Morin, P.; St-Coeur, P.D.; Doiron, J.A.; Cormier, M.; Poitras, J.J.; Surette, M.E.; Touaibia, M. Substituted caffeic and ferulic acid phenethyl esters: Synthesis, leukotrienes biosynthesis inhibition, and cytotoxic activity. *Molecules* **2017**, *22*, 124.

26. Borrelli, F.; Izzo, A.A.; Di Carlo, G.; Maffia, P.; Russo, A.; Maiello, F.M.; Capasso, F.; Mascolo, N. Effect of a propolis extract and caffeic acid phenethyl ester on formation of aberrant crypt foci and tumors in the rat colon. *Fitoterapia* **2002**, *73* (Suppl. 1), S38–S43. [CrossRef]

27. Xiang, D.; Wang, D.; He, Y.; Xie, J.; Zhong, Z.; Li, Z.; Xie, J. Caffeic acid phenethyl ester induces growth arrest and apoptosis of colon cancer cells via the beta-catenin/T-cell factor signaling. *Anti-Cancer Drug* **2006**, *17*, 753–762. [CrossRef] [PubMed]

28. Chen, M.F.; Wu, C.T.; Chen, Y.J.; Keng, P.C.; Chen, W.C. Cell killing and radiosensitization by caffeic acid phenethyl ester (CAPE) in lung cancer cells. *J. Radiat. Res.* **2004**, *45*, 253–260. [CrossRef] [PubMed]

29. Kudugunti, S.K.; Vad, N.M.; Ekogbo, E.; Moridani, M.Y. Efficacy of caffeic acid phenethyl ester (CAPE) in skin B16-F0 melanoma tumor bearing C57BL/6 mice. *Investig. New Drug* **2011**, *29*, 52–62. [CrossRef] [PubMed]

30. Wu, C.S.; Chen, M.F.; Lee, I.L.; Tung, S.Y. Predictive role of nuclear factor-kappaB activity in gastric cancer: A promising adjuvant approach with caffeic acid phenethyl ester. *J. Clin. Gastroenterol.* **2007**, *41*, 894–900. [CrossRef] [PubMed]

31. Chen, M.J.; Chang, W.H.; Lin, C.C.; Liu, C.Y.; Wang, T.E.; Chu, C.H.; Shih, S.C.; Chen, Y.J. Caffeic acid phenethyl ester induces apoptosis of human pancreatic cancer cells involving caspase and mitochondrial dysfunction. *Pancreatology* **2008**, *8*, 566–576. [CrossRef] [PubMed]

32. Lee, K.W.; Kang, N.J.; Kim, J.H.; Lee, K.M.; Lee, D.E.; Hur, H.J.; Lee, H.J. Caffeic acid phenethyl ester inhibits invasion and expression of matrix metalloproteinase in SK-Hep1 human hepatocellular carcinoma cells by targeting nuclear factor kappa B. *Genes Nutr.* **2008**, *2*, 319–322. [CrossRef] [PubMed]

33. Huang, M.T.; Ma, W.; Yen, P.; Xie, J.G.; Han, J.; Frenkel, K.; Grunberger, D.; Conney, A.H. Inhibitory effects of caffeic acid phenethyl ester (CAPE) on 12-O-tetradecanoylphorbol-13-acetate-induced tumor promotion in mouse skin and the synthesis of DNA, RNA and protein in HeLa cells. *Carcinogenesis* **1996**, *17*, 761–765. [CrossRef] [PubMed]

34. Dziedzic, A.; Kubina, R.; Kabala-Dzik, A.; Wojtyczka, R.D.; Morawiec, T.; Buldak, R.J. Caffeic acid reduces the viability and migration rate of oral carcinoma cells (SCC-25) exposed to low concentrations of ethanol. *Int. J. Mol. Sci.* **2014**, *15*, 18725–18741. [CrossRef] [PubMed]

35. Dziedzic, A.; Kubina, R.; Kabala-Dzik, A.; Tanasiewicz, M. Induction of cell cycle arrest and apoptotic response of head and neck squamous carcinoma cells (Detroit 562) by caffeic acid and caffeic acid phenethyl ester derivative. *Evid. Based Complement. Altern. Med.* **2017**, *2017*, 6793456. [CrossRef] [PubMed]

36. Onori, P.; DeMorrow, S.; Gaudio, E.; Franchitto, A.; Mancinelli, R.; Venter, J.; Kopriva, S.; Ueno, Y.; Alvaro, D.; Savage, J.; et al. Caffeic acid phenethyl ester decreases cholangiocarcinoma growth by inhibition of NF-kappaB and induction of apoptosis. *Int. J. Cancer* **2009**, *125*, 565–576. [CrossRef] [PubMed]

37. Kuo, H.C.; Kuo, W.H.; Lee, Y.J.; Lin, W.L.; Chou, F.P.; Tseng, T.H. Inhibitory effect of caffeic acid phenethyl ester on the growth of C6 glioma cells in vitro and in vivo. *Cancer Lett.* **2006**, *234*, 199–208. [CrossRef] [PubMed]

38. Watabe, M.; Hishikawa, K.; Takayanagi, A.; Shimizu, N.; Nakaki, T. Caffeic acid phenethyl ester induces apoptosis by inhibition of NFkappaB and activation of Fas in human breast cancer MCF-7 cells. *J. Biol. Chem.* **2004**, *279*, 6017–6026. [CrossRef] [PubMed]

39. Rzepecka-Stojko, A.; Kabała-Dzik, A.; Moździerz, A.; Kubina, R.; Wojtyczka, R.D.; Stojko, R.; Dziedzic, A.; Jastrzębska-Stojko, Ż.; Jurzak, M.; Buszman, E.; et al. Caffeic acid phenethyl ester and ethanol extract of propolis induce the complementary cytotoxic effect on triple-negative breast cancer cell lines. *Molecules* **2015**, *20*, 9242–9262. [CrossRef] [PubMed]

40. Liao, H.F.; Chen, Y.Y.; Liu, J.J.; Hsu, M.L.; Shieh, H.J.; Liao, H.J.; Shieh, C.J.; Shiao, M.S.; Chen, Y.J. Inhibitory effect of caffeic acid phenethyl ester on angiogenesis, tumor invasion, and metastasis. *J. Agric. Food Chem.* **2003**, *51*, 7907–7912. [CrossRef] [PubMed]

41. Wu, J.; Bukkapatnam, U.; Eckard, J.; Frenkel, K. Caffeic acid phenethyl ester (CAPE, a product of propolis) as an inhibitor of human breast cancer growth in a pre-clinical study and its effects on factors involved in cell cycle, angiogenesis, and drug resistance. In Proceedings of the AACR Annual Meeting, San Diego, CA, USA, 12–16 April 2008; Volume 68, p. 5710.

42. Jia, L.T.; Zhang, R.; Shen, L.; Yang, A.G. Regulators of carcinogenesis: Emerging roles beyond their primary functions. *Cancer Lett.* **2015**, *357*, 75–82. [CrossRef] [PubMed]

43. Carey, L.A. Directed therapy of subtypes of triple-negative breast cancer. *Oncologist* **2010**, *15* (Suppl. 5), 49–56. [CrossRef] [PubMed]

44. Bauer, K.R.; Brown, M.; Cress, R.D.; Parise, C.A.; Caggiano, V. Descriptive analysis of estrogen receptor (ER)-negative, progesterone receptor (PR)-negative, and HER2-negative invasive breast cancer, the so-called triple-negative phenotype. *Cancer* **2007**, *109*, 1721–1728. [CrossRef] [PubMed]

45. Chacón, R.D.; Costanzo, M.V. Triple-negative breast cancer. *Breat Cancer Res.* **2010**, *12* (Suppl. 2), S3. [CrossRef] [PubMed]

46. Foulkes, W.D.; Smith, I.E.; Reis-Filho, J.S. Triple-Negative Breast Cancer. *N. Engl. J. Med.* **2010**, *363*, 1938–1948. [CrossRef] [PubMed]

47. Hammond, M.E.; Hayes, D.F.; Dowsett, M.; Allred, D.C.; Hagerty, K.L.; Badve, S.; Fitzgibbons, P.L.; Francis, G.; Goldstein, N.S.; Hayes, M.; et al. American Society of Clinical Oncology/College of American Pathologists guideline recommendations for immunohistochemical testing of estrogen and progesterone receptors in breast cancer. *J. Clin. Oncol.* **2010**, *28*, 2784–2795. [CrossRef] [PubMed]

48. Pal, S.K.; Childs, B.H.; Pegram, M. Triple negative breast cancer: Unmet medical needs. *Breast Cancer Res. Treat.* **2011**, *125*, 627–636. [CrossRef] [PubMed]

49. Conlin, A.K.; Seidman, A.D. Taxanes in breast cancer: An update. *Curr. Oncol. Rep.* **2007**, *9*, 22–30. [CrossRef] [PubMed]

50. Jones, S.E. Metastatic breast cancer: The treatment challenge. *Clin. Breast Cancer* **2008**, *8*, 224–233. [CrossRef] [PubMed]

51. Schwartz, J.; Wong, S.T. Novel combinations for treating metastatic breast cancer: Improving the odds. Introduction. *Am. J. Health Syst. Pharm.* **2009**, *66* (Suppl. 6), S1–S2. [CrossRef] [PubMed]

52. Longley, D.B.; Johnston, P.G. Molecular mechanisms of drug resistance. *J. Pathol.* **2005**, *205*, 275–292. [CrossRef] [PubMed]

53. Mosmann, T. Rapid colorimetric assay for cellular growth and survival: Application to proliferation and cytotoxicity assays. *J. Immunol. Methods* **1983**, *65*, 55–63. [CrossRef]

54. Borenfreund, E.; Puerner, J. A simple quantitative procedure using monolayer cultures for cytotoxicity assays (HTD/NR90). *J. Tissue Cult. Methods* **1984**, *9*, 7–9. [CrossRef]

55. Skehan, P.; Storeng, R.; Scudiero, D.; Monks, A.; McMahon, J.; Vistica, D.; Warren, J.T.; Bokesch, H.; Kenney, S.; Boyd, M.R. New colorimetric cytotoxicity assay for anticancer-drug screening. *J. Natl. Cancer Inst.* **1990**, *82*, 1107–1112. [CrossRef] [PubMed]

56. Orellana, E.A.; Kasinski, A.L. Sulforhodamine B (SRB) assay in cell culture to investigate cell proliferation. *Bio-protocol* **2016**, *6*, E1984. [CrossRef] [PubMed]

57. Yarrow, J.C.; Perlman, Z.E.; Westwood, N.J.; Mitchison, T.J. A high-throughput cell migration assay using scratch wound healing, a comparison of image-based readout methods. *BMC Biotechnol.* **2004**, *4*, 21. [CrossRef] [PubMed]

58. Jonkman, J.E.; Cathcart, J.A.; Xu, F.; Bartolini, M.E.; Amon, J.E.; Stevens, K.M.; Colarusso, P. An introduction to the wound healing assay using live-cell microscopy. *Cell. Adhes. Migr.* **2014**, *8*, 440–451. [CrossRef] [PubMed]

59. Mukhtar, E.; Adhami, V.M.; Khan, N.; Mukhtar, H. Apoptosis and autophagy induction as mechanism of cancer prevention by naturally occurring dietary agents. *Curr. Drug Targets* **2012**, *13*, 1831–1841. [CrossRef] [PubMed]

60. Beutler, J.A. *Natural Products and Cancer Drug Discovery*; Springer: New York, NY, USA, 2013; p. 244.

61. Mates, J.M.; Segura, J.A.; Alonso, F.J.; Marquez, J. Natural antioxidants: Therapeutic prospects for cancer and neurological diseases. *Mini Rev. Med. Chem.* **2009**, *9*, 1202–1214. [CrossRef] [PubMed]

62. Mates, J.M.; Segura, J.A.; Alonso, F.J.; Marquez, J. Anticancer antioxidant regulatory functions of phytochemicals. *Curr. Med. Chem.* **2011**, *18*, 2315–2338. [CrossRef] [PubMed]

63. DiGianni, L.M.; Garber, J.E.; Winer, E.P. Complementary and alternative medicine use among women with breast cancer. *J. Clin. Oncol.* **2002**, *20* (Suppl. 18), S34–S38.

64. Crocetti, E.; Crotti, N.; Feltrin, A.; Ponton, P.; Geddes, M.; Buiatti, E. The use of complementary therapies by breast cancer patients attending conventional treatment. *Eur. J. Cancer* **1998**, *34*, 324–328. [CrossRef]

65. Sparber, A.; Bauer, L.; Curt, G.; Eisenberg, D.; Levin, T.; Parks, S.; Steinberg, S.M.; Wootton, J. Use of complementary medicine by adult patients participating in cancer clinical trials. *Oncol. Nurs. Forum* **2000**, *27*, 623–630. [PubMed]

66. Richardson, M.A.; Sanders, T.; Palmer, J.L.; Greisinger, A.; Singletary, S.E. Complementary/alternative medicine use in a comprehensive cancer center and the implications for oncology. *J. Clin. Oncol.* **2000**, *18*, 2505–2514. [CrossRef] [PubMed]

67. Morris, K.T.; Johnson, N.; Homer, L.; Walts, D. A comparison of complementary therapy use between breast cancer patients and patients with other primary tumor sites. *Am. J. Surg.* **2000**, *179*, 407–411. [CrossRef]

68. Simonetti, P.; Gardana, C.; Pietta, P. Plasma levels of caffeic acid and antioxidant status after red wine intake. *J. Agric. Food Chem.* **2001**, *49*, 5964–5968. [CrossRef] [PubMed]

69. Chavez, K.J.; Garimella, S.V.; Lipkowitz, S. Triple negative breast cancer cell lines: One tool in the search for better treatment of triple negative breast cancer. *Breast Dis.* **2010**, *32*, 35–48. [CrossRef] [PubMed]

70. Omene, C.; Kalac, M.; Wu, J.; Marchi, E.; Frenkel, K.; O'Connor, O.A. Propolis and its active component, caffeic acid phenethyl ester (CAPE), modulate breast cancer therapeutic targets via an epigenetically mediated mechanism of action. *J. Cancer Ther.* **2013**, *5*, 334–342.

71. Thomas, C.; Rajapaksa, G.; Nikolos, F.; Hao, R.; Katchy, A.; McCollum, C.W.; Bondesson, M.; Quinlan, P.; Thompson, A.; Krishnamurthy, S.; et al. ERbeta1 represses basal breast cancer epithelial to mesenchymal transition by destabilizing EGFR. *Breast Cancer Res.* **2012**, *14*, R148. [CrossRef] [PubMed]

72. Holliday, D.L.; Speirs, V. Choosing the right cell line for breast cancer research. *Breast Cancer Res.* **2011**, *13*, 215. [CrossRef] [PubMed]

73. Simmons, J.K.; Hildreth, B.E.; Supsavhad, W.; Elshafae, S.M.; Hassan, B.B.; Dirksen, W.P.; Toribio, R.E.; Rosol, T.J. Animal models of bone metastasis. *Vet. Pathol.* **2015**, *52*, 827–841. [CrossRef] [PubMed]

74. Bos, P.D.; Zhang, X.H.; Nadal, C.; Shu, W.; Gomis, R.R.; Nguyen, D.X.; Minn, A.J.; van de Vijver, M.J.; Gerald, W.L.; Foekens, J.A.; et al. Genes that mediate breast cancer metastatis to the brain. *Nature* **2009**, *459*, 1005–1009. [CrossRef] [PubMed]

75. Kang, Y.; Siegel, P.M.; Shu, W.; Drobnjak, M.; Kakonen, S.M.; Cordon-Cardo, C.; Guise, T.A.; Massagué, J. A multigenic program mediating breast cancer metastasis to bone. *Cancer Cell* **2003**, *3*, 537–549. [CrossRef]

76. Minn, A.J.; Gupta, G.P.; Siegel, P.M.; Bos, P.D.; Shu, W.; Giri, D.D.; Viale, A.; Olshen, A.B.; Gerald, W.L.; Massagué, J. Genes that mediate breast cancer metastasis to lung. *Nature* **2005**, *436*, 518–524. [CrossRef] [PubMed]

77. Minn, A.J.; Kang, Y.; Serganova, I.; Gupta, G.P.; Giri, D.D.; Doubrovin, M.; Ponomarev, V.; Gerald, W.L.; Blasberg, R.; Massagué, J. Distinct organ-specific metastatic potential of individual breast cancer cells and primary tumours. *J. Clin. Investig.* **2005**, *115*, 44–55. [CrossRef] [PubMed]

78. Jung, B.I.; Kim, M.S.; Kim, H.A.; Kim, D.; Yang, J.; Her, S.; Song, Y.S. Caffeic acid phenethyl ester, a component of beehive propolis, is a novel selective estrogen receptor modulator. *Phytother. Res.* **2010**, *24*, 295–300. [CrossRef] [PubMed]

79. Khoram, N.M.; Bigdeli, B.; Nikoofar, A.; Goliaei, B. Caffeic acid phenethyl ester increases radiosensitivity of estrogen receptor-positive and -negative breast cancer cells by prolonging radiation-induced DNA damage. *J. Breast Cancer* **2016**, *19*, 18–25. [CrossRef] [PubMed]

80. Lin, Y.H.; Chiu, J.H.; Tseng, W.S.; Wong, T.T.; Chiou, S.H.; Yen, S.H. Antiproliferation and radiosensitization of caffeic acid phenethyl ester on human medulloblastoma cells. *Cancer Chemother. Pharmacol.* **2006**, *57*, 525–532. [CrossRef] [PubMed]

81. Beauregard, A.P.; Harquail, J.; Lassalle-Claux, G.; Belbraouet, M.; Jean-Francois, J.; Touaibia, M.; Robichaud, G.A. CAPE analogs induce growth arrest and apoptosis in breast cancer cells. *Molecules* **2015**, *20*, 12576–12589. [CrossRef] [PubMed]

82. Rosendahl, A.H.; Perks, C.M.; Zeng, L.; Markkula, A.; Simonsson, M.; Rose, C.; Ingvar, C.; Holly, J.M.; Jernstrom, H. Caffeine and caffeic acid inhibit growth and modify estrogen receptor and insulin-like growth factor i receptor levels in human breast cancer. *Clin. Cancer Res.* **2015**, *21*, 1877–1887. [CrossRef] [PubMed]

83. Wadhwa, R.; Nigam, N.; Bhargava, P.; Dhanjal, J.K.; Goyal, S.; Grover, A.; Sundar, D.; Ishida, Y.; Terao, K.; Kaul, S.C. Molecular characterization and enhancement of anticancer activity of caffeic acid phenethyl ester by gamma cyclodextrin. *J. Cancer* **2016**, *7*, 1755–1771. [CrossRef] [PubMed]

84. Bonuccelli, G.; De Francesco, E.M.; de Boer, R.; Tanowitz, H.B.; Lisanti, M.P. NADH autofluorescence, a new metabolic biomarker for cancer stem cells: Identification of vitamin C and CAPE as natural products targeting "stemness". *Oncotarget* **2017**, *8*, 20667–20678. [CrossRef] [PubMed]

85. Buchegger, K.; Ili, C.; Riquelme, I.; Letelier, P.; Corvalán, A.H.; Brebi, P.; Huang, T.H.; Roa, J.C. Reprimo as a modulator of cell migration and invasion in the MDA-MB-231 breast cancer cell line. *Biol. Res.* **2016**, *49*. [CrossRef] [PubMed]

86. Bhat, K.; Sarkissyan, M.; Wu, Y.; Vadgama, J.V. GROα overexpression drives cell migration and invasion in triple negative breast cancer cells. *Oncol. Rep.* **2017**, *38*, 21–30. [CrossRef] [PubMed]

87. Liu, Z.; Chu, S.; Yao, S.; Li, Y.; Fan, S.; Sun, X.; Su, L.; Liu, X. CD74 interacts with CD44 and enhances tumorigenesis and metastasis via RHOA-mediated cofilin phosphorylation in human breast cancer cells. *Oncotarget* **2016**, *7*, 68303–68313. [CrossRef] [PubMed]

88. Wang, B.; Zhao, H.; Zhao, L.; Zhang, Y.; Wan, Q.; Shen, Y.; Bu, X.; Wan, M.; Shen, C. Up-regulation of OLR1 expression by TBC1D3 through activation of TNFα/NF-κB pathway promotes the migration of human breast cancer cells. *Cancer Lett.* **2017**, *408*, 60–70. [CrossRef] [PubMed]

89. Shigeoka, Y.; Igishi, T.; Matsumoto, S.; Nakanishi, H.; Kodani, M.; Yasuda, K.; Hitsuda, Y.; Shimizu, E. Sulindac sulfide and caffeic acid phenethyl ester suppress the motility of lung adenocarcinoma cells promoted by transforming growth factor-β through Akt inhibition. *J. Cancer Res. Clin. Oncol.* **2004**, *130*, 146–152. [CrossRef] [PubMed]

90. Natarajan, K.; Singh, S.; Burke, T.R.; Grunberger, D.; Aggarwal, B.B. Caffeic acid phenethyl ester is a potent and specific inhibitor of activation of nuclear transcription factor NF-kappa B. *Proc. Natl. Acad. Sci. USA* **1996**, *93*, 9090–9095. [CrossRef] [PubMed]

91. Pidugu, V.R.; Yarla, N.; Bishayee, A.; Kalle, A.M.; Satya, A.K. Novel histone deacetylase 8-selective inhibitor 1,3,4-oxadiazole-alanine hybrid induces apoptosis in breast cancer cells. *Apoptosis* **2017**. [CrossRef] [PubMed]

92. Kabała-Dzik, A.; Rzepecka-Stojko, A.; Kubina, R.; Jastrzębska-Stojko, Ż.; Stojko, R.; Wojtyczka, R.D.; Stojko, J. Comparison of two components of propolis: Caffeic acid (CA) and caffeic acid phenethyl ester (CAPE) induce apoptosis and cell cycle arrest of breast cancer cells MDA-MB-231. *Molecules* **2017**, *22*, 1554. [CrossRef] [PubMed]

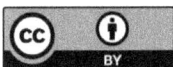

nutrients

MDPI

Review

The Dual Antioxidant/Prooxidant Effect of Eugenol and Its Action in Cancer Development and Treatment

Daniel Pereira Bezerra [1], Gardenia Carmen Gadelha Militão [2], Mayara Castro de Morais [3] and Damião Pergentino de Sousa [3,*]

[1] Instituto Gonçalo Moniz, Fundação Oswaldo Cruz (IGM-FIOCRUZ/BA), Salvador 40296-710, Bahia, Brazil; danielpbezerra@gmail.com
[2] Departamento de Fisiologia, Universidade Federal de Pernambuco, Recife 50670-901, Pernambuco, Brazil; gcgadelha@yahoo.com.br
[3] Departamento de Ciências Farmacêuticas, Universidade Federal da Paraíba, João Pessoa 58051-970, Paraíba, Brazil; mayaracastrodemorais@gmail.com
* Correspondence: damiao_desousa@yahoo.com.br; Tel.: +55-83-3209-8417

Received: 8 November 2017; Accepted: 12 December 2017; Published: 17 December 2017

Abstract: The formation of reactive oxygen species (ROS) during metabolism is a normal process usually compensated for by the antioxidant defense system of an organism. However, ROS can cause oxidative damage and have been proposed to be the main cause of age-related clinical complications and diseases such as cancer. In recent decades, the relationship between diet and cancer has been more studied, especially with foods containing antioxidant compounds. Eugenol is a natural compound widely found in many aromatic plant species, spices and foods and is used in cosmetics and pharmaceutical products. Eugenol has a dual effect on oxidative stress, which can action as an antioxidant or prooxidant agent. In addition, it has anti-carcinogenic, cytotoxic and antitumor properties. Considering the importance of eugenol in the area of food and human health, in this review, we discuss the role of eugenol on redox status and its potential use in the treatment and prevention of cancer.

Keywords: reactive oxygen species; metabolism; antitumor activity; antioxidant activity; phenylpropanoid; natural products; essential oils; clove; *Syzygium aromaticum*

1. Introduction

Reactive oxygen species (ROS) are a heterogeneous group of molecules that are, along with endogenous antioxidants, ubiquitously present in all organisms. They are implicated in various diseases including malignant transformations [1]. The term "oxidative stress" refers to an imbalance in which pro-oxidants overwhelm the capacity of antioxidant defense systems [2]; it has been shown to contribute to the development of some types of cancer [3].

The report of anticancer potential of aromatic compounds found in foods and plants have increased in the recent decades [4–8] and there are advanced studies of mechanisms of action and clinical approaches in progress. This chemical class of natural products show interesting potential as health promoting agents and, consequently, with application to improving the quality of life. These include the polyphenols that are important components of human diet. Interestingly, some of these compounds may act as either antioxidants or pro-oxidants to exert protective effects against cancer [9–11]. Eugenol (4-allyl-2-methoxyphenol) (Figure 1) is an aromatic phenylpropanoid phenol contained in clove (*Syzygium aromaticum*, Myrtaceae), which is well-known for its culinary uses. Eugenol also occurs in soybeans, mung beans [12], coffee [13], bananas [14] and in herbs such as nutmeg (*Myristica fragrans*, Myristicaceae), cinnamon (*Cinnamomum verum*, Lauraceae) and basil (*Ocimum basilicum*, Lamiaceae); however, *Syzygium aromaticum* can be considered the principal natural source of this compound (45% or 90% of the total oil) [15]. Clove has been used for a long time by civilizations because of its flavor and its properties make it important for culinary and medicinal uses. Eugenol has been included as a spicy flavoring in whisky, ice cream, baked goods and candy in restricted concentrations [16–18]. Eugenol has dual effect on the oxidative stress, which can action as an antioxidant or prooxidant agent. In addition, it has anti-carcinogenic, cytotoxic and antitumor properties. Considering the importance of eugenol in the area of food and human health, in this review, we discuss the role of eugenol on redox status and its potential use in the treatment and prevention of cancer. Searches were performed in the scientific literature database PubMed comprising all papers in English published until September 2017 using the following key words: eugenol with oxidant; antioxidant; cancer; cytotoxic; or antitumor. No exclusion criteria were performed.

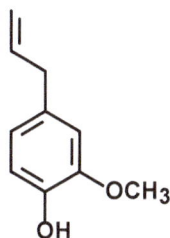

Figure 1. Chemical structure of eugenol.

2. Anti-Carcinogenic/Chemopreventive Effect of Eugenol and Its Relation to the Inhibition of Oxidative Stress

The ability to inhibit oxidative stress has been described as a protective effect against cancer formation (carcinogenesis or tumorigenesis); on the other hand, once a cancer has already formed, the antioxidant effect can contribute to the cancer's development, while the pro-oxidant effect can induce cancer cell death by several signaling pathways [19]. Interestingly, eugenol has been described as an agent with a double effect, antioxidant and pro-oxidant, presenting beneficial effects in the prevention of cancer formation and in cancer treatment (Figure 2). Despite some contradictory studies, there are many articles evaluating these biochemical and pharmacologic aspects.

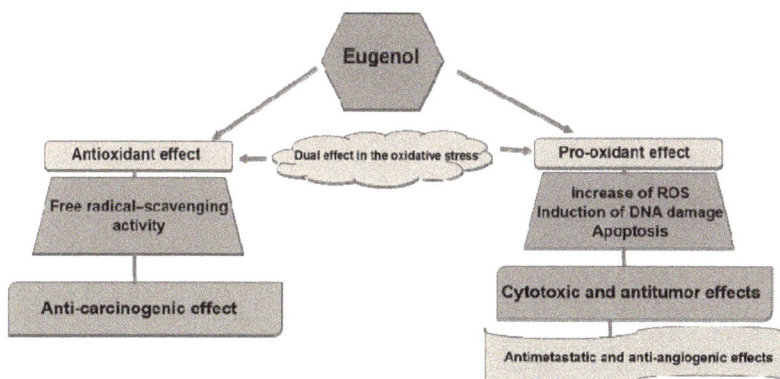

Figure 2. The dual effect of eugenol in the oxidative stress and its action in cancer development and treatment.

The anti-carcinogenic effect of eugenol had been investigated in several models [20–28]. The anti-carcinogenic effect of eugenol against skin carcinogenesis was investigated by Kaur et al. [20]. Skin cancer was initiated by applying 160 nmol 7,12-dimethylbenz[a]anthracene (DMBA) and promoted by twice weekly applications of 8.5 nmol 12-otetradecanoylphorbol-13-acetate (TPA) for 28 weeks and was followed by eugenol treatment. DMBA is a polycyclic aromatic hydrocarbon pro-carcinogen that requires metabolic conversion to its ultimate carcinogenic diol epoxide metabolites by oxidation, which is carried out through cytochrome P450 family 1 subfamily A member 1 (CYP1A1) and cytochrome P450 family 1 subfamily B member 1 (CYP1B1). Therefore, the carcinogenic effect of DMBA depends on the level of the oxidative metabolism of cytochrome P450 family 1. Two protocols were established: an anti-initiation protocol (topical application of 200 µL eugenol at 15% v/v in acetone one week before, one hour prior and two times after DMBA application); and an anti-promotion protocol (topical application of 30 µL eugenol at 15% v/v in acetone, 30 min prior to every TPA application). The treatment with eugenol did not prevent tumor formation but led to a reduction in tumor size. The control group presented tumor size of 9.7 g, and eugenol treatment showed tumor size of 5.6 g in the anti-initiation protocol and 2.8 g in the anti-promotion protocol. In addition, topical application of eugenol prior to TPA exposure led to the development of papillomatous keratoacanthoma with minimal cell proliferation but without squamous cell carcinoma. The anti-carcinogenic effect of eugenol was attributed to its anti-inflammatory activity, because some markers of inflammation, including inducible nitric oxide synthase (iNOS) and cyclooxygenase-2 (COX-2) expression and the levels of pro-inflammatory cytokines interleukin-6 (IL-6), tumor necrosis factor alpha (TNF-α) and prostaglandin E2 (PGE2), were reduced in DMBA/TPA-exposed animals after treatment with eugenol. Furthermore, eugenol was found to suppress the activation of nuclear factor kappa B (NF-κB) in mouse skin with TPA-induced inflammation [20].

Additionally, eugenol treatment (~100 mg/kg) inhibited the tumor formation in mouse skin model induced by application of DMBA as initiator and croton oil as promotor via radical scavenging activity of eugenol, downregulation of Myc (proto-oncogene), H-ras (harvey rat sarcoma virus oncogene) and Bcl-2 (B-cell lymphoma 2, apoptosis regulator) expression along with upregulation of p53, Bax (BCL2 associated X, apoptosis regulator) and active caspase-3 expression in the skin lesions [21,22]. Topical administration of eugenol also partially inhibited the benzo[a]pyrene-induced skin carcinogenesis in Swiss mice [23]. However, topical application of eugenol had minimal protection in reducing DMBA-induced skin carcinogenesis in Swiss mice [24].

The chemopreventive effect of eugenol on *N*-methyl-*N'*-nitro-*N*-nitrosoguanidine (MNNG)-induced gastric carcinogenesis in Wistar rats was also performed [25,26]. MNNG (150 mg/kg) was administered by intragastric intubation three times with a gap of two weeks in between the treatments and eugenol (100 mg/kg) was administered by intragastric route, three times per week starting on the day following the first exposure to MNNG and continued until the end of the experimental period. The incidence of gastric tumors in MNNG-treated rats was 100% with a mean tumor burden of 274.38 mm^3 and eugenol treatment decreased the tumor incidence to 16.66% with a tumor burden of 14.78 mm^3. Administration of eugenol induced apoptosis via the mitochondrial pathway by modulating the Bcl-2 family proteins, apoptotic protease activating factor 1 (Apaf-1), cytochrome c and caspases and inhibiting of invasion and angiogenesis as evidenced by changes in the activities of matrix metalloproteinases (MMP) and the expression of MMP-2 and -9, vascular endothelial growth factor (VEGF), vascular endothelial growth factor receptor 1 (VEGFR1), tissue inhibitor of metalloproteinase-2 (TIMP-2) and reversion-inducing-cysteine-rich protein with kazal motifs (RECK). Moreover, reduction in the NF-κB activation along with increasing of its inhibitor family members, IκB kinase α (IκBα) and inhibitor of kappa B (IKKβ), reduction of cyclin D1, cyclin B and proliferating cell nuclear antigen (PCNA) and increasing of p53, p21^{waf1} and growth arrest and DNA damage-inducible 45 (Gadd45) were observed in eugenol-treated animals [25,26].

Using MCF 10A breast epithelial cells and H-ras transfected MCF 10A (MCF 10A-ras) as a model of cancer progression, eugenol exhibited cytotoxicity in µM range to MCF 10A-ras cells but not in MCF 10A cells [27]. In addition, eugenol reduced the ATP generation and inhibited oxidative phosphorylation and fatty acid oxidation via downregulating of c-Myc/PGC-1β/ERRα signaling pathway and inhibiting ROS production in H-ras transfected MCF 10A breast epithelial cells, indicating that eugenol can prevent breast cancer progression by regulation of cellular energy metabolism [27]. On the other hand, eugenol treatment does not exert modifying effects on lung carcinogenesis induced by urethane [28]. No significant differences in the incidences and multiplicities of lung lesions were observed between eugenol and control groups. In this model of lung carcinogenesis, transgenic mice with the human prototype c-Ha-ras gene received a single intraperitoneal injection of 250 mg/kg urethane, followed by a diet containing 6000 ppm eugenol or basal diet for 26 weeks [28]. The Table 1 summarize the anti-carcinogenic effect of eugenol.

Table 1. Summary of anti-carcinogenic effect of eugenol.

Carcinogenesis Model	Carcinogen	Eugenol Administration	Effect	References
Skin carcinogenesis	DMBA + TPA	Topical	Reduction in tumor incidence and size; and/or development of papillomatous keratoacanthoma with minimal cell proliferation but without squamous cell carcinoma	[20]
Skin carcinogenesis	DMBA + croton oil	Topical	Inhibition of tumor formation ~60%	[21,22]
Skin carcinogenesis	benzo[a]pyrene	Topical	Inhibition of tumor formation ~50%	[23]
Skin Carcinogenesis	DMBA	Topical	Minimal protection	[24]
Gastric carcinogenesis	MNNG	Intragastric	Inhibition of tumor formation ~75%	[25,26]
Lung carcinogenesis	Urethane	Oral	No protection	[28]

DMBA: 7,12-dimethylbenz[a]anthracene; TPA: 12-otetradecanoylphorbol-13-acetate; MNNG: *N*-methyl-*N'*-nitro-*N*-nitrosoguanidine.

The anti-carcinogenic effect of eugenol can also be attributed to its antioxidant property. Eugenol has been reported to have antioxidant activity, as assessed by diverse models [12,29–35]. Eugenol reacts with 2,2-diphenyl-1-picrylhydrazyl (DPPH) and shows high DPPH free radical-scavenging activity [29–33]. The concentration of eugenol required for 50% DPPH scavenging (IC_{50}: half maximal inhibitory concentration) activity ranged from 98 to 138 μM [31,35]. Eugenol also exhibits effective antioxidant activity in the linoleic acid emulsion system by inhibiting lipid peroxidation at 91 μM. In addition, eugenol has ferric ion (Fe^{3+}) reducing ability and electron donor properties for neutralizing free radicals by forming stable products [31]. Eugenol inhibits malonaldehyde (MA) formation from cod liver oil by 91% at ~1 mM [12]. Furthermore, eugenol inhibits microsomal lipid peroxidation (IC_{50} about 80 μM) as well as iron and OH radical-initiated lipid peroxidation in rat liver mitochondria, with IC_{50} values of 10 and 14 μM, respectively. The antioxidant effect was determined by the inhibition of thiobarbituric acid-reactive substances (TBARS) formation [29,30].

The effect of eugenol on in vivo lipid peroxidation mediated by carbon tetrachloride (CCl_4) has also been evaluated [30]. The CCl_4 model has been used for many years to investigate the effect of antioxidants in the liver xenobiotic metabolism. When eugenol was given at 5 mg/kg orally at three different times—i.e., prior to (−1 h), along with (0 h), or after (+3 h)—in relation to the time of CCl_4 dosing (i.p. administration of 0.4 mg/kg), it prevented significantly the rise in serum glutamic-oxaloacetic transaminase (SGOT) activity, lipid peroxidation and liver necrosis. However, eugenol failed to prevent a decrease in glucose-6-phosphatase activity, suggesting that the damage to endoplasmic reticulum (ER) is not protected by eugenol. Thus, the protective action of eugenol can be explained by the interception of secondary radicals derived from ER lipids rather than interference with the primary radicals of CCl_4 (•CCl_3/CCl_3OO•) [30]. In addition, the in vivo antioxidant effect of eugenol on liver danger induced by thioacetamide (TA) was also performed [36]. TA is frequently used to produce liver danger in animals due to generation of ROS and instigation of oxidative stress, which causes liver damage. Adult male Wistar rats were treated with eugenol (10.7 mg/kg/day) orally for 15 days. TA was administered (300 mg/kg, i.p.) for the last two days at 24 h intervals and the rats were sacrificed on the 16th day. Pretreatment with eugenol controlled the levels of lipid peroxidation and protein oxidation products with consequent reduction of TBARS, lipid hydroperoxides and protein carbonyl formation in plasma and the liver. Increased expression of the COX-2 gene as well as increases in pro-inflammatory cytokine TNF-α and IL-6 plasma levels induced by TA was also partially reverted by eugenol pretreatment. The protective effect of eugenol can be attributed to the reduction of cytochrome P450 family 2 subfamily E member 1 (CYP2E1) activity, the main enzyme responsible for TA-induced hepatotoxicity and oxidative stress [36].

Genotoxicity and mutagenicity of xenobiotics are also involved in the carcinogenic process and may occur as a result of oxidative stress. Interestingly, the antimutagenic and anti-genotoxic effects of eugenol has been also reported. Eugenol suppressed the mutagenicity induced by furylfuramide, 4-nitroquinoline 1-oxide, aflatoxin B in *Salmonella typhimurium* [37]. Eugenol also inhibits detoxification enzymes and prevents DMBA-induced DNA damage in MCF-7 (human breast adenocarcinoma) cell line [38,39]. Eugenol at dose of 50–500 mg/kg administered by gavage prevents the genotoxicity-induced by cyclophosphamide, procarbazine, *N*-methyl-*N'*-nitro-N-nitrosoguanidine and urethane [40]. In addition, the mutagenicity of benzo[a]pyrene but not DMBA and aflatoxin B1, in the *S. typhimurium* mutagenicity assay was reduced in liver S-9 fractions prepared from rats treated orally with eugenol (1000 mg/kg) [41]. In contrast, eugenol causes intrachromosomal recombination in yeast *Saccharomyces cerevisiae* in logarithmic phase cultures [42] and although eugenol induces no mutagenesis in Ames test, it causes chromosomal aberrations and increased the incidence of sister chromatid exchanges in Chinese hamster ovary cells [43,44]. At μM range, eugenol is not able to prevent the DNA lesions induced by hydrogen peroxide (H_2O_2) [33]. However, eugenol protected the supercoiled pBR322 plasmid DNA oxidative damage induced by Fe^{2+} and H_2O_2 at mM range [35]. Moreover, eugenol, at concentrations above 50 μM, inhibited the DNA oxidative damage induced by hydroxyl radicals produced by Fenton reactions using Fe^{2+} and H_2O_2 [32].

3. Cytotoxic and Antitumor Effects of Eugenol and Its Relation to the Induction of Oxidative Stress

Controversial results have been found for the cytotoxic activity of eugenol. Some studies have shown that eugenol is capable of inducing cytotoxicity at concentrations in the μM range, whereas other studies show that eugenol is capable of inducing cytotoxic effects only at concentrations in the mM range. Nevertheless, eugenol is able to induce cytotoxicity to cancer cell lines with different histological types, including skin, breast, colon, prostate, cervical, hepatocellular, lung, oral squamous cells and leukemia. In addition, the ability to induce oxidative stress has been also ascribed to eugenol in cell-based assays.

Eugenol in the μM range inhibits the growth of melanoma cells—Sbcl2 (primary melanoma), WM3211 (primary radial growth phase), WM98-1 (primary vertical growth phase) and WM1205Lu (metastatic melanoma)—accompanied by cell cycle arrest at the S phase, followed by apoptosis [45]. Using cDNA array analysis, it was demonstrated that eugenol modulates expression of E2F family members. In addition, eugenol was able to inhibit the E2F1 transcriptional activity and, as overexpression of E2F1 restores melanoma cell proliferation, this indicates that eugenol targets E2F functions in melanoma cells [45]. In addition, eugenol in the μM range inhibits the growth of HL-60 (human promyelocytic leukemia), U-937 (human histiocytic lymphoma), HepG2 (human hepatocellular carcinoma), 3LL (Lewis mouse lung carcinoma) and SNU-C5 (human colon carcinoma) lines [46]. Eugenol-treated HL-60 cells display DNA fragmentation, ROS production, loss of mitochondrial transmembrane potential, bax translocation, Bcl-2 reduction, cytochrome c release and caspase-9 and -3 activation, suggesting that eugenol causes apoptotic cell death. Moreover, pretreatment of HL-60 cells with *N*-acetyl-L-cysteine (an antioxidant), Z-VAD-FMK (a pan caspase inhibitor) and Z-DEVD-FMK (a caspase-3 inhibitor) decreases the eugenol-induced apoptosis, indicating that eugenol activates the caspase- and ROS-mediated apoptosis pathways [46]. Moreover, treatment of HL-60 cells with eugenol, produced formation of three DNA adducts and incubation of HL-60 cells with the combination of 100 μM eugenol and 100 μM H_2O_2 potentiated the levels of DNA adduct in HL-60 cells. Oxidative base damage was also observed. The DNA adducts formed were inhibited by the addition of either ascorbic acid or glutathione [47]. Eugenol in the μM range is also cytotoxic to DU-145 (androgen-insensitive prostate cancer cells) and KB (oral squamous carcinoma cells) [48].

Using LNCaP (androgen responsive human prostate carcinoma) and PC-3 (androgen independent human prostate carcinoma) cell lines, eugenol induces cytotoxicity in the μM range and causes an increase in G_2/M phase [49]. Apoptotic cell death was not detected at the concentrations used; however, eugenol in combination with 2-methoxyestradiol causes apoptosis along with a reduction of the expression of anti-apoptotic protein Bcl-2 and enhancement of the expression of the pro-apoptotic protein Bax. The apoptosis induced by this combination is not affected in PC-3 cells with overexpression or lack of Bcl-2 but is associated with the loss of mitochondrial membrane potential [49]. Eugenol in μM concentrations causes cytotoxicity to MCF-7, T47-D (human breast carcinoma) and MDA-MB-231 (human breast adenocarcinoma) cells through down-regulation of E2F1 and its downstream anti-apoptosis target, surviving independently of the status of p53 and ERα [50]. Eugenol inhibits the breast cancer related oncogenes, NF-κB and cyclin D1 and up-regulates the cyclin-dependent kinase inhibitor p21^{WAF1} protein; On the other hand, eugenol was also cytotoxic to non-cancer cell line MCF 10A (human breast epithelial) with IC_{50} value of 2.2 μM [50]. Júnior et al. [51] also assessed the cytotoxicity of eugenol in the μM range on MDA-MB-231, MCF-7, SIHA (human cervix carcinoma), SK-Mel-28 (human melanoma) and A2058 (human melanoma) cells; it was accompanied by ROS production, causing G2/M phase block and, consequently, clastogenesis. Eugenol also induced downregulation of PCNA (proliferation cell nuclear antigen), decreased the mitochondria transmembrane potential and upregulated Bax [51].

Controversially, some studies have indicated that eugenol has no cytotoxic activity or has cytotoxicity only when present in the mM range [52–73]. In studies with HSG (human submandibular gland adenocarcinoma) and HSC-2 (human oral squamous cell carcinoma) cells, eugenol caused cytotoxicity when in the mM range but no ROS induction was observed [58,59]. On the other hand, Atsumi et al. [60] stated that eugenol caused a biphasic ROS production that was enhanced at 5–10 μM and decreased at 500 μM in HSG, treated with H_2O_2 plus horseradish peroxidase or with visible light irradiation. In HL-60 cells, eugenol presents IC_{50} of 0.38 mM that is accompanied by internucleosomal DNA fragmentation. The expression of the mRNAs and the activity of manganese superoxide dismutase and copper- and zinc-containing superoxide dismutase are inhibited by eugenol, suggesting that eugenol targets the oxidative stress in cancer cells. In contrast, eugenol-induced cytotoxicity is enhanced by *N*-acetyl-L-cysteine or glutathione treatment [58,61]. On the other hand, eugenol induces cytotoxicity and ROS generation in HSG cells in which glutathione or cysteine are protecting from damage [62,63].

Pisano et al. [64] demonstrated that eugenol has no cytotoxic effect at 100 μM in malignant melanoma cell lines WM266-4, SK-Mel-28, LCP-Mel, LCM-Mel, PNP-Mel, CN-MelA, 13443 and GR-Mel. In human melanoma G361 cells, eugenol in the mM range inhibits the viability of G361 cells. Eugenol-treated G361 cells present caspase-3 and -6 cleavage and activation. The caspase-3 substrates poly(ADP-ribose)polymerase (PARP) and DNA fragmentation factor 45 (DFF45) are cleaved in eugenol-induced apoptosis, suggesting induction of caspase-dependent apoptosis [65]. Interestingly, similar results were found in human osteosarcoma HOS cells, suggesting that eugenol can also induce caspase-dependent apoptosis pathways in HOS cells [66].

In a study with human cervical carcinoma cell line (HeLa), eugenol presented cytotoxicity in the mM range and in a synergistic combination with sulforaphane, downregulated the expression of Bcl-2, COX-2 and IL-β. It also produced a synergistic effect when combined with gemcitabine, causing downregulation of the expression of Bcl-2, COX-2 and IL-β [67,68]. Also, in the mM range, eugenol was cytotoxic and induced apoptosis to colon carcinoma cell lines HCT-15 and HT-29. The loss of the membrane mitochondrial potential and generation of ROS were accompanied in the eugenol-induced apoptosis. Augmented ROS generation resulted in the DNA fragmentation and activation of PARP, p53 and caspase-3 [69]. Eugenol in the mM range also inhibits the growth of human breast carcinoma MCF-7 cells, accompanied by cell shrinkage and an increase in the percentage of apoptotic cells and DNA fragments. A depleted level of intracellular glutathione and increased level of lipid peroxidation are also observed [70]. In another study with MCF-7 cells, eugenol presented an IC$_{50}$ value of 0.9 mM, increased the ROS production, decreased the ATP level and induced the loss of the mitochondrial membrane potential and release of the cytochrome c and lactate. Cell viability and ROS production were restored by pretreatment with the antioxidants. On the other hand, the eugenol effect was not affected in MCF-7 cells with overexpression of Bcl-2 [71]. Human oral squamous cell carcinoma cell line HSC-2 treated with a concentration of eugenol in the mM range presented metabolic changes including reduction of ATP utilization, oxidative stress and an increase in the polyamines and glycolytic metabolites [72]. In HepG2 and Caco-2 (human colon carcinoma) cells, the treatment with eugenol-loaded nanoemulsions and free eugenol caused increasing in the cell death by apoptosis and ROS generation [73]. The Table 2 summarize the in vitro cytotoxic effect of eugenol.

Table 2. Summary of in vitro cytotoxic effects of eugenol against cancer and non-cancer cell lines.

Cell Lines	Histological Type	Origin	IC$_{50}$ (µM)	References
Cancer cells				
Sbcl2	Primary melanoma	Human	~0.5	[45]
WM3211	Primary melanoma	Human	~0.5	[45]
WM98-1	Primary melanoma	Human	~0.5	[45]
WM1205Lu	Metastatic melanoma	Human	~0.5	[45]
SK-Mel-28	Melanoma	Human	7.2	[51]
A2058	Melanoma	Human	12.2	[51]
WM266-4	Melanoma	Human	>100	[64]
SK-Mel-28	Melanoma	Human	>100	[64]
LCP-Mel	Melanoma	Human	>100	[64]
LCM-Mel	Melanoma	Human	>100	[64]
PNP-Mel	Melanoma	Human	>100	[64]
CN-MelA	Melanoma	Human	>100	[64]
13443	Melanoma	Human	>100	[64]
GR-Mel	Melanoma	Human	>100	[64]
HSG	Submandibular gland adenocarcinoma	Human	~100	[59]
			396	[60]
T47-D	Breast carcinoma	Human	0.9	[50]
MDA-MB-231	Breast adenocarcinoma	Human	1.7	[50]
			15.1	[51]
			~1600	[71]
MCF-7	Breast adenocarcinoma	Human	1.5	[50]
			22.8	[51]
			~400	[70]
			900	[71]

Table 2. *Cont.*

Cell Lines	Histological Type	Origin	IC$_{50}$ (μM)	References
HCT-15	Colon adenocarcinoma	Human	300	[69]
HT-29	Colon adenocarcinoma	Human	500	[69]
Caco-2	Colon carcinoma	Human	~750	[73]
SNU-C5	Colon carcinoma	Human	129.4	[46]
LNCaP	Prostate adenocarcinoma	Human	~550	[49]
PC-3	Prostate carcinoma	Human	~180	[49]
DU-145	Prostate carcinoma	Human	30.4	[48]
SIHA	Cervical carcinoma	Human	18.3	[51]
HeLa	Cervical carcinoma	Human	500	[72]
HepG2	Hepatocellular carcinoma	Human	118.6	[46]
			~500	[73]
3LL	Lewis lung carcinoma	Mouse	89.6	[46]
KB	Oral squamous cell carcinoma	Human	28.5	[48]
HSC-2	Oral squamous cell carcinoma	Human	~700	[72]
HOS	Osteosarcoma	Human	1500	[66]
HL-60	Promyelocytic leukemia	Human	23.7	[46]
			380	[61]
U-937	Histocytic lymphoma	Human	39.4	[46]
Non-cancer cells				
MCF 10A	Breast epithelial	Human	2.2	[50]

IC$_{50}$: half maximal inhibitory concentration.

In vivo antitumor effects of eugenol have been also investigated [45,50,74]. Using B6D2F1 mice bearing B16 melanoma, eugenol treatment (125 mg/kg/i.p. of body weight twice a week) caused the in vivo antitumor effect [45]. On day 15, the size of tumors in the eugenol-treated group was 62% less than the control group, with an increase of 19% in the survival rate. At the end of the treatment, 50% of the animals in the control group presented metastases but no eugenol-treated animals showed any signs of invasion or metastasis [45]. Moreover, eugenol (100 mg/kg/i.p.) was able to inhibit the growth of the Ehrlich ascites model by 28.88% and inhibited 24.35% tumor growth in the Ehrlich solid tumor model [74].

In mice engrafted with human breast adenocarcinoma MDA-MB-231 cells subcutaneously, eugenol treatment with a dose of 100 mg/kg every two days for four weeks inhibited tumor growth [50]. Moreover, eugenol downregulated E2F1, survivin, NF-κB and cyclin D1 and increased the levels of p21^{WAF1}, Bax, cleaved PARP-1 and the active form of caspase-9 in tumor xenografts [50]. The Table 3 summarize the in vivo antitumor effect of eugenol. Regarding the antimetastatic potential of eugenol, it exerts inhibitory effects on matrix metallopeptidase 9 (MMP-9) via inhibition of extracellular signal-regulated kinase (ERK) phosphorylation in human fibrosarcoma HT1080 cells [32].

Table 3. Summary of in vivo antitumor effect of eugenol.

Tumor	Histological Type	Origin	Dose (mg/kg)	Treatment	Route	Inhibition Rate (%)	References
B16	Melanoma	Mouse	125	Twice a week	i.p.	62	[45]
Ehrlich (ascites model)	Carcinoma	Mouse	100	Every two days for four weeks	i.p.	28.9	[74]
Ehrlich (solid model)	Carcinoma	Mouse	100	Every two days for four weeks	i.p.	24.4	[74]
MDA-MB-231	Breast adenocarcinoma	Human	100	Every two days for four weeks	i.p.	~66	[50]

i.p.: intraperitoneal.

Although there are a large number of papers on the cytotoxic properties of eugenol, controversial results delay the completion of preclinical efficacy and safety studies as well as clinical trials. However, the ability of eugenol to induce oxidative stress, as observed in cell-based assays, appears to be related to its cytotoxic and antitumor effect. Other compounds with dual antioxidant and prooxidant effect have a dose/concentration-response relationship, for example, at low doses/concentrations present antioxidant effect and at high doses/concentrations show prooxidant effect [75–78]; however, we do not find this relationship with the data published with eugenol. Problems related to the degree of purity of the compound, its evaporation (for volatile compounds for example) during the experiments, the methods used to quantify these data (since different cellular and animal models may present divergent results and interpretations) and some laboratory and interpretation errors (including the use of cell lines contaminated with *Mycoplasma* sp., errors in cell line authentication, etc.) may contribute to explain these controversial results.

In relation to the structure-activity relationship of eugenol, the cytotoxicity of eugenol-related compounds has been associated with the activity of the production of phenoxyl radicals, their stability of the subsequent quinonemethide and the hydrophobicity [79]. In relation to the antioxidant activity, the number of hydroxyl groups in the phenol ring of eugenol enhanced it antioxidant action [31,80]. Moreover, the presence of bromine substituent in ortho-position to the OH-group increases its antioxidant activity [81].

4. Conclusions

The studies presented in this review reveal the therapeutic potential of eugenol in cancer prevention and treatment and the relationship with its antioxidant and pro-oxidant activities. The Figure 3 summarize the molecular mechanisms of eugenol. Therefore, the consumption of vegetables containing this compound in significant quantities might well be useful in inhibiting the free radicals responsible for tumor development. In addition, the data reported are in accordance with the scientific understanding that a better quality of life and increased longevity may be obtained via healthy food, with the health promoting effects of its bioactive constituents.

Nutrients **2017**, *9*, 1367

Eugenol

Anti-carcinogenic effect		Cytotoxic and antitumor effects	
↓iNOS	↓IL-β	↓NF-κB	↑ROS
↓COX-2	↓PGE2	↓E2F1	↑caspase-9
↓IL-6	↓PGC-1β	↓Bcl-2	↑caspase-3
↓TNF-α	↓H-ras	↓survivin	↑caspase-6
↓Myc	↓ERRα	↓MMP-2	↑Apaf-1
		↓MMP-9	↑Bax
		↓cyclin D1	↑Gadd45
		↓cyclin B	↑p53
		↓Cu/ZnSOD	↑p21^{WAFI}
		↓MnSOD	↑IκBα
		↓VEGF	↑IKKβ
		↓VEGFR1	↑RECK
		↓PCNA	↑TIMP-2

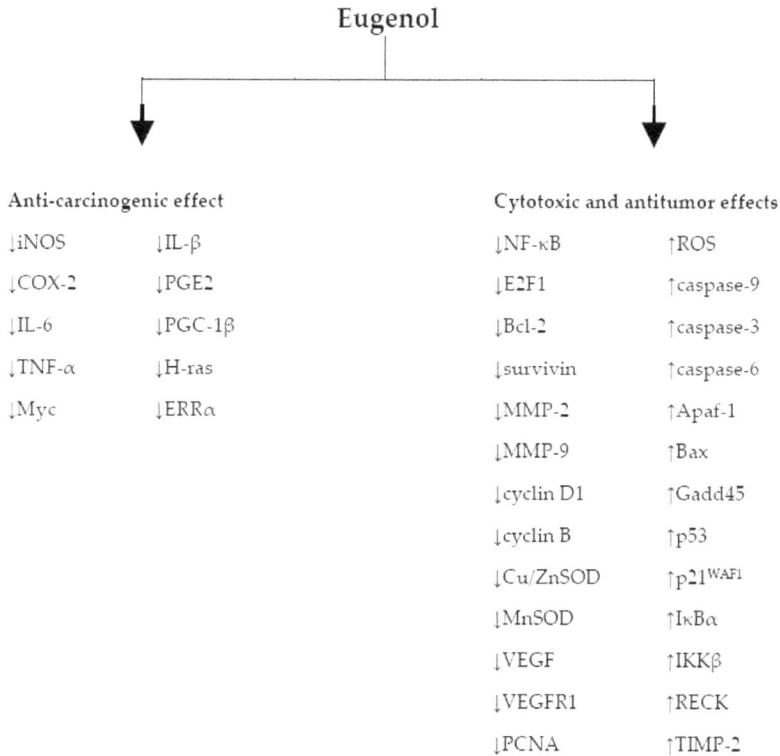

Figure 3. Molecular mechanisms of eugenol. ↑: upregulation; ↓: downregulation; Apaf-1: apoptotic protease activating factor 1; Bax: BCL2 associated X, apoptosis regulator; Bcl-2: B-cell lymphoma 2, apoptosis regulator; COX-2: cycloxygenase-2; Cu/ZnSOD: copper- and zinc-containing superoxide dismutase; ERRα: estrogen-related receptor alpha; Gadd45: growth arrest and DNA damage-inducible 45: IKKβ: IκB kinase α; IL-6: interleukin 6; iNOS: inducible nitric oxide synthase; IκBα: inhibitor of kappa B; MMP-2: matrix metalloproteinase-2; MMP-9: matrix metalloproteinase-9; MnSOD: manganese superoxide dismutase; NF-κB: nuclear factor-kappa B; PCNA: proliferating cell nuclear antigen; PGC-1β: peroxisome proliferator-activated receptor gamma coactivator 1-beta; PGE2: prostaglandin E2; RECK: reversion-inducing-cysteine-rich protein with kazal motifs; ROS: reactive oxygen species; TIMP-2: tissue inhibitor of metalloproteinase-2; TNF-α: tumor necrosis factor alpha; VEGF: vascular endothelial growth factor; VEGFR1: vascular endothelial growth factor receptor 1.

Acknowledgments: This work was supported by the Brazilian agencies: Conselho Nacional de Desenvolvimento Científico e Tecnológico (CNPq) and Coordenação de Aperfeiçoamento de Pessoal de Nível Superior (CAPES).

Author Contributions: Daniel Pereira Bezerra surveyed the data and wrote the pharmacological part of the review. Gardenia Carmen Gadelha Militão was responsible for the analysis of these data and wrote the pharmacological part. Damião Pergentino de Sousa wrote the chemical content, revised and planned the study. Mayara Castro de Morais was responsible for formatting the manuscript.

Conflicts of Interest: The authors declare no conflicts of interest.

Abbreviations

Apaf-1	Apoptotic protease activating factor 1
Bax	BCL2 associated X, apoptosis regulator
Bcl-2	B-cell lymphoma 2, apopstosis regulator
COX-2	Cyclooxygenase-2
CYP 1A1	Cytochrome P450 family 1 subfamily A member 1
CYP1B1	Cytochrome P450 family 1 subfamily B member 1
DFF45	DNA fragmentation factor 45
DMBA	7,12-dimethylbenz[a]anthracene
DNA	Deoxyribonucleic acid
DPPH	2,2-diphenyl-1-picrylhydrazyl
ER	Endoplasmic reticulum
Gadd45	Growth arrest and DNA damage-inducible 45
IC_{50}	Half maximal inhibitory concentration
IKKβ	Inhibitor of kappa B
IL-6	Interleukin-6
iNOS	Inducible nitric oxide synthase
IκBα	IκB Kinase α
MA	Malonaldehyde
MCF 10A-ras	H-ras transfected MCF 10A
MMP	Matrix metalloproteinases
MNNG	*N*-Methyl-*N'*-nitro-*N*-nitrosoguanidine
NF-κB	Nuclear factor kappa B
PARP	Poly(ADP-ribose)polymerase
PCNA	Proliferating cell nuclear antigen
PGE2	Prostaglandin E2
RECK	Reversion-inducing-cysteine-rich protein with kazal motifs
ROS	Reactive Oxygen Species
SGOT	Serum glutamic-oxaloacetic transaminase
TA	Thioacetamide
TBARS	Thiobarbituric acid-reactive substances
TIMP-2	Tissue inhibitor of metalloproteinase-2
TNF-α	Tumor necrosis factor alpha
TPA	12-otetradecanoylphorbol-13-acetate
VEGF	Vascular endothelial growth factor
VEGFR1	Vascular endothelial growth factor receptor 1

References

1. Selim, K.A.; Abdelrasoul, H.; Aboelmagd, M.; Tawila, A.M. The role of the MAPK signaling, topoisomerase and dietary bioactives in controlling cancer incidence. *Diseases* **2017**, *5*, 13. [CrossRef] [PubMed]
2. Gào, X.; Schöttker, B. Reduction-oxidation pathways involved in cancer development: A systematic review of literature reviews. *Oncotarget* **2017**, *8*, 51888–51906. [CrossRef] [PubMed]
3. Fiaschi, T.; Chiarugi, P. Oxidative stress, tumor microenvironment, and metabolic reprogramming: A diabolic liaison. *Int. J. Cell Biol.* **2012**, 762825. [CrossRef] [PubMed]
4. Bezerra, D.P.; Soares, A.K.; de Sousa, D.P. Overview of the role of vanillin on redox status and cancer development. *Oxid. Med. Cell Longev.* **2016**, 9734816. [CrossRef] [PubMed]
5. Carvalho, A.A.; Andrade, L.N.; De Sousa, E.B.; De Sousa, D.P. Antitumor phenylpropanoids found in essential oils. *Biomed. Res. Int.* **2015**, 392674. [CrossRef] [PubMed]
6. Sobral, M.V.; Xavier, A.L.; Lima, T.C.; De Sousa, D.P. Antitumor activity of monoterpenes found in essential oils. *Sci. World J.* **2014**, 953451. [CrossRef] [PubMed]
7. De Sousa, D.P. *Bioactive Essential Oils and Cancer*; Springer: New York, NY, USA, 2015.

8. Ferraz, R.P.; Bomfim, D.S.; Carvalho, N.C.; Soares, M.B.; da Silva, T.B.; Machado, W.J.; Prata, A.P.; Costa, E.V.; Moraes, V.R.; Nogueira, P.C.; et al. Cytotoxic effect of leaf essential oil of *Lippia gracilis* Schauer (Verbenaceae). *Phytomedicine* **2013**, *20*, 615–621. [CrossRef] [PubMed]

9. Khan, H.Y.; Zubair, H.; Ullah, M.F.; Ahmad, A.; Hadi, S.M. A prooxidant mechanism for the anticancer and chemopreventive properties of plant polyphenols. *Curr. Drug Targets* **2012**, *13*, 1738–1749. [CrossRef] [PubMed]

10. Forester, S.C.; Lambert, J.D. The role of antioxidant versus pro-oxidant effects of green tea polyphenols in cancer prevention. *Mol. Nutr. Food Res.* **2011**, *55*, 844–854. [CrossRef] [PubMed]

11. Assi, M. The differential role of reactive oxygen species in early and late stages of cancer. *Am. J. Physiol. Regul. Integr. Comp. Physiol.* **2017**, *313*, R646–R653. [CrossRef] [PubMed]

12. Lee, K.-G.; Shibamoto, T. Antioxidant properties of aroma compounds isolated from soybeans and mung beans. *J. Agric. Food Chem.* **2000**, *48*, 4290–4293. [CrossRef] [PubMed]

13. Charalambous, G. *The Quality of Foods and Beverages V2: Chemistry and Technology*, 1st ed.; Academic Press: New York, NY, USA, 1981; p. 408.

14. Jordán, M.J.; Tandon, K.; Shaw, P.E.; Goodner, K.L. Aromatic profile of aqueous banana essence and banana fruit by gas chromatography-mass spectrometry (GC-MS) and gas chromatography-olfactometry (GC-O). *J. Agric. Food Chem.* **2001**, *49*, 4813–4817. [CrossRef] [PubMed]

15. Kamatou, G.P.; Vermaak, I.; Viljoen, A.M. Eugenol-from the remote maluku islands to the international market place: A review of a remarkable and versatile molecule. *Molecules* **2012**, *17*, 6953–6981. [CrossRef] [PubMed]

16. Lee, K.-Y.M.; Patterson, A.; Piggot, J.R.; Richardson, G.D. Origins of flavour in whiskies and a revised flavour wheel: A review. *J. Inst. Brew.* **2001**, *107*, 287–313. [CrossRef]

17. Bohnert, H.J.; Nguyen, H.R.; Lewis, N.G. *Bioengineering and Molecular Biology of Plant Pathways*; Elsevier: San Diego, CA, USA, 2008.

18. Srinivasan, K. Antioxidant potential of spices and their active constituents. *Crit. Rev. Food Sci. Nutr.* **2014**, *54*, 352–372. [CrossRef] [PubMed]

19. Gorrini, C.; Harris, I.S.; Mak, T.W. Modulation of oxidative stress as an anticancer strategy. *Nat. Rev. Drug Discov.* **2013**, *12*, 931–947. [CrossRef] [PubMed]

20. Kaur, G.; Athar, M.; Alam, M.S. Eugenol precludes cutaneous chemical carcinogenesis in mouse by preventing oxidative stress and inflammation and by inducing apoptosis. *Mol. Carcinog.* **2010**, *49*, 290–301. [CrossRef] [PubMed]

21. Sukumaran, K.; Unnikrishnan, M.C.; Kuttan, R. Inhibition of tumour promotion in mice by eugenol. *Indian J. Physiol. Pharmacol.* **1994**, *38*, 306–308. [PubMed]

22. Pal, D.; Banerjee, S.; Mukherjee, S.; Roy, A.; Panda, C.K.; Das, S. Eugenol restricts DMBA croton oil induced skin carcinogenesis in mice: Downregulation of c-Myc and H-ras, and activation of p53 dependent apoptotic pathway. *J. Dermatol. Sci.* **2010**, *59*, 31–39. [CrossRef] [PubMed]

23. Van Duuren, B.L.; Goldschmidt, B.M. Cocarcinogenic and tumor-promoting agents in tobacco carcinogenesis. *J. Natl. Cancer Inst.* **1976**, *56*, 1237–1242. [CrossRef] [PubMed]

24. Azuine, M.A.; Amonkar, A.J.; Bhide, S.V. Chemopreventive efficacy of betel leaf extract and its constituents on 7,12-dimethylbenz(a)anthracene induced carcinogenesis and their effect on drug detoxification system in mouse skin. *Indian J. Exp. Biol.* **1991**, *29*, 346–351. [PubMed]

25. Manikandan, P.; Murugan, R.S.; Priyadarsini, R.V.; Vinothini, G.; Nagini, S. Eugenol induces apoptosis and inhibits invasion and angiogenesis in a rat model of gastric carcinogenesis induced by MNNG. *Life Sci.* **2010**, *86*, 936–941. [CrossRef] [PubMed]

26. Manikandan, P.; Vinothini, G.; Vidya Priyadarsini, R.; Prathiba, D.; Nagini, S. Eugenol inhibits cell proliferation via NF-κB suppression in a rat model of gastric carcinogenesis induced by MNNG. *Invest. New Drugs* **2011**, *29*, 110–117. [CrossRef] [PubMed]

27. Yan, X.; Zhang, G.; Bie, F.; Lv, Y.; Ma, Y.; Ma, M.; Wang, Y.; Hao, X.; Yuan, N.; Jiang, X. Eugenol inhibits oxidative phosphorylation and fatty acid oxidation via downregulation of c-Myc/PGC-1β/ERRα signaling pathway in MCF10A-ras cells. *Sci. Rep.* **2017**, *7*, 12920. [CrossRef] [PubMed]

28. Koujitani, T.; Yasuhara, K.; Tamura, T.; Onodera, H.; Takagi, H.; Takizawa, T.; Hirose, M.; Hayashi, Y.; Mitsumori, K. Lack of modifying effects of eugenol on development of lung proliferative lesions induced by urethane in transgenic mice carrying the human prototype c-Ha-ras gene. *J. Toxicol. Sci.* **2001**, *26*, 129–139. [CrossRef] [PubMed]

29. Ito, M.; Murakami, K.; Yoshino, M. Antioxidant action of eugenol compounds: Role of metal ion in the inhibition of lipid peroxidation. *Food Chem. Toxicol.* **2005**, *43*, 461–466. [CrossRef] [PubMed]

30. Nagababu, E.; Rifkind, J.M.; Boindala, S.; Nakka, L. Assessment of antioxidant activity of eugenol in vitro and in vivo. *Methods Mol. Biol.* **2010**, *610*, 165–180. [PubMed]

31. Gülçin, İ. Antioxidant activity of eugenol: A structure-activity relationship study. *J. Med. Food* **2011**, *14*, 975–985. [CrossRef] [PubMed]

32. Nam, H.; Kim, M.M. Eugenol with antioxidant activity inhibits MMP-9 related to metastasis in human fibrosarcoma cells. *Food Chem. Toxicol.* **2013**, *55*, 106–112. [CrossRef] [PubMed]

33. Horvathova, E.; Navarova, J.; Galova, E.; Sevcovicova, A.; Chodakova, L.; Snahnicanova, Z.; Melusova, M.; Kozics, K.; Slamenova, D. Assessment of antioxidative, chelating, and DNA-protective effects of selected essential oil components (eugenol, carvacrol, thymol, borneol, eucalyptol) of plants and intact *Rosmarinus officinalis* oil. *J. Agric. Food Chem.* **2014**, *62*, 6632–6639. [CrossRef] [PubMed]

34. Mahapatra, S.K.; Roy, S. Phytopharmacological approach of free radical scavenging and anti-oxidative potential of eugenol and *Ocimum gratissimum* Linn. *Asian Pac. J. Trop. Med.* **2014**, *7S1*, S391–S397. [CrossRef]

35. Zhang, L.L.; Zhang, L.F.; Xu, J.G.; Hu, Q.P. Comparison study on antioxidant, DNA damage protective and antibacterial activities of eugenol and isoeugenol against several foodborne pathogens. *Food Nutr. Res.* **2017**, *61*, 1353356. [CrossRef] [PubMed]

36. Yogalakshmi, B.; Viswanathan, P.; Anuradha, C.V. Investigation of antioxidant, anti-inflammatory and DNA-protective properties of eugenol in thioacetamide-induced liver injury in rats. *Toxicology* **2010**, *268*, 204–212. [CrossRef] [PubMed]

37. Miyazawa, M.; Hisama, M. Suppression of chemical mutagen-induced SOS response by alkylphenols from clove (*Syzygium aromaticum*) in the *Salmonella typhimurium* TA1535/pSK1002 umu test. *J. Agric. Food Chem.* **2001**, *49*, 4019–4025. [CrossRef] [PubMed]

38. Rompelberg, C.J.; Verhagen, H.; van Bladeren, P.J. Effects of the naturally occurring alkenylbenzenes eugenol and trans-anethole on drug-metabolizing enzymes in the rat liver. *Food Chem. Toxicol.* **1993**, *31*, 637–645. [CrossRef]

39. Han, E.H.; Hwang, Y.P.; Jeong, T.C.; Lee, S.S.; Shin, J.G.; Jeong, H.G. Eugenol inhibit 7,12-dimethylbenz[a]anthracene-induced genotoxicity in MCF-7 cells: Bifunctional effects on CYP1 and NAD(P)H: Quinone oxidoreductase. *FEBS Lett.* **2007**, *581*, 749–756. [CrossRef] [PubMed]

40. Abraham, S.K. Anti-genotoxicity of trans-anethole and eugenol in mice. *Food Chem. Toxicol.* **2001**, *39*, 493–498. [CrossRef]

41. Rompelberg, C.J.; Evertz, S.J.; Bruijntjes-Rozier, G.C.; van den Heuvel, P.D.; Verhagen, H. Effect of eugenol on the genotoxicity of established mutagens in the liver. *Food Chem. Toxicol.* **1996**, *34*, 33–42. [CrossRef]

42. Schiestl, R.H.; Chan, W.S.; Gietz, R.D.; Mehta, R.D.; Hastings, P.J. Safrole, eugenol and methyleugenol induce intrachromosomal recombination in yeast. *Mutat. Res.* **1989**, *224*, 427–436. [CrossRef]

43. Stich, H.F.; Stich, W.; Lam, P.P.S. Potentiation of genotoxicity by concurrent application of compounds found in betel quid: Arecoline, eugenol, quercetin, chlorogenic acid and Mn^{2+}. *Mutat. Res.* **1981**, *90*, 355–363. [CrossRef]

44. National Toxicology Program (NTP). Carcinogenesis Studies of Eugenol (CAS No. 97–53–0) in F344/N Rats and B6C3F1 Mice (Feed Studies). *Natl. Toxicol. Program Tech. Rep. Ser.* **1983**, *223*, 1–159.

45. Ghosh, R.; Nadiminty, N.; Fitzpatrick, J.E.; Alworth, W.L.; Slaga, T.J.; Kumar, A.P. Eugenol causes melanoma growth suppression through inhibition of E2F1 transcriptional activity. *J. Biol. Chem.* **2005**, *280*, 5812–5819. [CrossRef] [PubMed]

46. Yoo, C.B.; Han, K.T.; Cho, K.S.; Ha, J.; Park, H.J.; Nam, J.H.; Kil, U.H.; Lee, K.T. Eugenol isolated from the essential oil of Eugenia caryophyllata induces a reactive oxygen species-mediated apoptosis in HL-60 human promyelocytic leukemia cells. *Cancer Lett.* **2005**, *225*, 41–52. [CrossRef] [PubMed]

47. Bodell, W.J.; Ye, Q.; Pathak, D.N.; Pongracz, K. Oxidation of eugenol to form DNA adducts and 8-hydroxy-2′-deoxyguanosine: Role of quinone methide derivative in DNA adduct formation. *Carcinogenesis* **1998**, *19*, 437–443. [CrossRef] [PubMed]

48. Carrasco, A.; Espinoza, C.; Cardile, V.; Gallardo, C.; Cardona, W.; Lombardo, L.; Catalán, M.; Cuellar, F.; Russo, A. Eugenol and its synthetic analogues inhibit cell growth of human cancer cells. *J. Braz. Chem. Soc.* **2008**, *19*, 543–548. [CrossRef]

49. Ghosh, R.; Ganapathy, M.; Alworth, W.L.; Chan, D.C.; Kumar, A.P. Combination of 2-methoxyestradiol (2-ME2) and eugenol for apoptosis induction synergistically in androgen independent prostate cancer cells. *J. Steroid Biochem. Mol. Biol.* **2009**, *113*, 25–35. [CrossRef] [PubMed]

50. Al-Sharif, I.; Remmal, A.; Aboussekhra, A. Eugenol triggers apoptosis in breast cancer cells through E2F1/survivin down-regulation. *BMC Cancer* **2013**, *13*, 600. [CrossRef] [PubMed]

51. Júnior, P.L.; Câmara, D.A.; Costa, A.S.; Ruiz, J.L.; Levy, D.; Azevedo, R.A.; Pasqualoto, K.F.; de Oliveira, C.F.; de Melo, T.C.; Pessoa, N.D.; et al. Apoptotic effect of eugenol envolves G2/M phase abrogation accompanied by mitochondrial damage and clastogenic effect on cancer cell in vitro. *Phytomedicine* **2016**, *23*, 725–735. [CrossRef] [PubMed]

52. Young, S.C.; Wang, C.J.; Hsu, J.D.; Hsu, J.L.; Chou, F.P. Increased sensitivity of Hep G2 cells toward the cytotoxicity of cisplatin by the treatment of piper betel leaf extract. *Arch Toxicol.* **2006**, *80*, 319–327. [CrossRef] [PubMed]

53. Fujimoto, A.; Sakanashi, Y.; Matsui, H.; Oyama, T.; Nishimura, Y.; Masuda, T.; Oyama, Y. Cytometric analysis of cytotoxicity of polyphenols and related phenolics to rat thymocytes: Potent cytotoxicity of resveratrol to normal cells. *Basic Clin. Pharmacol. Toxicol.* **2009**, *104*, 455–462. [CrossRef] [PubMed]

54. Slamenová, D.; Horváthová, E.; Wsólová, L.; Sramková, M.; Navarová, J. Investigation of anti-oxidative, cytotoxic, DNA-damaging and DNA-protective effects of plant volatiles eugenol and borneol in human-derived HepG2, Caco-2 and VH10 cell lines. *Mutat. Res.* **2009**, *677*, 46–52. [CrossRef] [PubMed]

55. Jaganathan, S.K.; Supriyanto, E. Antiproliferative and molecular mechanism of eugenol-induced apoptosis in cancer cells. *Molecules* **2012**, *17*, 6290–6304. [CrossRef] [PubMed]

56. Koh, T.; Machino, M.; Murakami, Y.; Umemura, N.; Sakagami, H. Cytotoxicity of dental compounds towards human oral squamous cell carcinoma and normal oral cells. *In Vivo* **2013**, *27*, 85–95. [PubMed]

57. Sharma, U.K.; Sharma, A.K.; Gupta, A.; Kumar, R.; Pandey, A.; Pandey, A.K. Pharmacological activities of cinnamaldehyde and eugenol: Antioxidant, cytotoxic and anti-leishmanial studies. *Mol. Cell. Biol.* **2017**, *63*, 73–78. [CrossRef] [PubMed]

58. Fujisawa, S.; Atsumi, T.; Satoh, K.; Kadoma, Y.; Ishihara, M.; Okada, N.; Nagasaki, M.; Yokoe, I.; Sakagami, H. Radical generation, radical-scavenging activity, and cytotoxicity of eugenol-related compounds. *In Vitro Mol. Toxicol.* **2000**, *13*, 269–280.

59. Fujisawa, S.; Atsumi, T.; Ishihara, M.; Kadoma, Y. Cytotoxicity, ROS-generation activity and radical-scavenging activity of curcumin and related compounds. *Anticancer Res.* **2004**, *24*, 563–569. [PubMed]

60. Atsumi, T.; Fujisawa, S.; Tonosaki, K. A comparative study of the antioxidant/prooxidant activities of eugenol and isoeugenol with various concentrations and oxidation conditions. *Toxicol. In Vitro* **2005**, *19*, 1025–1033. [CrossRef] [PubMed]

61. Okada, N.; Hirata, A.; Murakami, Y.; Shoji, M.; Sakagami, H.; Fujisawa, S. Induction of cytotoxicity and apoptosis and inhibition of cyclooxygenase-2 gene expression by eugenol-related compounds. *Anticancer Res.* **2005**, *25*, 3263–3269. [PubMed]

62. Atsumi, T.; Iwakura, I.; Fujisawa, S.; Ueha, T. Reactive oxygen species generation and photo-cytotoxicity of eugenol in solutions of various pH. *Biomaterials* **2001**, *22*, 1459–1466. [CrossRef]

63. Fujisawa, S.; Atsumi, T.; Satoh, K.; Sakagami, H. Interaction between 2-ethoxybenzoic acid (EBA) and eugenol, and related changes in cytotoxicity. *J. Dent. Res.* **2003**, *82*, 43–47. [CrossRef] [PubMed]

64. Pisano, M.; Pagnan, G.; Loi, M.; Mura, M.E.; Tilocca, M.G.; Palmieri, G.; Fabbri, D.; Dettori, M.A.; Delogu, G.; Ponzoni, M.; et al. Antiproliferative and pro-apoptotic ctivity of eugenol-related biphenyls on malignant melanoma cells. *Mol. Cancer* **2007**, *6*, 8–20. [CrossRef] [PubMed]

65. Kim, G.C.; Choi, D.S.; Lim, J.S.; Jeong, H.C.; Kim, I.R.; Lee, M.H.; Park, B.S. Caspases-dependent apoptosis in human melanoma cell by eugenol. *Korean J. Anat.* **2006**, *39*, 245–253.

66. Shin, S.H.; Park, J.H.; Kim, G.C. The mechanism of apoptosis induced by eugenol in human osteosarcoma cells. *J. Korean Assoc. Oral Maxillofac. Surg.* **2007**, *33*, 20–27.

67. Hussain, A.; Brahmbhatt, K.; Priyani, A.; Ahmed, M.; Rizvi, T.A.; Sharma, C. Eugenol enhances the chemotherapeutic potential of gemcitabine and induces anticarcinogenic and anti-inflammatory activity in human cervical cancer cells. *Cancer Biother. Radiopharm.* **2011**, *26*, 519–527. [CrossRef] [PubMed]

68. Hussain, A.; Priyani, A.; Sadrieh, L.; Brahmbhatt, K.; Ahmed, M.; Sharma, C. Concurrent sulforaphane and eugenol induces differential effects on human cervical cancer cells. *Integr. Cancer Ther.* **2012**, *11*, 154–165. [CrossRef] [PubMed]

69. Jaganathan, S.K.; Mazumdar, A.; Mondhe, D.; Mandal, M. Apoptotic effect of eugenol in human colon cancer cell lines. *Cell Biol. Int.* **2011**, *35*, 607–615. [CrossRef] [PubMed]

70. Vidhya, N.; Devaraj, S.N. Induction of apoptosis by eugenol in human breast cancer cells. *Indian J. Exp. Biol.* **2011**, *49*, 871–878. [PubMed]

71. Al Wafai, R.; El-Rabih, W.; Katerji, M.; Safi, R.; El Sabban, M.; El-Rifai, O.; Usta, J. Chemosensitivity of MCF-7 cells to eugenol: Release of cytochrome-c and lactate dehydrogenase. *Sci. Rep.* **2017**, *7*, 43730. [CrossRef] [PubMed]

72. Koh, T.; Murakami, Y.; Tanaka, S.; Machino, M.; Onuma, H.; Kaneko, M.; Sugimoto, M.; Soga, T.; Tomita, M.; Sakagami, H. Changes of metabolic profiles in an oral squamous cell carcinoma cell line induced by eugenol. *In Vivo* **2013**, *27*, 233–243. [PubMed]

73. Majeed, H.; Antoniou, J.; Fang, Z. Apoptotic effects of eugenol-loaded nanoemulsions in human colon and liver cancer cell lines. *Asian Pac. J. Cancer Prev.* **2014**, *15*, 9159–9164. [CrossRef] [PubMed]

74. Jaganathan, S.K.; Mondhe, D.; Wani, Z.A.; Pal, H.C.; Mandal, M. Effect of honey and eugenol on ehrlich ascites and solid carcinoma. *J. Biomed. Biotechnol* **2010**, 989163:1–989163:5. [CrossRef] [PubMed]

75. Osseni, R.A.; Rat, P.; Bogdan, A.; Warnet, J.M.; Touitou, Y. Evidence of prooxidant and antioxidant action of melatonin on human liver cell line HepG2. *Life Sci.* **2000**, *68*, 387–399. [CrossRef]

76. Schwartz, J.L. The dual roles of nutrients as antioxidants and prooxidants: Their effects on tumor cell growth. *J. Nutr.* **1996**, *126*, 1221S–1227S. [PubMed]

77. Shi, M.; Xu, B.; Azakami, K.; Morikawa, T.; Watanabe, K.; Morimoto, K.; Komatsu, M.; Aoyama, K.; Takeuchi, T. Dual role of vitamin C in an oxygen-sensitive system: Discrepancy between DNA damage and cell death. *Free Radic Res.* **2005**, *39*, 213–220. [CrossRef] [PubMed]

78. Chakraborthy, A.; Ramani, P.; Sherlin, H.J.; Premkumar, P.; Natesan, A. Antioxidant and pro-oxidant activity of Vitamin C in oral environment. *Indian J. Dent. Res.* **2014**, *25*, 499–504. [CrossRef] [PubMed]

79. Fujisawa, S.; Atsumi, T.; Kadoma, Y.; Sakagami, H. Antioxidant and prooxidant action of eugenol-related compounds and their cytotoxicity. *Toxicology* **2002**, *177*, 39–54. [CrossRef]

80. Kim, D.O.; Lee, C.Y. Comprehensive study on vitamin C equivalent antioxidant capacity (VCEAC) of various polyphenolics in scavenging a free radical and its structural relationship. *Crit. Rev. Food Sci. Nutr.* **2004**, *44*, 253–273. [CrossRef] [PubMed]

81. Mahboub, R.; Memmou, F. Antioxidant activity and kinetics studies of eugenol and 6-bromoeugenol. *Nat. Prod. Res.* **2015**, *29*, 966–971. [CrossRef] [PubMed]

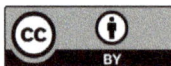

nutrients

MDPI

Review

Batzella, Crambe and Monanchora: Highly Prolific Marine Sponge Genera Yielding Compounds with Potential Applications for Cancer and Other Therapeutic Areas

Amr El-Demerdash [1,2,*], Atanas G. Atanasov [3,4,*], Anupam Bishayee [5,*], Mamdouh Abdel-Mogib [2], John N. A. Hooper [6] and Ali Al-Mourabit [1]

[1] Institut de Chimie des Substances Naturelles, CNRS UPR 2301, Univ. Paris-Sud, University of Paris-Saclay, 1, Avenue de la Terrasse, 91198 Gif-Sur-Yvette, France; Ali.ALMOURABIT@cnrs.fr
[2] Organic Chemistry Division, Chemistry Department, Faculty of Science, Mansoura University, Mansoura 35516, Egypt; mmdhbdlmgb@gmail.com
[3] Institute of Genetics and Animal Breeding of the Polish Academy of Sciences, 05-552 Jastrzebiec, Poland
[4] Department of Pharmacognosy, University of Vienna, 1090 Vienna, Austria
[5] Department of Pharmaceutical Sciences, College of Pharmacy, Larkin University, 18301 N. Miami Avenue, Miami, FL 33169, USA
[6] Queensland Museum, P.O. Box 3300, South Brisbane, QLD BC 4101, Australia; john.hooper@qm.qld.gov.au
[*] Correspondence: eldemerdash555@gmail.com (A.E.-D.); atanas.atanasov@univie.ac.at (A.G.A.); abishayee@ularkin.org or abishayee@gmail.com (A.B.); Tel.: +0033-758-490-229 (A.E.-D.); Tel.: +0048-227-367-022 (A.G.A.); Tel.:+1-305-760-7511 (A.B.)

Received: 1 November 2017; Accepted: 22 December 2017; Published: 2 January 2018

Abstract: Pyrroloquinoline and guanidine-derived alkaloids present distinct groups of marine secondary metabolites with structural diversity that displayed potentialities in biological research. A considerable number of these molecular architectures had been recorded from marine sponges belonging to different marine genera, including *Batzella*, *Crambe*, *Monanchora*, *Clathria*, *Ptilocaulis* and New Caledonian starfishes *Fromia monilis* and *Celerina heffernani*. In this review, we aim to comprehensively cover the chemodiversity and the bioactivities landmarks centered around the chemical constituents exclusively isolated from these three marine genera including *Batzella*, *Crambe* and *Monanchora* over the period 1981–2017, paying a special attention to the polycyclic guanidinic compounds and their proposed biomimetic landmarks. It is concluded that these marine sponge genera represent a rich source of novel compounds with potential applications for cancer and other therapeutic areas.

Keywords: marine sponges; Poecilosclerida; Batzella; *Crambe*; *Monanchora*; guanidine alkaloids; pyrroloquinoline alkaloids; bioactivities; biomimetic synthesis

1. Introduction

As a result of the rise of many current medical challenges, including hepatitis, parasitic infection, lifestyle-induced diseases, such as diabetes, hypertension, many forms of cancer, multi-drug resistance pathogens and other diseases, searching for new bioactive compounds with novel modes of action is necessary. Marine natural products represent potent, promising and sustainable sources for biomedications [1]. Up to present time, eight marine-derived drugs were approved for market pipelines for the treatment of some of these current medical challenges [2,3]. Marine sponges (phylum Porifera), even though they are the most primitive class within the animal kingdom, are considered renewable powerful suppliers for bioactives. The marine genera belonging to the order Poecilosclerida, *Batzella* (family Chondropsidae), *Crambe* and *Monanchora* (family Crambeidae), are rich in the production of highly physiologically active pyrroloquinoline and guanidine-derived alkaloids [4–6], with a vast scope of biological potentialities including cytotoxic and antiviral [7–12], HIV-1 inhibitors [13,14], enzyme inhibitors [15], receptor antagonist [16], Ca^{2+} channel blocker [17], antifungal [18] and antimicrobial [19–21]. These interesting compounds are considered taxonomic markers in particular for some Poecilosclerida and Axinellida marine sponge genera [5]. Their complex molecular architectures and potent biological activities have made them for years ideal target molecules for synthetic applications [22–28]. Beside the production of guanidine-derived architectures, some deep-water species of *Batzella* produced pyrroloquinoline-derived alkaloids, which raises a chemotaxonomic question about the systematic relatedness of this genus (family Chondropsidae) to other genera like *Crambe* and *Monanchora* (family Crambeidae). A chemosystematic exploration has revealed that *Batzella* sponges containing cyclic guanidine alkaloids are chemically and taxonomically similar, and perhaps synonymous with, *Monanchora* and *Crambe*. However, the deep-water *Batzella* sponges produced pyrroloquinoline alkaloids is taxonomically unrelated to the *Batzella* previously mentioned. Chemically, it is almost similar to the *Zyzzya* and *Latrunculia* marine sponges but their phylogenetic relationship is still undetermined [29]. Systematically, the World Porifera Database accepts nine valid species of *Batzella* [30], nine valid species in the genus *Crambe* [31] and fourteen valid species currently in the genus *Monanchora* [32]. To the best of our knowledge, previous chemical investigations of *Batzella* was centered on only a single unidentified species from Madagascar [33], for the genus *Crambe* only one identified species, the type species *Crambe crambe* from the Mediterranean [34] and finally five identified *Monanchora* species including *Monanchora ungiculata* [35], *Monanchora dianchora* [36], *Monanchora pulchra* [37], *Monanchora arbuscula* [38] and *Monanchora unguifera* [35] in addition to one unidentified species of *Monanchora* n. sp. [39].

2. Chemistry and Biology of Natural Products Isolated from *Batzella*, *Crambe* and *Monanchora*

In this review, we provide comprehensive insights on the previous chemical and biological reports for the metabolites of the three marine genera. To facilitate the handling of this survey, the isolated natural compounds are classified by their polycyclic skeleton coupled with their recorded biological potentialities whenever applicable.

2.1. Piperidine Iminosugars Alkaloids

(+)-Batzellasides A–C (**1–3**), three alkylated piperidine iminosugars were isolated from a Madagascar sponge, *Batzella* sp. and represented the first naturally occurring marine iminosugars. These compounds demonstrated inhibition of the growth of *Staphylococcus epidermidis* with MICs (Minimum Inhibitory Concentration) that were under 6.3 µM [33] (Figure 1).

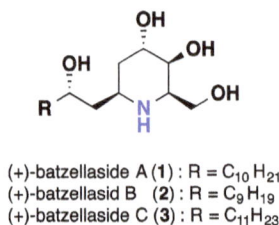

(+)-batzellaside A (**1**) : R = $C_{10}H_{21}$
(+)-batzellasid B (**2**) : R = C_9H_{19}
(+)-batzellaside C (**3**) : R = $C_{11}H_{23}$

Figure 1. Isolated iminosugars **1–3** from *Batzella* sp.

2.2. Bicyclic Guanidine Alkaloids

Eleven bicyclic guanidine metabolites including five bearing crambescin type A (**4–8**), three bearing crambescin type B (**9–11**) and further three possessing crambescin type C (**12–14**) were recorded from the Mediterranean sponge *Crambe crambe*. Their structures were established using NMR and careful HRMS/MS data analyses for the complete assignment of the alkyl chain lengths. These compounds demonstrated cytotoxic activity against neuronal cell lines in micromolar range [34,40,41]. Additional homologue crambescin A (**15**), the only known bicyclic compound reported from the Caribbean sponge *Batzella* sp. Compound **15** displayed potent cytotoxicity against proliferating Vero cells and HIV gp120-human CD4 binding inhibition activity with $IC_{50} > 100$ μM [14]. Further bicyclic compounds including dehydrocrambine A (**16**) recorded from *Monanchora* sp. that inhibits HIV-1 fusion [42]. Monanchorin (**17**), a guanidine alkaloid with unusual bicyclic skeleton from *Monanchora ungiculata* showed very weak cytotoxic activity with $IC_{50} = 11.3$ μM against IC2 murine mast cell lines [35]. The simple pyrimidine monalidine A (**18**), an anti-parasitic bicyclic guanidine alkaloid, was recently recorded from *Monanchora arbuscula* [43]. Urupocidins A (**19**) and B (**20**), bisguanidine alkaloids possessing unusual *N*-alkyl-*N*-hydroxyguanidine motif, were isolated from *Monanchora pulchra*. Urupocidin A (**19**) increases nitric oxide production in murine macrophages via inducing iNOS expression [44]. Recently, seven cytotoxic guanidine alkaloids were described from a French Polynesian *Monanchora* n. sp. including three bicyclic architectures possessing a free carboxylic acid group monanchoradins A–C (**21–23**) and four bicyclic compounds bearing crambescin A2 type skeleton with a short butyl-guanidine side chain including dehydrocrambescin A2 418 (**24**), (−)-crambescin A2 392 (**25**), (−)-crambescin A2 406 (**26**) and (−)-crambescin A2 420 (**27**) along with monalidine A (**18**). Most of these compounds showed antiproliferative and cytotoxic activities against several cancer cell lines including KB, HCT-116, HL-60, MRC-5 and B16-F10, with IC_{50} values in the micromolar range. The bicyclic analogue monanchoradin A (**21**) that bearing a carboxylic acid functionality was found to be less potent, however, it is still in the nanomolar range. On the other hand, the bicyclic compounds **24–27** bearing the butyl-guanidine terminus were found more potent, in particular (−)-crambescin A2 420 (**27**) that was found to be the most active with $IC_{50} = 0.03$ μM against KB cancer cell lines [39]. Moreover, the simple compound **18** showed potent antiproliferative and cytotoxic activities against KB, HCT-116, MDA-435, HL-60 and MRC-5 with an IC_{50} values 0.2/0.4, 0.84/0.74, 0.32/0.86, 1.3/1.3, 0.55/0.60 μM respectively. It is worth noting that the bicyclic (−)-crambescin compounds **25–27** are enantiomers for the antipodal bicyclic (+)-crambescins, recently isolated from the marine sponge *Pseudaxinella reticulata* (now known as *Dragmacidon reticulatum*, family Axinellidae) and their recording draws important insights about chirality and its dependence on the species of sponge [45] (Figure 2).

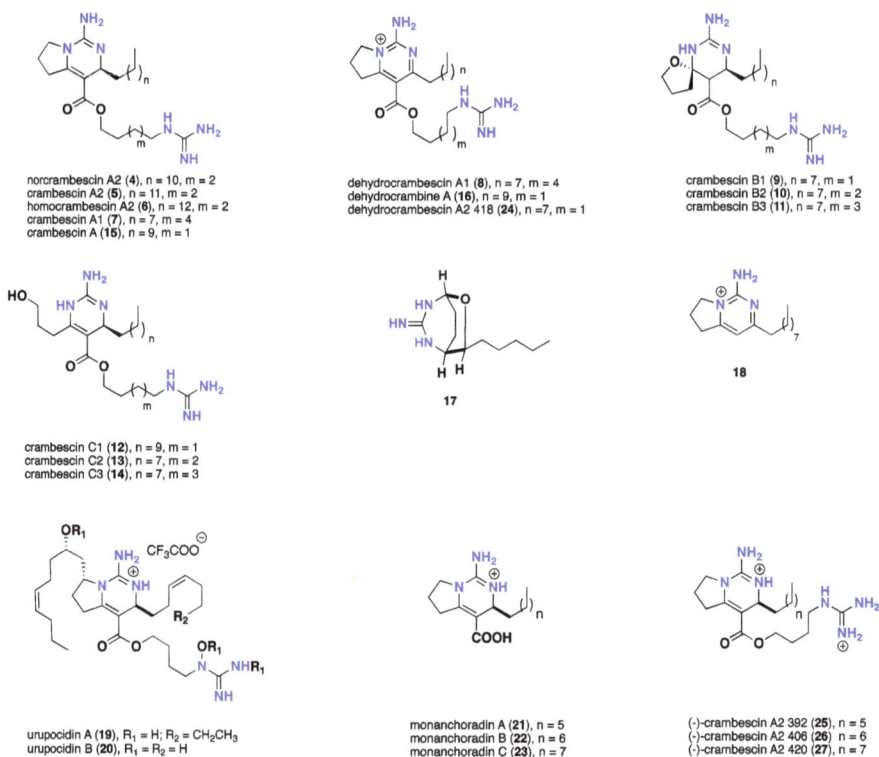

Figure 2. Isolated bicyclic guanidine alkaloids **4–27**.

2.3. Tricyclic Guanidine Alkaloids Bearing Ptilocaulin

Four tricyclic compounds including 8a,8b-dehydroptilocaulin (**28**), 8a,8b-dehydro-8-hydroxyptilocaulin (**29**), 1,8a;8b,3a-didehydro-8-hydroxyptilocaulin (**30**) and mirabilin B (**31**) were recorded from the Bahamas marine sponge, *Batzella* sp. [46]. (+)-Ptilocaulin (**32**), an antimicrobial and cytotoxic tricyclic guanidine alkaloid, in addition to isoptilocaulin (**33**) and (+)-8-hydroxyptilocaulin (**34**), were obtained from *Monanchora arbuscula* [38,47]. Moreover, (+)-ptilocaulin (**32**), exhibited antimicrobial activity against an oxacillin-resistant strain of *Staphylococcus aureus* with IC_{50} = 1.3 µM [48]. Further three tricyclic guanidine alkaloids, including 1, 8a; 8b; 3a-didehydro-8β-hydroxyptilocaulin (**35**), 1, 8a; 8b, 3a-didehydro-8α hydroxyptilocaulin (**36**) and mirabilin B (**31**), were described from *Monanchora unguifera* [49]. The mixture of **35** and **36** was active against the malaria parasite *Plasmodium falciparum* with an IC_{50} = 3.8 µM. Furthermore, mirabilin B (**31**) exhibited antifungal activity against *Cryptococcus neoformans* with an IC_{50} = 7.0 µM and antiprotozoal activity against *Leishmania donovani* with an IC_{50} = 17 µM [49]. The tricyclic guanidines **31–36** were identified from a Brazilian specimen of *Monanchora arbuscula* and were tested for their cytotoxicity against four cancer cell lines including HL-60, MDA-MB-435, HCT-8 and SF-295. The two compounds (+)-ptilocaulin (**32**) and (+)-8-hydroxyptilocaulin (**34**) displayed cytotoxicity with IC_{50} values ranging from 5.8–40.0 and 7.9–61.5 µM respectively. However, the other compounds **31**, **35** and **36** exhibited no activity. Additionally, compounds **32** and **34** were tested for their hemolytic activity against potential damage of mouse erythrocytes plasma membrane, where they displayed effective concentrations with EC_{50} values of 577.95 and 352.91 µM respectively [50]. Further anti-parasitic tricyclic guanidine alkaloid arbusculidine A (**37**) was reported recently from *Monanchora arbuscula* [43] (Figure 3).

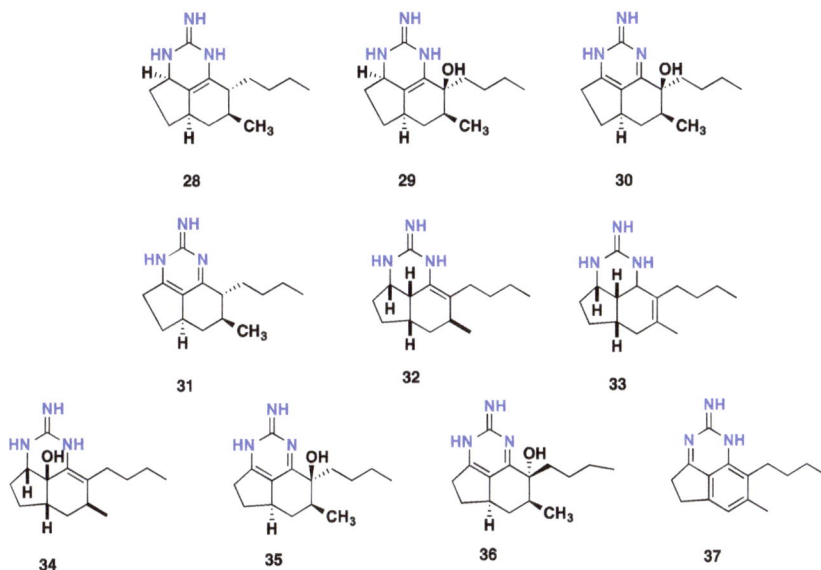

Figure 3. Isolated tricyclic guanidine alkaloids 28–37.

2.4. Tricyclic Pyrroloquinoline Alkaloids

Seven highly functionalized pyrroloquinoline alkaloids including three compounds named batzellines A–C (**38–40**) and four compounds named isobatzellines A–D (**41–44**) were isolated from the deep-water Bahama's sponge *Batzella* sp. The isobatzellines A–D (**41–44**) showed in vitro cytotoxicity against P388 leukemia cell with IC$_{50}$ values 0.42, 2.6, 12.6 and 20 µM and moderate antifungal activity against *Candida albicans* with IC$_{50}$ 3.1, 25, 50 and 25 µM respectively [7,51,52]. Further brominated compounds incorporating the pyrroloiminoquinone moiety, trivially named discorhabdins P, S, T and U (**45–48**) were obtained from a deep-water marine sponge of the genus *Batzella*. Discorhabdin P (**45**) inhibited CaN and CPP32 with IC$_{50}$ values of 0.55 and 0.37 µM respectively. It also showed in vitro cytotoxicity against the cultured murine P-388 tumor cell line and human lung carcinoma A-549 cell line, with IC$_{50}$ values of 0.025 and 0.41 µM, respectively [53]. Compounds **46–48** displayed in vitro cytotoxicity against cultured murine P-388 tumor cells, with IC$_{50}$ values of 3.08, >5 and 0.17 µM, respectively. Further cytotoxicity was also observed for A-549 human lung adeno-carcinoma cells, with IC$_{50}$ values of >5, >5 and 0.17 µM and for PANC-1 human pancreatic cells with IC$_{50}$ values of 2.6, 0.7 and 0.069 µM, respectively [54]. A comprehensive review on their therapeutic applications has been reported [55]. Additionally, secobatzellines A–B (**49–50**), two simple pyrroloiminoquinone enzyme inhibitors were recorded from a deep-water marine sponge of the genus *Batzella*. Secobatzelline B (**50**) is an artifact compound that was obtained during the purification process. Secobatzelline A (**49**) inhibited calcineurin (CaN) and CPP32 with IC$_{50}$ values of 0.55 and 0.02 µM. Moreover, secobatzelline B (**50**) inhibited calcineurin (CaN) IC$_{50}$ values of 2.21 µM. Furthermore, compounds **49** and **50** displayed cytotoxicity in vitro against the cultured murine P-388 tumor cell line, with IC$_{50}$ values of 0.06, 1.22 µM and against human lung carcinoma A-549 cell line, with IC$_{50}$ values of 0.04, 2.86 µM [56]. A huge number of synthetic aminoiminoquinone and aminoquinones analogues were prepared and tested as capase inhibitors [57]. Furthermore, a comprehensive evaluation for the cytotoxic activity of compounds **38–39**, **41–44** and **49–50** were determined against four different pancreatic cell lines Panc-1, AsPC-1, BxPC-3 and MIA-PaCa2 as well as in the Vero cell line, an epithelial cell line from the kidney tissue of an African green monkey [58] (Figure 4).

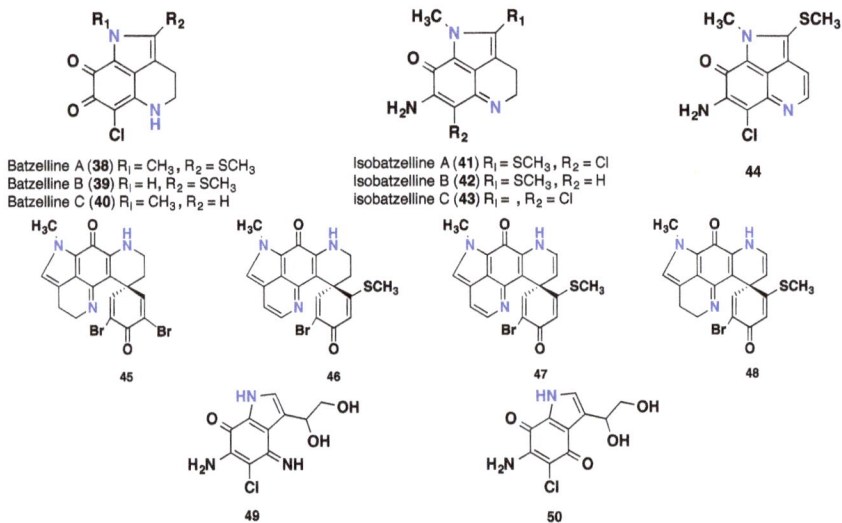

Figure 4. Isolated pyrroloquinoline alkaloids **38–50** from *Batzella* sp.

2.5. Polycyclic Alkaloids Bearing Batzelladine

Batzelladines represent a distinct class of particular guanidine-derived alkaloids that usually contain two main guanidinic moieties. Chemically, they are esters compounds that bear a principle tricyclic ring system named clathriadic acid that acting as an acidic portion bonded to another clathriadic acid molecule or crambescin A bicyclic system as an alcoholic part. Such a unique class of marine alkaloids is assumed to be synthesized biomimetically from different modes of cyclization between a polyketide-derived chain and a putative guanidine precursor affording these structurally complex metabolites [59]. These natural compounds are known for their potent bioactivities [13,14]. A considerable number of bioactive batzelladines were recorded from *Batzella* sponges. Batzelladines A–E (**51–55**), five potential inhibitors of HIV gpl20-human CD4 binding were recorded from the Caribbean sponge *Batzella* sp. [13,14]. Batzelladines F–I (**56–59**), four inducers of p56lck-CD4 dissociation, were isolated from *Batzella* sp. collected from Jamaica [60]. Batzelladine J (**60**) was isolated from the Caribbean *Monanchora unguifera* [61]. A further six guanidines—including batzelladines K–N (**61–64**), batzelladine C (**53**) and dehydrobatzelladine C (**65**)—were discovered from Jamaican *Monanchora unguifera* with activities against several cancer cell lines, protozoa, HIV-1 and AIDS [14,62,63]. Batzelladine C (**53**) displayed anti-HIV-1 activity at an EC$_{50}$ of 7.7 µM [63]. Four batzelladines **66–69** containing crambescin A bicyclic system in addition to dihomodehydrobatzelladine (**70**) were reported from the Caribbean *Monanchora arbuscula*. These compounds displayed mild antitumor activity with GI$_{50}$ (3–7 µM) against three cancer cell lines, lung carcinoma A549, colon carcinoma HT-29 and breast MDA-MB-231, in addition to antimalarial activity against protozoa [64]. Norbatzelladine L (**71**) was isolated from unidentified species, *Monanchora* sp. that displayed MNTC (maximum non-toxic concentration) at 2.5 µg mL^{-1} against HSV-1, with 97% of inhibition in the viral adsorption phase. Furthermore, it displayed cytotoxicity against several human cancer cell lines including leukemia, colorectal, breast, melanoma and glioblastoma [65,66]. Two anti-infective tricyclic members with unique stereochemical features—named merobatzelladines A–B (**72–73**)—were isolated from *Monanchora* sp. Merobatzelladines A–B exhibited moderate antimicrobial activity against *Vibrio anguillarum* with inhibitory zones of 9–10 mm on application of 50 µg of a sample to a paper disk of 6 mm diameter.

Moreover, **72–73** also inhibited *Tripanosoma bruceibrucei* (GUT at 3.1) with IC_{50} = 0.24 µg mL^{-1} each. Furthermore, they display moderate inhibitory activity against the K1 strain of *Plasmodium falciparum* with an IC_{50} = 0.48 µM and 0.97 µM, respectively [67]. Four anti-parasitic batzelladines (**74–77**) against *Trypanosoma cruzi* and *Leishmania infantum* were recently recorded from *Monanchora arbuscula* [43,68]. Numerous synthetic batzelladines and their derivatives showed potent activities against HIV-1 and AIDS opportunistic infectious pathogens, inhibition of HIV-1 envelope-mediated fusion [69], inhibitors of HIV-1 Nef interactions with p53, actin and p56^{lck} [70], antimalarial, antileishmanial, antimicrobial and antiviral (HIV-1) activities [71], inhibitors against HIV-1 reverse transcriptase (RT) [72] and antileishmanial [73] (Figures 5 and 6).

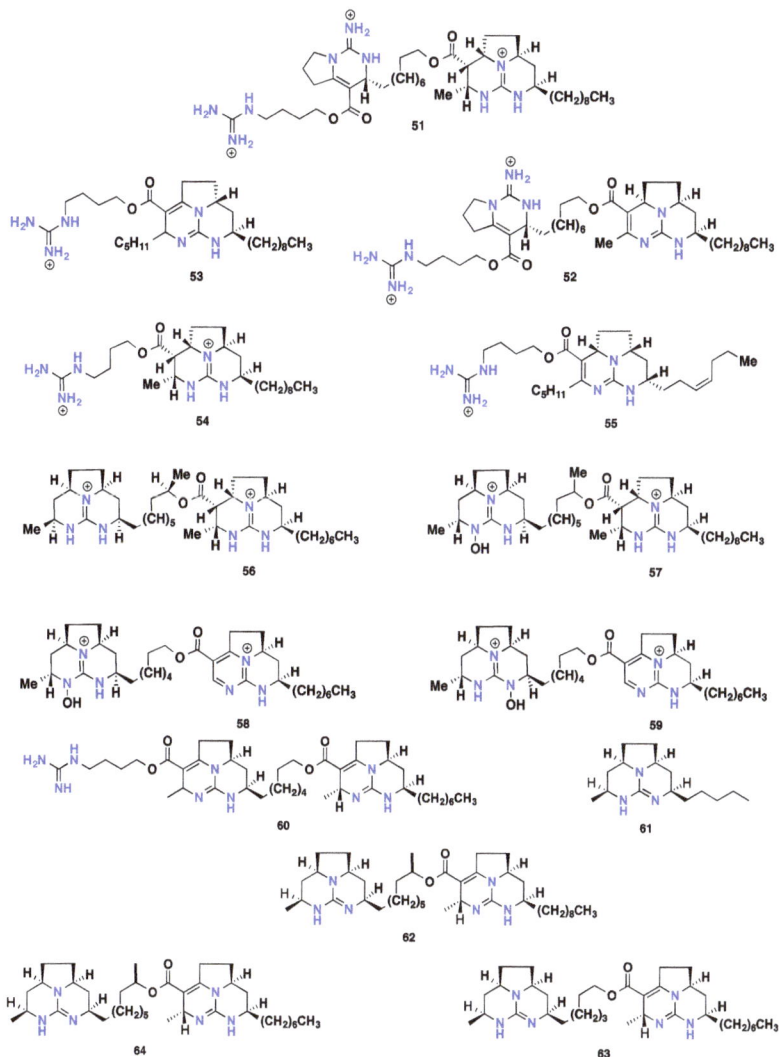

Figure 5. Isolated batzelladine alkaloids **51–64**.

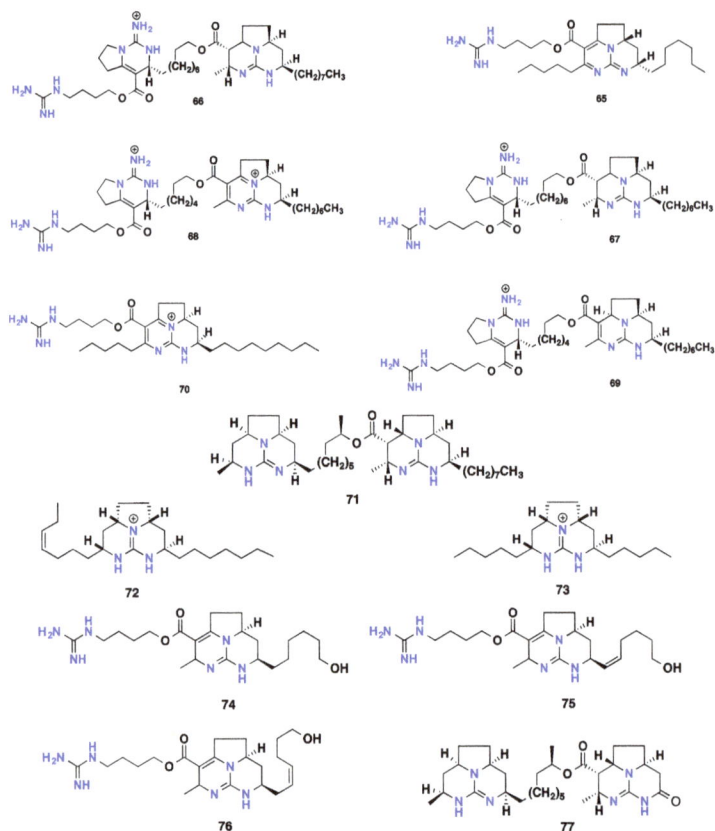

Figure 6. Isolated batzelladine alkaloids **65–77**.

2.6. Pentacyclic Alkaloids Bearing Crambescidin

Crambescidines are pentacyclic guanidine-derived alkaloids that represent recognizable complex marine metabolites. Chemically, they bear a common core of (5,6,8b)-triazaperhydroacenaphthalene in their molecules (trivially named as *vessel*) that coupled with a linear ω-hydroxy fatty acid (spermidine or hydroxyspermidine). These compounds vary from one to another in the length of the internal polymethylene chain and the oxidation degree of the two-spiro rings within the pentacyclic core. This group of compounds covers the major secondary metabolites recorded from these three genera. Since the discovery of the parent antiviral and cytotoxic marine metabolite ptilomycalin A (**78**) by Kashman and co-workers [74] from *Ptilocaulis spiculifer* (family Axinellidae) and *Hemimycale* sp. (family Hymedesmiidae) collected from the Red Sea coast in 1989, renewable efforts led to the discovery of further crambescidin analogues. Crambescidin 800 (**79**), crambescidin 816 (**80**), crambescidin 830 (**81**) and crambescidin 844 (**82**) were recorded from the Mediterranean marine sponge *Crambe crambe* [75]. These compounds demonstrated antiviral and cytotoxic activity against *Herpes simplex* virus, type1 (HSV-1) and cytotoxic activity against L1210 murine leukemia cells. Compounds **79**, **80** and **82** showed complete inhibition for HSV-1 and 98% of L1210 cell growth at concentration of $IC_{50} = 0.1$ μM. Furthermore, crambescidin 816 (**80**) displayed potent Ca^{2+} antagonist activity and inhibited the acetylcholine-induced contraction of guinea pig ileum within very low concentrations [17], however, recent novel evidence showed that compound **80** partially blocked CaV and NaV channels in neurons, proposes that this compound might be included in decreasing the neurotransmitter release and synaptic transmission within the central nervous system [76]. Further, recent study proved that crambescidin 816 (**80**) could be stored into specialized sponge cells where it can be dispersed into the water affording a chemical umbrella surrounding the *Crambe crambe* sponge [77]. Recently, Botana and co-workers [78] reported important insights about the mechanism of the neurons cytotoxic activity of crambescidin 816 (**80**) in primary cultures of cortical neurons. These results showed that compound **80** is responsible for the decreasing of neuronal viability and hence provided a dose-dependent increase in cytosolic Ca^{2+} level that was also linked to the presence of Ca^{2+} in the extracellular media. Crambescidins **78**, **79** and **80** were recorded also from *Batzella* sp. [14]. 13,14,15-isocrambescidin 800 (**83**) with *trans*-ring junction within the pentacyclic core and crambidine (**84**) were discovered from *Crambe crambe* [17,79]. Surprisingly, compound **83** was found to be a less potent cytotoxic against L1210 cells compared to other crambescidines and there was no observed antiviral activity against HSV-1. This observation could be attributed to the enclosed ionic pocket feature found in **78** and related crambescidins and lacking in **83** [80]. Additional crambescidin analogues with a chlorinated spermidine motif including crambescidin 818 (**85**), crambescidin 834 (**86**), crambescidin 673 (**87**), crambescidin 687 (**88**) and 13,14,15-isocrambescidin 657 (**89**) without a spermidine unit were recorded from the FABMS guided isolation of *Crambe crambe* extracts. The ADMET predictor revealed that ptilomycalin and crambescidin 800 (**78–79**) possess three features of the Lipinski guidelines. Additionally, **78** showed low flexibility and a low tendency to permeate into cell membranes. However, compound **79** displayed low permeability, low flexibility and less tendency to permeate the cell membranes [81] Compounds **87**, **88** and **89** exhibited in vitro cytotoxicity against L1210 murine leukemia five times compared to compound **80**. Furthermore, they displayed antimicrobial activity against *Rhodotorula glutinis* [82,83]. Crambescidin 800 (**79**), crambescidin 359 (**90**) and crambescidin 431 (**91**) have been isolated from *Monanchora unguiculata* [62]. Crambescidin 826 (**92**) and fromiamycalin (**93**) were recorded from *Monanchora* sp. They inhibited HIV-1 envelope-mediated fusion in vitro with an IC_{50}'s = 1–3 µM [14,42]. Indeed **78**, **79** and **93** displayed high cytotoxic activity against CEM 4 infected by HIV-1 with CC-50 of 0.11 µg mL^{-1}, without cytoprotective effects, at a dose of <0.1 µM [84]. The antifungal **78** inhibits melanogenesis of *Cryptococcus neoformans* in vitro through the inhibition of the biosynthesis of laccase in the melanin biosynthetic pathway with an IC_{50} value of 7.3 µM [85]. Additionally, **79** induced a morphological change with neurite outgrowth in neuro 2A cells at concentration of 0.03–0.1 µM and recorded to induce the differentiation of K562 chronic myelogenous leukemia (CML) cells into erythroblasts accompanied by cell cycle arrest at the S-phase as well [86]. Further pentacyclic members were described, including crambescidin acid (**94**) from *Monanchora ungiculata* [35] and crambescidic acid (**95**) from *Monanchora unguifera* [61]. Crambescidin 359 (**90**) and 16-β-hydroxycrambescidin 359 (**96**) were obtained from *Monanchora unguifera* [63]. Ptilomycalin D (**97**) showed cytotoxicity against cancer cell line P-388 with IC_{50} = 0.1 µM in addition to **78** and **95** were reported from *Monanchora dianchora* [36]. Monanchocidins A–E (**98–102**) are five unusual pentacyclic guanidine alkaloids with a morpholine modified spermidine motif from *Monanchora pulchra*. These compounds exhibited potent cytotoxic activities against HL-60 human leukemia cells with IC_{50} values of 540, 200, 110, 830 and 650 µM respectively [37]. Monanchocidin A (**97**) showed anti-migratory activity against several human cancer cell lines where it is able to prevent local expansion and metastatic spread of cancer cells [87]. Moreover, it could be a promising new compound for overcoming resistance to standard therapies in genitourinary malignancies by the induction of autophagy and lysosomal membrane permeabilization [88]. Monanchomycalins A–B (**103–104**), two pentacyclic with a modified spiro five-membered ring, showed potent cytotoxicity against HL-60 human leukemia cells with the IC_{50} values 120 and 140 nM, respectively, were isolated from *Monanchora pulchra* [89]. Recently, compound **104** was recorded to inhibit of the TRPV1, TRPV2 and TRPV3 channels with EC_{50} values 6.02, 2.84 and 3.25 µM, respectively, however it displayed no activity against the TRPA1 receptor [90]. Moreover, monanchomycalin C (**105**) exhibited cytotoxicity against human breast cancer cell lines

MAD-MB-231 with an IC$_{50}$ of 8.2 µM, isolated from *Monanchora pulchra* [91]. Normonanchocidins A–B and D (**106–108**) were isolated from *Monanchora pulchra*. Compound **106** and a mixture of **107** and **108** (1:1) displayed cytotoxic activities against human leukemia THP-1 cells with IC$_{50}$ values of 2.1 µM and 3.7 µM and against cervix epithelial carcinoma HeLa cells with IC$_{50}$ of 3.8 µM and 6.8 µM, respectively [92]. Recently, further three cytotoxic pentacyclic guanidine compounds including crambescidin 786 (**109**), crambescidin 814 (**110**) and 20-norcrambescidic acid (**111**) along with pentacyclic analogues **79, 90, 92** and **95** were isolated from a French Polynesian sponge *Monanchora* n. sp. The isolated compounds showed potent antiproliferative and cytotoxic activities against KB, HCT-116, HL-60, MRC-5 and B16-F10 cancer cells. Compounds **109, 110** and **111** exhibited cytotoxicity against KB cell lines with an IC$_{50}$ values 0.3 µM, 5 nM and 0.5 µM, respectively. The two crambescidin **95** and **111** where the (*anchor*) motif is terminated with the carboxylic acid functionality displayed potent cytotoxic activity against KB cell lines with IC$_{50}$ = 0.55 µM, however, they still less active compared with analogues possessing spermidine terminus. Furthermore, crambescidin 800 (**79**) exhibited the highest cytotoxic activity, while shorter pentacyclic homologue **109** along with the longer one **110** were found less active. These observations might highlight the impact of the polymethylene chain length within the (*anchor*) motif as a spacer for two site interactions. Crambescidin 359 (**90**), possessing only a pentacyclic core, showed no activity against KB cell lines and this correlates with the importance of the spermidine part for cytotoxicity. Regarding the B16-F10 murine melanoma cells, crambescidins **79, 92** and **110** exhibited moderate activity with IC$_{50}$ values of 0.2, 0.8 and 0.2 µM respectively. The discovery of 20-norcrambescidic acid (**111**) with this new pentacyclic motif carries some biogenesis impacts and raises some important insights about the variation in the oxidation degree and the mode of cyclization within the pentacyclic core [39]. A further two new hybrid pentacyclic guanidines monanchoxymycalin A–B (**112–113**) were obtained from the Far-Eastern marine sponge *Monanchora pulchra*. They displayed cytotoxic activities against cervical epithelioid carcinoma HeLa cells and breast adenocarcinoma MDA-MB231 cells [93]. Additionally, ptilomycalins E–H (**114–117**)—with guanidinic modified spermidine—were recorded from the Madagascar marine sponge *Monanchora unguiculata*. They displayed promising antimalarial activity against *Plasmodium falciparum* with IC$_{50}$ values 0.38, 0.30 and 0.27 µM respectively [94,95] (Figures 7 and 8).

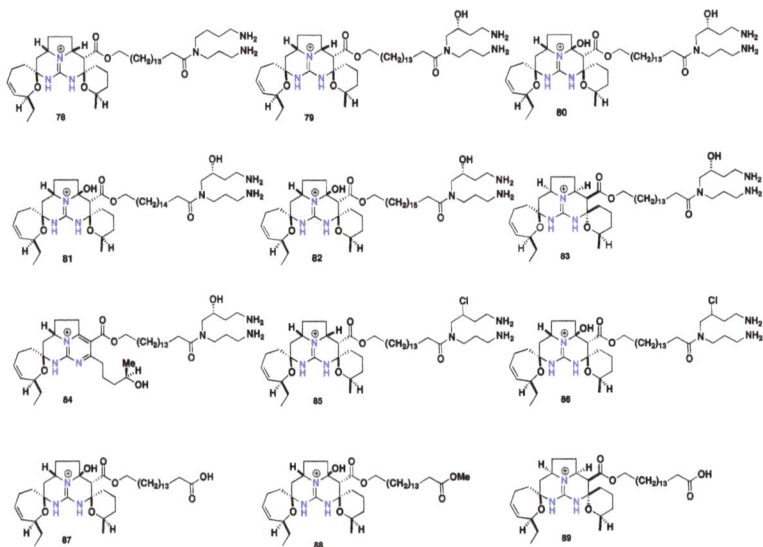

Figure 7. Isolated pentacyclic crambescidin alkaloids **78–89**.

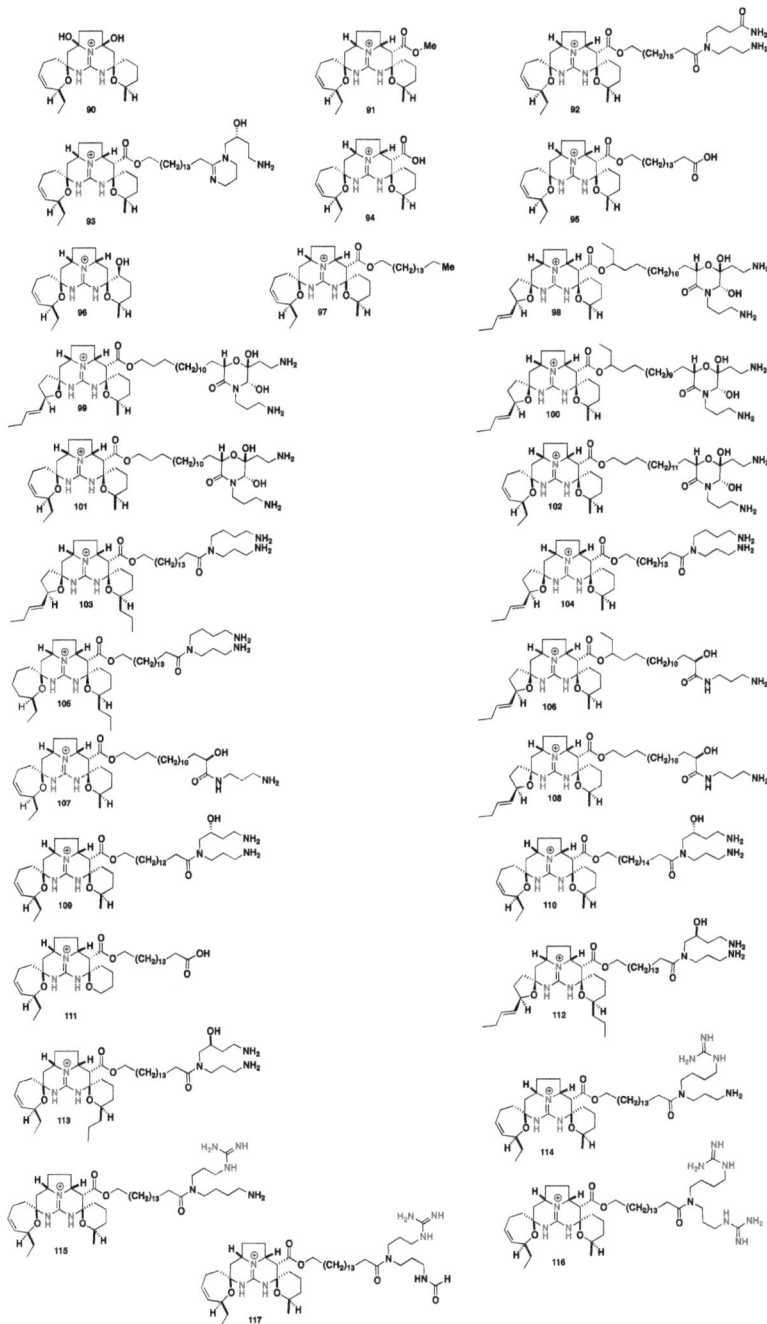

Figure 8. Isolated pentacyclic crambescidin alkaloids **90–117**.

2.7. Acyclic Guanidine Alkaloids

Small number of open chain guanidine-derived alkaloids was recorded. Pulchranin A (**118**), was described as the first marine non-peptide inhibitor of TRPV-1 channels with an EC_{50} value 41.2 μM, in addition two other acyclic members pulchranins B–C (**119–120**) reported from the Far-Eastern marine sponge *Monanchora pulchra*. Compounds **119** and **120** exhibited moderate inhibition against TRPV1 with EC_{50} value 95 and 183 μM respectively and were even less potent against TRPV3 and TRPA1 receptors [96,97]. Moreover, two synthetic derivatives—dihydropulchranin A (**121**) and hexadecylguanidine (**122**)—were prepared and studied for their TRPV channel-regulating activities. Compound **121** showed activity as an inhibitor of rTRPV1 and hTRPV3 receptors with EC_{50} values of 24.3 and 59.1 μM, respectively, while compound **122** was found not active against those receptors [98]. Additionally, recent studies revealed that pulchranin A (**118**) exhibited cytotoxic properties and prevented EGF-induced neoplastic transformation in vitro [99]. Further, acyclic analogue unguiculin A (**123**) with a modified bis-guanidine spermidine motif was isolated from the Madagascar marine sponge *Monanchora unguiculata*. It displayed antimalarial activity against the parasite *Plasmodium falciparum* with IC_{50} value of 6.04 μM [94,95]. Recently, a further two acyclic bis-guanidine alkaloids—named unguiculins B–C (**124–125**), beside unguiculin A (**123**)—were discovered from the French Polynesian *Monanchora* n. sp. sponge. These compounds displayed potent cytotoxic activity against KB cell lines with IC_{50} values 0.19/0.22, 0.08/0.09 and 0.03/0.03 μM respectively. Such activity might be attributed to the two terminal guanidines ends. Moreover, unguiculin C (**125**), the shorter homologue was found the most active. This could be concluded of how the chain and its length can play an important role as a spacer between two sites of interaction. Moreover, unguiculin B (**124**) showed further cytotoxicity against HCT-116, HL-60 and MRC-5 cell lines with IC_{50} values 3.6/3.6, >10/>10 and 9.6/11.4 μM respectively [100,101] (Figure 9).

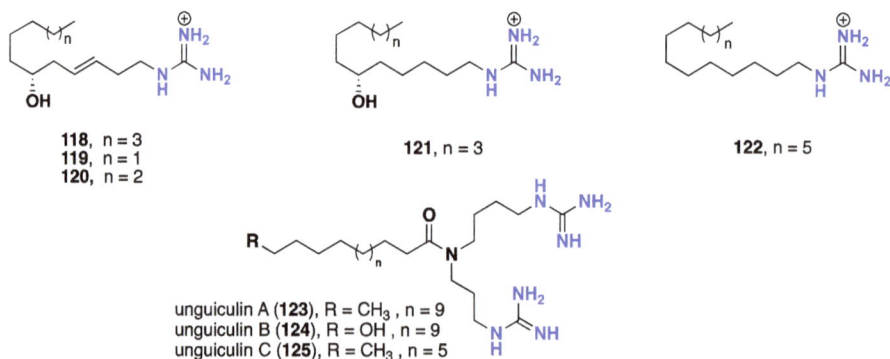

118, n = 3
119, n = 1
120, n = 2

121, n = 3

122, n = 5

unguiculin A (**123**), R = CH$_3$, n = 9
unguiculin B (**124**), R = OH , n = 9
unguiculin C (**125**), R = CH$_3$, n = 5

Figure 9. Isolated acyclic guanidine alkaloids **118–125**.

2.8. Terpenoid Compounds

Marine sponges belong to *Monanchora* genus have also produced a small number of terpenoid metabolites and classical sterols [102]. Nine sesterterpenoids **126–134** were isolated from the Korean *Monanchora* sp. along with four phorbaketals **135–138**. These compounds were investigated for their cytotoxic activity against four human cancer cell lines—A498, ACHN, MIA-paca and PANC-1—where some of them showed potent cytotoxicity [103]. Seven cytotoxic 5α,8α-epidioxy sterols **139–145** were also described from *Monanchora* sp. These sterols showed moderate cytotoxicity against several human carcinoma cell lines including renal (A-498), pancreatic (PANC-1 and MIAPaCa-2) and colorectal (HCY-116) cancer cell lines [104]. Monanchosterols A–B (**146–147**) were identified from a South Korean *Monanchora* sp. and described as the first examples of naturally occurring steroids bearing a rearranged bicyclo [4.3.1] A/B ring system. Moreover, Monanchosterols A–B (**146–147**) exhibited significant inhibition of mRNA expression of Il-60 without notable cytotoxicity to the cells in a dose-dependent manner [105] (Figure 10).

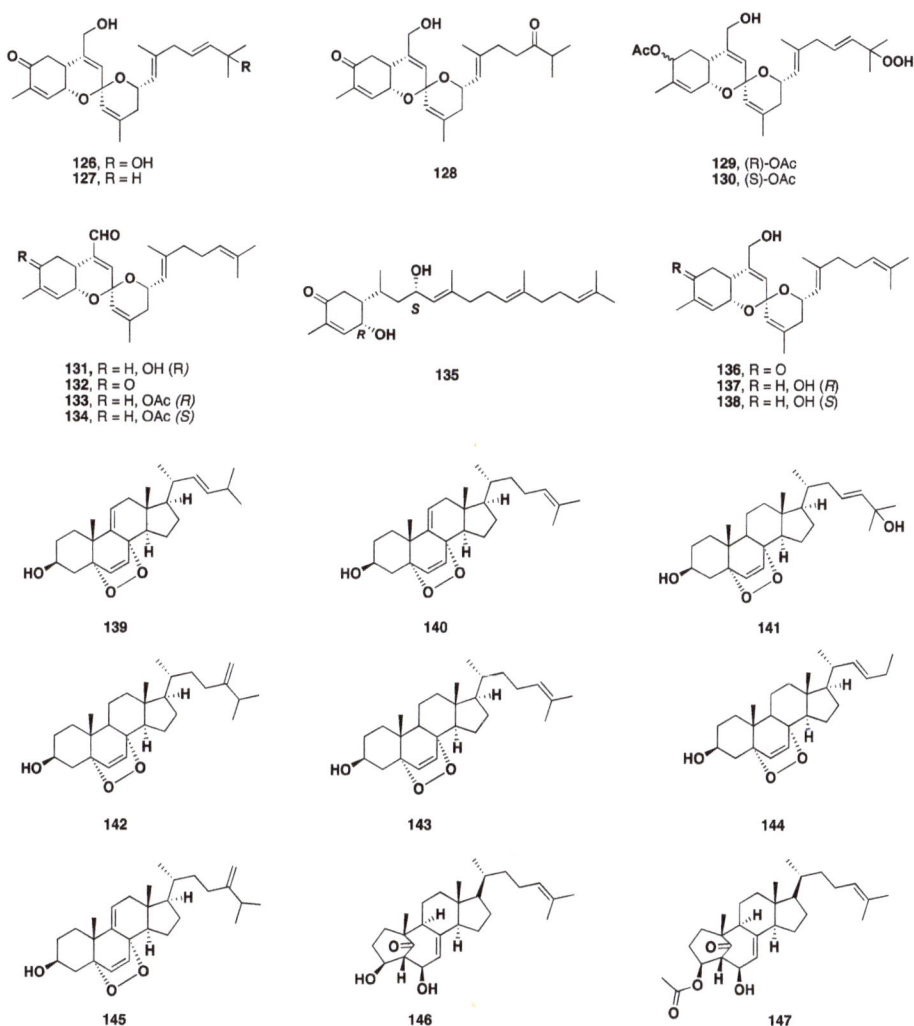

Figure 10. Isolated terpenoid and steroidal metabolites **126–147** isolated from *Monanchora* sp.

3. Biomimetic Landmarks of Polycyclic Guanidinium Motifs

The bio-mechanistic studies along with the structural analyses for the different polycyclic guanidine alkaloids revealed two important insights; the first is chemical; where they are sharing the same biogenesis routs. A second is ecological; where marine sponges that produced such metabolites could be systematically classified under the same order. Generally, the different polycyclic guanidinic moieties could be biomimetically synthesized by way of the double aza Michael strategy, by the addition of free guanidine to α, β unsaturated polyketide chains (Figure 11) [59].

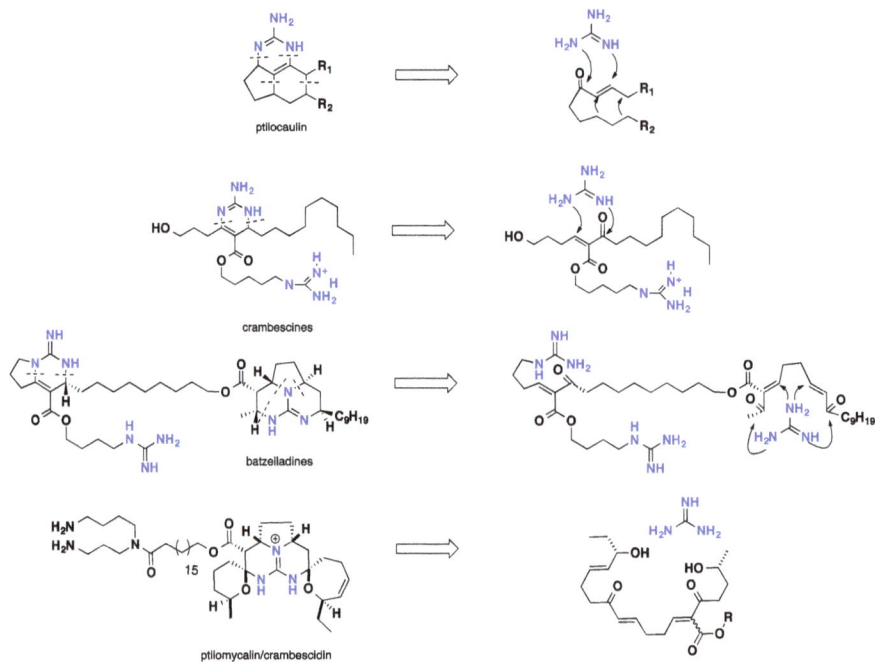

Figure 11. Structural analysis of different polycyclic guanidine alkaloids.

3.1. Bicyclic Compounds Possessing Crambescins Type A, B and C

Snider and his team had several contributions towards the biomimetic synthesis of the polycyclic guanidinic motifs. The bicyclic crambescin alkaloids possess three different cyclic moieties—crambescin type A with tetrahydropyrrolo [1,2-c] pyrimidine nucleus, crambescin type B possesses an oxa-6,8-diazaspiro [4.5] motif, while crambescin type C displays a tetrahydropyrimidin fragment. Crambescins type B and C were isolated exclusively from the Mediterranean marine sponge *Crambe crambe* [34,40,41]. A postulated strategy showed that these three guanidinium cores could be constructed biomimetically through a conjugated Michael addition of guanidine to *enone* ester. This strategy seems pertinent since it gathers the formation of three different atom arrangements from one unified precursor (Figure 12) [106].

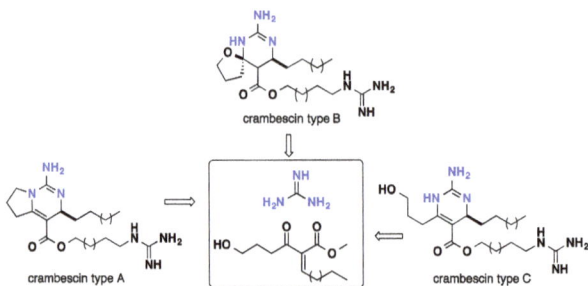

Figure 12. Proposed retrosynthetic analysis of the bicyclic alkaloids.

The less basic *O*-methylisourea was chosen as guanidine precursor instead of free guanidines. The condensation of *O*-methylisourea with previously prepared enone (**148**) followed by acid hydrolysis and desilylation afforded the corresponding dihydropyrimidine intermediate (**149**). In presence of methanolic ammonium acetate saturated with ammonia, **150** afforded the key compound **150**, corresponding to crambescin type C. Subsequently, **150** was transformed to compound **151**, corresponding to crambescin type A by mesylation, hydrogenolysis and cyclization. Compound **152** possesses crambescin type B was obtained by cyclization of **150** under basic condition (Figure 13) [106].

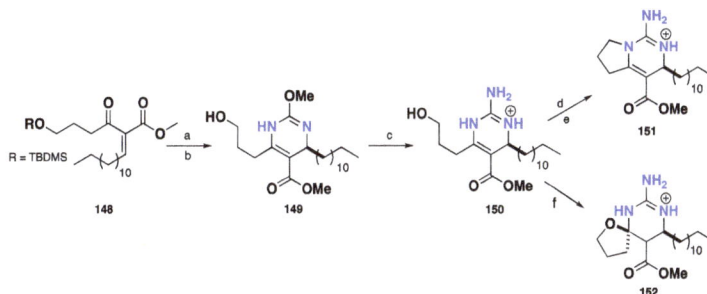

Figure 13. a: 2 equiv. *O*-methylisourea and 7 equiv. NaHCO$_3$ in DMF for 12 h at 60 °C, 79%; **b**: hydrolysis, TBAF, THF, 12 h, rt, 90%; **c**: NH$_4$OAc (1.5 equiv.), MeOH saturated with NH$_3$ at 60 °C for 2 days, 61%; **d**: MsCl, Et$_3$N in DCM for 30 min, 0 °C, 6 h, rt; **e**: Et$_3$N in CHCl$_3$, reflux, 12 h, 90%; **f**: Et$_3$N in CHCl$_3$, Δ, 12 h.

Based on the previous biomimetic approach, Berlinck and co-workers [43] accomplished the biomimetic synthesis of the cytotoxic and anti-parasitic monalidine A (**18**). 1,3-diketone **153** was introduced for condensation with guanidine free base to afford the corresponding pyrimidine **154** in 25% yield. Subsequently, the key intermediate **152** was cyclized using the Mitsunobu modified protocol to afford **18** as hydrochloride salt in a 67% yield (Figure 14).

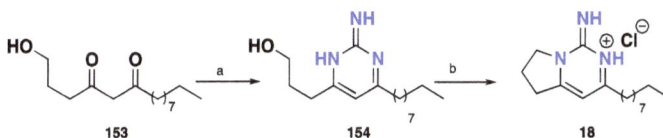

Figure 14. a: Guanidine hydrochloride, *t*-BuOK, CF$_3$CH$_2$OH, 30 min, then **154**, rt, 48 h, 25%; **b**: Ph$_3$P, imidazole, I$_2$, CH$_2$Cl$_2$, −18 °C, 6 h, 67%.

3.2. Tricyclic Possessing Ptilocaulin/Batzelladine

(±)-Ptilocaulin (**32**) was first synthesized biomimetically as a racemic mixture via Michael addition strategy by addition of free guanidine to *enone* **155** followed by intramolecular enamine formation. (−)-Ptilocaulin (**156**) was formed as a kinetic product where the guanidine was added to the less hindered top convex face of *enone* **155**, whereas (+)-ptilocaulin (**32**) was obtained as a thermodynamic adduct as the guanidine was added to the more hindered bottom side of *enone* **155**. This strategy highlights and proves a unique unified biosynthetic route for ptilocaulins and related tricyclic guanidinic analogues (Figure 15) [107–109].

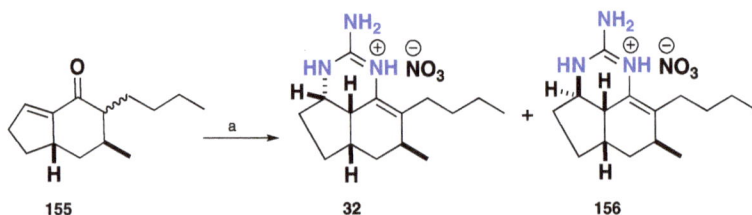

Figure 15. a: Guanidine, PH, reflux 25 h, then HNO$_3$ (1% aq), 35%.

The tricyclic guanidinium framework of batzelladine K (**61**) was biomimetically synthesized through the addition of free guanidine to a *bis-enone* **157** affording the pyrrolidine-dione **158**, which was subsequently introduced to cyclization followed by iminium ion formation giving rise to the full fused tricyclic guanidinium core. A subsequent reduction afforded **61**. A unified synthetic strategy was applied to ptilocaulin (**32**), isoptilocaulin (**33**) and batzelladine K (**61**), which indicated that these classes of tricyclic guanidines are subjected to the same biomimetic gate (Figure 16) [71,110,111].

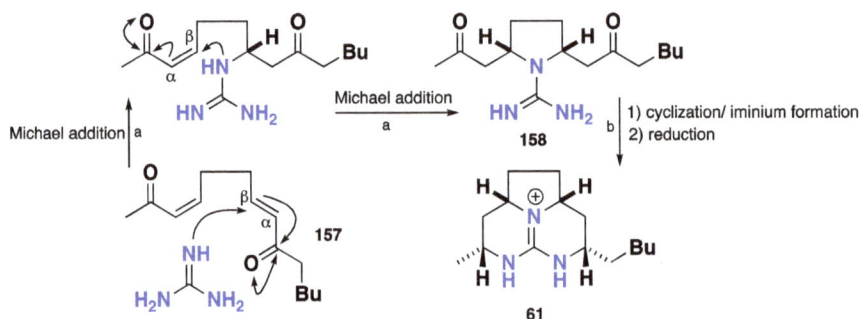

Figure 16. a: Guanidine, DMF, 0 °C, then 25 °C, 5 h **b**: 0 °C, MeOH-H$_2$O (2:1), NaBH$_4$ (6 equiv.), 25 °C, 16 h, 25%.

3.3. Pentacyclic Possessing Ptilomycalins, Crambescidins and Monanchomycalins

Numerous total syntheses of the pentacyclic guanidinium core of ptilomycalin A (**78**), crambescidin 800 (**79**) and crambescidin 359 (**95**) were biomimetically achieved [23,112,113]. A biomimetic synthesis of the methyl ester of the pentacyclic nucleus of **78** was conducted through a conjugated condensation of *O*-methylisourea as protected guanidine strategy with double Michael acceptor *bis-enone* **159** as α-β unsaturated polyketide framework. Subsequently, desilylation under acidic conditions provided the first seven-membered spiroaminal ring within the intermediate **160**. Later, the second six-membered spiroaminal ring was achieved under basic conditions followed by subsequently aminal formation affording the ptilomycalin A pentacyclic framework **161** (*vessel*) in one single biomimetic step (Figure 17).

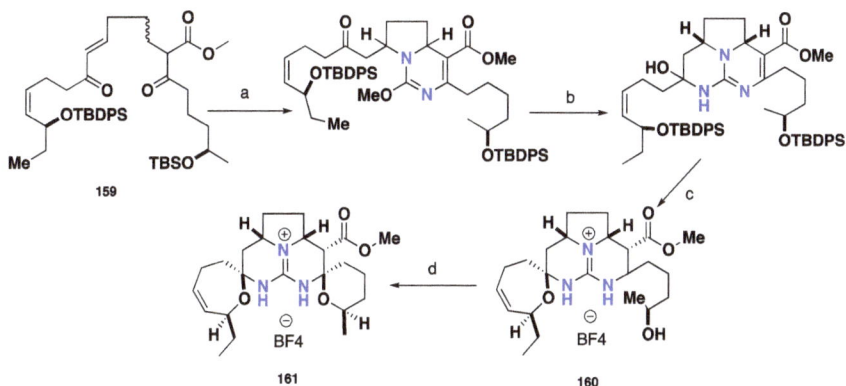

Figure 17. a: *O*-methylisourea, *i*-Pr$_2$EtN, DMSO, 80 °C, 1.5 h (52%, 4:l, H$_{10}$, H$_{13}$ *trans*: H$_{10}$, H$_{13}$ *cis*); **b**: NH$_3$, NH$_4$OAc, *t*-BuOH, 60 °C, 40 h (72%, 1:1, H$_{10}$, H$_{13}$ *cis* β: H$_{10}$, H$_{13}$ *cis* α); **c**: 3:7 HF-CH$_3$CN, −30 °C, 3d; **d**: Et$_3$N, MeOH, 60 °C, 20 h (78%).

Recently, a detailed biomimetic gate was proposed illustrating the biogenesis of different pentacyclic guanidinium cores. The pentacyclic core of monanchomycalin A (**103**), suggests polyketide-like biogenesis, followed by spermidine-spermidine condensations. Two different precursors were employed, including either nine acetate units as in monanchomycalin B (**104**) and other known pentacyclic members, or ten acetate and one propionate units as in monanchomycalin A (**103**). To finish the pentacyclic guanidinium polyketide framework (*vessel*), a cyclization key-step developed by adding guanidine to *bis*-α, β unsaturated chain followed by imine-enamine tautomerization (transformation (**a**)). Further conversions including the allylic oxidation (transformation (**b**)) to afford putative intermediates (III and/or IV) followed by cyclization-elimination (**c**) and (**d**) to generate monanchomycalins A–B (103–104) and related pentacyclic analogues. Moreover, the interconversion of the presumptive intermediates III and IV (transformation (**e**)) through allylic rearrangement like reactions also might be possible (Figure 18) [89].

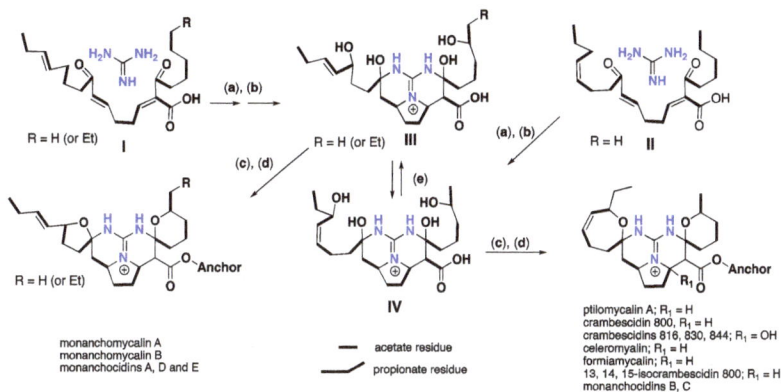

Figure 18. Proposed conversions (**a–e**) and hypothetical biogenesis of different pentacyclic guanidine alkaloids.

Recently, Guzii and collaborators [96] proposed biogenetic correlations linking between the acyclic guanidine alkaloid pulchranin A (**118**) and the pentacyclic crambescidins and monanchomycalins

A–B (**103**–**104**). This proposed biogenetic rout could unify the variation in the oxidation degree for the left-hand side spiroaminal rings (Figure 19).

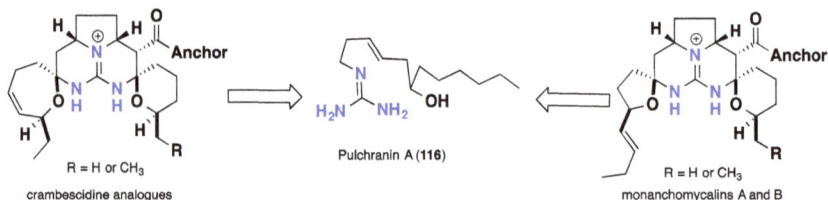

Figure 19. Pulchranin A (**118**), as a biosynthetic precursor for pentacyclic compounds (**103**–**104**).

4. Conclusions

In conclusion, we have presented complete and comprehensive up-to date literature survey exclusively dedicated to the chemistry, biology and insights on the most leading biomimetic syntheses of guanidine derived natural products isolated from marine sponges of three genera *Batzella*, *Crambe* and *Monanchora*. One hundred forty-seven marine natural products were recorded with distinct structural diversities that afforded wide scope of bioactivities. For their chemodiversity, along with their displayed biological potentialities, they still present promising and attractive marine species that are worth attracting the worldwide interest of natural products chemists and pharmacologists.

Acknowledgments: This work was supported by the mission sector of the Ministry of High Education of the Arab Republic of Egypt (Egyptian Cultural Bureau in Paris, France); Amr El-Demerdash's was granted and completely funded. Many thanks to Ali Al-Mourabit and his research team at the ICSN-CNRS for hosting, supervising and supplying with research facilities.

Author Contributions: Amr El-Demerdash wrote the first draft of the manuscript. Atanas G. Atanasov, Anupam Bishayee, Mamdouh Abdel-Mogib, John N. A. Hooper and Ali Al-Mourabit critically revised and improved the manuscript. All the authors read and approved the final version of the manuscript.

Conflicts of Interest: The authors declare no conflict of interest.

Abbreviations

The following abbreviations are used in this manuscript:

ADMET	absorption, distribution, metabolism and excretion–toxicity in pharmacokinetics
EC50	Half maximal effective concentration
GI50	Half maximal growth inhibition
gp120	glycoprotein 120
HIV-1	Human immunodeficiency virus 1
HSV-1	*Herpes simplex* virus 1
IC50	Half maximal inhibitory concentration
MIC	Minimum inhibitory concentration

References

1. Montaser, R.; Luesch, H. Marine natural products: A new wave of drugs. *Future Med. Chem.* **2011**, *3*, 1475–1489. [CrossRef] [PubMed]
2. Martins, A.; Vieira, H.; Gaspar, H.; Santos, S. Marketed marine natural products in the pharmaceutical and cosmeceutical Industries: Tips for success. *Mar. Drugs* **2014**, *12*, 1066–1101. [CrossRef] [PubMed]
3. Rangel, M.; Falkenberg, M. An overview of the marine natural products in clinical trials and on the market. *J. Coast. Life Med.* **2015**, *3*, 421–428. [CrossRef]
4. Shanmugam, A.; Vairamani, S. Biologically active metabolites from sponges and their activities. In *Marine Sponges: Chemicobiological and Biomedical Applications*; Pallela, R., Ehrlich, H., Eds.; Springer: Berlin, Germany, 2016; pp. 115–142; ISBN 978-81-322-2794-6.

5. Sfecci, E.; Lacour, T.; Amad, P.; Mehiri, M. Polycyclic guanidine alkaloids from Poecilosclerida marine sponges. *Mar. Drugs* **2016**, *14*, 77. [CrossRef] [PubMed]
6. Berlinck, R.G.S. Some aspects of guanidine secondary metabolites. *Prog. Chem. Nat. Prod.* **1995**, 119–295. [CrossRef]
7. Sun, H.H.; Sakemi, S.; Burres, N.; McCarthy, P. Isobatzellines A, B, C and D. cytotoxic and antifungal pyrroloquinoline alkaloids from the marine sponge *Batzella* sp. *J. Org. Chem.* **1990**, *55*, 4964–4966. [CrossRef]
8. Jares-Erijman, E.A.; Sakai, R.; Rinehart, K.L. Crambescidins: New antiviral and cytotoxic compounds from the sponge *Crambe crambe*. *J. Org. Chem.* **1991**, *6*, 5712–5715. [CrossRef]
9. Gochfeld, D.J.; El-Sayed, K.A.; Yousaf, M.; Hu, J.F.; Bartyzel, P.; Dunbar, D.C.; Wilkins, S.P.; Zjawiony, J.K.; Schinazi, R.F.; Schlueter, W.S.; et al. Marine natural products as lead anti-HIV agents. *Mini Rev. Med. Chem.* **2003**, *3*, 401–424. [CrossRef] [PubMed]
10. Zhou, X.; Liu, J.; Yang, B.; Lin, X.; Yang, X.; Liu, Y. Marine natural products with anti-HIV activities in the last decade. *Curr. Med. Chem.* **2013**, *20*, 953–973. [CrossRef] [PubMed]
11. Rubiolo, J.A.; López-Alonso, H.; Roel, M.; Vieytes, M.R.; Thomas, O.; Ternon, E.; Vega, F.V.; Botana, L.M. Mechanism of cytotoxic action of crambescidin-816 on human liver-derived tumour cells. *Br. J. Pharmacol.* **2014**, *171*, 1655–1667. [CrossRef] [PubMed]
12. El-Sayed, K.A. Natural products as antiviral agents. *Stud. Nat. Prod. Chem.* **2000**, *24*, 473–572.
13. Mai, S.H.; Nagulapalli, V.K.; Patil, A.D.; Truneh, A.; Westley, J.W. Marine Compounds as HIV Inhibitors. U.S. Patent Application No. WO9301193 (A1), 21 January 1993.
14. Patil, A.D.; Kumar, N.V.; Kokke, W.; Bean, M.F.; Freyer, A.J.; Brosse, C.D.; Mai, S.; Truneh, A.; Faulkner, D.J.; Carte, B.; et al. Novel alkaloids from the sponge *Batzella* sp. Inhibitors of HIV gp120-Human CD4 Binding. *J. Org. Chem.* **1995**, *60*, 1182–1188. [CrossRef]
15. Nakao, Y.; Fusetani, N. Enzyme inhibitors from marine invertebrates. *J. Nat. Prod.* **2007**, *70*, 689–710. [CrossRef] [PubMed]
16. Carté, B.K. Marine natural products as a source of novel pharmacological agents. *Curr. Opin. Biotechnol.* **1993**, *4*, 275–279. [CrossRef]
17. Berlinck, R.G.S.; Braekman, J.C.; Daloze, D.; Bruno, I.; Riccio, R.; Ferri, S.; Spampinato, S.; Speroni, E. Polycyclic guanidine alkaloids from the marine sponge *Crambe crambe* and Ca^{2+} channel blocker activity of crambescidin 816. *J. Nat. Prod.* **1993**, *56*, 1007–1015. [CrossRef] [PubMed]
18. Rubiolo, J.A.; Ternon, E.; Lopez-Alonso, H.; Thomas, O.; Vega, F.V.; Vieytes, M.R.; Botana, L. Crambescidin-816 Acts as a fungicidal with more potency than crambescidin 800 and 830, Inducing cell cycle arrest, increased cell size and apoptosis in *Saccharomyces cerevisiae*. *Mar. Drugs* **2013**, *11*, 4419–4434. [CrossRef] [PubMed]
19. Amad, P.; Charroin, C.; Baby, C.; Vacelet, J. Antimicrobial activities of marine sponges from the Mediterranean Sea. *Mar. Biol.* **1987**, *94*, 271–275. [CrossRef]
20. Sun, X.; Sun, S.; Ference, C.; Zhu, W.; Zhou, N.; Zhang, Y.; Zhou, K. A potent antimicrobial compound isolated from *Clathria cervicornis*. *Bioorg. Med. Chem. Lett.* **2015**, *25*, 67–69. [CrossRef] [PubMed]
21. Mishra, A.; Batra, S. Thiourea and guanidine derivatives as antimalarial and antimicrobial agents. *Curr. Med. Chem.* **2013**, *13*, 2011–2025. [CrossRef]
22. Shimokawa, J.; Ishiwata, T.; Shirai, K.; Koshino, H.; Tanatani, A.; Nakata, T.; Hashimoto, Y.; Nagasawa, K. Total synthesis of (+)-Batzelladine A.; (−)-Batzelladine D and identification of their target protein. *Chem. Eur. J.* **2005**, *11*, 6878–6888. [CrossRef] [PubMed]
23. Moore, C.G.; Murphy, P.J.; Williams, H.L.; McGown, A.T.; Smith, N.K. Synthetic studies towards ptilomycalin A: Total synthesis of crambescidin 359. *Tetrahedron Lett.* **2007**, *63*, 11771–11780. [CrossRef]
24. Sekine, M.; Iijima, Y.; Iwamoto, O.; Nagasawa, K. Synthesis of (+)-Batzelladine K. *Heterocycles* **2010**, *80*, 395–408. [CrossRef]
25. Wierzejska, J.; Ohshima, M.; Inuzuka, T.; Sengoku, T.; Takahashi, M.; Yoda, H. Total synthesis and absolute stereochemistry of (+)-batzellaside B.; its C8-epimer, a new class of piperidine alkaloids from the sponge *Batzella* sp. *Tetrahedron Lett.* **2011**, *52*, 1173–1175. [CrossRef]
26. Babij, N.R.; Wolfe, J.P. Asymmetric total synthesis of (+)-Merobatzelladine B. *Angew. Chem. Int. Ed.* **2012**, *51*, 4128–4130. [CrossRef] [PubMed]
27. Ma, Y.; De, S.; Chen, C. Syntheses of cyclic guanidine-containing natural products. *Tetrahedron* **2015**, *71*, 1145–1173. [CrossRef] [PubMed]

28. Parr, B.T.; Economou, C.; Herzon, S.B.A. Concise synthesis of (+)-batzelladine B from simple pyrrole-based starting materials. *Nature* **2015**, *525*, 507–510. [CrossRef] [PubMed]

29. Van Soest, R.W.M.; Braekman, J.C.; Faulkner, D.J.; Hajdu, E.; Harper, M.K.; Vacelet, J. The genus *Batzella*: A chemosystematic problem. *Bull. Inst. R. Sci. Nat. Belg.* **1996**, *66*, 89–101.

30. World Porifera Database. 2017. Available online: http://www.marinespecies.org/porifera/porifera.php?p= taxdetails&id=168731 (accessed on 20 March 2017).

31. World Porifera Database. 2017. Available online: http://www.marinespecies.org/porifera/porifera.php?p= taxdetails&id=131931 (accessed on 20 March 2017).

32. World Porifera Database. 2017. Available online: http://www.marinespecies.org/porifera/porifera.php?p= taxdetails&id=169014 (accessed on 20 March 2017).

33. Segraves, N.L.; Crews, P.A. Madagascar sponge *Batzella* sp. as a source of alkylated iminosugars. *J. Nat. Prod.* **2005**, *68*, 118–121. [CrossRef] [PubMed]

34. Berlinck, R.G.S.; Braekman, J.C.; Daloze, D.; Bruno, I.; Riccio, R.; Rogeau, D.; Amade, P. Crambines C1 and C2: Two further cytotoxic guanidine alkaloids from the sponge *Crambe crambe*. *J. Nat. Prod.* **1992**, *55*, 528–532. [CrossRef] [PubMed]

35. Meragelman, K.M.; McKee, T.C.; McMahon, J.B. Monanchorin, a bicyclic alkaloid from the sponge *Monanchora ungiculata*. *J. Nat. Prod.* **2004**, *67*, 1165–1167. [CrossRef] [PubMed]

36. Bensemhoun, J.; Bombarda, I.; Aknin, M.; Vacelet, J.; Gaydou, E.M. Ptilomycalin D, a polycyclic guanidine alkaloid from the marine sponge *Monanchora dianchora*. *J. Nat. Prod.* **2007**, *70*, 2033–2035. [CrossRef] [PubMed]

37. Makarieva, T.N.; Tabakmaher, K.M.; Guzii, A.G.; Denisenko, V.A.; Dmitrenok, P.S.; Shubina, L.K.; Kuzmich, A.S.; Lee, H.S.; Stonik, V.A. Monanchocidins B–E: Polycyclic guanidine alkaloids with potent antileukemic activities from the sponge *Monanchora pulchra*. *J. Nat. Prod.* **2011**, *74*, 1952–1958. [CrossRef] [PubMed]

38. Tavares, R.; Daloze, D.; Braekman, J.C.; Hajdu, E.; van Soest, R.W.M. 8b-hydroxyptilocaulin, a hew guanidine alkaloid from the sponge *Monanchora arbuscula*. *J. Nat. Prod.* **1995**, *58*, 1139–1142. [CrossRef]

39. El-Demerdash, A.; Moriou, C.; Martin, M.T.; Rodrigues-Stien, A.; Petek, S.; Demoy-Schnider, M.; Hall, K.; Hooper, J.N.A.; Debitus, C.; Al-Mourabit, A. Cytotoxic guanidine alkaloids from a French Polynesian *Monanchora* n. sp. sponge. *J. Nat. Prod.* **2016**, *79*, 1929–1937. [CrossRef] [PubMed]

40. Berlinck, R.G.S.; Braekman, J.C.; Daloze, D.; Hallenga, K.; Ottinger, R. Two new guanidine alkaloids from the Mediterranean sponge *Crambe crambe*. *Tetrahedron Lett.* **1990**, *31*, 6531–6534. [CrossRef]

41. Bondu, S.; Genta-Jouve, G.; Leiros, M.; Vale, C.; Guigonis, J.M.; Botana, L.M.; Thomas, O.P. Additional bioactive guanidine alkaloids from the Mediterranean sponge *Crambe crambe*. *RSC Adv.* **2012**, *2*, 2828–2835. [CrossRef]

42. Chang, L.C.; Whittaker, N.F.; Bewley, C.A. Crambescidin 826 and Dehydrocrambine A: New polycyclic guanidine alkaloids from the marine sponge *Monanchora* sp. that inhibit HIV-1 Fusion. *J. Nat. Prod.* **2003**, *66*, 1490–1494. [CrossRef] [PubMed]

43. Santos, M.F.C.; Harper, P.M.; Williams, D.E.; Mesquita, J.T.; Pinto, E.G.; Da Costa-Silva, T.A.; Hajdu, E.; Ferreira, A.G.; Santos, R.A.; Murphy, P.J.; et al. Anti-parasitic guanidine and pyrimidine alkaloids from the marine sponge *Monanchora arbuscula*. *J. Nat. Prod.* **2015**, *78*, 1101–1112. [CrossRef] [PubMed]

44. Makarieva, T.N.; Ogurtsova, E.K.; Deisenko, V.A.; Dmitrenok, P.S.; Tabakmakher, K.M.; Guzii, A.G.; Pislyagin, E.A.; Es'kov, A.A.; Kozhemyako, V.B.; Aminin, D.L.; et al. Urupocidin A: A new, inducing iNOS sxpression bicyclic guanidine alkaloid from the marine sponge *Monanchora pulchra*. *Org. Lett.* **2014**, *16*, 4292–4295. [CrossRef] [PubMed]

45. Jamison, M.T.; Molinski, T.F. Antipodal crambescin A2 homologues from the marine sponge *Pseudaxinella reticulata*. Antifungal structure–activity relationships. *J. Nat. Prod.* **2015**, *78*, 557–561. [CrossRef] [PubMed]

46. Patil, A.D.; Freyer, A.J.; Offen, P.; Bean, M.F.; Johnson, R.K. Three new tricyclic guanidine alkaloids from the sponge *Batzella* sp. *J. Nat. Prod.* **1997**, *60*, 704–707. [CrossRef]

47. Harbour, G.C.; Tymiak, A.A.; Rinehart, K.L.; Shaw, P.D.; Hughes, R.G.; Mizsak, S.A.; Coats, J.H.; Zurenko, G.E.; Li, L.H.; Kuentzel, S.L. Ptilocaulin and isoptilocaulin, antimicrobial and cytotoxic Cyclic guanidines from the Caribbean Sponge *ptilocaulis* aff. *P. spiculifer* (Lamarck, 1814). *J. Am. Chem. Soc.* **1981**, *103*, 5604–5606. [CrossRef]

48. Kossuga, M.H.; Delira, S.P.; Nascimento, A.M.; Gambardella, M.T.P.; Berlinck, R.G.S.; Torres, Y.R.; Nascimento, G.G.F.; Pimenta, E.F.; Silva, M.; Thiemann, O.H.; et al. Isolation and biological activities

of secondary metabolites from the sponges *Monanchora* aff. *arbuscula*, *Aplysina* sp. *Petromica ciocalyptoides* and *Topsentia ophiraphidies*, from the ascidian *Didemnum ligulum* and from the octocoral *Carijoa riisei*. *Quim. Nova* **2007**, *30*, 1194–1202. [CrossRef]

49. Hua, H.M.; Peng, J.; Fronczek, F.R.; Kelly, M.; Hamann, M.T. Crystallographic and NMR studies of antiinfective tricyclic guanidine alkaloids from the sponge *Monanchora unguifera*. *Bioorg. Med. Chem.* **2004**, *12*, 6461–6464. [CrossRef] [PubMed]

50. Ferreira, E.G.; Wilke, D.V.; Jimenez, P.C.; De oliveira, J.R.; Pessoa, O.D.L.; Silveria, E.R.; Viana, F.A.; Pessoa, C.; Maraes, M.O.; Hajdu, E.; et al. Guanidine alkaloids from *Monanchora arbuscula*: Chemistry and antitumor potential. *Chem. Biodivers.* **2011**, *8*, 1433–1445. [CrossRef]

51. Sakemi, S.; Sun, H.H.; Jefford, C.W.; Bemardinelli, G. Batzellines A, B and C. Novel pyrroloquinoline alkaloids from the sponge *Batzella* sp. *Tetrahedron Lett.* **1989**, *30*, 2517–2520. [CrossRef]

52. Sun, H.H.; Sakemi, S.I. Pyrroloquinoline Alkaloids, Batzellines and Isobatzellines from Marine Sponge and Methods of Use. U.S. Patent Application No. US5028613 (A), 2 July 1991.

53. Gunasekera, S.P.; McCarthy, P.J.; Longley, R.E.; Pomponi, S.A.; Wright, A.E.; Lobkovsky, E.; Clardy, J. Discorhabdin P, a new enzyme inhibitor from a deep-water Caribbean sponge of the genus *Batzella*. *J. Nat. Prod.* **1999**, *62*, 173–175. [CrossRef] [PubMed]

54. Gunasekera, S.P.; Zuleta, I.A.; Longley, R.E.; Wright, A.E.; Pomponi, S.A. Discorhabdins S, T and U, new cytotoxic pyrroloiminoquinones from a deep-water Caribbean sponge of the genus *Batzella*. *J. Nat. Prod.* **2003**, *66*, 1615–1617. [CrossRef] [PubMed]

55. Gunaskera, S.P.; McCarthy, P.J.; Pomponi, S.A.; Wright, A.E.; Longley, R.E. Discorhabdin Compounds and Methods of Use. U.S. Patent Application No. US6057333 (A), 2 May 2000.

56. Gunasekera, S.P.; McCarthy, P.J.; Longley, R.E.; Pomponi, S.A.; Wright, A.E. Secobatzellines A and B, two new enzyme inhibitors from a deep-water Caribbean sponge of the genus *Batzella*. *J. Nat. Prod.* **1999**, *62*, 1208–1211. [CrossRef] [PubMed]

57. Gunasekera, S.P.; McCarthy, P.J.; Longley, R.E.; Pomponi, S.A.; Wright, A.E. Aminoiminoquinone and Aminoquinine Alkaloid Compounds as Capase Inhibitors. U.S. Patent No. WO2000002858 (A1), 20 January 2000.

58. Guzman, E.A.; Johnson, J.D.; Carrier, M.K.; Meyer, C.I.; Pitts, T.P.; Gunasekera, S.P.; Wright, A.E. Selective cytotoxic activity of the marine-derived batzelladine compounds against pancreatic cancer cell lines. *Anti-Cancer Drugs* **2009**, *20*, 149–155. [CrossRef] [PubMed]

59. Capon, R.J.; Miller, M.; Rooney, F. Clathrins A–C: Metabolites from a southern Australian marine sponge *Clathria* species. *J. Nat. Prod.* **2001**, *64*, 643–644. [CrossRef] [PubMed]

60. Patil, A.D.; Freyer, A.J.; Taylor, P.B.; Carté, B.; Zuber, G.; Johnson, R.K.; Faulkner, D.J. Batzelladines F–I, novel alkaloids from the sponge *Batzella* sp.: Inducers of p56lck-CD4 dissociation. *J. Org. Chem.* **1997**, *62*, 1814–1819. [CrossRef]

61. Gallimore, W.A.; Kelly, M.; Scheuer, P.J. Alkaloids from the sponge *Monanchora unguifera*. *J. Nat. Prod.* **2005**, *68*, 1420–1423. [CrossRef] [PubMed]

62. Braekman, J.C.; Daloze, D.; Tavares, R.; Hajdu, E.; van Soest, R.W.M. Novel polycyclic guanidine alkaloids from two marine sponges of the genus *Monanchora*. *J. Nat. Prod.* **2000**, *63*, 193–196. [CrossRef] [PubMed]

63. Hua, H.M.; Peng, J.; Dunber, D.C.; Schinazi, R.F.; Andrews, A.G.C.; Cuevas, C.; Fernandez, L.F.G.; Kelly, M.; Hamann, M.T. Batzelladine alkaloids from the caribbean sponge *Monanchora unguifera* and the significant activities against HIV-1 and AIDS opportunistic infectious pathogens. *Tetrahedron* **2007**, *63*, 11179–11188. [CrossRef]

64. Laville, R.; Thomas, O.P.; Berrue, F.; Marquez, D.; Vacelet, J.; Amade, P. Bioactive guanidine alkaloids from two Caribbean marine sponges. *J. Nat. Prod.* **2009**, *72*, 1589–1594. [CrossRef] [PubMed]

65. Kohon, L.; Porto, P.; Binachi, B.; santos, M.; Berlinck, R.G.S.; Arns, C. Nor-batzelladine L from the sponge *Monanchora* sp. displays antiviral activity against *Herpes Simplex* virus type 1. *Planta Med.* **2012**, *78*, CL27. [CrossRef]

66. Pessoa, C.; dos Santos, M.F.C.; Berlinck, R.G.S.; Ferreira, P.M.P.; Cavalcanti, B.C. Cytotoxic batzelladine L from the Brazilian marine sponge *Monanchora arbuscula*. *Planta Med.* **2013**, *79*, PK6. [CrossRef]

67. Takishima, S.; Ishiyama, A.; Iwatsuki, M.; Otoguro, K.; Yamada, H.; Omura, S.; Kobayashi, K.; Van Soest, R.W.M.; Matsunaga, S. Merobatzelladines A and B, anti-infective tricyclic guanidines from a marine sponge *Monanchora* sp. *Org. Lett.* **2009**, *11*, 2655–2658. [CrossRef] [PubMed]

68. Martins, L.F.; Mesquita, J.T.; Pinto, E.G.; Thais, A.; Costa-Silva, T.A.; Borborema, S.E.T.; Junior, A.J.G.; Neves, B.J.; Andrade, C.H.; Al Shuhaib, Z.; et al. Analogues of marine guanidine alkaloids are in vitro effective against *Trypanosoma cruzi* and selectively *eliminate Leishmania* (L.) *infantum* Intracellular amastigotes. *J. Nat. Prod.* **2016**, *79*, 2202–2210. [CrossRef] [PubMed]

69. Bewley, C.A.; Ray, S.; Cohen, F.; Collins, S.K.; Overman, L.E. Inhibition of HIV-1 envelope-mediated fusion by synthetic batzelladine analogues. *J. Nat. Prod.* **2004**, *67*, 1319–1324. [CrossRef] [PubMed]

70. Olszewski, A.; Sato, K.; Aron, Z.D.; Cohen, F.; Harris, A.; McDougall, B.R.; Robinson, W.E.; Overman, L.E.; Weiss, G.A. Guanidine alkaloid analogues as inhibitors of HIV-1 Nef interactions with p53, actin and p56lck. *Proc. Natl. Acad. Sci. USA* **2004**, *101*, 14079–14084. [CrossRef] [PubMed]

71. Ahmed, N.; Brahmbhatt, K.G.; Khan, S.I.; Jacob, M.; Tekwani, B.L.; Sabde, S.; Mitra, D.; Singh, I.; Khan, I.A.; Bhutani, K.K. Synthesis and biological evaluation of tricyclic guanidine analogues of batzelladine K for antimalarial, antileishmanial, antibacterial, antifungal and anti-HIV activities. *Chem. Biol. Drug Des.* **2013**, *81*, 491–498. [CrossRef] [PubMed]

72. Bennett, E.L.; Black, G.P.; Browne, P.; Hizi, A.; Jaffar, M.; Leyland, J.P.; Martin, C.; Oz-Gleenberg, I.; Murphy, P.J.; Roberts, T.D.; et al. Synthesis and biological activity of analogues of batzelladine F. *Tetrahedron* **2013**, *69*, 3061–3066. [CrossRef]

73. Tempone, A.G.; Martins, L.F.; Pinto, E.G.; Mesquita, J.T.; Bennett, E.L.; Black, G.P.; Murphy, P.J. Synthetic marine guanidines are effective antileishmanial compounds by altering the plasma membrane permeability. *Planta Med.* **2014**, *80*, P1L154. [CrossRef]

74. Kashman, Y.; Hirsh, S.; McConnell, O.J.; Ohtani, I.; Kusumi, T.; Kakisawa, H. Ptilomycalin A: A novel polycyclic guanidine alkaloid of marine origin. *J. Am. Chem. Soc.* **1989**, *111*, 8925–8926. [CrossRef]

75. Rinehart, K.L.; Jares-Erijman, E.A. Crambescidins: New Antiviral and Cytotoxic Compounds from the Sponge Crambe crambe. U.S. Patent Application No. 5756734 (A), 26 May 1998.

76. Martin, V.; Vale, C.; Bondu, S.; Thomas, O.P.; Vieytes, M.R.; Botana, L.M. Differential effects of crambescins and crambescidin 816 in voltage-gated sodium, potassium and calcium channels in neurons. *Chem. Res. Toxicol.* **2013**, *26*, 169–178. [CrossRef] [PubMed]

77. Ternon, E.; Zarate, L.; Chenesseau, S.; Croué, J.; Dumollard, R.; Marcelino, T.; Suzuki, M.T.; Thomas, O.P. Spherulization as a process for the exudation of chemical cues by the encrusting sponge *Cramb crambe*. *Sci. Rep.* **2016**, *6*, 29474. [CrossRef] [PubMed]

78. Mendez, A.G.; Juncal, B.; Silva, S.B.L.; Thomas, O.P.; Vàzquez, V.M.; Alfonso, A.; Vieytes, M.R.; Vale, C.; Botana, L.M. The marine guanidine alkaloid crambescidin 816 induces calcium influx and cytotoxicity in primary cultures of cortical neurons through glutamate receptors. *ACS Chem. Neurosci.* **2017**, *8*, 1608–1617. [CrossRef] [PubMed]

79. Jares-Erijman, E.A.; Ingrum, A.L.; Carney, J.R.; Rinehart, K.L.; Sakai, R. Polycyclic guanidine-containing compounds from the Mediterranean sponge *Crambe crambe*: The structure of 13,14,15-isocrambescidin 800 and the absolute stereochemistry of the pentacyclic guanidine moieties of the crambescidins. *J. Org. Chem.* **1993**, *58*, 4805–4808. [CrossRef]

80. Heys, L.; Moore, C.G.; Murphy, P.J. The guanidine metabolites of *Ptilocaulis spiculifer* and related compounds; isolation and synthesis. *Chem. Soc. Rev.* **2000**, *29*, 57–67. [CrossRef]

81. Gogineni, V.; Schinazi, R.F.; Hamann, M.T. Role of marine natural products in the genesis of antiviral agents. *Chem. Rev.* **2015**, *115*, 9655–9705. [CrossRef] [PubMed]

82. Shi, J.G.; Sun, F.; Rinehart, K.L. Crambescidin Compounds. U.S. Patent Application No. WO1998046575 (A1), 22 October 1998.

83. Rinehart, K.L.; Shi, J.G.; Sun, F. Crambescidin Compounds. U.S. Patent Application No. US006028077 (A), 22 February 2000.

84. Palagiano, E.; De Marino, S.; Minale, L.; Riccio, R.; Zollo, F.; Iorizzi, M.; Carre, J.; Debitus, C.; Lucarain, L.; Provost, J. Ptilomycalin A, crambescidin 800 and related new highly cytotoxic guanidine alkaloids from the starfishes *Fromia monilis* and *Celerina heffernani*. *Tetrahedron* **1995**, *51*, 3675–3682. [CrossRef]

85. Dalisay, D.S.; Saludes, J.P.; Molinski, T.F. Ptilomycalin A inhibits laccase and melanization in *Cryptococcus neoformans*. *Bioorg. Med. Chem.* **2011**, *19*, 6654–6657. [CrossRef] [PubMed]

86. Aoki, S.; Kong, D.; Matsui, K.; Kobayashi, M. Erythroid differentiation in K562 chronic myelogenous cells induced by crambescidin 800, a pentacyclic guanidine alkaloid. *Anticancer Res.* **2004**, *24*, 2325–2330. [PubMed]

87. Dyshlovoy, S.A.; Venz, S.; Hauschild, J.; Tabakmakher, K.M.; Otte, K.; Madanchi, R.; Walther, R.; Guzii, A.G.; Makarieva, T.N.; Shubina, L.K.; et al. Anti-migratory activity of marine alkaloid monanchocidin A, proteomics-based discovery and confirmation. *Proteomics* **2016**, *16*, 1590–1603. [CrossRef] [PubMed]

88. Dyshlovoy, S.A.; Hauschild, J.; Amann, K.; Tabakmakher, K.M.; Venz, S.; Walther, R.; Guzii, A.G.; Makarieva, T.N.; Shubina, L.K.; Fedorov, S.N.; et al. Marine alkaloid monanchocidin A overcomes drug resistance by induction of autophagy and lysosomal membrane permeabilization. *Oncotarget* **2015**, *6*, 17328–17341. [CrossRef] [PubMed]

89. Makarieva, T.N.; Tabakmakher, K.M.; Guzii, A.G.; Denisenko, V.A.; Dmitrenko, P.S.; Kuzmich, A.S.; Lee, H.S.; Stonik, V.A. Monanchomycalins A and B, unusual guanidine alkaloids from the sponge *Monanchora pulchra*. *Tetrahedron Lett.* **2012**, *53*, 4228–4231. [CrossRef]

90. Korolkova, Y.; Makarieva, T.; Tabakmakher, K.; Shubina, L.; Kudryashova, E.; Andreev, Y.; Mosharova, I.; Lee, H.S.; Lee, Y.J.; Kozlov, S. Marine cyclic guanidine alkaloids monanchomycalin B and urupocidin A act as inhibitors of TRPV1, TRPV2 and TRPV3 but not TRPA1 receptors. *Mar. Drugs* **2017**, *15*, 87. [CrossRef] [PubMed]

91. Tabakmakher, K.M.; Denisenko, V.A.; Guzii, A.G.; Dmitrenko, P.S.; Dyshlovoy, S.A.; Lee, H.S.; Makarieva, T.N. Monanchomycalin C, a new pentacyclic guanidine alkaloid from the Far-Eastern marine sponge *Monanchora pulchra*. *Nat. Prod. Commun.* **2013**, *8*, 1399–1402. [PubMed]

92. Tabakmakher, K.M.; Makarieva, T.N.; Denisenko, V.A.; Guzii, A.G.; Dmitrenko, P.S.; Kuzmich, A.S.; Stonik, V.A. Normonanchocidins A, B and D, new pentacyclic guanidine alkaloids from the Far-Eastern marine sponge *Monanchora pulchra*. *Nat. Prod. Commun.* **2015**, *10*, 913–916. [PubMed]

93. Tabakmakher, K.M.; Makarieva, T.N.; Shubina, L.K.; Denisenko, V.A.; Popov, R.S.; Kuzmich, A.S.; Lee, H.S.; Stonik, V.A. Monanchoxymycalins A and B, new hybrid pentacyclic guanidine alkaloids from the Far-Eastern marine sponge *Monanchora pulchra*. *Nat. Prod. Commun.* **2016**, *11*, 1817–1820.

94. Campos, P.E.; Queiroz, E.F.; Marcourt, L.; Wolfender, J.M.; Sanchez, A.S.; Illien, B.; Al-Mourabit, A.; Gauvin-Bialecki, A. Isolation and identification of new secondary metabolites from the marine sponge *Monanchora unguiculata*. *Planta Med.* **2016**, *81*, P580. [CrossRef]

95. Campos, P.E.; Wolfender, J.M.; Queiroz, E.F.; Marcourt, L.; Al-Mourabit, A.; Frederich, M.; Bordignon, A.; De Voogd, N.; Illien, B.; Gauvin-Bialecki, A. Unguiculin A and ptilomycalins E–H, antimalarial guanidine alkaloids from the marine sponge *Monanchora unguiculata*. *J. Nat. Prod.* **2017**, *80*, 1404–1410. [CrossRef] [PubMed]

96. Guzii, A.G.; Makarieva, T.N.; Korolkova, Y.V.; Andreev, Y.A.; Mosharova, I.V.; Tabakmaher, K.M.; Denisenko, V.A.; Dmitrenok, P.S.; Ogurtsova, E.K.; Antonov, A.S.; et al. Pulchranin A, isolated from the Far-Eastern marine sponge, *Monanchora pulchra*: The first marine non-peptide inhibitor of TRPV-1 channels. *Tetrahedron Lett.* **2013**, *54*, 1247–1250. [CrossRef]

97. Makarieva, T.N.; Ogurtsova, E.K.; Korolkova, Y.V.; Andreev, Y.A.; Mosharova, I.V.; Tabakmaher, K.M.; Guzii, A.G.; Denisenko, V.A.; Dmitrenok, P.S.; Lee, H.S.; et al. Pulchranins B and C, new acyclic guanidine alkaloids From the Far-Eastern marine sponge *Monanchora pulchra*. *Nat. Prod. Commun.* **2013**, *8*, 1229–1232. [PubMed]

98. Ogurtsova, E.K.; Makarieva, T.N.; Korolkova, Y.V.; Andreev, Y.A.; Mosharova, I.V.; Denisenko, V.A.; Dmitrenok, P.S.; Lee, Y.I.; Grishin, E.V.; Stonik, V.A. New derivatives of natural acyclic guanidine alkaloids with TRPV receptor-regulating properties. *Nat. Prod. Commun.* **2015**, *10*, 1171–1173. [PubMed]

99. Dyshlovoy, S.A.; Tabakmakher, K.M.; Hauschild, J.; Shchekateva, R.K.; Otte, K.; Guzii, A.G.; Makarieva, T.N.; Kudryashova, E.K.; Fedorov, S.N.; Shubina, L.K.; et al. Guanidine alkaloids from the marine sponge *Monanchora pulchra* show cytotoxic properties and prevent EGF-Induced neoplastic transformation in vitro. *Mar. Drugs* **2016**, *14*, 133. [CrossRef] [PubMed]

100. El-Demerdash, A. Isolation of Bioactive Marine Natural Products and Bio-Inspired Synthesis of Fused Guanidinic Tricyclic Analogues. Unpublished Ph.D. Thesis, University of Paris-Saclay, Paris, France, May 2016.

101. El-Demerdash, A.; Moriou, C.; Martin, M.T.; Petek, S.; Debitus, C.; Al-Mourabit, A. Unguiculins A–C: Cytotoxic bis-guanidine alkaloids from the French Polynesian sponge, *Monanchora* n. sp. *Nat. Prod. Res.* **2017**, 1–6. [CrossRef] [PubMed]

102. Kapustina, I.I.; Tabakmakher, K.M.; Makar'eva, T.N. Sterols from the toxin containing Far-Eastern sponge *Monanchora pulchra*. *Chem. Nat. Compd.* **2012**, *47*, 1025–1027. [CrossRef]

103. Wang, W.; Mun, B.; Lee, Y.; Reddy, M.V.; Park, Y.; Lee, J.; Kim, H.; Hahn, D.; Chin, J.; Ekins, M.; et al. Bioactive sesterterpenoids from a Korean sponge *Monanchora* sp. *J. Nat. Prod.* **2013**, *76*, 170–177. [CrossRef] [PubMed]

104. Mun, B.; Wang, W.; Kim, H.; Hahn, D.; Tang, I.; Won, D.H.; Kim, E.H.; Lee, J.; Han, C.; Kim, H.; et al. Cytotoxic 5a,8a-epidioxy sterols from the marine sponge *Monanchora* sp. *Arch. Pharm. Res.* **2015**, *38*, 18–25. [CrossRef] [PubMed]

105. Wang, W.; Lee, T.G.; Patil, R.S.; Mun, B.; Yang, I.; Kim, H.; Hahn, D.; Won, D.H.; Lee, J.; Lee, Y.; et al. Monanchosterols A and B, bioactive bicyclo [4.3.1] steroids from a Korean sponge *Monanchora* sp. *J. Nat. Prod.* **2015**, *78*, 368–373. [CrossRef] [PubMed]

106. Snider, B.B.; Shi, Z.J. Biomimetic synthesis of the bicyclic guanidine moieties of crambines A and B. *J. Org. Chem.* **1992**, *57*, 2526–2528. [CrossRef]

107. Snider, B.B.; Faith, W.C. The total synthesis of (±)-ptilocaulin. *Tetrahedron Lett.* **1983**, *24*, 861–864. [CrossRef]

108. Snider, B.B.; Faith, W.C. Total synthesis of (+)- and (−)-ptilocaulin. *J. Am. Chem. Soc.* **1984**, *106*, 1443–1445. [CrossRef]

109. Yu, M.; Pochapsky, S.; Snider, B.B. Synthesis of 7-Epineoptilocaulin, mirabilin B and isoptilocaulin. A unified biosynthetic proposal for the ptilocaulin and batzelladine alkaloids. Synthesis and structure revision of netamines E and G. *J. Org. Chem.* **2008**, *73*, 9065–9074. [CrossRef] [PubMed]

110. Black, G.P.; Murphy, P.J.; Walshe, N.D.A.; Hibbs, D.E.; Hursthouse, M.B.; Malik, K.M.A. A short synthetic route to the tricyclic guanidinium core of the batzelladine alkaloids. *Tetrahedron Lett.* **1996**, *37*, 6943–6946. [CrossRef]

111. Ahmed, N.; Brahmbhatt, K.G.; Singh, I.P.; Bhutani, K.K. Total synthesis of (±) batzelladine K: A biomimetic approach. *Synthesis* **2010**, *15*, 2567–2570. [CrossRef]

112. Snider, B.B.; Shi, Z. Biomimetic synthesis of the pentacyclic nucleus of ptilomycalin A. *J. Am. Chem. Soc.* **1994**, *116*, 549–557. [CrossRef]

113. Moore, C.G.; Murphy, P.J.; Williams, H.L.; McGown, A.T.; Smith, N.K. A synthesis of crambescidin 359. *Tetrahedron Lett.* **2003**, *44*, 251–254. [CrossRef]

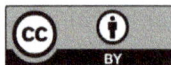

Review

Potential Anticancer Properties of Osthol: A Comprehensive Mechanistic Review

Yalda Shokoohinia [1,2], Fataneh Jafari [1], Zeynab Mohammadi [3], Leili Bazvandi [3], Leila Hosseinzadeh [1], Nicholas Chow [4], Piyali Bhattacharyya [5], Mohammad Hosein Farzaei [1,*], Ammad Ahmad Farooqi [6], Seyed Mohammad Nabavi [7], Mükerrem Betül Yerer [8] and Anupam Bishayee [9,*]

[1] Pharmaceutical Sciences Research Center, School of Pharmacy, Kermanshah University of Medical Sciences, Kermanshah 67146, Iran; yshokoohinia@kums.ac.ir (Y.S.); fataneh.jafari@yahoo.com (F.J.); lhosseinzadeh90@yahoo.com (L.H.)
[2] Department of Pharmacognosy and Biotechnology, School of Pharmacy, Kermanshah University of Medical Sciences, Kermanshah 67146, Iran
[3] Students Research Committee, School of Pharmacy, Kermanshah University of Medical Sciences, Kermanshah 67146, Iran; zeynabmohamadi47@yahoo.com (Z.M.); leilibazvandi@yahoo.com (L.B.)
[4] Department of Clinical and Administrative Sciences, College of Pharmacy, Larkin University, Miami, FL 33169, USA; NChow@ularkin.org
[5] School of Health Sciences, University of Turabo, Gurabo, PR 00778, USA; pbhattacharyya@suagm.edu
[6] Laboratory for Translational Oncology and Personalized Medicine, Rashid Latif Medical College, Lahore 54000, Pakistan; ammadfarooqi@rlmclahore.com
[7] Applied Biotechnology Research Center, Baqiyatallah University of Medical Sciences, Tehran 1435916471, Iran; Nabavi208@gmail.com
[8] Department of Pharmacology, Faculty of Pharmacy, University of Erciyes, 38039 Kayseri, Turkey; eczbetul@yahoo.com
[9] Department of Pharmaceutical Sciences, College of Pharmacy, Larkin University, Miami, FL 33169, USA
* Correspondence: mh.farzaei@gmail.com (M.H.F.); abishayee@ularkin.org or abishayee@gmail.com (A.B.) Tel.: +98-831-427-6493 (M.H.F.); +1-305-760-7511 (A.B.)

Received: 21 November 2017; Accepted: 29 December 2017; Published: 3 January 2018

Abstract: Cancer is caused by uncontrolled cell proliferation which has the potential to occur in different tissues and spread into surrounding and distant tissues. Despite the current advances in the field of anticancer agents, rapidly developing resistance against different chemotherapeutic drugs and significantly higher off-target effects cause millions of deaths every year. Osthol is a natural coumarin isolated from Apiaceaous plants which has demonstrated several pharmacological effects, such as antineoplastic, anti-inflammatory and antioxidant properties. We have attempted to summarize up-to-date information related to pharmacological effects and molecular mechanisms of osthol as a lead compound in managing malignancies. Electronic databases, including PubMed, Cochrane library, ScienceDirect and Scopus were searched for in vitro, in vivo and clinical studies on anticancer effects of osthol. Osthol exerts remarkable anticancer properties by suppressing cancer cell growth and induction of apoptosis. Osthol's protective and therapeutic effects have been observed in different cancers, including ovarian, cervical, colon and prostate cancers as well as chronic myeloid leukemia, lung adenocarcinoma, glioma, hepatocellular, glioblastoma, renal and invasive mammary carcinoma. A large body of evidence demonstrates that osthol regulates apoptosis, proliferation and invasion in different types of malignant cells which are mediated by multiple signal transduction cascades. In this review, we set spotlights on various pathways which are targeted by osthol in different cancers to inhibit cancer development and progression.

Keywords: osthol; cancer; phytochemicals; natural product; malignancies; apoptosis

1. Introduction

Cancer is a multifaceted and therapeutically challenging disease and rapidly emerging pre-clinical and clinical studies have started to shed light on the molecular mechanisms which underlie cancer development and progression [1]. Based on the United States National Cancer Institute's categorization, diverse types of cancer include myeloma, carcinoma, leukemia, lymphoma and central nervous system cancer depending on cell type involved [2].

In the next couple of decades, the prevalence of cancer is predicted to rise to 70%, amounting to 22 million cases. The most common sites of cancer diagnosed in 2012 were lung, breast, prostate, colon, stomach, cervix and liver carcinomas. One-third of cancer deaths can be attributed to five life style and nutritive factors, such as overweight, low fresh and fiber food intake, absence of physical activity as well as tobacco and alcohol use [1]. Moreover, malignancies affect the psychological well-being (e.g., depression, anxiety, distress and somatization) of patients and their caregivers [3].

The goals of cancer treatment are to destroy tumors or to markedly prolong survival and improve a patient's quality of life [1]. Deregulations in spatio-temporally controlled signaling mechanisms, including nuclear factor kappa-light-chain-enhancer of activated B cells (NF-κB) [4], activator protein-1 (Ap-1) [4,5] and mitogen-activated protein kinase (MAPK) signaling pathways, played contributory role in carcinogenesis and drug resistance [6–8]. Additionally, microtubules have been targeted to disrupt the normal function of the mitotic spindle [9]. Although chemotherapy and radiotherapy are greatly efficient approaches in the treatment of cancer, malignant cells continue to develop resistance to these treatments [4].

Natural products, containing bioactive secondary metabolites, have beneficial effects on human health [10,11] and the active ingredients are strong candidates to be lead compounds for the development of new drugs [12]. From 1930 to 2012, 183 drugs were approved as antitumor agents; 30% of these were obtained from natural sources, 57% were natural agents with semisynthetic modifications and 34% had natural product mimetic pharmacophores [13]. Although targeted therapies, such as monoclonal antibodies, have greatly improved, the perfect treatment of several cancers, such as leukemia, gastrointestinal and breast cancers, remain to be achieved through new therapies [10]. Natural products exert anticancer effects through various mechanisms such as alteration of cell cycle [4,14] interference with microtubules [15], topoisomerase inhibitory activities [16], immunomodulatory effects [17] and chemopreventive effects [18] achieved by modulation of various oncogenic signaling molecules and pathways [19–21].

Coumarins are derivatives of 2H-1-benzopyran-2-one which can be obtained mainly from cyclization of a C-2 oxygenated *cis*-cinnamic acid. These compounds are widely found in plants in the form of free coumarins or their glycosides [22]. Coumarins naturally occurr with several molecular structures, especially in the Apiaceae [23,24] and Rutaceae families, as well as many other plant families, including Asteraceae, Poaceae and Rubiaceae [22]. Coumarins have various biological properties related to their chemical structure [25–27]. Some coumarins have vasorelaxant activity in coronary vessels and some other showed hypotensive [22], antiviral [28], antileishmanial [29] anti-inflammatory [30] and antispasmodic [31] effects. Furanocoumarins are also widely used in the treatment of leucoderma and psoriasis due to their photosensitivity properties [32,33]. Some hydroxy- and methoxy-coumarins are able to absorb ultraviolet radiation and are commonly used in sunblock creams [22].

Coumarins have prominent anticancer properties with low adverse effects based on the functional groups in the original structure [34,35]. They can affect different cellular pathways, including suppression of angiogenesis, several types of heat shock proteins (HSPs) and cell proliferation as well as inhibition of the enzymes chiefly involved in the pathophysiology of cancer, such as telomerase, monocarboxylate transporters, carbonic anhydrase, aromatase and sulfatase [35,36].

Osthol (osthole), 7-methoxy-8-(3-methyl-2-butenyl)-2H-1-benzopyran-2-one, a natural coumarin obtained from *Cnidium* spp. and other Apiaceous plants [37], has been found to exert health-promoting effects [38]. *Cnidium monnieri* fruits rich in osthol are popularly used in traditional Chinese medicine [39].

Osthol is a prenylated coumarin with a wide range of pharmacological effects, such as neuroprotective [40], spasmolytic [41] immunomodulatory [42], osteogenic [43], hepatoprotective [44], vasorelaxant [45], antimicrobial [45], antiviral [46] and antileishmanial properties [47], many of which could be implicated in the primary or secondary prevention of cancer. In this review, we aim to provide a critical and mechanistic insight into the biological and pharmacological properties of osthol that are useful in the treatment of cancer.

2. Literature Search Methodology

Electronically available databases, including PubMed, Science Direct, Cochrane library and Scopus, were searched for cellular, animal or human studies which assessed the anticancer effects of osthol. We have followed the preferred reporting items for systematic review and meta-analysis (PRISMA) criteria which are preferred for reporting systematic reviews. Relevant and high-quality publications were collected for the years 1966–2017 (up to January). Unpublished results were not included. Only English language papers were included in this review. The search terms were "osthol" or "osthole" in title and abstract. Results from primary search were screened by two independent investigators. Included articles were checked for verification of scientific name of source plant, the dose of administration, type of cancer as well as type of cell line for cellular studies and the animal model for animal studies. Results were reviewed for significant effects on proliferation, apoptosis, pro-inflammatory cytokines, oxidative markers, antioxidant enzymes and tissue damage biomarkers.

From total 1354 results, 676 reports were excluded because of duplication and 17 were omitted as they were review papers. Additionally, two were ruled out since they were not in English and 31 were excluded because the subject was on other compounds rather than osthol. Among 628 retrieved studies, 355 were excluded out as they were analytical and phytochemical aspects of osthol rather than pharmacological effects; 273 reports on pharmacological effects of osthol were retrieved amongst which 248 were omitted since they assessed pharmacological effects of osthol other than anticancer properties. Twenty five reports including one in vivo and 24 in vitro studies were finally included. Figure 1 shows a flow diagram of the selective procedure for literature included in this review.

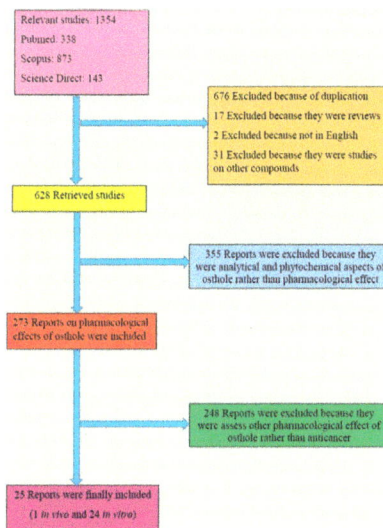

Figure 1. Study selection diagram.

3. Cellular and Molecular Mechanisms of Anticancer Effects of Osthol

A comprehensive review of the reported literature on anticancer activity of osthol indicated that this therapeutic agent could potentially exert anticancer and antitumor activity via several mechanisms, including cell cycle inhibition, apoptosis induction, anti-angiogenesis, inhibition of metastasis, and suppression of cell proliferation and cell migration (Figure 2). Based on the type of cancer, the effective dose and the mechanism of action could be different. A detailed data on the anticancer mechanism of osthol is presented below and Table 1.

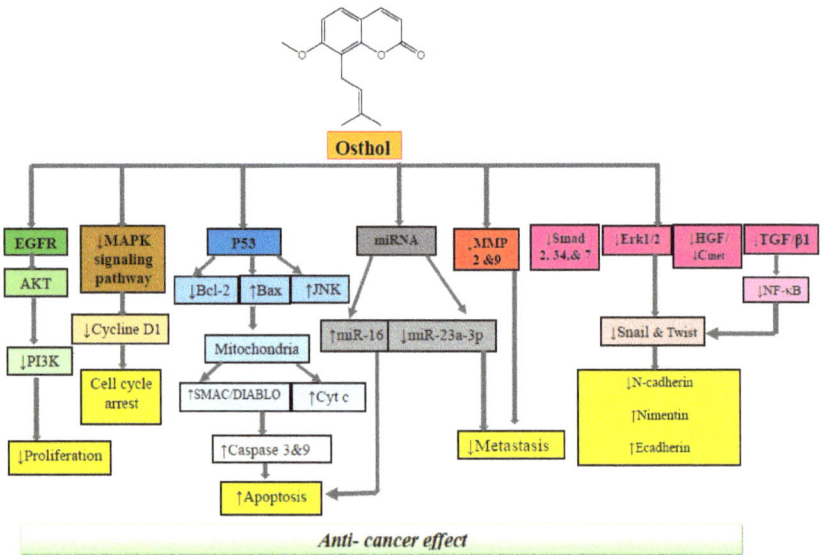

Figure 2. Molecular mechanisms underlying anticancer effect of osthol. EGFR, epidermal growth factor receptor; Akt, AKR mouse thymoma kinase; MAPK, mitogen-activated protein kinase; RNA, ribonucleic acid; MMP, matrix metalloprotease; HGF, hepatocyte growth factor; TGF, tumor growth factor; NF-κB, nuclear factor-κB.

Table 1. Pharmacological mechanisms of osthol involved in its anticancer activities.

Type of Cancer	Conc. or Dose	Cancer Model Used	Anticancer Effects and Mechanisms	Reference
Colon	1, 3 & 10 mM	In vitro (HCT116 & SW480 cells)	↓Cell motility; ↑apoptosis; ↑phosphorylation of p53 on Ser15 (p-p53); ↑acetylation of p53; ↑ROS; ↑JNK	[48]
Prostate	100 mM	In vitro (PC3 cells)	↑Apoptosis; ↓Bcl-; ↑Bax; ↑Smac/DIABLO	[49]
Prostate	20~80 μM	In vitro (AIPC, DU145 & PC3 cells)	↓TGF-β, ↓Akt, JNK& ERK ↓miR-23a-3p	[50]
Breast	15 mM	In vitro (MDA-MB-231 & 4T1)	↓TbetaRII; ↓Smad2; ↓Smad3; ↓Smad4	[51]
Breast	20 mM	In vitro (MCF-7, MDA-MB-453, MDA-MB-231 & BT-20 cells)	↓c-Met signaling; ↓FASN; ↓HGF- induced EMT; ↓c-Met protein levels; ↓cell migration; ↓invasion; ↓c-Met/Akt/mTOR	[52]

Table 1. *Cont.*

Type of Cancer	Conc. or Dose	Cancer Model Used	Anticancer Effects and Mechanisms	Reference
Breast	5, 10, 24, 40 & 80 mM	In vitro (MDA-MB-231, MCF-7, HBL-100 & HER2-overexpressing human cancer cell lines)	↓proliferation; ↑apoptosis; ↓FASN; ↓Akt; ↓mTOR; ↑paclitaxel-induced cytotoxicity	[53]
Breast	5.25 mg/kg	In vivo (Mice treated orally twice weekly)	↑IL-8; ↑M-CSF; ↑PTHrP; ↓OPG/RANKL	[54]
Breast	20–90 mM	In vitro (MDA-231BO cells)	↓Cell viability; ↓proliferation; ↑apoptosis; ↓TGF-β/Smads	[54]
Brain	50, 100 & 200 mM	In vitro (U87 cells)	↓proliferation; ↑apoptosis; ↑miR16; ↓MMP9	[55]
Brain	25, 50 & 100 mM	In vitro (Rat glioma cells)	↓Proliferation; ↓PI3K/Akt/MAPK	[56]
Brain	10–100 mM	In vitro (GBM8401 cells)	↓EMT; ↓Akt and GSK3β; ↓Snail; ↓Twist; ↓I3K/Akt	[57]
Brain	100 mM	In vitro (SKNMC cells)	↑Apoptosis by ↑Bcl; ↑Bax; ↑Smac/DIABLO	[49]
Lung	50, 100 & 150 mM	In vitro (A549 cells)	↑G2/M arrest; ↑apoptosis; ↓Cyclin B1; ↓p-Cdc2; ↓Bcl-2; ↑Bax, ↓PI3K/Akt signaling pathway	[58]
Lung	20, 40, 60 mM 80 mM	In vitro (A549 cells)	↓MMP-2; ↓MMP-9	[58]
Lung	5–20 mM	In vitro (A549 cells)	↓NF-κB mediated snail activation; ↓invasion; ↓migration; ↓adhesion	[59]
Lung	100 mM	In vitro (H1299 cells)	↑Apoptosis; ↓Bcl; ↑Bax; ↑Smac/DIABLO	[49]
Leukemia	5 mM 15 mM	In vitro (K562/ADM cells)	↓MDR in myelogenous leukemia	[60]
Leukemia	30 mg/kg for 8 days	In vivo (CDF1 female mice transplanted with P-388 D1 cells)	↑Apoptosis; ↓P-388 D1 cells	[61]
Cervix	77.96 mM 64.94 mM	In vitro (HeLa cells)	↑Apoptosis	[61]
Ovary	20, 40, 80, 120, 160 and 200	In vitro (A2780 & OV2008 cells)	↓Cells proliferation; ↑apoptosis	[62]
Ovary	5, 10, 24, 40 mM 80 mM	In vitro (SKOV3 human cancer cells)	↓FASN; ↓proliferation; ↑apoptosis; ↓Akt; ↓mTOR; ↑paclitaxel-induced cytotoxicity	[53]
Renal	20–30 mM	In vitro (Caki & U251MG cells)	↑Apoptosis; ↓MMP level; ↑cytochrome *c*; ↓c-FLIP	[63]
Liver	20, 40, 80, 120, 160 or 200 mM	In vitro (SMCC-7721, MHCC-97H, HCC-LM3 & BEL-7402 cells)	↓Proliferation; ↑DNA damage; ↓migration; ↓Cdc2; ↓cyclin B1; ↑ERCC1	[64]

Arrows (↑ and ↓) show increase and decrease in the obtained variables, respectively. H1299, human non-small cell lung carcinoma; GSK3β, glycogen synthase kinase 3-β; EMT, epithelial-mesenchymal transition; Akt, AKR mouse thymoma kinase; PI3K, phosphatidylinositol-3-kinase; IGF, insulin-like growth factor; EGFR, epidermal growth factor receptor; COX-2, cyclooxygenase 2; TPK, tyrosine protein kinase; VEGF, vascular endothelial growth factor; NF-κB, nuclear factor kappa-light-chain-enhancer of activated B cells; MAPK, mitogen-activated protein kinase; ROS, reactive oxygen species; JNK, c-Jun N-terminal kinase; c-MET, cellular mesenchymal to epithelial transition factor; mTOR, mammalian target of rapamycin; MDR, multiple drug resistance; Bax: BCL2-Associated X Protein; TGFβRII, transforming growth factor-β receptor, type II; GMP, guanosine monophosphate.

3.1. Colon Cancer

Epidemiological and scientific studies have considerably enhanced our understanding of the evolutionary process underpinning colon cancer development and progression. Metastasis of primary tumors affects the survival of patients [65]. In a study conducted by Huang et al. [48] using HCT116 and SW480 human colon cancer cell lines, osthol demonstrated specific antitumor effect with concentrations of 1, 3 and 10 µM (Table 1). Osthol significantly decreased cell motility in both cell lines through activation of pro-apoptotic signaling pathways and up-regulation of p53 expression; p53 protein has a main role in the regulation of several genes involved in growth inhibition process, apoptosis, cell cycle arrest as well as DNA repair [66]. Apoptosis-induction capacity has been accepted as a mechanism of action for the antitumor drugs [12]; therefore, considerable effort is being directed towards the development of potential medicines that induce apoptosis in tumor cells.

Apoptosis can occur in two main pathways: the mitochondrial (intrinsic) pathway and the death receptor (extrinsic) pathway [67]. In the intrinsic pathway, the mitochondria have a principle role. It is characterized by cytochrome c release from the mitochondrial which activates a family of cysteine protease enzymes, caspases. This process is controlled by the Bcl-2 family of proteins. This family is an essential member of the programmed cell death process, acting to either inhibit (Bcl-2 and Bcl-xl) or promote (Bax and Bcl-xS) cell death [68]. The elevation of the Bax/Bcl-2 ratio, which has a pivotal contribution in apoptosis, is considered as one of the important mechanisms of osthol in the induction of apoptosis and disturbance in permeability of mitochondrial membranes in cancer cells. Osthol exerted apoptotic effect on colon cancer cell line via several mechanisms, including enhancement of the p53 phosphorylation on Ser15 (p-p53) and p53 acetylation on Lys379 (acetylp53). The p53 protein, acting as a tumor suppressor, plays key roles in activating apoptosis through sensing both intrinsic and extrinsic stresses [69]. Moreover, p53 protein has a significant participation in the regulation of cell cycle arrest, and DNA repair, activating c-Jun N-terminal kinase (JNK) pathway, generation of ROS, modulating PI3K/Akt signaling pathway as well as promoting G2/M arrest. Another mechanism which is involved in pro-apoptotic activity of osthol is p53-independent apoptosis process via stimulating JNK and reactive oxygen species (ROS) formation as summarized in Figure 2 [48].

3.2. Prostate Cancer

Genome sequencing and gene expression analyses have highlighted essential roles of epigenetic and genetic changes in prostate carcinogenesis. Almost all prostate cancers are adenocarcinomas. Mounting evidences have suggested that prostate cancer is found more often in African-American men in comparison to white men [70]. In a cellular study performed by Shokoohinia et al. [18], potential anticancer effect of osthol was assessed on PC3 human prostate cancer cell line. Results of this investigation suggested that osthol acts as a powerful cytotoxic agent against PC3 cells. Caspase activation through intrinsic or extrinsic pathway was significantly involved in the induction of apoptotic cell death. Osthol could remarkably boost the expression of caspase-9 and caspase-3 in PC3 cells. This natural coumarin also activated apoptosis by down-regulation of the antiapoptotic agent, Bcl-2, and up-regulation of the proapoptotic gene Bax (BCL2-Associated X Protein) as well as Smac/DIABLO, a mitochondrial protein released in response to apoptosis stimuli and suppresses the activity apoptosis inhibitors; thus, can facilitate apoptosis [67].

It has previously been convincingly revealed that ectopic expression of miR-23a-3p in DU145 cells induced considerable reversal of osthol-mediated reduction in invasive potential of prostate cancer cells. Detailed mechanistic insights suggested that osthol markedly downregulated miR-23a-3p in DU145 cells [50].

3.3. Breast Cancer

Breast cancer is a common malignancy responsible for cancer-related deaths in females around the world, and accordingly, exploring therapeutic approaches in order to suppressing this disease is immediately vital [71]. In an in vitro study reported by Ye et al. [51] on MDA-MB-231 and 4T1, two invasive mammary carcinoma cell lines, osthol at 15 µM showed inhibitory effect on cell proliferation and invasion. Results showed that osthol in combination with platycodin D, a triterpene saponin, could dramatically reduce tumor growth factor-β receptor II (TGFβRII), Smad2, Smad3 and Smad4 gene or protein expressions and efficiently suppressed TGF-β-induced Smad2 and Smad3 phosphorylation. The latter is the main mechanism of osthol in the reduction of proliferation and invasion of breast cancer cells. Hepatocyte growth factor (HGF) is able to induce epithelial–mesenchymal passage in cancerous cells which can result in cancer cell migration. In an in vitro study performed by Hung et al. [48], a series of human breast cancer cells, such as MDA-MB-453, MDA-MB-23, BT-20 and MCF-7, were treated with osthol. It has been observed that osthol significantly suppressed HGF-induced cell distribution, invasion and migration in MCF-7 cell cultures. Abnormal stimulation of the HGF/c-Met (cellular mesenchymal to epithelial transition factor) pathway has a remarkable role in the progression of various models of cancers as well as advancement of tumor invasion and metastatic system. Osthol inhibited HGF-induced c-Met phosphorylation along with a reduction in the total c-Met protein expression in MCF-7 cells which is intervened by C75 (pharmacological inhibitor) of fatty acid synthase (FASN).

In addition to the effects of osthol in breast cancer, this compound reduces the metastasis of this cancer to the bone marrow. In an in vivo study [54], the researchers used a mouse model to investigate the preventive effect of osthol against the metastasis of human breast cancer cells to the bone. Results showed that osthol blocked breast cancer cell growth, migration and invasion, along with enhancement of apoptosis of breast cancer cells.

Osteoprotegerin (OPG) is a soluble decoy receptor which lacks a trans-membrane domain. It protects the skeleton from excessive bone resorption. Mechanistically, it was shown that OPG interacted with receptor activator of nuclear factor-κB ligand (RANKL) and prevented its structural binding with RANK. The role of osthol in prevention of bone marrow metastasis is mediated by the regulation of OPG/RANKL cascade in the interactions between osteoblasts and breast cancer cells and also suppressing TGF-β/Smads pathway which has a pivotal role in breast cancer bone metastasis. However, many researchers are trying to find strategies to suppress tumor growth as well as tumor metastasis [72].

3.4. Brain Cancer

Glioma, a highly relapsing type of tumor, represents 44.6% of central nervous system tumors and has a high rate of morbidity [73]. In vitro investigation by Lin et al. [55] on glioma cell line U87 showed a significant inhibition of proliferation and augmentation of apoptosis at concentrations of 50, 100 and 200 µM of osthol. Mechanistically, it has been shown that osthol upregulated miR-16 in the U87 cells. These effects were mediated through up-regulation of expression miR-16 and down-regulation of matrix metalloprotease (MMP)-9 expression [74]. MicroRNAs (miRNAs) are a class of non-coding, small molecule RNAs and act as regulators of gene expression [55]. Ding et al. [56] investigated the anticancer effect of osthol on C6 rat glioma cell. Results showed that osthol apparently prevented glioma cell proliferation. This natural compound was also able to induce apoptosis by up-regulating the expression of pro-apoptotic proteins as well as reduction of anti-apoptotic factors expression. Furthermore, the compound could inhibit C6 cell migration and invasion. Results showed that inhibition occurred through phosphatidylinositol-3-kinase (PI3K)/AKR mouse thymoma kinase (Akt) and MAPK signaling pathway [75]. MAPK pathway was significantly involved in regulation of the phospho-proteome of brain tumors. MAPK activation can also induce cell-cycle arrest via cyclin D1 activation and reduction of apoptosis through modulation of the BCL-2-family [76]. Several proteins control cell proliferation processes, amongst which cyclin-dependent kinases (CDKs) are the most important ones. A CDK binds a regulatory protein called cyclin. This complex (CDK-cyclin) has a modulatory role in cell cycle progression and drive cells to enter the next phase at the appropriate time. Increased cyclin D1 expression has been involved in several types of cancer. Osthol is demonstrated to reduce D1 expression. The PI3K/Akt signaling pathway is involved in regulation of cancer development and progression mainly through triggering an increase in phosphorylated levels of Akt [77].

Glioblastoma multiform (GBM) is a progressive type of brain tumor in adults. Recent treatment approaches for GBM include surgical resection, radiotherapy and chemotherapy [78,79]. An in vitro study on insulin-like growth factor (IGF)-1-induced GBM8401 cells exposed to different concentration of osthol showed that this natural agent can reverse IGF-1-induced morphological changes, mediated by increasing epithelial marker expression and reducing mesenchymal marker expression. It has been found that IGF-1 can result in the conversion of GBM8401 cells to fibroblastic phenotype and in this condition the intercellular space becomes expanded. In addition, a wound-healing experiment indicated that osthol could suppress IGF-1-induced migration of GBM8401 cells. Suppression of MMP-2 and MMP-9 plays a significant role in the inhibition of IGF-1-induced cell migration in GBM8401 cells. Osthol reduced the phosphorylation of Akt and glycogen synthase kinase 3β (GSK3β) and regained the GSK3β activity [57]. Pretreatment with IGF-1 can lead to phosphorylation of Akt and Erk1/2 involved in expression of Snail and Twist. Osthol can remarkably suppress the IGF-1-induced down-regulation of ZO-1 and β-catenin as well as up regulation of vimentin, N-cadherin, Snail and Twist in a dose- and time-dependent manner. Suppressing Snail and Twist expression which is characteristic of mesenchymal tumor areas, is one of the main mechanism of osthol in inhibiting the induction of EMT in epithelial neoplasms [80]. One of the mechanisms by which the growth suppressive effect of osthol suppresses the growth of the malignant cells is mediated via the effects of osthol on the PI3K/Akt mTOR pathway. EMT is the critical step for metastatically competent brain cancer cells to spread and invade distant sites. This process is mediated through growth factors. It is interesting that osthol is able to inhibit IGF-1-induced EMT through PI3K/Akt pathway inhibition in human brain cancer cells [81].

3.5. Lung Cancer

Lung cancer is the leading cause of cancer-related deaths all over the world, and non-small cell lung cancer (NSCLC) is responsible for about 80% of all cases [82,83]. In an in vitro study by Xu et al. [84], A549 human lung cancer cells were exposed to osthol at various concentrations. Osthol significantly reduced cell growth and arrested the cells in G_2/M phase. It has been revealed that the osthol cellular mechanism of action includes down-regulation of cyclin B1, p-Cdc2 and Bcl-2 expressions and up-regulation of Bax expression in A549 cells. Osthol could also suppress the PI3K/Akt signaling pathway which might be one of the molecular mechanisms by which the compound exerts anticancer effects. In another study by Xu et al. [58], the effects of various concentration of osthol on the migratory and invasive potential of A549 cells were evaluated. Osthol dose-dependently exerted inhibitory effects on lung cancer cells and effectively suppressed proliferation, migration and invasion of cancerous cells. Cellular mechanisms which are essential for these effects were associated with the inhibition of MMP-2 and MMP-9 expression in the human lung cancer cells which have a significant role in cell invasion and migration. Moreover, Feng et al. [59] investigated the effect of osthol on adenocarcinomic human alveolar basal epithelial cells (A549). The cancerous cells were treated with osthol in 5–20 mM for 48 h. Results showed that osthol extremely suppressed TGF-β1-induced epithelial-to-mesenchymal transition (EMT), adhesion, invasion and migration in A549 which is mediated by adjusting NF-κB and Snail signaling pathways. This molecule can interact with cell adhesion molecules which are involved in angiogenesis. The process of angiogenesis is under regulation of several pro-angiogenic genes as well as growth factors including epidermal growth factor (EGF), vascular endothelial growth factor (VEGF), basic fibroblast growth factor (bFGF), platelet derived growth factors (PDGF), angiopoetin-1 and 2 and MMPs [81].

3.6. Leukemia

Chronic myeloid leukemia (CML) is a type of hematologic malignancy [85]. Multidrug resistance (MDR) has an important role in CML chemotherapy failure through drug resistance [86]. Wang et al. [60] showed that osthol has a remarkable effect on CML. In this research, K562/ADM cells were treated with osthol for 24 h. The potential of osthol to overcome MDR caused by P-glycoprotein (P-gp) was measured by the CCK-8 assay in the K562/ADM cell line. Results demonstrated that osthol remarkably reduced P-gp expression through suppression of the PI3K/Akt signaling pathway which is associated with modulation of MDR mediated by P-gp in different types of leukemia. The authors concluded that the PI3K/Akt signaling pathway is a key mechanism triggered in the reversal effect of osthol in the MDR.

Chou et al. [61] evaluated pharmacological properties of osthol against human leukemia via in vivo and in vitro assessments. P-388 D1 murine leukemia cells were intraperitoneally administered into CDF1 female mice (BALB/c female × DBA/2 male). CDF1 mice with leukemia received osthol (30 mg/kg, orally) once a day for a period of nine days. Data clearly suggested that osthol significantly prolonged lifespan of P-388 D1 tumor-bearing mice by more than 37.5% in comparison to solvent-treated animals. Importantly, survival of one mouse of the osthol-treated group was noted to be more than 60 days.

3.7. Cervical Cancer

A common type of malignancy in women all over the world is cervical cancer [87]. In an in vitro study that utilized HeLa human cervical cancer cells, osthol concentration- and time-dependently suppressed cell growth. Furthermore, cytotoxic effects were non-significant in coumarin-treated primary cultured normal cervical fibroblasts which indicates its specific pharmacological effects on cancer cells. It has been revealed that osthol performs its anticancer potential on cervical cancer cells by elevating DNA fragmentation as well as activation of poly (ADP-ribose) polymerase (PARP) which has an essential contribution in programmed cell death resulting in induction of apoptosis in HeLa cells [61].

3.8. Ovarian Cancer

Ovarian cancer is considered as the most lethal gynecologic cancer [88] in women. Epidemiological studies demonstrated that the proportion of ovarian cancer patients who experienced a five-year survival rate is less than 50% post-diagnosis. The main therapeutic approach for ovarian cancer patients is cytoreductive surgery along with paclitaxel-based chemical agents [88,89]. Clinical evidence reported good primary response in many cases; however, there are still remarkable challenges such as multi-chemotherapy drug resistance. In an in vitro study reported by Jiang et al. [62] uncontrolled proliferation and migration of ovarian cancer cells, including OV2008 and A2780, were assessed. Osthol remarkably reduced cell viability of ovarian cancer cells; whereas no toxicity was detected in normal ovarian cells. Subsequent to treatment with osthol, migratory potential, expression levels and functionalities of MMP-9 and MMP-2 were noted to be significantly suppressed in wound healing and trans-well assays. This natural coumarin repressed cells proliferation via promoting G_2/M phase cell cycle arrest and activation of apoptosis process in malignant cells. It has been suggested that other underlying mechanisms of its anticancer action were the enhancement of the apoptotic protein caspase-3, caspase-9 and Bax/Bcl-2.

3.9. Renal Cancer

In an in vitro study, Min et al. [63] showed that osthol increased TNF-related apoptosis-inducing ligand (TRAIL)-mediated cell death in Caki cell line. Induction of apoptotic cell death by osthol (20–30 µM for 24 h) is mediated by regulation of the FLICE like inhibitory protein (c-FLIP) expression in human renal carcinoma cells. c-FLIP overexpression markedly inhibited apoptosis; however, osthol significantly reduced c-FILP levels and sensitized resistant cells to TRAIL. Also, osthol significantly decreased MMP levels and synergistic treatment with TRAIL induced an increase in cytosolic accumulation of cytochrome c. These findings provided evidence that osthol worked synergistically with TRAIL and induced apoptosis in TRAIL-resistant cell lines. Moreover, osthol blocks the growth and invasion of bladder cancer cells by inhibiting the expression of the angiogenesis-related proteins COX-2, VEGF, MMP-2 and NF-κB. Future studies must converge on detailed investigation of osthol-mediated regulation of the TRAIL pathway in resistant cancer cells. We still have insufficient information about regulation of death receptors (DR4 and DR5) by osthol in cancer cells.

3.10. Liver Cancer

In an in vitro study, Lin et al. [64] reported that osthol reduced hepatocellular carcinoma (HCC) cell proliferation. The chemotherapeutic potential of osthol on HCC cell proliferation was mediated through induction of DNA damage and cell cycle arrest as well as inhibition of migration of HCC cells. It remarkably suppressed the cell cycle in the G_2/M phase by blocking the expression of Cdc2. Cyclin-dependent kinase 1 (CDK1)-cyclin B, also known as cell division control protein kinase 2 (Cdc2)-cyclin B is a member of cyclin-dependent kinases with a significant role in regulation of the cell cycle. It has been found that down-regulation of MMP-2 and MMP-9 is involved in suppression of migration of HCC cells by this natural agent. Finally, the authors demonstrated that osthole inhibited EMT by increasing epithelial biomarkers E-cadherin and β-catenin and simultaneously repressing the levels of N-cadherin and vimentin. This phytoconstituents also damaged DNA by induction of DNA excision repair protein (ERCC) 1 expression enhancing epithelial biomarkers E-cadherin and β-catenin, and reducing mesenchymal N-cadherin are among the main cellular factors which have a key role in suppression of EMT by osthol [90]. These cellular pathways suggest an interesting chemotherapeutic effect of osthol on HCC. The interaction of DNA and other coumarins have been reported previously [91].

3.11. Protectice Effect against Toxicity of Chemotherpy

The positive effects of osthol in modulating cancer include direct anticarcinogenic activity along with protective effects against side effects of conventional chemotherapeutic agents. One of the chemotherapeutic drugs that are used for treatment of several types of cancers is doxorubicin [55] which shows several adverse effects due to its inherent pro-oxidant activity. Protective effects of osthol against doxorubicin-induced oxidative stress and apoptosis in the neuronal cell line (PC12) has been confirmed. The protective mechanisms of osthol include enhancement of mitochondrial membrane potential, elevation of Bax/Bcl-2 ratio, improvement in loss of cell viability, suppression of intracellular reactive oxygen species (ROS) generation as well as increases in mitochondrial membrane potential in PC12 cells [18,92]. Fatty acid synthase (FASN) is the only enzyme engaged in long-chain saturated fatty acid synthesis and is implicated in cancer progression by regulating lipid raft function. Thus, one of the molecular pathways by which osthol performs its protective action against cancer progression is its potent inhibitory effect on FASN [53].

4. Toxicity of Osthol

Reviewing current literature can help to collect information regarding the bio-efficacy and safety of the administration of significant phytochemicals in the prevention and management of different malignancies and their relevant complications. Since osthol safety has been investigated, the no-observed adverse-effect level (NOAEL) of osthol for both male and female rats is considered to be less than 5 mg/kg [93]. We suggest to perform randomized, controlled, trials with adequate sample size in order to validate the safety and efficacy of osthol in managing patients with malignancies.

5. Conclusions and Future Directions

Osthol is a natural coumarin isolated from Umbelliferae plants with a wide range of pharmacological effects. The goal of the present review was to provide a summary of current knowledge on the anticancer effects of osthol as a lead compound in malignancy therapy along with in-depth molecular mechanisms. This natural phytochemical suppresses the activation of different apoptotic proteins such as caspase-3 and caspase-9, Smac/DIABLO, poly-ADP ribose polymerase and survivin, which are associated with the intrinsic pathways of apoptosis. Osthol is demonstrated to induce apoptosis in different carcinoma cell lines through up-regulation of p53 expression. It has also been shown that osthol induces apoptosis through a mechanism independent of the tumor-suppressing properties of p53. This effect of osthol seems to be promising since the compound demonstrated antitumor effects in several types of cancers in which a p53 regulatory system is involved [94]. It also can diminish metastasis via different molecular mechanisms such as reducing the expression of Smad 2, 3 and 4, C75, and inhibition of the HGF/c-Met signaling pathway as well as HGF-induced c-Met phosphorylation. Osthol also has a stimulatory effect on the extrinsic apoptotic pathway by increasing levels of caspase-8 (unique to the extrinsic pathway). Furthermore, ability of osthol to inhibit NF-κB-mediated cell survival pathway plays an important contribution in its pro-apoptotic properties, as summarized in Figure 2.

Results obtained from studies evaluating anticancer potential of osthol have confirmed its protective and therapeutic effect on various types of malignancies including ovarian cancer, cervical cancer, chronic myeloid leukemia, lung adenocarcinoma cells, glioma as well as glioblastoma multiform cells, invasive mammary carcinoma cells, colon cancer, and prostate cancer. Recent investigations, mentioned previously, have suggested that osthol has a significant action in the brain by protecting neurons. Additionally, the ability of osthol in penetrating the blood–brain barrier indicates its potential as a future drug for chemotherapy of brain tumors.

Based on the insights gleaned from decades of research, it seems clear that a "one size fits all" approach will not be effective in clinical settings. There has been a paradigm shift in our understanding about the heterogeneous nature of cancer, and accordingly, researchers are now focusing on multi-targeted approaches. Osthol has emerged as a promising phytochemical reportedly involved in the regulation of different signaling pathways. However, we have just started to scratch the surface of information related to the potential of osthol to target multiple proteins and signaling pathways. We still need to have a better understanding of how osthol regulates specific signaling pathways, such as VEGF/VEGFR, PDGF/PDGFR and SHH/GLI pathways, and exert differential modulation of oncogenic and tumor suppressor microRNAs.

Numerous studies presented here clearly suggest that osthol possesses the potential to act in an inhibitory role in the progression of malignancies. A large body of evidence demonstrated that osthol regulates apoptosis, proliferation and invasion in different types of malignant cells which is mediated by multiple cellular signaling pathways. However, the mechanisms of function of osthol toward various cancers are not the same. As it was mentioned, osthol possesses antioxidant activity, causing inhibition of ROS overproduction in different cells. ROS can activate several pathways involved in metastasis and possess critical roles in invasion and invadopodia formation; moreover, ROS also possess prominent roles on signaling cascades relating to resistance to apoptosis, neovascularization, and proliferation. Therefore, ROS contribute in various mechanisms [95–98], and reduction of ROS using antioxidants is a promising way to inhibit different cancers. Based on the different roles of ROS in cancer cells and their contribution in different mechanistic pathways, the function of antioxidants such as osthol in excretion of anticancer activity could be probably different. Regarding the remarkable pharmacological functions of osthol in the protection and treatment of malignancies as described above, this natural compound is becoming a significant natural structure for drug discovery. Furthermore, mechanistic investigations for exploring precise intracellular mechanisms of osthol in defending and fighting against cancer are recommended. Also, well-designed randomized clinical trials are important to evaluate the safety and efficacy of osthol in patients with different types of cancers.

Acknowledgments: Authors are grateful to the deputy of Research, Kermanshah University of Medical Sciences, Kermanshah, Iran for the grant No. 93487.

Author Contributions: Y.S., M.H.F. and L.H. designed the structure of the paper and drafted the manuscript. F.J., Z.M., L.B. performed the literature search and contributed in writing the manuscript. A.B., P.B., N.C., M.B.Y., A.A.F. and S.M.N. reviewed and revised the manuscript. All authors had full access to the final version of the manuscript and gave their approval before publishing.

Conflicts of Interest: The authors declare no conflict of interest.

References

1. World-Health-Organization. Cancer: Fact Sheet No. 297. 2015. Available online: http://www.who.int (accessed on 2 October 2016).
2. Jena, J.; Ranjan, R.; Ranjan, P.; Sarangi, M.K. A Study on Natural Anticancer Plants. *Int. J. Pharm. Chem. Sci.* **2012**, *1*, 365–368.
3. Padmaja, G.; Vanlalhruaii, C.; Rana, S.; Nandinee, D.; Hariharan, M. Care givers' depression, anxiety, distress, and somatization as predictors of identical symptoms in cancer patients. *J. Cancer Res. Ther.* **2016**, *12*, 53–57. [CrossRef] [PubMed]
4. Safarzadeh, E.; Sandoghchian, S.S.; Baradaran, B. Herbal medicine as inducers of apoptosis in cancer treatment. *Adv. Pharm. Bull.* **2014**, *4*, 421–427. [PubMed]
5. Hemalswarya, S.; Doble, M. Potential synergism of natural products in the treatment of cancer. *Phytother. Res.* **2006**, *20*, 239–249. [CrossRef] [PubMed]
6. Cragg, G.M.; Newman, D.J. Plants as a source of anti-cancer agents. *J. Ethnopharmacol.* **2005**, *100*, 72–79. [CrossRef] [PubMed]
7. Guan, X.; Sun, Z.; Chen, X.; Wu, H.; Zhang, X. Inhibitory effects of Zengshengping fractions on DMBA-induced buccal pouch carcinogenesis in hamsters. *Chin. Med. J.* **2012**, *125*, 332–337. [CrossRef] [PubMed]
8. Sadeghi-Aliabadi, H.; Aliasgharluo, M.; Fattahi, A.; Mirian, M.; Ghanadian, M. In vitro cytotoxic evaluation of some synthesized COX-2 inhibitor derivatives against a panel of human cancer cell lines. *Res. Pharm. Sci.* **2013**, *8*, 298–303. [PubMed]
9. Mukhtar, E.; Adhami, V.M.; Mukhtar, H. Targeting microtubules by natural agents for cancer therapy. *Mol. Cancer Ther.* **2014**, *13*, 275–284. [CrossRef] [PubMed]
10. Basmadjian, C.; Zhao, Q.; Bentouhami, E.; Djehal, A.; Nebigil, C.G.; Johnson, R.A.; Serova, M.; De Gramont, A.; Faivre, S.; Raymond, E.; et al. Cancer wars: Natural products strike back. *Front. Chem.* **2014**, *2*, 20. [CrossRef] [PubMed]
11. Vergara, D.; De Domenico, S.; Tinelli, A.; Stanca, E.; Del Mercato, L.L.; Giudetti, A.M.; Simeone, P.; Guazzelli, N.; Lessi, M.; Manzini, C.; et al. Anticancer effects of novel resveratrol analogues on human ovarian cancer cells. *Mol. BioSyst.* **2017**, *13*, 1131–1141. [CrossRef] [PubMed]
12. Ahmadi, F.; Derakhshandeh, K.; Jalalizadeh, A.; Mostafaie, A.; Hosseinzadeh, L. Encapsulation in PLGA-PEG enhances 9-nitro-camptothecin cytotoxicity to human ovarian carcinoma cell line through apoptosis pathway. *Res. Pharm. Sci.* **2015**, *10*, 161–168. [PubMed]
13. Newman, D.J.; Giddings, L.-A. Natural products as leads to antitumor drugs. *Phytochem. Rev.* **2014**, *13*, 123–137. [CrossRef]
14. Farzaei, M.H.; Bahramsoltani, R.; Rahimi, R. Phytochemicals as adjunctive with conventional anticancer therapies. *Curr. Pharm. Des.* **2016**, *22*, 4201–4218. [CrossRef] [PubMed]
15. Nobili, S.; Lippi, D.; Witort, E.; Donnini, M.; Bausi, L.; Mini, E.; Capaccioli, S. Natural compounds for cancer treatment and prevention. *Pharmacol. Res.* **2009**, *59*, 365–378. [CrossRef] [PubMed]
16. Ashley, R.E.; Osheroff, N. Natural products as topoisomerase II poisons: Effects of thymoquinone on DNA cleavage mediated by human topoisomerase IIα. *Chem. Res. Toxicol.* **2014**, *27*, 787–793. [CrossRef] [PubMed]
17. Schafer, G.; Kaschula, C.H. The immunomodulation and anti-inflammatory effects of garlic organosulfur compounds in cancer chemoprevention. *Anti-Cancer Agents Med. Chem.* **2014**, *14*, 233–240. [CrossRef]
18. Shokoohinia, Y.; Hosseinzadeh, L.; Moieni-Arya, M.; Mostafaie, A.; Mohammadi-Motlagh, H.-R. Osthole attenuates doxorubicin-induced apoptosis in PC12 cells through inhibition of mitochondrial dysfunction and ROS production. *BioMed Res. Int.* **2014**, *2014*, 156848. [CrossRef] [PubMed]
19. Bishayee, A.; Sethi, G. Bioactive natural products in cancer prevention and therapy: Progress and promise. *Semin. Cancer Biol.* **2016**, *40–41*, 1–3. [CrossRef] [PubMed]

20. Block, K.I.; Gyllenhaal, C.; Lowe, L.; Amedei, A.; Amin, A.R.; Amin, A.; Aquilano, K.; Arbiser, J.; Arreola, A.; Arzumanyan, A. Designing a broad-spectrum integrative approach for cancer prevention and treatment. *Semin. Cancer Biol.* **2015**, *35*, S276–S304. [CrossRef] [PubMed]

21. Shanmugam, M.K.; Lee, J.H.; Chai, E.Z.P.; Kanchi, M.M.; Kar, S.; Arfuso, F.; Dharmarajan, A.; Kumar, A.P.; Ramar, P.S.; Looi, C.Y. Cancer prevention and therapy through the modulation of transcription factors by bioactive natural compounds. *Semin. Cancer Biol.* **2016**, *40–41*, 35–47. [CrossRef] [PubMed]

22. Waksmundzka-Hajnos, M.; Sherma, J.; Kowalska, T. *Thin Layer Chromatography in Phytochemistry*; CRC Press: Boca Raton, FL, USA, 2008.

23. Sajjadi, S.; Zeinvand, H.; Shokoohinia, Y. Isolation and identification of osthol from the fruits and essential oil composition of the leaves of *Prangos asperula* Boiss. *Res. Pharm. Sci.* **2009**, *4*, 19–23.

24. Sajjadi, S.E.; Shokoohinia, Y.; Hemmati, S. Isolation and identification of furanocoumarins and a phenylpropanoid from the acetone extract and identification of volatile constituents from the essential oil of *Peucedanum pastinacifolium*. *Chem. Nat. Compd.* **2012**, *48*, 668–671. [CrossRef]

25. Ahmadi, F.; Valadbeigi, S.; Sajjadi, S.; Shokoohinia, Y.; Azizian, H.; Taheripak, G. Grandivittin as a natural minor groove binder extracted from Ferulago macrocarpa to ct-DNA, experimental and in silico analysis. *Chem. Biol. Interact.* **2016**, *258*, 89–101. [CrossRef] [PubMed]

26. Venugopala, K.-N.; Rashmi, V.; Odhav, B. Review on natural coumarin lead compounds for their pharmacological activity. *BioMed Res Int.* **2013**, *2013*, 963248. [CrossRef] [PubMed]

27. Shokoohinia, Y.; Gheibi, S.; Kiani, A.; Sadrjavadi, K.; Nowroozi, A.; Shahlaei, M. Multi-spectroscopic and molecular modeling investigation of the interactions between prantschimgin and matrix metalloproteinase 9 (MMP9). *Luminescence* **2015**, *31*, 587–593. [CrossRef] [PubMed]

28. Ghannadi, A.; Fattahian, K.; Shokoohinia, Y.; Behbahani, M.; Shahnoush, A. Anti-viral evaluation of sesquiterpene coumarins from *Ferula assa-foetida* against HSV-1. *Iran. J. Pharm. Res.* **2014**, *13*, 523–530. [PubMed]

29. Sajjadi, S.E.; Eskandarian, A.-A.; Shokoohinia, Y.; Yousefi, H.-A.; Mansourian, M.; Asgarian-Nasab, H.; Mohseni, N. Antileishmanial activity of prenylated coumarins isolated from *Ferulago angulata* and *Prangos asperula*. *Res. Pharm. Sci.* **2016**, *11*, 324–331. [CrossRef] [PubMed]

30. Kiani, A.; Almasi, K.; Shokoohinia, Y.; Sadrjavadi, K.; Nowroozi, A.; Shahlaei, M. Combined spectroscopy and molecular modeling studies on the binding of galbanic acid and MMP9. *Int. J. Biol. Macromol.* **2015**, *81*, 308–315. [CrossRef] [PubMed]

31. Sadraei, H.; Shokoohinia, Y.; Sajjadi, S.E.; Mozafari, M. Antispasmodic effects of *Prangos ferulacea* acetone extract and its main component osthole on ileum contraction. *Res. Pharm. Sci.* **2013**, *8*, 137–144. [PubMed]

32. Ceska, O.; Chaudhary, S.; Warrington, P.; Ashwood-Smith, M. Photoactive furocoumarins in fruits of some umbellifers. *Phytochemistry* **1986**, *26*, 165–169. [CrossRef]

33. Ranjbar, S.; Shokoohinia, Y.; Ghobadi, S.; Bijari, N.; Gholamzadeh, S.; Moradi, N.; Ashrafi-Kooshk, M.R.; Aghaei, A.; Khodarahmi, R. Studies of the interaction between isoimperatorin and human serum albumin by multispectroscopic method: Identification of possible binding site of the compound using esterase activity of the protein. *Sci. World J.* **2013**, *2013*, 305081. [CrossRef] [PubMed]

34. Bijari, N.; Shokoohinia, Y.; Ashrafi-Kooshk, M.R.; Ranjbar, S.; Parvaneh, S.; Moieni-Arya, M.; Khodarahmi, R. Spectroscopic study of interaction between osthole and human serum albumin: Identification of possible binding site of the compound. *J. Lumin.* **2013**, *143*, 328–336. [CrossRef]

35. Thakur, A.; Singla, R.; Jaitak, V. Coumarins as anticancer agents: A review on synthetic strategies, mechanism of action and SAR studies. *Eur. J. Med. Chem.* **2015**, *101*, 476–495. [CrossRef] [PubMed]

36. Geisler, J.; Sasano, H.; Chen, S.; Purohit, A. Steroid sulfatase inhibitors: Promising new tools for breast cancer therapy? *J. Steroid Biochem. Mol. Biol.* **2011**, *125*, 39–45. [CrossRef] [PubMed]

37. Jelodarian, Z.; Shokoohinia, Y.; Rashidi, M.; Ghiasvand, N.; Hosseinzadeh, L.; Iranshahi, M. New polyacetylenes from *Echinophora cinerea* (Boiss.) Hedge et Lamond. *Nat. Prod. Res.* **2017**, *31*, 2256–2263. [CrossRef] [PubMed]

38. You, L.; Feng, S.; An, R.; Wang, X. Osthole: A promising lead compound for drug discovery from a traditional Chinese medicine (TCM). *Nat. Prod. Commun.* **2009**, *4*, 297–302. [PubMed]

39. Zhang, Q.; Qin, L.; He, W.; Van Puyvelde, L.; Maes, D.; Adams, A.; Zheng, H.; De Kimpe, N. Coumarins from *Cnidium monnieri* and their antiosteoporotic activity. *Planta Med.* **2007**, *73*, 13–19. [CrossRef] [PubMed]

40. Wang, S.-J.; Lin, T.-Y.; Lu, C.-W.; Huang, W.-J. Osthole and imperatorin, the active constituents of *Cnidium monnieri* (L.) Cusson, facilitate glutamate release from rat hippocampal nerve terminals. *Neurochem. Int.* **2008**, *53*, 416–423. [CrossRef] [PubMed]

41. Sadraei, H.; Shokoohinia, Y.; Sajjadi, S.; Ghadirian, B. Antispasmodic effect of osthole and *Prangos ferulacea* extract on rat uterus smooth muscle motility. *Res. Pharm. Sci.* **2012**, *7*, 141–149. [PubMed]

42. Resch, M.; Steigel, A.; Chen, Z.-L.; Bauer, R. 5-Lipoxygenase and cyclooxygenase-1 inhibitory active compounds from *Atractylodes lancea*. *J. Nat. Prod.* **1998**, *61*, 347–350. [CrossRef] [PubMed]

43. Zhang, W.; Ma, D.; Zhao, Q.; Ishida, T. The effect of the major components of *Fructus Cnidii* on osteoblasts in vitro. *J. Acupunct. Meridian Stud.* **2010**, *3*, 32–37. [CrossRef]

44. Huang, R.; Chen, C.; Huang, Y.; Hsieh, D.; Hu, C.; Chang, C. Osthole increases glycosylation of hepatitis B surface antigen and suppresses the secretion of hepatitis B virus in vitro. *Hepatology* **1996**, *24*, 508–515. [CrossRef] [PubMed]

45. Guh, J.-H.; Yu, S.-M.; Ko, F.-N.; Wu, T.-S.; Teng, C.-M. Antiproliferative effect in rat vascular smooth muscle cells by osthole, isolated from *Angelica pubescens*. *Eur. J. Pharmacol.* **1996**, *298*, 191–197. [CrossRef]

46. Gholamzadeh, S.; Behbahani, M.; Fattahi, A.; Sajjadi, S.; Shokoohinia, Y. Antiviral evaluation of coumarins from *Prangos ferulacea* L. (Lindl). *Res. Pharm. Sci.* **2012**, *7*, S783.

47. Kermani, E.-K.; Sajjadi, S.-E.; Hejazi, S.-H.; Arjmand, R.; Saberi, S.; Eskandarian, A.-A. Anti-Leishmania activity of osthole. *Pharmacog. Res.* **2016**, *8* (Suppl. 1), S1. [CrossRef] [PubMed]

48. Huang, S.-M.; Tsai, C.-F.; Chen, D.-R.; Wang, M.-Y.; Yeh, W.-L. p53 is a key regulator for osthole-triggered cancer pathogenesis. *BioMed Res. Int.* **2014**, *2014*, 175247. [CrossRef] [PubMed]

49. Shokoohinia, Y.; Hosseinzadeh, L.; Alipour, M.; Mostafaie, A.; Mohammadi-Motlagh, H.-R. Comparative evaluation of cytotoxic and apoptogenic effects of several coumarins on human cancer cell lines: Osthole induces apoptosis in p53-deficient H1299 cells. *Adv. Pharmacol. Sci.* **2014**, *2014*, 847574. [CrossRef] [PubMed]

50. Wen, Y.-C.; Lee, W.-J.; Tan, P.; Yang, S.-F.; Hsiao, M.; Lee, L.-M.; Chien, M.-H. By inhibiting snail signaling and miR-23a-3p, osthole suppresses the EMT-mediated metastatic ability in prostate cancer. *Oncotarget* **2015**, *6*, 21120–21136. [CrossRef] [PubMed]

51. Ye, Y.; Han, X.; Guo, B.; Sun, Z.; Liu, S. Combination treatment with platycodin D and osthole inhibits cell proliferation and invasion in mammary carcinoma cell lines. *Environ. Toxicol. Pharmacol.* **2013**, *36*, 115–124. [CrossRef] [PubMed]

52. Hung, C.-M.; Kuo, D.-H.; Chou, C.-H.; Su, Y.-C.; Ho, C.-T.; Way, T.-D. Osthole suppresses hepatocyte growth factor (HGF)-induced epithelial-mesenchymal transition via repression of the c-Met/Akt/mTOR pathway in human breast cancer cells. *J. Agric. Food Chem.* **2011**, *59*, 9683–9690. [CrossRef] [PubMed]

53. Lin, V.C.-H.; Chou, C.-H.; Lin, Y.-C.; Lin, J.-N.; Yu, C.-C.; Tang, C.-H.; Lin, H.-Y.; Way, T.-D. Osthole suppresses fatty acid synthase expression in HER2-overexpressing breast cancer cells through modulating Akt/mTOR pathway. *J. Agric. Food Chem.* **2010**, *58*, 4786–4793. [CrossRef] [PubMed]

54. Wu, C.; Sun, Z.; Guo, B.; Ye, Y.; Han, X.; Qin, Y.; Liu, S. Osthole inhibits bone metastasis of breast cancer. *Oncotarget* **2017**, *8*, 58480–58493. [CrossRef] [PubMed]

55. Lin, K.; Gao, Z.; Shang, B.; Sui, S.; Fu, Q. Osthole suppresses the proliferation and accelerates the apoptosis of human glioma cells via the upregulation of microRNA-16 and downregulation of MMP-9. *Mol. Med. Rep.* **2015**, *12*, 4592–4597. [CrossRef] [PubMed]

56. Ding, D.; Wei, S.; Song, Y.; Li, L.; Du, G.; Zhan, H.; Cao, Y. Osthole exhibits anti-cancer property in rat glioma cells through inhibiting PI3K/Akt and MAPK signaling pathways. *Cell. Physiol. Biochem.* **2013**, *32*, 1751–1760. [CrossRef] [PubMed]

57. Lin, Y.-C.; Lin, J.-C.; Hung, C.-M.; Chen, Y.; Liu, L.-C.; Chang, T.-C.; Kao, J.-Y.; Ho, C.-T.; Way, T.-D. Osthole inhibits insulin-like growth factor-1-induced epithelial to mesenchymal transition via the inhibition of PI3K/Akt signaling pathway in human brain cancer cells. *J. Agric. Food Chem.* **2014**, *62*, 5061–5071. [CrossRef] [PubMed]

58. Xu, X.-M.; Zhang, Y.; Qu, D.; Feng, X.-W.; Chen, Y.; Zhao, L. Osthole suppresses migration and invasion of A549 human lung cancer cells through inhibition of matrix metalloproteinase-2 and matrix metallopeptidase-9 in vitro. *Mol. Med. Rep.* **2012**, *6*, 1018–1022. [CrossRef] [PubMed]

59. Feng, H.; Lu, J.-J.; Wang, Y.; Pei, L.; Chen, X. Osthole inhibited TGF β-induced epithelial–mesenchymal transition (EMT) by suppressing NF-κB mediated Snail activation in lung cancer A549 cells. *Cell Adhes. Migr.* **2017**, *11*, 464–475. [CrossRef] [PubMed]

60. Wang, H.; Jia, X.-H.; Chen, J.-R.; Wang, J.-Y.; Li, Y.-J. Osthole shows the potential to overcome P-glycoprotein-mediated multidrug resistance in human myelogenous leukemia K562/ADM cells by inhibiting the PI3K/Akt signaling pathway. *Oncol. Rep.* **2016**, *35*, 3659–3668. [CrossRef] [PubMed]

61. Chou, S.Y.; Hsu, C.S.; Wang, K.T.; Wang, M.C.; Wang, C.C. Antitumor effects of Osthol from *Cnidium monnieri*: An in vitro and in vivo study. *Phytother. Res.* **2007**, *21*, 226–230. [CrossRef] [PubMed]

62. Jiang, G.; Liu, J.; Ren, B.; Tang, Y.; Owusu, L.; Li, M.; Zhang, J.; Liu, L.; Li, W. Anti-tumor effects of osthole on ovarian cancer cells in vitro. *J. Ethnopharmacol.* **2016**, *193*, 368–376. [CrossRef] [PubMed]

63. Min, K.-J.; Han, M.; Kim, S.; Park, J.-W.; Kwon, T.K. Osthole enhances TRAIL-mediated apoptosis through downregulation of c-FLIP expression in renal carcinoma Caki cells. *Oncol. Rep.* **2017**, *37*, 2348–2354. [CrossRef] [PubMed]

64. Lin, Z.-K.; Liu, J.; Jiang, G.-Q.; Tan, G.; Gong, P.; Luo, H.-F.; Li, H.-M.; Du, J.; Ning, Z.; Xin, Y. Osthole inhibits the tumorigenesis of hepatocellular carcinoma cells. *Oncol. Rep.* **2017**, *37*, 1611–1618. [CrossRef] [PubMed]

65. Friend, S. p53: A glimpse at the puppet behind the shadow play. *Science* **1994**, *265*, 334–336. [CrossRef] [PubMed]

66. Livingstone, L.R.; White, A.; Sprouse, J.; Livanos, E.; Jacks, T.; Tlsty, T.D. Altered cell cycle arrest and gene amplification potential accompany loss of wild-type p53. *Cell* **1992**, *70*, 923–935. [CrossRef]

67. Hosseinzadeh, L.; Behravan, J.; Mosaffa, F.; Bahrami, G.; Bahrami, A.R.; Karimi, G. Effect of curcumin on doxorubicin-induced cytotoxicity in H9c2 cardiomyoblast cells. *Iran. J. Basic Med. Sci.* **2011**, *14*, 49–56.

68. Elmore, S. Apoptosis: A review of programmed cell death. *Toxicol. Pathol.* **2007**, *35*, 495–516. [CrossRef] [PubMed]

69. Amaral, J.D.; Xavier, J.M.; Steer, C.J.; Rodrigues, C.M. The role of p53 in apoptosis. *Discov. Med.* **2010**, *9*, 145–152. [PubMed]

70. Mao, H.L.; Liu, P.S.; Zheng, J.F.; hai Zhang, P.; Zhou, L.G.; Xin, G.; Liu, C. Transfection of Smac/DIABLO sensitizes drug-resistant tumor cells to TRAIL or paclitaxel-induced apoptosis in vitro. *Pharmacol. Res.* **2007**, *56*, 483–492. [CrossRef] [PubMed]

71. Jemal, A.; Bray, F.; Center, M.M.; Ferlay, J.; Ward, E.; Forman, D. Global cancer statistics. *CA Cancer J. Clin.* **2011**, *61*, 69–90. [CrossRef] [PubMed]

72. De Cicco, P.; Panza, E.; Armogida, C.; Ercolano, G.; Taglialatela-Scafati, O.; Shokoohinia, Y.; Camerlingo, R.; Pirozzi, G.; Calderone, V.; Cirino, G.; et al. The hydrogen sulfide releasing molecule acetyl deacylasadisulfide inhibits metastatic melanoma. *Front. Pharmacol.* **2017**, *8*, 65. [CrossRef] [PubMed]

73. Sun, Y.-C.; Wang, J.; Guo, C.-C.; Sai, K.; Wang, J.; Chen, F.-R.; Yang, Q.-Y.; Chen, Y.-S.; Wang, J.; To, T.S.-S.; et al. MiR-181b sensitizes glioma cells to teniposide by targeting MDM2. *BMC Cancer* **2014**, *14*, 611. [CrossRef] [PubMed]

74. Gheibi, S.; Shokohinia, Y.; Kiani, A.; Sadrjavadi, K.; Nowroozi, A.; Shahlaei, M. Molecular insight into the Grandivitin-matrix metalloproteinase 9 interactions. *J. Photochem. Photobiol. B* **2016**, *162*, 493–499. [CrossRef] [PubMed]

75. Tatevossian, R.G.; Lawson, A.R.; Forshew, T.; Hindley, G.F.; Ellison, D.W.; Sheer, D. MAPK pathway activation and the origins of pediatric low-grade astrocytomas. *J. Cell. Physiol.* **2010**, *222*, 509–514. [CrossRef] [PubMed]

76. Balmanno, K.; Cook, S. Tumour cell survival signalling by the ERK1/2 pathway. *Cell Death Differ.* **2009**, *16*, 368–377. [CrossRef] [PubMed]

77. Luo, J.; Manning, B.D.; Cantley, L.C. Targeting the PI3K-Akt pathway in human cancer: Rationale and promise. *Cancer Cell* **2003**, *4*, 257–262. [CrossRef]

78. Buckner, J.C. Factors influencing survival in high-grade gliomas. In *Seminars in Oncology*; WB Saunders: Philadelphia, PA, USA, 2003; Volume 30, pp. 10–14.

79. Chen, Y.-H.; Hung, M.-C.; Shyu, W.-C. Role of cancer stem cells in brain tumors. *Biomedicine* **2012**, *2*, 84–91. [CrossRef]

80. Zhang, X.; Chen, T.; Zhang, J.; Mao, Q.; Li, S.; Xiong, W.; Qiu, Y.; Xie, Q.; Ge, J. Notch1 promotes glioma cell migration and invasion by stimulating β-catenin and NF-κB signaling via AKT activation. *Cancer Sci.* **2012**, *103*, 181–190. [CrossRef] [PubMed]

81. Wilken, R.; Veena, M.S.; Wang, M.B.; Srivatsan, E.S. Curcumin: A review of anti-cancer properties and therapeutic activity in head and neck squamous cell carcinoma. *Mol. Cancer* **2011**, *10*, 12. [CrossRef] [PubMed]

82. Jemal, A.; Siegel, R.; Ward, E.; Hao, Y.; Xu, J.; Murray, T.; Thun, M.J. Cancer statistics, 2008. *CA Cancer J. Clin.* **2008**, *58*, 71–96. [CrossRef] [PubMed]

83. Parkin, D.M.; Bray, F.; Ferlay, J.; Pisani, P. Global cancer statistics, 2002. *CA Cancer J. Clin.* **2005**, *55*, 74–108. [CrossRef] [PubMed]

84. Xu, X.; Zhang, Y.; Qu, D.; Jiang, T.; Li, S. Osthole induces G2/M arrest and apoptosis in lung cancer A549 cells by modulating PI3K/Akt pathway. *J. Exp. Clin. Cancer Res.* **2011**, *30*, 33. [CrossRef] [PubMed]

85. Mathisen, M.S.; Kantarjian, H.M.; Cortes, J.; Jabbour, E. Mutant BCR-ABL clones in chronic myeloid leukemia. *Haematologica* **2011**, *96*, 347–349. [CrossRef] [PubMed]

86. Souza, P.S.; Vasconcelos, F.C.; De Souza Reis, F.R.; De Moraes, G.N.; Maia, R.C. P-glycoprotein and survivin simultaneously regulate vincristine-induced apoptosis in chronic myeloid leukemia cells. *Int. J. Oncol.* **2011**, *39*, 925–933. [PubMed]

87. Echelman, D.; Feldman, S. Management of cervical precancers: A global perspective. *Hematol. Oncol. Clin. N. Am.* **2012**, *26*, 31–44. [CrossRef] [PubMed]

88. Mei, L.; Chen, H.; Wei, D.M.; Fang, F.; Liu, G.J.; Xie, H.Y.; Wang, X.; Zou, J.; Han, X.; Feng, D. Maintenance chemotherapy for ovarian cancer. *Curr. Oncol. Rep.* **2013**, *5*, 454–458.

89. Park, J.T.; Chen, X.; Trope, C.G.; Davidson, B.; Shih, I.-M.; Wang, T.-L. Notch3 overexpression is related to the recurrence of ovarian cancer and confers resistance to carboplatin. *Am. J. Pathol.* **2010**, *177*, 1087–1094. [CrossRef] [PubMed]

90. Wells, A.; Grahovac, J.; Wheeler, S.; Ma, B.; Lauffenburger, D. Targeting tumor cell motility as a strategy against invasion and metastasis. *Trends Pharmacol. Sci.* **2013**, *34*, 283–289. [CrossRef] [PubMed]

91. Ahmadi, F.; Shokoohinia, Y.; Javaheri, S.; Azizian, H. Proposed binding mechanism of galbanic acid extracted from *Ferula assa–foetida* to DNA. *J. Photochem. Photobiol. B* **2017**, *166*, 63–73. [CrossRef] [PubMed]

92. Shokoohinia, Y.; Khajouei, S.; Ahmadi, F.; Ghiasvand, N.; Hosseinzadeh, L. Protective effect of bioactive compounds from *Echinophora cinerea* against cisplatin-induced oxidative stress and apoptosis in the PC12 cell line. *Iran. J. Basic Med. Sci.* **2017**, *20*, 438–445. [PubMed]

93. Shokoohinia, Y.; Bazargan, S.; Miraghaee, S.; Javadirad, E.; Hosseinzadeh, L. Safety assessment of osthole isolated from *Prangos ferulacea*: Acute and subchronic toxicities and modulation of cytochrome P450. *Jundishapur J. Nat. Pharm. Prod.* **2017**. [CrossRef]

94. Davatgaran-Taghipour, Y.; Masoomzadeh, S.; Farzaei, M.H.; Bahramsoltani, R.; Karimi-Soureh, Z.; Rahimi, R.; Abdollahi, M. Polyphenol nanoformulations for cancer therapy: Experimental evidence and clinical perspective. *Int. J. Nanomed.* **2017**, *12*, 2689–2702. [CrossRef] [PubMed]

95. Peiris-Pagès, M.; Martinez-Outschoorn, U.E.; Sotgia, F.; Lisanti, M.P. Metastasis and oxidative stress: Are antioxidants a metabolic driver of progression? *Cell Metabol.* **2015**, *22*, 956–958. [CrossRef] [PubMed]

96. Panieri, E.; Santoro, M.M. ROS homeostasis and metabolism: A dangerous liaison in cancer cells. *Cell Death Dis.* **2016**, *7*, e2253. [CrossRef] [PubMed]

97. Nelson, K.K.; Melendez, J.A. Mitochondrial redox control of matrix metallopro-teinases. *Free Radic. Biol. Med.* **2004**, *37*, 768–784. [CrossRef] [PubMed]

98. Morry, J.; Ngamcherdtrakul, W.; Yantasee, W. Oxidative stress in cancer and fibrosis: Opportunity for therapeutic intervention with antioxidant compounds, enzymes, and nanoparticles. *Redox Biol.* **2017**, *11*, 240–253. [CrossRef] [PubMed]

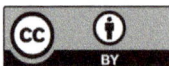

nutrients

MDPI

Review

Soy Consumption and the Risk of Prostate Cancer: An Updated Systematic Review and Meta-Analysis

Catherine C. Applegate [1], Joe L. Rowles III [1], Katherine M. Ranard [1], Sookyoung Jeon [1] and John W. Erdman Jr. [1,2,*]

[1] Division of Nutritional Sciences, University of Illinois at Urbana-Champaign, Urbana, IL 61801, USA; cca2@illinois.edu (C.C.A.); jrowles2@illinois.edu (J.L.R.); ranard2@illinois.edu (K.M.R.); sjeon17@illinois.edu (S.J.)
[2] Department of Food Science and Human Nutrition, University of Illinois at Urbana-Champaign, Urbana, IL 61801, USA
* Correspondence: jwerdman@illinois.edu; Tel.: +1-217-333-2527; Fax: +1-217-333-9368

Received: 29 November 2017; Accepted: 28 December 2017; Published: 4 January 2018

Abstract: Prostate cancer (PCa) is the second most commonly diagnosed cancer in men, accounting for 15% of all cancers in men worldwide. Asian populations consume soy foods as part of a regular diet, which may contribute to the lower PCa incidence observed in these countries. This meta-analysis provides a comprehensive updated analysis that builds on previously published meta-analyses, demonstrating that soy foods and their isoflavones (genistein and daidzein) are associated with a lower risk of prostate carcinogenesis. Thirty articles were included for analysis of the potential impacts of soy food intake, isoflavone intake, and circulating isoflavone levels, on both primary and advanced PCa. Total soy food ($p < 0.001$), genistein ($p = 0.008$), daidzein ($p = 0.018$), and unfermented soy food ($p < 0.001$) intakes were significantly associated with a reduced risk of PCa. Fermented soy food intake, total isoflavone intake, and circulating isoflavones were not associated with PCa risk. Neither soy food intake nor circulating isoflavones were associated with advanced PCa risk, although very few studies currently exist to examine potential associations. Combined, this evidence from observational studies shows a statistically significant association between soy consumption and decreased PCa risk. Further studies are required to support soy consumption as a prophylactic dietary approach to reduce PCa carcinogenesis.

Keywords: prostate cancer; soy; isoflavones; epidemiology; cohort; case-control

---

1. Introduction

Prostate cancer (PCa) is the second most commonly diagnosed cancer in men worldwide. According to the International Agency for Research on Cancer's GLOBOCAN database, 1.1 million men were diagnosed with PCa in 2012, accounting for 15% of all cancers in men [1]. Incidence rates are lowest in Asian countries, where soy foods are regularly consumed as part of a normal diet. Several studies have reviewed the inverse association seen between soy food intake and PCa incidence in Asian populations, proposing that soy isoflavones act as weak hormones to exert a protective physiological effect against the development of PCa [2–5]. Indeed, the soy isoflavones, genistein and daidzein, have been shown to accumulate in prostatic tissue [6], where they may be cytotoxic to cancer cells [7]. These effects may occur as a result of both non-hormonal and hormonal action. For example, genistein upregulates tumor suppressor genes in PCa cells [8] and suppresses prostate carcinogenesis in an estrogen receptor (ER) wild-type mouse model, when compared to ER knock-out mouse models [9].

This hypothesis has further been supported by four previous meta-analyses of epidemiological studies, all of which showed a protective association between soy consumption and PCa [10–13]. However, these meta-analyses did not integrate and evaluate all available existing studies pertaining to both dietary soy food intake and circulating levels of isoflavones. Our current analysis broadens the included categories of soy food and isoflavone measurements, allowing for a more complete review of the literature. We include a larger number of studies and an in-depth analysis on the relationship between total soy food intake, fermented and unfermented soy food intakes, individual and combined dietary isoflavones, and circulating individual and combined isoflavones and the risk of PCa. Furthermore, no previous meta-analysis has explored potential links between soy foods and advanced PCa. Because soy isoflavones have also been linked to inhibiting PCa cell motility and invasion [14] and reducing inflammatory markers in men with PCa [15], we also evaluated the impact of soy on the risk of advanced PCa.

2. Materials and Methods

2.1. Study Selection Criteria

This meta-analysis was conducted following PRISMA and Meta-analysis of Observational Studies in Epidemiology (MOOSE) guidelines [16,17]. Studies fitting the following criteria were included in this meta-analysis: (a) examined the relationship between soy and PCa risk by using randomized control trials and/or cohort, cross-sectional, retrospective, prospective and case-control studies; (b) methodology was reported in replicable detail; (c) examined the association between soy and PCa risk; (d) reported relative risk ratios with 95% confidence intervals for the reported exposure categories; (e) were written in English; and (f) were peer-reviewed publications.

2.2. Literature Search

We conducted a thorough literature search of PubMed, Web of Science, and the Cochrane Library, using a combination of the following key words and their variants: prostate cancer, prostate neoplasm, soy, soymilk, soy milk, isoflavone, bean curd, tofu, soy protein, daidzein and genistein (up to 25 May 2017). The keyword search yielded a comprehensive list of titles and abstracts of articles that were screened for relevance against the listed study selection criteria. These screened articles were evaluated in full text for study inclusion. Finally, we conducted a reference list search (i.e., backward search) and works cited search (i.e., forward search) from the articles identified as meeting the inclusion criteria. The studies identified through this process were further assessed using the same inclusion criteria, with this process being repeated until all relevant articles were identified. Three authors (CA, JR3 and KR) individually considered all articles obtained in full text for inclusion or exclusion, and any discrepancies were discussed and resolved.

2.3. Data Extraction and Quality Assessment

The following information was extricated from each article: name of first author; year of publication; location of study; study period; number of cases, controls and total number of participants in the study; age of participants; total years of follow-up; exposure values of soy (serum/plasma and/or intake); relative risk ratios for PCa; adjustments made for any covariates; and study type. The term RR (relative risk) will be used in this study as a general term to denote the following: relative odds (cumulative incidence data), rate ratio (incidence-rate data) and odds ratios (OR; case-control data). Study quality was examined using the Newcastle–Ottawa Scale, which is a validated scale used to assess the quality for case-control and non-randomized cohorts in a meta-analysis [18]. This scale evaluates each study based on the following three categories: selection of cases and controls, comparability of studies, and exposure of the main variable (soy, genistein, daidzein, or total isoflavones). We regarded scores of 1–3, 4–6 and 7–9 as low, medium and high quality, respectively. The resulting quality score was included as a measurement of the strength of the evidence presented in each study and was not used to determine the inclusion or exclusion of studies. The significance of the study quality was analyzed in the subgroup analysis.

2.4. Statistical Analysis

STATA/IC version 14.2 (StataCorp LP, College Station, TX, USA) was used to analyze the data. Because OR is nearly equivalent to RR when considering low incidence of diseases [19], RR and 95% confidence intervals (CI) were used as a measure of the effect size for all included studies. Heterogeneity amongst studies was determined using the I^2 statistic [20]. Fixed and random (DerSimonian–Laird) effects models were used, depending on the I^2 result, as markers of study heterogeneity [20]. An I^2 value of less than 50% ($I^2 < 50\%$) signified low-to-moderate heterogeneity between studies, so a fixed effect model was used to determine RR estimates. An I^2 value of greater than or equal to 50% ($I^2 \geq 50\%$) signified moderate-to-substantial heterogeneity between studies, so a random effects model was used to determine RR estimates. When results from fixed and random effects models were conflicting and studies showed moderate heterogeneity ($I^2 = 30$–60%), we presented the latter as it represents a more conservative approach [21,22].

Because studies reported different exposure categories as tertiles, quartiles or quintiles, we used the study specific RR for the highest quantile of dietary soy intake and/or circulating (serum or plasma) isoflavone concentrations. Potential publication bias was assessed by using funnel plots [23,24], Egger's linear regression test [25], and Begg's rank correlation test of asymmetry [26]. We also performed sensitivity analyses to evaluate whether the pooled results could have been affected by excluding a single study at a time. Subgroup analyses were performed on study type, study location, study quality, and individual covariate adjustment. A *p*-value of less than 0.05 was considered statistically significant for all analyses.

3. Results

3.1. Literature Search

In total, 3356 articles were identified from the library search engines. After removing duplicates and adding articles identified from reference lists, 2531 articles remained. Of the 2531 articles that were screened by abstract, 39 articles were found to contain potentially relevant information and were evaluated by full text review. Upon reviewing the full text articles for the aforementioned inclusion criteria, 30 articles were included in the final analysis [27–56]. Of these 30 articles, 24 [27–34,36–43,45–49,52,53,55] included information regarding dietary soy intake and nine [29,35,40,42,44,50,51,54,56] included information regarding circulating isoflavone levels (Figure 1).

3.2. Study Characteristics

Of the 30 articles included for analysis, fifteen [28–30,32,34,37–39,41,42,47–49,52,56] articles were case-control studies, eight [27,31,33,36,43,45,46,53] articles were cohort studies, and seven [35,40,44,50,51,54,55] articles were nested case-control studies (NCC). The total number of study participants included was 266,699, and the total number of PCa cases reported was 21,612. Twelve [27,32,35–37,39,41,42,44,47,49,56] articles reported data from Asia, ten [31,33,34,38,43,45,46,48,52,53] articles reported data from North America, and eight [28–30,40,50,51,54,55] articles reported data from Europe. The study characteristics are summarized in Table 1. Articles analyzing soy intake from the diet used lifestyle questionnaires or validated food frequency questionnaires (FFQs) to collect usual dietary intake. All articles reported results using risk estimates as RR or OR.

Quality scores were assigned to each article using the criteria outlined by the Newcastle–Ottawa scales for case-control and cohort studies. The average score for case-control studies was 6.93 (standard deviation = 0.7); 6 was the lowest score and 8 was the highest score given. Cohort and NCC studies received an average score of 7.73 (standard deviation = 0.7); 6 was the lowest score and 9 was the highest score given. Individual quality assessment scores are provided in Appendix A (Table A1).

3.3. Soy Intake and PCa Risk

Twenty-four articles evaluated dietary soy and soy isoflavone intake and PCa risk. These articles were further divided into groups that analyzed risk pertaining to total soy (n = 16) [27,29,31–34,36,37,39, 41,43,45–47,49,52], unfermented soy food (n = 11) [27,31,33,34,37,39,43,46,47,49,52], fermented soy food (n = 8) [27,32,36,37,41,45–47], genistein (n = 10) [30,36–38,40–42,45,48,55], daidzein (n = 10) [30,36–38,40–42,45,48,55], total isoflavones (n = 6) [28–30,45,53,55], tofu (n = 5) [27,37,43,46,47], miso (n = 3) [27,36,46], soy milk (n = 2) [31,49], and natto (n = 1) [47] intakes. Funnel plots used to explore publication bias are shown in Appendix A (Figure 1).

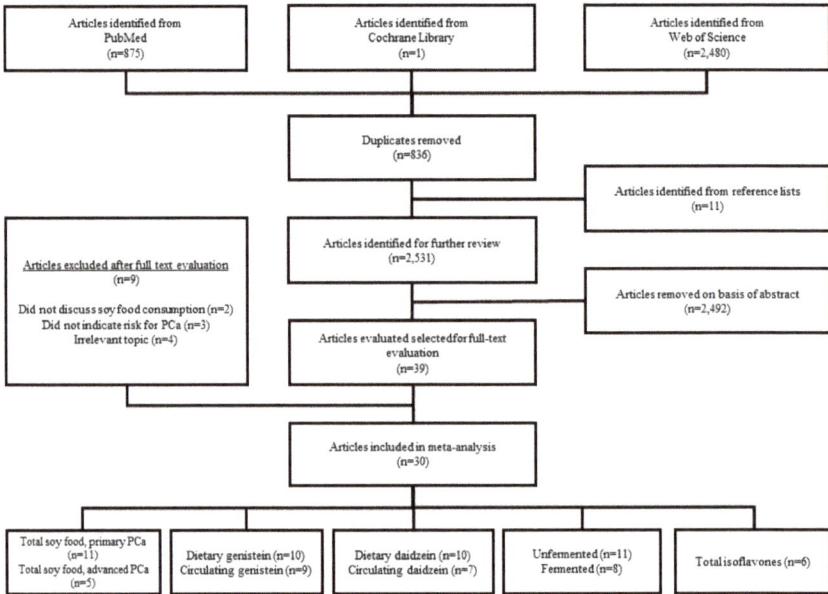

Figure 1. Literature search and study selection flow chart.

Articles that reported soy intake as either a combination of multiple soy food items or as a single soy food item were classified as total soy intake. Sixteen articles reported the association between total soy intake and PCa risk. The pooled RR for this association was 0.71 (95% CI: 0.58–0.85, p < 0.001) (Figure 2A). Neither Begg's correlation test (p = 0.300) nor Egger's linear regression test (p = 0.052) for bias were significant. Heterogeneity amongst studies was analyzed using the I^2 index to show high variation between studies (68.9%).

When selecting articles for evaluating the association between unfermented or fermented soy food intake and PCa risk, studies had to have explicitly stated which soy food items were being reported. Examples of commonly reported unfermented soy foods included soy milk, tofu and soybeans; fermented soy foods included miso and natto. The pooled RR for unfermented soy foods and risk of PCa was 0.65 (95% CI: 0.56–0.83, p < 0.001), and the pooled RR for fermented soy foods and risk of PCa was 0.86 (95% CI: 0.66–1.13, p = 0.218) (Figure 2B,C, respectively). Neither Begg's correlation test (p = 0.161 and p = 0.902, respectively) nor Egger's linear regression test (p = 0.117 and p = 0.670, respectively) for bias were significant. The I^2 index showed high heterogeneity amongst studies included in the unfermented (60.3%) and fermented (66.6%) groups.

Table 1. Characteristics of included studies.

Author, Year	Country	Exposure	Exposure Type	Cases/Sample	Study Type	Study Period (Years)	Adjustments	Participant Age Range, Mean (SD)	Exposure Measurement (Intake or Circulating)
Allen, 2004 [27]	Japan	Total soy, miso, tofu	Diet	196/18,115	Cohort	1950–1996	Age, education, geographic area, city of residence, radiation dose	51–89 Cases: 75	Tofu, miso: T1 < 2x/week, T3 = almost daily; Total soy: T1 = low, T3 = high
Bosetti, 2006 [28]	Italy	Total isoflavones	Diet	1294/2745	Case–Control	1991–2002	Age, BMI, FHPC, education, energy, study center	46–74 Cases: 66 Controls: 63	Q1 ≤ 14.7 µg/day, Q5 > 32.2 µg/day
Heald, 2007 [29]	Scotland	Total isoflavones, total soy	Diet	437/920	Case–Control	1998–2001	Age, smoking, FHPC, energy, family history of breast cancer, Carstairs Deprivation Index, smoking and energy intake:BMR ratio	50–74 Cases: 67.2 (5.5) Controls: 66.0 (5.4)	Isoflavones (µg/day): Q1 < 581.1, Q4 > 1982.2 Soy food: no, yes
		Genistein, daidzein, total isoflavones	Serum				Age, smoking, FHPC, family history of breast cancer, Carstairs Deprivation Index		Genistein (nmol/L): Q1 < 14.23, Q4 > 64.53; Daidzein (nmol/L): Q1 < 8.26, Q4 > 29.11; Isoflavones (nmol/L): Q1 < 25.57, Q4 > 98.86
Hedelin, 2006 [30]	Sweden	Total isoflavones, genistein, daidzein	Diet	1499/2629	Case–Control	2001–2002	Age, energy	35–79 Cases: 66.8 Controls: 67.8	Total isoflavones (µg/day): Q1 ≤ 1.0, Q4 ≥ 2.6; Genistein (µg/day): Q1 ≤ 0.27, Q4 ≥ 1.08; Daidzein (µg/day): Q1 ≤ 0.49, Q4 ≥ 1.11
Jacobsen, 1998 [31]	USA	Soy milk	Diet	225/12,395	Cohort	1976–1992	Age	≥25	Never, <daily, 1x/day, >1x/day
Jian, 2004 [32]	China	Total soy	Diet	130/404	Case–Control	2001–2002	Age, BMI, FHPC, education, PA, energy, geographic area, marital status, income, fresh vegetables and fruit consumption, tea drinking	Cases: 74.7 (7.1) Controls: 71.4 (7.2)	T1 = 0 g/day, T3 > 4.00 g/day
Kirsh, 2007 [33]	USA	Total soy	Diet	1338/29,361	Cohort	1993–2001	Age, BMI, smoking, FHPC, PA, energy, ethnicity, geographic area, supplemental vitamin E, total fat intake, red meat intake, diabetes, aspirin use, previous number of PCa screening examinations	63.3	Q1 = 0 servings/month, Q4 > 0.5 servings/month
Kolonel, 2000 [34]	USA, Canada	Total soy	Diet	1619/3237	Case–Control	1987–1991	Age, education, energy, ethnicity, geographic area	≥65	Q1 < 0.1 g/day, Q5 > 39.4 g/day
Kurahashi, 2007 [36]	Japan	Total soy, miso, genistein, daidzein	Diet	307/43,509	Cohort	1995–2004	Age, geographic area	45–74	Total soy (g/day): Q1 < 46.6, Q4 ≥ 107.4; Miso (mL/day): Q1 < 110.0, Q4 ≥ 356.0; Genistein (mg/day): Q1 < 13.2, Q4 ≥ 32.8; Daidzein (mg/day): Q1 < 8.5, Q4 ≥ 20.4

Table 1. *Cont.*

Author, Year	Country	Exposure	Exposure Type	Cases/Sample	Study Type	Study Period (Years)	Adjustments	Participant Age Range, Mean (SD)	Exposure Measurement (Intake or Circulating)
Kurahashi, 2008 [35]	Japan	Genistein, daidzein	Plasma	201/603	Nested Case-Control	1990–2005	Smoking; alcohol; marital status; intake of green tea, protein, fiber, green or yellow vegetables	40–69 Cases: 58.6 (6.4) Controls: 58.4 (6.6)	Genistein (ng/mL): T1 < 57, T3 ≥ 151.7 Daidzein (ng/mL): T1 < 22, T3 ≥ 61.5
Lee, 2003 [37]	China	Total soy, tofu, genistein, daidzein	Diet	133/398	Case-Control	1989–1992	Age, energy	50–89	Total soy (g/day): Q1 < 27.5, Q4 >111.8 Tofu (g/day): T1 < 14.3, T3 > 34.5 Genistein (mg/day): Q1 < 17.9, Q4 > 62.0 Daidzein (mg/day): Q1 < 10.0, Q4 > 36.3
Lewis, 2009 [38]	USA	Genistein, daidzein	Diet	478/860	Case-Control	1998–2004	Age, BMI, smoking, FHPC, education, energy	Controls: 62.0 (10.7) Incident cases: 63.3 (8.2) Prevalent cases: 66.9 (8.1)	Genistein (mcg/day): L ≤ 196.0, U > 196.1 Daidzein (mcg/day): L ≤ 77.0, U > 77.1
Li, 2008 [39]	China	Total soy	Diet	28/308	Case-Control	1998–2000	BMI, smoking, education, alcohol, food frequency	Cases: 71.39 (6.03) Control: 71.14 (5.78)	T1 ≤ 2x/week T3 ≥ 1x/day
Low, 2006 [40]	Europe	Genistein, daidzein	Diet	85/241	Nested Case-Control	1993–1997	BMI, FHPC, energy	45–75	Genistein average (95% CI) cases (ug/day): 287.7 (255.5–323.9); controls: 310.2 (283.0–339.9) Daidzein average (95% CI) cases (ug/day): 224.4 (198.1–254.2); controls: 249.2 (227.8–272.5)
			Plasma						Genistein average (95% CI) cases (ng/mL): 4.8 (3.6–6.4): controls: 4.4 (3.7–5.4) Daidzein average (95% CI) cases (ng/mL): 2.4 (1.8–3.1); controls: 2.4 (2.0–2.9)
Nagata, 2007 [41]	Japan	Total soy, genistein, daidzein	Diet	200/400	Case-Control	1996–2003	Smoking, energy	59–73	Total soy (isoflavones) (mg/day): Q1 < 30.5, Q4 ≥ 89.9 Genistein (mg/day): Q1 < 1.1, Q4 ≥ 2.5 Daidzein (mg/day): Q1 < 0.8, Q4 ≥ 1.9

Table 1. *Cont.*

Author, Year	Country	Exposure	Exposure Type	Cases/Sample	Study Type	Study Period (Years)	Adjustments	Participant Age Range, Mean (SD)	Exposure Measurement (Intake or Circulating)
Nagata, 2016 [42]	Japan	Genistein, daidzein	Diet	56/112	Case-Control	2011–2014	Age, BMI, smoking, alcohol, energy	Cases: 64.7 (6.6) Controls: 63.6 (9.1)	Genistein (mg/day): T1 < 17.57, T3 ≥ 36.31, Daidzein (mg/day): T1 < 11.56, T3 ≥ 21.86
		Genistein, daidzein	Serum						Genistein (ng/mL): T1 < 57.10, T3 ≥ 144.50 Daidzein (ng/mL): T1 < 18, T3 ≥ 51.7
Nomura, 2004 [43]	USA	Tofu	Diet	222/5826	Cohort	1971–1995	Age, BMI, smoking, alcohol, energy, arm muscle area	Not given	Q1 = 0 g/week, Q5 > 240 g/week
Ozasa, 2004 [44]	Japan	Genistein, daidzein	Serum	52/203	Nested Case-Control	1988–1999	Age	≥40 Cases: 69.4 Controls: 68.7	Genistein (nM): T1 < 239, T3 > 682 Daidzein (nM): T1 < 89, T3 > 239
Park, 2008 [45]	USA	Total soy, total isoflavones, genistein, daidzein	Diet	4404/82,483	Cohort	1993–1996	Time since cohort entry, ethnicity, FHPC, education, BMI, smoking, energy	45–75	Total soy (g/1000 kcal): T1: 0, T2: 0.1–2.8, T3: ≥2.8; Genistein (mg/1000 kcal): Q1 < 0.7, Q2: 0.7–1.2, Q3: 1.2–1.9, Q4: 1.9–3.1, Q5 > 3.1; Daidzein (mg/1000 kcal): Q1 < 0.7, Q2: 0.7–1.3, Q3: 1.3–2.0, Q4: 2.0–3.2, Q5 > 3.2; Total isoflavones (mg/1000 kcal): Q1 < 1.6, Q2: 1.6–2.9, Q3: 2.9–4.5, Q4: 4.5–7.2, Q5 ≥ 7.2
Severson, 1989 [46]	USA	Miso, tofu	Diet	174/7999	Cohort	1965–1986	Age	≥46	Miso: T1 ≤ 1x/week, T3 ≥ 5x/week; Tofu: T1 ≤ 1x/week, T3 ≥ 5x/week
Sonoda, 2004 [47]	Japan	Total soy, natto, tofu	Diet	140/280	Case-Control	1996–2002	Smoking, energy	59–73	Total soy (g/day): Q1 ≤ 77.0, Q4 ≥ 187.2; Tofu (g/day): Q1 ≤ 19.7, Q4 ≥ 96.4; Natto (g/day): Q1 ≤ 5.7, Q4 ≥ 40.0
Strom, 1999 [48]	USA	Genistein, daidzein	Diet	83/190	Case-Control	1996–1998	Age, FHPC, alcohol, energy	Cases: 61 (6.6) Controls: 60.6 (6.9)	Genistein mean (µg/day): cases: 19.8; controls: 29.7 Daidzein mean (µg/day): cases: 14.2; controls: 22.8
Sung, 1999 [49]	China	Soy milk	Diet	90/270	Case-Control	1995–1996	None	≥50	Yes, No

Table 1. *Cont.*

Author, Year	Country	Exposure	Exposure Type	Cases/Sample	Study Type	Study Period (Years)	Adjustments	Participant Age Range, Mean (SD)	Exposure Measurement (Intake or Circulating)
Travis, 2009 [51]	Europe	Genistein, daidzein	Plasma	950/1992	Nested Case-Control	1992–2003	BMI, smoking, education, PA, alcohol, marital status	43–76 Cases: 60.4 (5.8) Controls: 60.1 (5.8)	Genistein (ng/mL): Q1 ≤ 0.30, Q5 ≥ 7.00 Daidzein (ng/mL): Q1 ≤ 0.30, Q5 ≥ 4.10
Travis, 2012 [50]	Europe	Genistein	Plasma	655/1310	Nested Case-Control	1992–2006	BMI, smoking, education, PA, alcohol, marital status	43–76 Cases: 60.4 (5.8) Controls: 60.1 (5.8)	Genistein (ng/mL): Q1 ≤ 0.30, Q5 ≥ 6.10
Villenueve, 1999 [52]	Canada	Total soy	Diet	1623/3246	Case-Control	1994–1997	Age, geographic area	50–74	None, some
Wang, 2014 [53]	USA	Total isoflavones	Diet	3974/43,268	Cohort	1999–2009	Age	50–74	Q1 < 0.029 mg/day, Q5 ≥ 0.144 mg/day
Ward, 2008 [54]	Europe	Total isoflavones, genistein, daidzein	Plasma	194/1006	Nested Case-Control	1993–2006	Age, energy	40–79	Total isoflavones median (ng/mL): 10.3 Genistein median (ng/mL): 6.9 Daidzein median (ng/mL): 2.5
Ward, 2010 [55]	Europe	Total isoflavones, genistein, daidzein	Diet	204/1016	Nested Case-Control	1993–2006	Age	40–79	Total isoflavones mean cases (µg/day): 948.6; controls: 1088 Genistein: mean cases (µg/day): 546.6; controls: 638.2 Daidzein: mean cases (µg/day): 314.9; controls: 355.2
Wu, 2015 [56]	China	Genistein	Plasma	46/100	Case-Control	2012–2013	Age	70.1 (8.9) Cases: 72.5 (8.4) Control: 68.0 (8.8)	<640.2 nmol/L, >640.0 nmol/L

Abbreviations: body mass index (BMI), family history of prostate cancer (FHPC), basal metabolic rate (BMR), physical activity (PA).

Ten articles reported soy intake as a measurement based on the calculation of genistein and daidzein present in soy foods. The pooled RR for genistein and risk of PCa was 0.90 (95% CI: 0.84–0.97, $p = 0.008$), and the pooled RR for daidzein and risk of PCa was 0.84 (95% CI: 0.73–0.97, $p = 0.018$) (Figure 2D,E, respectively). Begg's correlation test was significant for genistein but was not significant for daidzein ($p = 0.049$ and $p = 0.210$, respectively), and Egger's linear regression test was significant for both measurements ($p = 0.009$ and $p = 0.039$, respectively). The I^2 index showed moderate heterogeneity between studies included in the genistein (31.0%) and daidzein (50.5%) groups.

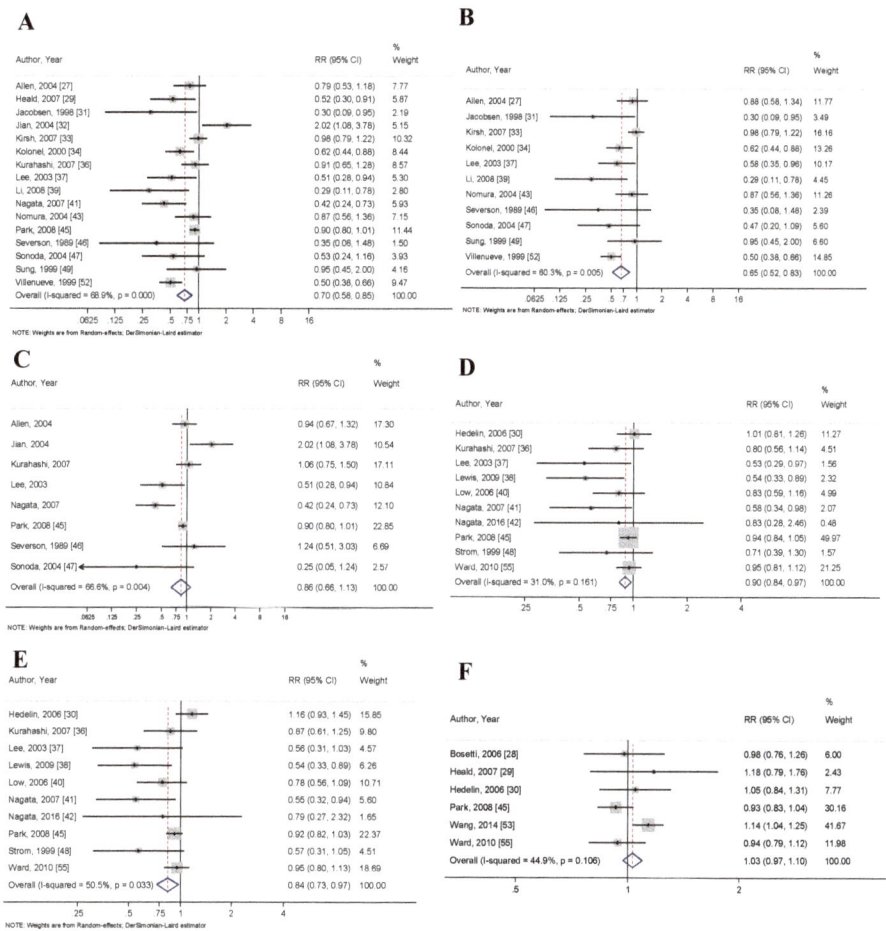

Figure 2. Forest plots for (**A**) total soy intake and risk of prostate cancer; (**B**) unfermented soy intake and risk of prostate cancer; (**C**) fermented soy intake and risk of prostate cancer; (**D**) genistein intake and risk of prostate cancer; (**E**) daidzein intake and risk of prostate cancer; and (**F**) total isoflavone intake and risk of prostate cancer. These associations were indicated as a relative risk (RR) estimate with the corresponding 95% confidence interval (CI).

Six articles reported isoflavone intake without disclosing the sources of the isoflavones. These studies were analyzed separately, so as not to interfere with measurements based solely on soy intake because isoflavones are found in other food items, such as seed sprouts and pulses. The pooled RR for isoflavone intake and PCa risk was 1.03 (95% CI: 0.97–1.09, $p = 0.313$) (Figure 2F). Neither Begg's correlation test (p = 0.707) nor Egger's linear regression test (p = 0.802) for bias were significant. The I^2 index showed moderate heterogeneity between studies (44.9%). Notably, the inclusion of these studies in the total soy analysis did not significantly change the RR of dietary soy intake and PCa risk.

Finally, articles were further stratified into specific soy food groups, which included tofu, miso and soy milk. Few studies were available to accurately represent meta-analysis data on these points, so RR are reported here, but not included in further subgroup analyses. The pooled RR for tofu and PCa risk was 0.73 (95% CI: 0.57–0.94, p = 0.013), the pooled RR for miso and PCa risk was 1.01 (95% CI: 0.80–1.28, p = 0.919), and the pooled RR for soy milk and PCa risk was 0.58 (95% CI: 0.19–1.78, p = 0.343). None of the groups were significant for bias using Begg's correlation test (p = 0.221, p = 0.296, and p = 1.000, respectively) or Egger's linear regression test (p = 0.093, p = 0.497, and p = NA, respectively). The I^2 index showed low heterogeneity amongst the studies included in the tofu (4.5%) and miso (0.0%) groups and high heterogeneity amongst studies included in the soy milk (63.1%) group.

3.4. Circulating Isoflavones and PCa Risk

Nine articles measured circulating isoflavone concentrations and their associations with PCa risk. Specifically, these articles reported RR data for circulating genistein (n = 9) [29,35,40,42,44,50,51,54,56], circulating daidzein (n = 7) [29,35,40,42,44,51,54], and total circulating isoflavones (n = 2) [29,54]. The pooled RR for circulating genistein and PCa risk was 0.87 (95% CI: 0.69–1.10, p = 0.236) (Figure 3A), the pooled RR for circulating daidzein and PCa risk was 0.92 (95% CI: 0.78–1.08) (Figure 3B), and the RR for circulating isoflavones and PCa risk was 1.01 (95% CI: 0.93–1.10, p = 0.738). None of the studies were significant for bias using Begg's correlation test (p = 0.175, p = 0.368, and p = 1.00, respectively) or Egger's linear regression test (p = 0.228, p = 0.197, and p = NA, respectively). The I^2 index showed high heterogeneity amongst the studies included in the circulating genistein (76.8%) and circulating daidzein (58.1%) groups and low heterogeneity amongst the circulating isoflavone group (0.0%). Funnel plots used to explore publication bias are shown in Appendix A (Figure 2).

3.5. Subgroup Analysis

Articles reporting total soy intake and PCa risk had a pooled RR of 0.61 (95% CI: 0.45–0.82, p = 0.001) for case-control studies and a pooled RR of 0.90 (95% CI: 0.82–0.99, p = 0.022) for cohort and NCC studies. Studies conducted in both North America (p = 0.009) and Europe (p = 0.021) were significantly associated with a reduced PCa risk, whereas studies conducted in Asia (p = 0.064) were not. A complete subgroup analysis can be found in Table 2. Cumulative meta-analyses first demonstrated that soy food intake was significantly associated with the reduced risk of PCa in 1998 and has remained significant over time, and with the inclusion of additional studies within the field (Figure 3).

Articles reporting unfermented soy food intake and PCa risk had a pooled RR of 0.55 (95% CI: 0.46–0.66, p < 0.001) for case-control studies and a pooled RR of 0.91 (95% CI: 0.76–1.08, p = 0.267) for cohort studies. Studies were conducted in both North America (p = 0.014) and Asia (p = 0.005), and there was a significantly reduced risk of PCa in both continents. Studies of medium quality were significantly associated with a lower PCa risk (p < 0.001).

The pooled RR for articles reporting dietary genistein intake and PCa risk was 0.81 (95% CI: 0.68–0.96, p = 0.016) for case-control studies and a pooled RR of 0.93 (95% CI: 0.85–1.01, p = 0.077) for cohort and NCC studies. Studies conducted in Asia (p = 0.004) showed a significantly reduced risk of PCa, while studies conducted in North America (p = 0.145) and Europe (p = 0.419) did not. Mid quality studies were significantly associated with a reduced risk of PCa (p = 0.007).

The pooled RR for articles reporting dietary daidzein intake and PCa risk was 0.68 (95% CI: 0.47–1.00, p = 0.052) for case-control studies and a pooled RR of 0.91 (95% CI: 0.84–1.00, p = 0.042) for cohort and NCC studies. Studies conducted in Asia (p = 0.012) showed a significantly reduced risk of PCa, while studies conducted in North America (p = 0.094) and Europe (p = 0.799) did not. High quality studies were significantly associated with a reduced risk of PCa (p = 0.042).

There was no significant association for case-control or NCC studies and risk of PCa for articles evaluating circulating levels of genistein. Only studies conducted in Asia ($p = 0.031$) were significantly associated with a decreased risk of PCa, while studies conducted in Europe ($p = 0.784$) showed no significant association with circulating genistein levels and PCa risk.

Articles evaluating dietary isoflavones, fermented soy intake, and circulating levels of daidzein showed no significant associations on risk of PCa when studies were grouped by design or by continent. Finally, no studies significantly affected any of the pooled RRs when conducting sensitivity analyses for each group.

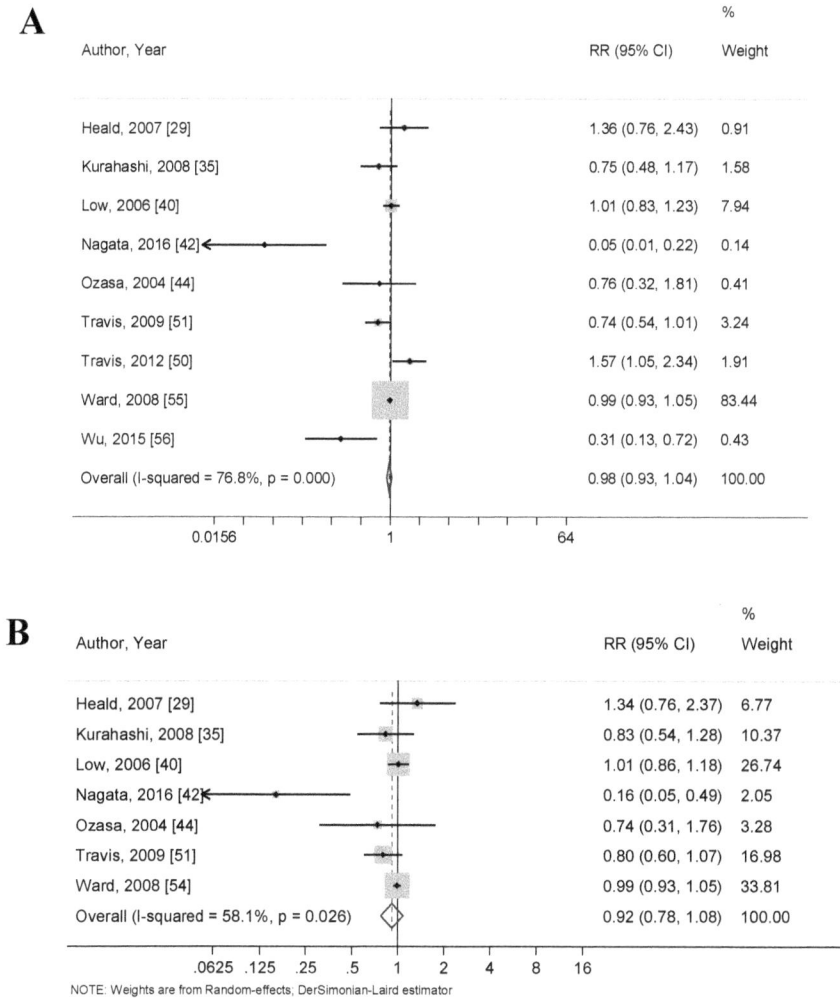

Figure 3. Forest plots for (**A**) circulating genistein and risk of prostate cancer; and (**B**) circulating daidzein and risk of prostate cancer. These associations were indicated as a relative risk (RR) estimate with the corresponding 95% confidence interval (CI).

Table 2. Subgroup analysis of included studies. Bold values indicate $p < 0.05$.

	Total Dietary Soy				Dietary Unfermented Soy				Dietary Fermented Soy			
	No. of Studies	RR (95% CI)	p-Value	I² (%)	No. of Studies	RR (95% CI)	p-Value	I² (%)	No. of Studies	RR (95% CI)	p-Value	I² (%)
Overall Model	16	0.71 (0.58–0.85)[†]	**<0.001**	68.9	11	0.66 (0.52–0.83)[†]	**<0.001**	60.3	8	0.86 (0.66–1.13)[†]	0.281	66.6
Study Type												
Case-control	9	0.61 (0.45–0.82)[†]	**0.001**	63.2	6	0.55 (0.46–0.66)	**<0.001**	0.0	4	0.64 (0.27–1.50)[†]	0.300	82.3
Cohort	7	0.90 (0.82–0.99)	**0.022**	2.7	5	0.91 (0.76–1.08)	0.267	30.6	4	0.92 (0.83–1.02)	0.123	0.0
Continent												
North America	7	0.72 (0.56–0.92)[†]	**0.009**	74.7	6	0.65 (0.47–0.92)[†]	**0.014**	73.4	2	0.91 (0.81–1.02)[†]	0.090	0.0
Europe	1	0.52 (0.30–0.91)	**0.021**	0.0	-	-	-	-	-	-	-	-
Asia	8	0.71 (0.50–1.02)[†]	0.064	67.3	5	0.68 (0.52–0.89)	**0.005**	35.4	6	0.79 (0.51–1.23)[†]	0.302	75.5
Adjustments												
High quality	12	0.72 (0.58–0.90)[†]	**0.003**	73.4	8	0.61 (0.45–0.82)[†]	**0.001**	69.2	5	1.00 (0.73–1.37)[†]	0.994	63.1
Mid quality	4	0.66 (0.50–0.87)	**0.003**	60.5	3	0.81 (0.58–1.13)	0.217	0.0	3	0.56 (0.27–1.17)[†]	0.124	74.0
Age												
Adjusted	11	0.73 (0.57–0.93)[†]	**0.010**	69.7	8	0.68 (0.52–0.88)[†]	**0.003**	65.6	5	1.03 (0.72–1.47)[†]	0.892	59.8
Unadjusted	5	0.61 (0.39–0.96)[†]	**0.032**	32.1	3	0.56 (0.35–0.92)	**0.021**	47.5	3	0.56 (0.28–1.15)[†]	0.115	0.0
BMI												
Adjusted	5	0.95 (0.73–1.22)[†]	0.661	66.2	3	0.78 (0.50–1.23)[†]	0.282	64.6	2	1.27 (0.58–2.78)[†]	0.552	83.8
Unadjusted	11	0.61 (0.53–0.71)[†]	**<0.001**	32.0	8	0.59 (0.50–0.70)[†]	**<0.001**	18.0	6	0.73 (0.50–1.07)[†]	0.103	63.3
Smoking												
Adjusted	7	0.71 (0.56–0.91)[†]	**0.007**	66.3	4	0.71 (0.46–1.10)[†]	0.122	62.2	3	0.56 (0.28–1.15)[†]	0.115	78.7
Unadjusted	9	0.72 (0.53–0.96)[†]	**0.027**	66.9	7	0.60 (0.51–0.71)[†]	**<0.001**	27.1	5	1.03 (0.72–1.47)[†]	0.892	59.8
FHPC												
Adjusted	4	0.95 (0.72–1.24)[†]	0.690	71.6	1	0.98 (0.79–1.22)	0.855	0.0	2	1.27 (0.58–2.78)[†]	0.552	83.8
Unadjusted	12	0.63 (0.55–0.72)	**<0.001**	41.5	10	0.61 (0.52–0.72)	**<0.001**	32.0	5	0.73 (0.50–1.07)[†]	0.103	63.3
Energy												
Adjusted	9	0.76 (0.61–0.95)[†]	**0.016**	69.7	5	0.74 (0.57–0.97)[†]	**0.029**	53.2	5	0.72 (0.43–1.22)[†]	0.221	79.2
Unadjusted	7	0.62 (0.45–0.86)[†]	**0.004**	57.1	6	0.57 (0.39–0.83)[†]	**0.004**	50.6	3	1.01 (0.80–1.28)	0.919	0.0
Education												
Adjusted	5	0.82 (0.58–1.16)[†]	0.263	74.7	3	0.64 (0.41–0.99)[†]	**0.045**	56.1	3	1.06 (0.76–1.47)[†]	0.741	67.7
Unadjusted	11	0.64 (0.50–0.82)[†]	**<0.001**	63.4	8	0.66 (0.48–0.89)[†]	**0.007**	65.5	5	0.66 (0.39–1.11)[†]	0.116	68.2
PA												
Adjusted	2	1.32 (0.66–2.66)[†]	0.433	78.1	1	0.98 (0.79–1.22)	0.855	0.0	1	2.02 (1.08–3.78)[†]	**0.028**	0.0
Unadjusted	14	0.64 (0.52–0.78)[†]	**<0.001**	63.6	10	0.61 (0.52–0.72)	**<0.001**	32.0	7	0.79 (0.62–1.02)[†]	0.071	58.1
Alcohol												
Adjusted	2	0.55 (0.19–1.59)[†]	0.270	74.4	2	0.55 (0.19–1.59)[†]	0.270	74.7	-	-	-	-
Unadjusted	14	0.71 (0.58–0.87)[†]	**0.001**	70.4	9	0.66 (0.51–0.85)[†]	**0.002**	62.3	8	0.86 (0.66–1.13)[†]	0.281	66.6
Geographic area												
Adjusted	6	0.83 (0.61–1.13)[†]	0.237	80.1	4	0.72 (0.51–1.02)[†]	0.064	80.7	3	1.16 (0.81–1.67)[†]	0.416	55.2
Unadjusted	10	0.59 (0.45–0.79)[†]	**<0.001**	60.9	7	0.63 (0.48–0.82)	**0.001**	28.1	5	0.64 (0.41–1.02)[†]	0.061	68.9
Marital status												
Adjusted	1	2.02 (1.08–3.78)[†]	**0.028**	0.0	-	-	-	-	1	2.02 (1.08–3.78)	**0.028**	0.0
Unadjusted	15	0.67 (0.56–0.81)[†]	**<0.001**	58.5	11	0.66 (0.52–0.83)[†]	**<0.001**	60.3	7	0.79 (0.62–1.02)[†]	0.071	58.1
Ethnicity												
Adjusted	3	0.86 (0.71–1.04)[†]	0.124	58.6	2	0.80 (0.51–1.25)[†]	0.319	78.7	-	-	-	-
Unadjusted	13	0.65 (0.50–0.84)[†]	**0.001**	62.6	9	0.61 (0.51–0.73)	**<0.001**	39.5	8	0.86 (0.66–1.13)[†]	0.281	66.6

Table 2. *Cont.*

	Dietary Isoflavones				Dietary Genistein				Dietary Daidzein			
	No. of studies	RR (95% CI)	p-Value	I² (%)	No. of studies	RR (95% CI)	p-Value	I² (%)	No. of studies	RR (95% CI)	p-Value	I² (%)
Overall Model	6	1.03 (0.97–1.09)	0.313	44.9	10	0.90 (0.84–0.97)	0.008	31.0	10	0.84 (0.73–0.97)†	0.018	50.5
Study Type												
Case-control	3	1.04 (0.89–1.22)	0.604	0.0	6	0.81 (0.68–0.96)	0.016	49.5	6	0.68 (0.47–1.00)†	0.052	70.1
Cohort/NCC	3	1.01 (0.87–1.17)†	0.928	76.3	4	0.93 (0.85–1.01)	0.077	0.0	4	0.91 (0.84–1.00)	0.042	0.0
Continent												
North America	2	1.03 (0.85–1.26)	0.757	86.2	3	0.76 (0.53–1.10)†	0.145	62.0	3	0.71 (0.47–1.06)†	0.094	68.2
Europe	4	1.00 (0.89–1.12)	0.961	0.0	3	0.95 (0.84–1.08)	0.419	0.0	3	0.98 (0.80–1.18)†	0.799	51.7
Asia	-	-	-	-	4	0.69 (0.53–0.89)	0.004	0.0	4	0.72 (0.55–0.93)	0.012	0.0
Adjustments												
High quality	5	1.02 (0.91–1.14)†	0.780	55.8	8	0.90 (0.83–0.98)	0.011	25.1	8	0.88 (0.81–0.96)	0.004	28.1
Mid quality	1	1.05 (0.84–1.31)	0.667	0.0	2	0.81 (0.47–1.38)†	0.430	72.5	2	0.83 (0.40–1.72)†	0.620	84.4
Age												
Adjusted	5	1.08 (1.00–1.16)	0.042	8.1	7	0.89 (0.79–1.00)	0.046	36.6	7	0.83 (0.66–1.03)†	0.092	56.7
Unadjusted	1	0.93 (0.83–1.04)	0.207	0.0	3	0.91 (0.83–1.01)	0.077	42.4	3	0.81 (0.64–1.03)†	0.088	51.0
BMI												
Adjusted	2	0.94 (0.85–1.04)	0.224	0.0	4	0.91 (0.82–1.00)	0.058	39.0	4	0.89 (0.80–0.98)	0.018	38.7
Unadjusted	4	1.09 (1.01–1.18)	0.029	19.6	6	0.90 (0.80–1.01)	0.063	38.2	6	0.83 (0.66–1.05)†	0.116	61.2
Smoking												
Adjusted	2	0.95 (0.85–1.06)	0.322	21.5	4	0.73 (0.51–1.04)†	0.080	59.6	4	0.71 (0.50–1.01)†	0.059	59.4
Unadjusted	4	1.08 (1.00–1.16)	0.055	27.8	6	0.91 (0.81–1.01)	0.086	10.8	6	0.88 (0.73–1.06)†	0.178	51.1
FHPC												
Adjusted	3	0.95 (0.86–1.05)	0.331	0.0	4	0.90 (0.82–1.00)	0.043	45.7	4	0.76 (0.59–0.98)†	0.032	55.9
Unadjusted	3	1.09 (1.00–1.18)	0.040	44.0	6	0.90 (0.80–1.02)	0.089	33.5	6	0.88 (0.71–1.09)†	0.228	52.0
Energy												
Adjusted	4	0.97 (0.88–1.06)	0.477	0.0	8	0.90 (0.82–0.98)	0.015	42.7	8	0.78 (0.63–0.96)†	0.017	60.6
Unadjusted	2	1.05 (0.87–1.27)†	0.600	71.2	2	0.92 (0.79–1.07)	0.283	0.0	2	0.93 (0.80–1.09)	0.393	0.0
Education												
Adjusted	2	0.94 (0.85–1.04)	0.224	0.0	2	0.75 (0.44–1.28)†	0.296	78.2	2	0.75 (0.45–1.24)†	0.261	76.3
Unadjusted	4	1.09 (1.01–1.18)	0.029	19.6	8	0.89 (0.80–0.99)	0.033	15.5	8	0.91 (0.82–1.02)	0.104	49.8
PA												
Adjusted	-	-	-	-	-	-	-	-	-	-	-	-
Unadjusted	6	1.03 (0.97–1.10)	0.313	44.9	10	0.90 (0.84–0.97)	0.008	31.0	10	0.84 (0.73–0.97)†	0.018	50.5
Alcohol												
Adjusted	-	-	-	-	2	0.74 (0.44–1.25)	0.255	0.0	2	0.62 (0.36–1.05)†	0.075	0.0
Unadjusted	6	1.03 (0.97–1.10)	0.313	44.9	8	0.91 (0.84–0.98)	0.012	43.5	8	0.86 (0.74–0.99)†	0.042	56.0
Geographic area												
Adjusted	-	-	-	-	1	0.80 (0.56–1.14)	0.219	0.0	1	0.87 (0.61–1.25)†	0.447	0.0
Unadjusted	6	1.03 (0.97–1.10)	0.313	44.9	9	0.91 (0.84–0.98)	0.015	36.4	9	0.83 (0.71–0.97)†	0.022	55.9
Marital status												
Adjusted	-	-	-	-	1	0.90 (0.84–0.97)	0.008	31.0	-	-	-	-
Unadjusted	6	1.03 (0.97–1.10)	0.313	44.9	9	0.90 (0.84–0.97)	0.008	31.0	10	0.84 (0.73–0.97)†	0.018	50.5
Ethnicity												
Adjusted	1	0.93 (0.83–1.04)	0.207	0.0	1	0.94 (0.85–1.05)	0.256	0.0	1	0.92 (0.83–1.03)	0.134	0.0
Unadjusted	5	1.08 (1.00–1.16)	0.042	8.1	9	0.87 (0.78–0.97)	0.009	33.2	9	0.79 (0.65–0.96)†	0.019	55.6

Table 2. Cont.

	Circulating Genistein				Circulating Daidzein			
	No. of studies	RR (95% CI)	p-Value	I² (%)	No. of studies	RR (95% CI)	p-Value	I² (%)
Overall Model	9	0.87 (0.69–1.10)†	0.236	76.8	7	0.92 (0.78–1.08)†	0.310	58.1
Study Type								
Case-control	3	0.31 (0.06–1.65)†	0.170	90.4	2	0.49 (0.06–3.92)†	0.502	90.9
Cohort	-	-	-	-	-	-	-	-
Nested Case-control	6	0.97 (0.83–1.13)†	0.668	52.0	5	0.98 (0.93–1.04)	0.490	0.0
Continent								
North America	-	-	-	-	-	-	-	-
Europe	5	1.02 (0.87–1.21)†	0.784	58.7	4	0.99 (0.93–1.04)	0.657	6.8
Asia	4	0.37 (0.15–0.92)†	0.031	79.1	3	0.52 (0.22–1.23)†	0.137	72.5
Adjustments								
High quality	9	0.87 (0.69–1.10)†	0.236	76.8	7	0.92 (0.78–1.08)†	0.310	58.1
Mid quality	-	-	-	-	-	-	-	-
Age								
Adjusted	5	0.41 (0.13–1.29)†	0.128	85.6	4	0.77 (0.44–1.35)†	0.362	74.3
Unadjusted	4	0.97 (0.72–1.29)†	0.814	69.9	3	0.95 (0.83–1.08)	0.397	13.1
BMI								
Adjusted	4	0.78 (0.45–1.34)†	0.368	87.6	3	0.72 (0.44–1.16)†	0.177	82.7
Unadjusted	5	0.84 (0.60–1.17)†	0.309	60.5	4	0.99 (0.93–1.05)	0.706	0.0
Smoking								
Adjusted	4	0.73 (0.34–1.57)†	0.424	88.2	3	0.66 (0.30–1.47)†	0.307	81.9
Unadjusted	5	0.90 (0.74–1.10)†	0.272	55.6	4	0.99 (0.93–1.05)	0.682	0.0
FHPC								
Adjusted	2	1.04 (0.86–1.26)	0.670	0.00	2	1.03 (0.89–1.2)	0.699	0.0
Unadjusted	7	0.73 (0.51–1.05)†	0.087	81.9	5	0.77 (0.58–1.06)†	0.115	69.1
Energy								
Adjusted	2	0.99 (0.94–1.05)	0.779	0.0	2	0.99 (0.94–1.05)	0.796	0.0
Unadjusted	7	0.69 (0.42–1.13)†	0.140	81.4	5	0.76 (0.50–1.15)†	0.195	64.0
Education								
Adjusted	2	1.07 (0.51–2.23)†	0.866	88.2	1	0.80 (0.60–1.07)	0.131	0.0
Unadjusted	7	0.80 (0.60–1.07)†	0.126	76.8	6	0.94 (0.78–1.14)†	0.528	59.6
PA								
Adjusted	2	1.07 (0.51–2.23)†	0.866	88.2	1	0.80 (0.60–1.07)	0.131	0.0
Unadjusted	7	0.80 (0.60–1.07)†	0.126	76.8	6	0.94 (0.78–1.14)†	0.528	59.6
Alcohol								
Adjusted	3	0.55 (0.20–1.51)†	0.244	91.6	2	0.39 (0.08–1.88)†	0.243	86.5
Unadjusted	6	0.93 (0.77–1.12)†	0.437	51.0	5	0.99 (0.94–1.05)	0.757	0.0
Geographic area								
Adjusted	-	-	-	-	-	-	-	-
Unadjusted	9	0.87 (0.69–1.10)†	0.236	76.8	7	0.92 (0.78–1.08)†	0.310	58.1
Marital status								
Adjusted	2	1.07 (0.51–2.23)†	0.866	88.2	1	0.80 (0.60–1.07)	0.131	0.0
Unadjusted	7	0.80 (0.60–1.07)†	0.126	76.8	6	0.94 (0.78–1.14)†	0.528	59.6
Ethnicity								
Adjusted	-	-	-	-	-	-	-	-
Unadjusted	9	0.87 (0.69–1.10)†	0.236	76.8	7	0.92 (0.78–1.08)†	0.310	58.1

† Signifies that results are estimated by DerSimonian–Laird random effects model. Abbreviations: relative risk (RR), confidence interval (CI), number (No.), body mass index (BMI), family history of prostate cancer (FHPC), physical activity (PA).

3.6. Soy and Advanced PCa Risk

Seven [34–36,43,45,50,53] studies reported the risk of advanced PCa with soy intake and circulating isoflavone levels. Of these seven studies, four [34,43,45,53] studies were conducted in North America, two [35,36] studies were conducted in Asia, and one [50] study was conducted in Europe. Only one [34] was a case-control study, two [35,50] were NCC studies, and four [36,43,45,53] were cohort studies. Five [34,36,43,45,53] studies reported a risk of advanced PCa with dietary soy food intake and two [35,50] studies reported a risk of advanced PCa with circulating isoflavones. For studies that reported dietary soy food intake, the pooled RR was 0.87 (95% CI: 0.74–1.06, p = 0.119) (Figure 4A). Neither Begg's correlation test (p = 1.00) nor Egger's linear regression test (p = 0.548) for bias were significant. The I^2 index showed moderate heterogeneity between studies (45.7%). Funnel plots, used to explore publication bias, are shown in Appendix A (Figure 4).

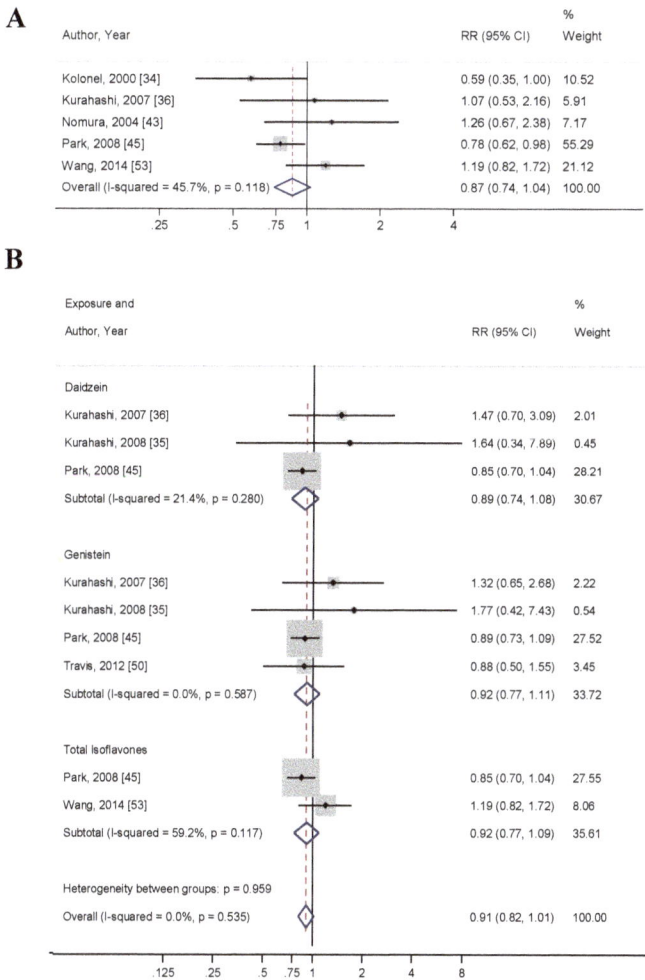

Figure 4. Forest plots for (**A**) total soy intake and risk of advanced prostate cancer; and (**B**) isoflavone exposure and risk of advanced prostate cancer. These associations were indicated as a relative risk (RR) estimate with the corresponding 95% confidence interval (CI).

When stratifying groups by combining dietary and circulating measurements of isoflavones, the pooled RR for genistein and PCa risk ($n = 4$) was 0.92 (95% CI: 0.77–1.11, $p = 0.381$), the pooled RR for daidzein and PCa risk ($n = 3$) was 0.89 (95% CI: 0.74–1.10, $p = 0.227$), and the pooled RR for total isoflavones and PCa risk ($n = 2$) was 0.91 (95% CI: 0.82–1.01, $p = 0.337$) (Figure 4B). The I^2 index showed moderate heterogeneity amongst studies reporting genistein and daidzein dietary and circulating levels (33.7% and 30.7%, respectively), while there was substantially high heterogeneity between the studies reporting total isoflavone measurements (100.0%).

4. Discussion

This updated systematic review and meta-analysis provides a thorough evaluation regarding the association between soy food intake and PCa risk. Using the current pool of scientific literature, our results support the existing evidence, which indicates that total soy food intake is associated with a reduced risk of PCa ($p < 0.001$). This population-based evidence corroborates observations in both in vitro and in vivo studies, which have shown that soy isoflavones inhibit PCa development and growth [57–59]. In agreement with this, we found that both genistein and daidzein intake were inversely associated with the risk of PCa ($p = 0.008$ and $p = 0.018$, respectively). These results support our finding that total soy food consumption is associated with decreased PCa risk, as genistein and daidzein are likely found in similar food products.

Soybeans and soy food products contain isoflavones—predominantly genistein and daidzein—mainly as β-glycosides [60]. During digestion, these glycosides are hydrolyzed to their aglycone forms by intestinal or bacterial β-glucosidases [60]. By removing the sugar molecule, the isoflavones are smaller and more hydrophobic, allowing them to more readily diffuse into enterocytes [61]. After absorption and first pass metabolism, aglycones are re-conjugated in the liver to their glycosidic or other conjugated forms and distributed to tissues via systemic circulation [61]. Once within cells, isoflavones act as weak estrogen receptor (ER) agonists or antagonists, depending on the cell type and concentration of estrogen present [61]. Prostatic tissues have higher concentrations of ER-β, to which genistein preferentially binds, with an affinity similar to that of the endogenously-produced estrogen, 17β-estradiol [62]. Increased presence and activation of ER-β is associated with reduced cell proliferation and reduced PCa histological grade [63,64]. This effect has been shown to occur, in part, by reducing the levels of prostate-specific antigen (PSA), cyclin D1, and cyclin-dependent kinase 4 (CDK4) in an ER-dependent manner [57,58]. Interestingly, ER-β expression is often lost during prostate carcinogenesis, so the ability of genistein to bind to ER-β may be a key factor in the inhibition of prostate carcinogenesis. Additional mechanisms of the effects of soy isoflavones on PCa cellular proliferation, apoptosis, and differentiation have been reviewed in depth by Mahmoud et al. (2014) [65].

We also analyzed the potential relationship between unfermented or fermented soy food products and risk of PCa. We found that unfermented soy food products were associated with a decreased risk of PCa ($p < 0.001$), while fermented soy food products had no associations with PCa risk ($p = 0.281$). More studies provided food intake data for unfermented soy food products than fermented soy food products (11 studies versus 8 studies, respectively). While this meta-analysis failed to demonstrate a significant association between fermented foods and the risk of PCa, it should be recognized that there was wider variation in results reported by these studies than there was for studies using unfermented and other soy foods. This wider variation could have impacted the risk outcomes. Some concerns have been expressed in the literature regarding the effects of soy fermentation on the risk of developing certain cancers, such as gastric cancer [66]. Due to this association, Yan and Spitznagel chose to not include fermented soy foods in their 2005 meta-analysis [10]. However, during fermentation, β-glucosidases, secreted by fermentative bacteria, cleave glycosidic linkages via a similar process that digestive enzymes in the small intestine and gut microbiota cleave these linkages [60,61,67]. Isoflavones are present in fermented foods, such as tempeh and miso, predominantly as aglycones, with few isoflavones retaining their side-chains. The ratio is reversed for nonfermented foods, but some naturally occurring plant β-glucosidase activity allows for continuous side-chain cleavage to yield aglycones [60]. The more bioavailable aglycone form is readily absorbed from the intestines, rendering this conversion from a glycosylated isoflavone to its aglycone counterpart essential for maximal isoflavone absorption. These similar enzymatic processes yield common aglycone products for intestinal absorption, regardless of whether these processes occur before digestion during the fermentation of soy foods or during the digestion of unfermented soy foods.

Circulating levels of genistein and daidzein were not associated with the risk of PCa ($p = 0.236$ and $p = 0.310$, respectively) despite the elevation of circulating genistein and daidzein levels after consumption of these isoflavones. However, peak circulating isoflavone levels can occur as soon as 30 min or as long as 6 h after feeding, depending on the specific isoflavones and foods consumed [61,68]. Mean half-life values vary as well; the average half-life for free genistein is 3.2 h and the average half-life for free daidzein is 4.2 h [69]. Because isoflavones can exist with multiple side-chains (e.g., glucose, sulfate, acetyl, or malonyl-CoA groups) and as different metabolites, accurately measuring in vivo pharmacokinetics is challenging. Thus, the amount of time between isoflavone consumption and blood collection may substantially affect measurement outcomes, which can impact the reliability of blood isoflavone measurements as markers of soy food intake. Due to these factors, an association may have been missed for these circulating isoflavones.

No association was seen when we examined six articles that did not disclose the source of isoflavones measured from participants' dietary intakes. For example, Bosetti et al. (2006) indicated that isoflavones were measured from the FFQ, primarily based on consumption of soy and soy products, but also from "vegetable or bean soups and pulses" [28]. Because isoflavones are found in other food sources and supplements, such as clover and alfalfa seeds and sprouts, garbanzo beans, and other pulses, we independently analyzed studies that did not explicitly indicate that measurements were taken from soy food sources. As such, total dietary isoflavones were not significantly associated with risk of PCa ($p = 0.313$). While most dietary isoflavones are consumed from soy food products, examining the sources and types of isoflavones that were included in these analyses could provide insight as to why no association was observed. Notably, this analysis was based on the information found from a limited number of articles, so additional studies could strengthen these observations.

To our knowledge, this is the first meta-analysis to investigate the risk associations between soy and advanced PCa. Advanced PCa is defined as poorly differentiated, aggressive, and metastatic disease. Advanced PCa is often difficult to treat, as patients are typically less responsive to therapy. It is therefore imperative to identify other ways to prevent disease progression, such as through dietary modification. Relatively few studies have examined the relationship between diet and advanced PCa or reported information pertaining to stage or grade of PCa. Our results do not show a significant reduction in the risk of advanced PCa with total soy intake ($p = 0.119$) or dietary and circulating levels of genistein ($p = 0.381$), daidzein ($p = 0.227$), or total isoflavones ($p = 0.337$), perhaps due to the lack of studies. Two double-blinded, randomized, placebo-controlled clinical trials have supplemented isoflavones in men awaiting radical prostatectomy. One study reported higher apoptotic activity in tumors of men treated with isoflavones when compared to tumors of the men in the placebo group [70], while the other study showed modulation of both cell cycle and apoptotic genes in the prostate tissues of men in the treatment group, when compared to tissues of men in the placebo group [71]. More studies are needed to further explore this promising relationship and to identify whether soy can protect against advanced PCa.

Few studies have analyzed individual soy foods and their relationships with PCa risk. Tofu was the most investigated soy food found in the literature. Tofu showed a significant protective association with PCa ($p = 0.013$). This result is consistent with the result shown by Hwang et al. (2009) [11]. More studies are needed to understand the role of individual soy foods in PCa risk.

The research design of studies did not seem to bias our results, as case-control and cohort studies both reported significant and null results. It is important to note that case-control studies are generally considered to have a higher risk of bias than cohort studies; however, significant measurement error can occur for both cohort and case-control studies when evaluating a single exposure variable. To accurately account for all reported estimates of soy exposure and PCa risk, both study designs were included in the analysis. To this end, sensitivity analyses conducted for each subgroup showed that no studies significantly altered results or heterogeneity within subgroups. Separating results by continent showed that total soy intake was only associated with a decreased risk of PCa in North America (p = 0.009) and Europe (p = 0.021), although only one study was included in the European group. However, when looking at the individual dietary isoflavones, genistein and daidzein, Asia was the only continent to show a significant risk reduction for PCa (p = 0.004 and p = 0.012, respectively). Similarly, Asia was the only continent to show a significant association between circulating genistein and risk of PCa (p = 0.031). Both North America (p = 0.014) and Asia (p = 0.005) showed a reduced risk of PCa when only considering unfermented soy foods. The variability in these associations makes it difficult to draw conclusions about whether ethnic differences, preparation methods, or eating patterns exist in soy food or isoflavone consumption and PCa risk.

Because differences in overall dietary composition or other unmeasured lifestyle factors could contribute to increased or decreased disease risk, the results from this study and others showing that soy intake is associated with a reduced risk of PCa should be interpreted with caution. Our study was limited in that our results relied on the reporting of the studies included in this analysis and may have been affected by several factors. For example, studies relying on dietary recall or FFQ reporting are subject to recall bias by participants. Soy food intake measurements could be inconsistently reported or nutrient analyses may differ based on the amount and type of soy food or the database used to collect nutrient information. In addition, not all studies accounted for potential confounding variables, such as family history of prostate cancer (FHPC), body mass index (BMI), smoking, or energy intake. The subgroup analyses in this study attempted to account for these limitations by highlighting some of these differences between studies, to account for variability in data adjustments and selection bias created by study design (i.e., whether the study was case-control or NCC/cohort).

In addition to attempting to address these study limitations, our analysis delved deeper into potential confounding factors, through meta-regression, to determine whether study quality, length, or the sample size impacted significant results of the study. None of these factors were found to impact our results, and as such were not included in our results. We also reported both dietary intakes and circulating levels of isoflavones to create a more comprehensive review of the existing literature. Finally, we analyzed any associations between soy and advanced PCa, which has not previously been reported.

As the second most commonly diagnosed cancer in men worldwide, it is important to identify modifiable factors, such as diet, that may impact the risk of developing PCa. The current study provides an updated systematic review and meta-analysis of the available literature describing the associations between soy food consumption and PCa risk. Of the four meta-analyses previously published, all showed that soy intake was associated with a reduced risk for PCa. Our study further enhances this association by including additional studies for analysis, grouping soy foods by type of food and by isoflavone intake, adding groups of circulating isoflavone concentrations, and by evaluating the potential relationship between soy food intake and advanced PCa risk.

Author Contributions: C.C.A., J.L.R., J.W.E. designed the study, C.C.A., J.L.R., K.M.R., S.J. conducted the research, C.C.A., J.L.R., K.M.R., J.W.E. analyzed the data, C.C.A. wrote the manuscript. All authors edited and approved the manuscript.

Conflicts of Interest: The authors declare no conflict of interest.

Appendix A

Table A1. Quality assessment of included studies.

Source	Selection				Comparability [5]	Exposure			Total [9]
Author, Year	Definition [1]	Representative [2]	Selection [3]	Definition [4]		Ascertainment [6]	Method [7]	Rate [8]	
Allen, 2004 [27]	0	★	0	★	★	★	★	★	6
Bosetti, 2006 [28]	★	★	0	★	★★	0	★	★	7
Heald, 2007 [29]	★	★	★	★	★★	★	★	0	8
Hedelin, 2006 [30]	★	★	0	★	★	★	★	0	6
Jacobsen, 1998 [31]	★	★	0	★	★	★	★	★	7
Jian, 2004 [32]	★	★	0	★	★★	0	★	★	7
Kirsh, 2007 [33]	★	★	0	★	★★	★	★	★	8
Kolonel, 2000 [34]	★	★	★	★	★	0	★	★	7
Kurahashi, 2007 [36]	★	★	0	★	★	★	★	★	7
Kurahashi, 2008 [35]	★	★	★	★	★	★	★	★	8
Lee, 2003 [37]	★	★	0	★	★	★	★	★	7
Lewis, 2009 [38]	★	★	0	★	★★	0	★	★	7
Li, 2008 [39]	★	★	★	★	★	0	★	★	7
Low, 2006 [40]	★	★	★	★	★★	★	★	★	9
Nagata, 2007 [41]	★	★	0	★	★	0	★	★	6
Nagata, 2016 [42]	★	★	0	★	★	★	★	★	7
Nomura, 2004 [43]	★	★	0	★	★	★	★	★	7
Ozasa, 2004 [44]	★	★	★	★	★	★	★	★	8
Park, 2008 [45]	★	★	0	★	★★	★	★	★	8
Severson, 1989 [46]	★	★	★	★	★	★	★	★	8
Sonoda, 2004 [47]	★	★	0	★	★	0	★	★	6
Strom, 1999 [48]	★	★	0	★	★★	0	★	★	7
Sung, 1999 [49]	★	★	0	★	★	0	★	★	6
Travis, 2009 [51]	★	★	★	★	★	★	★	★	8
Travis, 2012 [50]	★	★	★	★	★	★	★	★	8
Villenueve, 1999 [52]	★	★	0	★	★★	★	★	★	8
Wang, 2014 [53]	★	★	0	★	★★	★	★	★	8
Ward, 2008 [54]	★	★	★	★	★	★	★	★	8
Ward, 2010 [55]	★	★	0	★	★★	★	★	★	8
Wu, 2015 [56]	★	★	0	★	★★	★	★	★	8

[1] Indicates that cases are independently validated for case-control studies (0, 1 star); [2] cases are from a representative population or drawn from the same community as the non-exposed cohort (0, 1); [3] community controls or structured interview for cohort studies (0, 1); [4] controls have no history of prostate cancer (endpoint) (0, 1); [5] study controls for most important factor (age) and family history of prostate cancer (0, 1, 2); [6] structured interview where blind to case/control status for case-control studies, record linkage or independent blind assessment for cohort studies (0, 1); [7] same method of ascertainment for cases and controls or follow-up was long enough for outcomes to occur (4 years) (0, 1); [8] same non-response rate or <20% lost to follow up (0, 1); [9] total: minimum equals 1; maximum equals 9 stars.

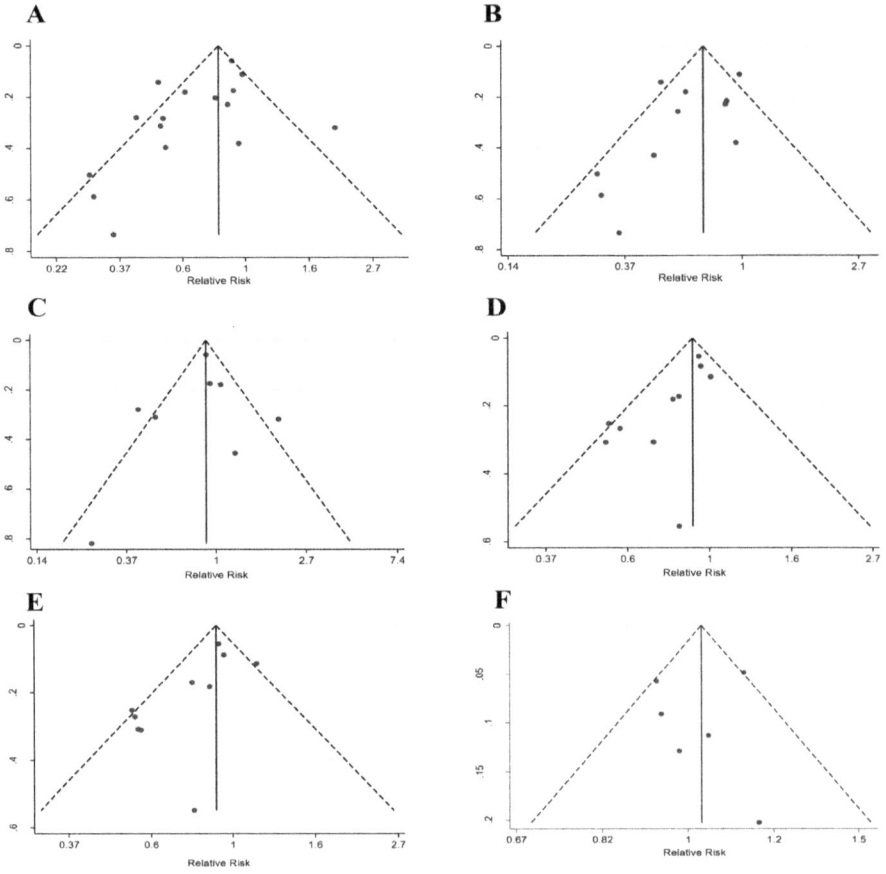

Figure 1. Funnel plots for (**A**) total soy intake and risk of prostate cancer; (**B**) unfermented soy intake and risk of prostate cancer; (**C**) fermented soy intake and risk of prostate cancer; (**D**) genistein intake and risk of prostate cancer; (**E**) daidzein intake and risk of prostate cancer; and (**F**) total isoflavone intake and risk of prostate cancer.

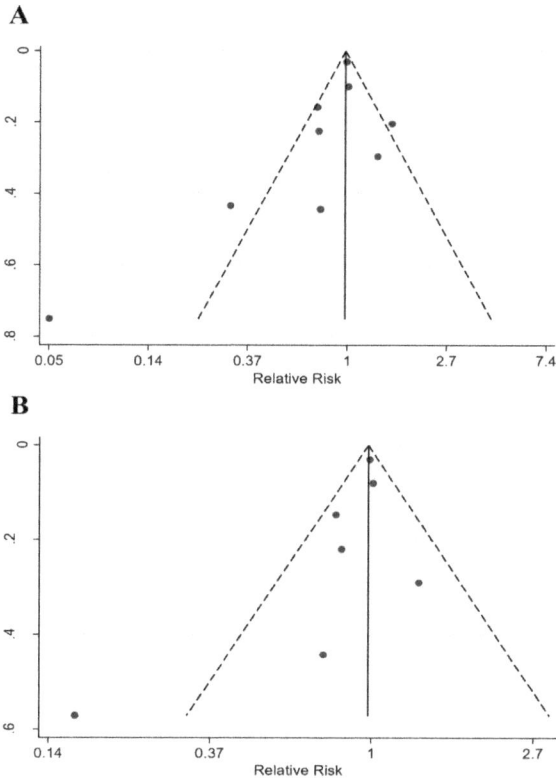

Figure 2. Funnel plots for (**A**) circulating genistein and risk of prostate cancer and (**B**) circulating daidzein and risk of prostate cancer.

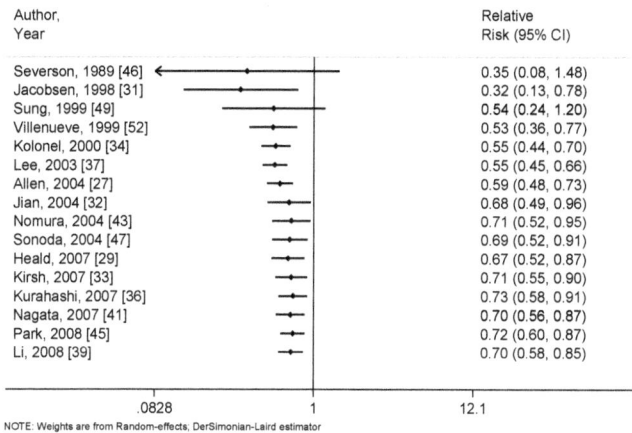

Figure 3. Forest plot for total soy intake and risk of prostate cancer by year of study publication. These associations were indicated as a relative risk (RR) estimate with the corresponding 95% confidence interval (CI).

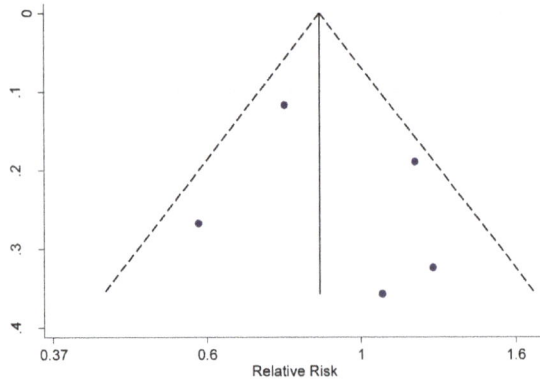

Figure 4. Funnel plot for total soy intake and risk of advanced prostate cancer.

References

1. GLOBOCAN. Cancer Fact Sheets: Prostate Cancer. Available online: http://globocan.iarc.fr/old/FactSheets/cancers/prostate-new.asp (accessed on 1 September 2017).
2. Adlercreutz, H.; Mazur, W. Phyto-oestrogens and Western diseases. *Ann. Med.* **1997**, *29*, 95–120. [CrossRef] [PubMed]
3. Andres, S.; Abraham, K.; Appel, K.E.; Lampen, A. Risks and benefits of dietary isoflavones for cancer. *Crit. Rev. Toxicol.* **2011**, *41*, 463–506. [CrossRef] [PubMed]
4. Messina, M.J. Legumes and soybeans: Overview of their nutritional profiles and health effects. *Am. J. Clin. Nutr.* **1999**, *70* (Suppl. 3), 439S–450S. [PubMed]
5. Valachovicova, T.; Slivova, V.; Sliva, D. Cellular and physiological effects of soy flavonoids. *Mini-Rev. Med. Chem.* **2004**, *4*, 881–887. [CrossRef] [PubMed]
6. Gardner, C.D.; Oelrich, B.; Liu, J.P.; Feldman, D.; Franke, A.A.; Brooks, J.D. Prostatic soy isoflavone concentrations exceed serum levels after dietary supplementation. *Prostate* **2009**, *69*, 719–726. [CrossRef] [PubMed]
7. Hsu, A.; Bray, T.M.; Helferich, W.G.; Doerge, D.R.; Ho, E. Differential effects of whole soy extract and soy isoflavones on apoptosis in prostate cancer cells. *Exp. Biol. Med.* **2010**, *235*, 90–97. [CrossRef] [PubMed]
8. Chiyomaru, T.; Fukuhara, S.; Hidaka, H.; Majid, S.; Saini, S.; Arora, S.; Guoren, D.; Shahryari, V.; Inik, C.; Tanaka, Y.; et al. Genistein up-regulates tumor suppressor microRNA-574-3p in prostate cancer. *PLoS ONE* **2013**, *8*, e58929. [CrossRef] [PubMed]
9. Slusarz, A.; Jackson, G.A.; Day, J.K.; Shenouda, N.S.; Bogener, J.L.; Browning, J.D.; Fritsche, K.L.; MacDonald, R.S.; Besch-Williford, C.L.; Lubahn, D.B.; et al. Aggressive prostate cancer is prevented in ERalphaKO mice and stimulated in ERbetaKO TRAMP mice. *Endocrinology* **2012**, *153*, 4160–4170. [CrossRef] [PubMed]
10. Yan, L.; Spitznagel, E.L. Meta-analysis of soy food and risk of prostate cancer in men. *Int. J. Cancer* **2005**, *117*, 667–669. [CrossRef] [PubMed]
11. Hwang, Y.; Kim, S.; Jee, S.; Kim, Y.; Nam, C. Soy food consumption and risk of prostate cancer: A meta-analysis of observational studies. *Nutr. Cancer* **2009**, *61*, 598–606. [CrossRef] [PubMed]
12. Zhang, M.; Wang, K.; Chen, L.; Yin, B.; Song, Y. Is phytoestrogen intake associated with decreased risk of prostate cancer? A systematic review of epidemiological studies based on 17,546 cases. *Andrology* **2016**, *4*, 745–756. [CrossRef] [PubMed]
13. Zhang, Q.; Feng, H.; Qluwakemi, B.; Wang, J.; Yao, S.; Cheng, G.; Xu, H.; Qiu, H.; Zhu, L.; Yuan, M. Phytoestrogens and risk of prostate cancer: An updated meta-analysis of epidemiologic studies. *Int. J. Food Sci. Nutr.* **2017**, *68*, 28–42. [CrossRef] [PubMed]
14. Pavese, J.M.; Krishna, S.N.; Bergan, R.C. Genistein inhibits human prostate cancer cell detachment, invasion, and metastasis. *Am. J. Clin. Nutr.* **2014**, *100* (Suppl. 1), 431S–436S. [CrossRef] [PubMed]

15. Lesinski, G.B.; Reville, P.K.; Mace, T.A.; Young, G.S.; Ahn-Jarvis, J.; Thomas-Ahner, J.; Vodovotz, Y.; Ameen, Z.; Grainger, E.; Riedl, K.; et al. Consumption of soy isoflavone enriched bread in men with prostate cancer is associated with reduced proinflammatory cytokines and immunosuppressive cells. *Cancer Prev. Res.* **2015**, *8*, 1036–1044. [CrossRef] [PubMed]

16. Moher, D.; Liberati, A.; Tetzlaff, J.; Altman, D.G.; Group, P. Preferred reporting items for systematic reviews and meta-analyses: The PRISMA statement. *J. Clin. Epidemiol.* **2009**, *62*, 1006–1012. [CrossRef] [PubMed]

17. Stroup, D.F.; Berlin, J.A.; Morton, S.C.; Olkin, I.; Williamson, G.D.; Rennie, D.; Moher, D.; Becker, B.J.; Sipe, T.A.; Thacker, S.B.; et al. Meta-analysis of observational studies in epidemiology: A proposal for reporting. Meta-analysis Of Observational Studies in Epidemiology (MOOSE) group. *JAMA* **2000**, *283*, 2008–2012. [CrossRef] [PubMed]

18. Stang, A. Critical evaluation of the Newcastle-Ottawa scale for the assessment of the quality of nonrandomized studies in meta-analyses. *Eur. J. Epidemiol.* **2010**, *25*, 603–605. [CrossRef] [PubMed]

19. Egger, M.; Smith, G.D.; Phillips, A.N. Meta-analysis: Principles and procedures. *BMJ* **1997**, *315*, 1533–1537. [CrossRef] [PubMed]

20. Higgins, J.P.; Thompson, S.G. Quantifying heterogeneity in a meta-analysis. *Stat. Med.* **2002**, *21*, 1539–1558. [CrossRef] [PubMed]

21. Jackson, D.; White, I.R.; Thompson, S.G. Extending DerSimonian and Laird's methodology to perform multivariate random effects meta-analyses. *Stat. Med.* **2010**, *29*, 1282–1297. [CrossRef] [PubMed]

22. Chen, H.; Manning, A.K.; Dupuis, J. A method of moments estimator for random effect multivariate meta-analysis. *Biometrics* **2012**, *68*, 1278–1284. [CrossRef] [PubMed]

23. Peters, J.L.; Sutton, A.J.; Jones, D.R.; Abrams, K.R.; Rushton, L. Contour-enhanced meta-analysis funnel plots help distinguish publication bias from other causes of asymmetry. *J. Clin. Epidemiol.* **2008**, *61*, 991–996. [CrossRef] [PubMed]

24. Sterne, J.A.C.; Egger, M. Funnel plots for detecting bias in meta-analysis: Guidelines on choice of axis. *J. Clin. Epidemiol.* **2001**, *54*, 1046–1055. [CrossRef]

25. Egger, M.; Davey Smith, G.; Schneider, M.; Minder, C. Bias in meta-analysis detected by a simple, graphical test. *BMJ* **1997**, *315*, 629–634. [CrossRef] [PubMed]

26. Begg, C.B.; Mazumdar, M. Operating characteristics of a rank correlation test for publication bias. *Biometrics* **1994**, *50*, 1088–1101. [CrossRef] [PubMed]

27. Allen, N.E.; Sauvaget, C.; Roddam, A.W.; Appleby, P.; Nagano, J.; Suzuki, G.; Key, T.J.; Koyama, K. A prospective study of diet and prostate cancer in Japanese men. *Cancer Causes Control* **2004**, *15*, 911–920. [CrossRef] [PubMed]

28. Bosetti, C.; Bravi, F.; Talamini, R.; Parpinel, M.; Gnagnarella, P.; Negri, E.; Montella, M.; Lagiou, P.; Franceschi, S.; La Vecchia, C.; et al. Flavonoids and prostate cancer risk: A study in Italy. *Nutr. Cancer* **2006**, *56*, 123–127. [CrossRef] [PubMed]

29. Heald, C.L.; Ritchie, M.R.; Bolton-Smith, C.; Morton, M.S.; Alexander, F.E. Phyto-oestrogens and risk of prostate cancer in Scottish men. *Br. J. Nutr.* **2007**, *98*, 388–396. [CrossRef] [PubMed]

30. Hedelin, M.; Klint, A.; Chang, E.T.; Bellocco, R.; Johansson, J.-E.; Andersson, S.-W.; Heinonen, S.-M.; Adlercreutz, H.; Adami, H.-O.; Gronberg, H.; et al. Dietary phytoestrogen, serum enterolactone and risk of prostate cancer: The cancer prostate Sweden study (Sweden). *Cancer Causes Control* **2006**, *17*, 169–180. [CrossRef] [PubMed]

31. Jacobsen, B.K.; Knutsen, S.F.; Fraser, G.E. Does high soy milk intake reduce prostate cancer incidence? The Adventist Health Study (United States). *Cancer Causes Control* **1998**, *9*, 553–557. [CrossRef] [PubMed]

32. Jian, L.; Zhang, D.H.; Lee, A.H.; Binns, C.W. Do preserved foods increase prostate cancer risk? *Br. J. Cancer* **2004**, *90*, 1792–1795. [CrossRef] [PubMed]

33. Kirsh, V.A.; Peters, U.; Mayne, S.T.; Subar, A.F.; Chatterjee, N.; Johnson, C.C.; Hayes, R.B.; Prostate, L.C. Prospective study of fruit and vegetable intake and risk of prostate cancer. *J. Natl. Cancer Inst.* **2007**, *99*. [CrossRef] [PubMed]

34. Kolonel, L.N.; Hankin, J.H.; Whittemore, A.S.; Wu, A.H.; Gallagher, R.P.; Wilkens, L.R.; John, E.M.; Howe, G.R.; Dreon, D.M.; West, D.W.; et al. Vegetables, fruits, legumes and prostate cancer: A multiethnic case-control study. *Cancer Epidemiol. Biomark. Prev.* **2000**, *9*, 795–804.

35. Kurahashi, N.; Iwasaki, M.; Inoue, M.; Sasazuki, S.; Tsugane, S. Plasma isoflavones and subsequent risk of prostate cancer in a nested case-control study: The Japan Public Health Center. *J. Clin. Oncol.* **2008**, *26*, 5923–5929. [CrossRef] [PubMed]

36. Kurahashi, N.; Iwasaki, M.; Sasazuki, S.; Otani, T.; Inoue, M.; Tsugane, S. Soy product and isoflavone consumption in relation to prostate cancer in Japanese men. *Cancer Epidemiol. Biomark. Prev.* **2007**, *16*, 538–545. [CrossRef] [PubMed]

37. Lee, M.M.; Gomez, S.L.; Chang, J.S.; Wey, M.; Wang, R.T.; Hsing, A.W. Soy and isoflavone consumption in relation to prostate cancer risk in China. *Cancer Epidemiol. Biomark. Prev.* **2003**, *12*, 665–668.

38. Lewis, J.E.; Soler-Vila, H.; Clark, P.E.; Kresty, L.A.; Allen, G.O.; Hu, J.J. Intake of plant foods and associated nutrients in prostate cancer risk. *Nutr. Cancer* **2009**, *61*, 216–224. [CrossRef] [PubMed]

39. Li, X.M.; Li, J.; Tsuji, I.; Nakaya, N.; Nishino, Y.; Zhao, X.J. Mass screening-based case-control study of diet and prostate cancer in Changchun, China. *Asian J. Androl.* **2008**, *10*, 551–560. [CrossRef] [PubMed]

40. Low, Y.L.; Taylor, J.I.; Grace, P.B.; Mulligan, A.A.; Welch, A.A.; Scollen, S.; Dunning, A.M.; Luben, R.N.; Khaw, K.T.; Day, N.E.; et al. Phytoestrogen exposure, polymorphisms in COMT, CYP19, ESR1, and SHBG genes, and their associations with prostate cancer risk. *Nutr. Cancer* **2006**, *56*, 31–39. [CrossRef] [PubMed]

41. Nagata, Y.; Sonoda, T.; Mori, M.; Miyanaga, N.; Okumura, K.; Goto, K.; Naito, S.; Fujimoto, K.; Hirao, Y.; Takahashi, A.; et al. Dietary isoflavones may protect against prostate cancer in Japanese men. *J. Nutr.* **2007**, *137*, 1974–1979. [PubMed]

42. Nagata, Y.; Sugiyama, Y.; Fukuta, F.; Takayanagi, A.; Masumori, N.; Tsukamoto, T.; Akasaka, H.; Ohnishi, H.; Saitoh, S.; Miura, T.; et al. Relationship of serum levels and dietary intake of isoflavone, and the novel bacterium *Slackia* sp. strain NATTS with the risk of prostate cancer: A case-control study among Japanese men. *Int. Urol. Nephrol.* **2016**, *48*, 1453–1460. [CrossRef] [PubMed]

43. Nomura, A.M.Y.; Hankin, J.H.; Lee, J.; Stemmermann, G.N. Cohort study of tofu intake and prostate cancer: No apparent association. *Cancer Epidemiol. Biomark. Prev.* **2004**, *13*, 2277–2279.

44. Ozasa, K.; Nakao, M.; Watanabe, Y.; Hayashi, K.; Miki, T.; Mikami, K.; Mori, M.; Sakauchi, F.; Washio, M.; Ito, Y.; et al. Serum phytoestrogens and prostate cancer risk in a nested case-control study among Japanese men. *Cancer Sci.* **2004**, *95*, 65–71. [CrossRef] [PubMed]

45. Park, S.-Y.; Murphy, S.P.; Wilkens, L.R.; Henderson, B.E.; Kolonel, L.N. Legume and isoflavone intake and prostate cancer risk: The multiethnic cohort study. *Int. J. Cancer* **2008**, *123*, 927–932. [CrossRef] [PubMed]

46. Severson, R.K.; Nomura, A.M.; Grove, J.S.; Stemmermann, G.N. A prospective study of demographics, diet, and prostate cancer among men of Japanese ancestry in Hawaii. *Cancer Res.* **1989**, *49*, 1857–1860. [PubMed]

47. Sonoda, T.; Nagata, Y.; Mori, M.; Miyanaga, N.; Takashima, N.; Okumura, K.; Goto, K.; Naito, S.; Fujimoto, K.; Hirao, Y.; et al. A case-control study of diet and prostate cancer in Japan: Possible protective effect of traditional Japanese diet. *Cancer Sci.* **2004**, *95*, 238–242. [CrossRef] [PubMed]

48. Strom, S.S.; Yamamura, Y.; Duphorne, C.M.; Spitz, M.R.; Babaian, R.J.; Pillow, P.C.; Hursting, S.D. Phytoestrogen intake and prostate cancer: A case-control study using a new database. *Nutr. Cancer* **1999**, *33*, 20–25. [CrossRef] [PubMed]

49. Sung, J.F.C.; Lin, R.S.; Pu, Y.; Chen, Y.; Chang, H.C.; Lai, M. Risk factors for prostate carcinoma in Taiwan: A case-control study in a Chinese population. *Cancer* **1999**, *86*, 484–491. [CrossRef]

50. Travis, R.C.; Allen, N.E.; Appleby, P.N.; Price, A.; Kaaks, R.; Chang-Claude, J.; Boeing, H.; Aleksandrova, K.; Tjonneland, A.; Johnsen, N.F.; et al. Prediagnostic concentrations of plasma genistein and prostate cancer risk in 1,605 men with prostate cancer and 1,697 matched control participants in EPIC. *Cancer Causes Control* **2012**, *23*, 1163–1171. [CrossRef] [PubMed]

51. Travis, R.C.; Spencer, E.A.; Allen, N.E.; Appleby, P.N.; Roddam, A.W.; Overvad, K.; Johnsen, N.F.; Olsen, A.; Kaaks, R.; Linseisen, J.; et al. Plasma phyto-oestrogens and prostate cancer in the European Prospective Investigation into Cancer and Nutrition. *Br. J. Cancer* **2009**, *100*, 1817–1823. [CrossRef] [PubMed]

52. Villenueve, P.J.; Johnson, K.C.; Krieger, N.; Mao, Y. Risk Factors for Prostate Cancer: Results from the Canadian National Enhanced CancerSurveillance System. *Cancer Causes Control* **1999**, *10*, 355–367. [CrossRef]

53. Wang, Y.; Stevens, V.L.; Shah, R.; Peterson, J.J.; Dwyer, J.T.; Gapstur, S.M.; McCullough, M.L. Dietary Flavonoid and Proanthocyanidin Intakes and Prostate Cancer Risk in a Prospective Cohort of US Men. *Am. J. Epidemiol.* **2014**, *179*, 974–986. [CrossRef] [PubMed]

54. Ward, H.; Chapelais, G.; Kuhnle, G.G.C.; Luben, R.; Khaw, K.-T.; Bingham, S. Lack of prospective associations between plasma and urinary phytoestrogens and risk of prostate or colorectal cancer in the European prospective into Cancer-Norfolk study. *Cancer Epidemiol. Biomark. Prev.* **2008**, *17*, 2891–2894. [CrossRef] [PubMed]

55. Ward, H.A.; Kuhnle, G.G.; Mulligan, A.A.; Lentjes, M.A.; Luben, R.N.; Khaw, K.T. Breast, colorectal, and prostate cancer risk in the European Prospective Investigation into Cancer and Nutrition-Norfolk in relation to phytoestrogen intake derived from an improved database. *Am. J. Clin. Nutr.* **2010**, *91*, 440–448. [CrossRef] [PubMed]

56. Wu, Y.; Zhang, L.; Na, R.; Xu, J.; Xiong, Z.; Zhang, N.; Dai, W.; Jiang, H.; Ding, Q. Plasma genistein and risk of prostate cancer in Chinese population. *Int. Urol. Nephrol.* **2015**, *47*, 965–970. [CrossRef] [PubMed]

57. Rice, L.; Handayani, R.; Cui, Y.; Medrano, T.; Samedi, V.; Baker, H. Soy isoflavones exert differential effects on androgen responsive genes in LNCaP human prostate cancer cells. *J. Nutr.* **2007**, *137*, 964–972. [PubMed]

58. Kang, N.H.; Shin, H.C.; Oh, S.; Lee, K.H.; Lee, Y.B.; Choi, K.C. Soy milk digestion extract inhibits progression of prostate cancer cell growth via regulation of prostate cancerspecific antigen and cell cycle-regulatory genes in human LNCaP cancer cells. *Mol. Med. Rep.* **2016**, *14*, 1809–1816. [CrossRef] [PubMed]

59. Zuniga, K.; Clinton, S.; Thomas-Ahner, J.M.; Erdman, J.W. The effect of tomato powder, soy germ, or a combination on prostate carcinogenesis in TRAMP mice. *FASEB J.* **2012**, *26*, 376.

60. Murphy, P.A.; Song, T.; Buseman, G.; Barua, K.; Beecher, G.; Trainer, D.; Holden, J. Isoflavones in retail and institutional soy foods. *J. Agric. Food Chem.* **1999**, *47*, 2697–2704. [CrossRef] [PubMed]

61. Larkin, T.; Price, W.E.; Astheimer, L. The key importance of soy isoflavone bioavailability to understanding health benefits. *Crit. Rev. Food Sci. Nutr.* **2008**, *48*, 538–552. [CrossRef] [PubMed]

62. Morito, K.; Hirose, T.; Kinjo, J.; Hirakawa, T.; Okawa, M.; Nohara, T.; Ogawa, S.; Inoue, S.; Muramatsu, M.; Masamune, Y. Interaction of phytoestrogens with estrogen receptors alpha and beta. *Biol. Pharm. Bull.* **2001**, *24*, 351–356. [CrossRef] [PubMed]

63. Heldring, N.; Pike, A.; Andersson, S.; Matthews, J.; Cheng, G.; Hartman, J.; Tujague, M.; Ström, A.; Treuter, E.; Warner, M.; et al. Estrogen Receptors: How Do They Signal and What Are Their Targets. *Physiol. Rev.* **2007**, *87*, 905–931. [CrossRef] [PubMed]

64. Warner, M.; Huang, B.; Gustafsson, J.-A. Estrogen Receptor β as a Pharmaceutical Target. *Trends Pharmacol. Sci.* **2017**, *38*, 92–99. [CrossRef] [PubMed]

65. Mahmoud, A.M.; Yang, W.; Bosland, M.C. Soy isoflavones and prostate cancer: A review of molecular mechanisms. *J. Steroid Biochem. Mol. Biol.* **2014**, *140*, 116–132. [CrossRef] [PubMed]

66. Wu, A.H.; Yang, D.; Pike, M.C. A meta-analysis of soyfoods and risk of stomach cancer: The problem of potential confounders. *Cancer Epidemiol. Biomark. Prev.* **2000**, *9*, 1051–1058.

67. Islam, M.A.; Punt, A.; Spenkelink, B.; Murk, A.J.; Rolaf van Leeuwen, F.X.; Rietjens, I.M. Conversion of major soy isoflavone glucosides and aglycones in in vitro intestinal models. *Mol. Nutr. Food Res.* **2014**, *58*, 503–515. [CrossRef] [PubMed]

68. Messina, M. Soy and Health Update: Evaluation of the Clinical and Epidemiologic Literature. *Nutrients* **2016**, *8*, 754. [CrossRef] [PubMed]

69. Busby, M.G.; Jeffcoat, A.R.; Bloedon, L.T.; Koch, M.A.; Black, T.; Dix, K.J.; Heizer, W.D.; Thomas, B.F.; Hill, J.M.; Crowell, J.A.; et al. Clinical characteristics and pharmacokinetics of purified soy isoflavones: Single-dose administration to healthy men. *Am. J. Clin. Nutr.* **2002**, *75*, 126–136. [PubMed]

70. Jarred, R.A.; Keikha, M.; Dowling, C.; McPherson, S.J.; Clare, A.M.; Husband, A.J.; Pedersen, J.S.; Frydenberg, M.; Risbridger, G.P. Induction of apoptosis in low to moderate-grade human prostate carcinoma by red clover-derived dietary isoflavones. *Cancer Epidemiol. Biomark. Prev.* **2002**, *11*, 1689–1696.

71. Hamilton-Reeves, J.M.; Banerjee, S.; Banerjee, S.K.; Holzbeierlein, J.M.; Thrasher, J.B.; Kambhampati, S.; Keighley, J.; Van Veldhuizen, P. Short-term soy isoflavone intervention in patients with localized prostate cancer: A randomized, double-blind, placebo-controlled trial. *PLoS ONE* **2013**, *8*, e68331. [CrossRef] [PubMed]

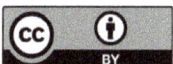

nutrients

MDPI

Article

Resveratrol and Pterostilbene Exhibit Anticancer Properties Involving the Downregulation of HPV Oncoprotein E6 in Cervical Cancer Cells

Kaushiki Chatterjee [1,2], Dina AlSharif [2], Christina Mazza [2], Palwasha Syar [2], Mohamed Al Sharif [2] and Jimmie E. Fata [1,2,*]

[1]   Doctoral Program in Biology, CUNY Graduate Center, New York, NY 10016, USA;
       kaushiki.chatterjee@csi.cuny.edu
[2]   Department of Biology, College of Staten Island, New York, NY 10314, USA; dina95usa@aol.com (D.A.);
       Christinamazza19@gmail.com (C.M.); palwashasyar@yahoo.com (P.S.);
       Alsharif.mohamed@hotmail.com (M.A.S.)
*   Correspondence: jimmie.fata@csi.cuny.edu; Tel.: +1-718-982-3862

Received: 3 January 2018; Accepted: 12 February 2018; Published: 21 February 2018

Abstract: Cervical cancer is one of the most common cancers in women living in developing countries. Due to a lack of affordable effective therapy, research into alternative anticancer compounds with low toxicity such as dietary polyphenols has continued. Our aim is to determine whether two structurally similar plant polyphenols, resveratrol and pterostilbene, exhibit anticancer and anti-HPV (Human papillomavirus) activity against cervical cancer cells. To determine anticancer activity, extensive in vitro analyses were performed. Anti-HPV activity, through measuring E6 protein levels, subsequent downstream p53 effects, and caspase-3 activation, were studied to understand a possible mechanism of action. Both polyphenols are effective agents in targeting cervical cancer cells, having low IC50 values in the μM range. They decrease clonogenic survival, reduce cell migration, arrest cells at the S-phase, and reduce the number of mitotic cells. These findings were significant, with pterostilbene often being more effective than resveratrol. Resveratrol and to a greater extent pterostilbene downregulates the HPV oncoprotein E6, induces caspase-3 activation, and upregulates p53 protein levels. Results point to a mechanism that may involve the downregulation of the HPV E6 oncoprotein, activation of apoptotic pathways, and re-establishment of functional p53 protein, with pterostilbene showing greater efficacy than resveratrol.

Keywords: cervical cancer; resveratrol; pterostilbene; HPV E6; p53; cell cycle

1. Introduction

Cervical cancer is one of the most prevalent cancers affecting women worldwide. It is the second most common cancer in developing countries and 11th in developed countries—these regional differences are often attributed to the lack of Pap smears, a preventative procedure often absent in underdeveloped areas [1,2]. It is widely accepted that the etiological factor that causes cervical cancer is chronic infection of the human papilloma virus (HPV), which is considered the most common sexually transmitted infection [3]. Every year about 500,000 women acquire the disease and 75% are from the developing countries [4]. Moreover, recent evidence indicates that HPV infection is on the rise in men, leading to higher incidences of penile and oropharyngeal cancer [5]. HPVs can be clinically classified as "low-risk" (LR-HPV) or "high-risk" (HR-HPV) depending on the relative tendency of the HPV lesions to transform into malignancy. HPV 16 and HPV 18 are the two most important cancer-causing, high-risk HPV [6]. HPV progression to cancer is dependent on prolonged infection by these high risk HPV viruses. The progression of HPV lesions to a neoplastic stage is dependent on several co-factors. Although there are approved HPV vaccines and drugs available, a problem is the affordability of these drugs in low income areas [7]. Two such vaccines are Cervarix® and Gardasil® [8], which renders prophylactic actions against cervical lesions associated with the most common oncogenic HPV types, 16/18, but effective therapeutic measures for post-infection lesions are currently not available. The major concern for the common chemotherapeutic medicines like cisplatin and paclitaxel are their adverse side effects [9,10]. The development of natural chemoprotective drugs that effectively target HPV infection could drastically reduce the incidence and progression of cervical cancer worldwide if they are not cost inhibitive and have low side effects.

Of the varied groups of naturally occurring antioxidants, polyphenols have gained increased importance in cervical cancer since they have displayed potent antitumor properties in a number of cancers by targeting several pathways that are involved in cancer progression [11,12]. The current article uses cervical cancer cells to compare the tumor-inhibitory effects and mechanism of action of two such polyphenols, resveratrol and pterostilbene. Both resveratrol and pterostilbene are stilbenes, which is a class of natural polyphenolic compounds that have been studied for their anticarcinogenic activities. Resveratrol (3,4,5-trihydroxy-trans-stilbene) has been isolated from grapes, red wine, purple grape juice, peanuts, berries, and some medicinal plants [13]. Resveratrol is a widely studied stilbene compound having very low toxicity in the human system, and it is also known to modulate several pathways that are directly linked to cancer progression [14]. Both in vitro and in vivo cancer studies have shown resveratrol to inhibit cell proliferation and angiogenesis along with inducing pro-apoptotic properties [15]. The potential problem of using resveratrol as a chemoprotective agent is that it has low systemic bioavailability, which might lower its efficacy in the human system [16]. In order to overcome this, several efforts are being made to develop resveratrol derivatives with higher systemic bioavailability [17]. Pterostilbene (trans-3,5-dimethoxy-4-hydroxystilbene) is a naturally derived dimethylether analogue of resveratrol. Pterostilbene is believed to be produced in plants as a defense mechanism against some external microbial or fungal infection and is therefore considered a phytoalexin [18]. It has been isolated from grapevine leaves and blueberries [19]. Recently, pterostilbene has gained much attention as a possible anticancer agent, showing no toxicity in humans up to a dose of 250 mg/day [20].

Although the chemical structure of pterostilbene is closely related to resveratrol, the substitution of the hydroxyl group with a methoxy group in pterostilbene is believed to make the molecule more stable as well as increase its capacity to enter cells [21]. In addition, clinical studies have shown that the half-life and oral bioavailability of pterostilbene are significantly greater than those of resveratrol [20]. Studies on colon cancer cell lines have shown pterostilbene to be more potent than resveratrol in inhibiting DNA synthesis and in decreasing the expression of inflammatory genes responsible for cancer progression [22]. Although studies in other types of carcinomas show the potential efficacy of resveratrol and pterostilbene, there has been no study to the best of our knowledge that explores an anticancer mechanism that is specific for HPV-positive carcinoma. An in silico docking study has shown that resveratrol interacts with the p53 binding site of E6 residues [23]. E6 is a vital HPV oncoprotein essential for cervical cancer progression. E6 binds to tumor suppressor protein p53 and targets it for degradation by the ubiquitin proteasome pathway [24], thus causing uncontrolled cell proliferation. Here, we set out to compare the relative effectiveness of resveratrol against pterostilbene on cervical cancer cells, paying particular attention to their comparative IC_{50} values, changes in the levels of the HPV oncoprotein E6 and its target p53, as well as their comparative pro-apoptotic and anti-migratory capacities.

2. Materials and Methods

2.1. Cell Culture

Human cervical carcinoma HeLa cells were obtained from a commercial supplier (American Type Culture Collection, Manassas, VA, USA) and were cultured in Dulbecco's Modified Eagle

Medium: Nutrient Mixture F-12 (DMEM/F-12) (HyClone, GE Healthcare Life Sciences, Manassas, VA, USA), supplemented with 10% fetal calf serum (HyClone, GE Healthcare Life Sciences) and 0.1% Penicillin-Streptomycin Solution (HyClone). Cells were incubated in a 37 °C incubator with 5% CO_2.

2.2. Determination of IC$_{50}$ Using WST-1 Assay

Seven thousand cells were plated on 96-well plates and allowed to grow for 24 h. Resveratrol (Acros, #430075000) or pterostilbene (TCI, #P1924) was serially diluted from 10–120 μM into DMEM/F-12 plus $1\times$ insulin-transferrin-selenium (ITS) supplement (Invitrogen). Cells were treated with dilutions (in triplicate) for 24 h prior to performing a WST-1 (Water Soluble Tetrazolium salt-1) cell viability assay. The WST assay involved aspiration of the medium after treatment and rinsing three times with equal volumes of $1\times$ Phosphate Buffered Saline (PBS), followed by the addition of 80 μL of 10% WST-1 (Clontech, Mountain View, CA, USA) in DMEM to each well. The plate was then incubated at 37 °C for 1 h and absorbance monitored at 440 nm using a plate reader. Results obtained were analyzed using GraphPad Prism 5 software to determine the IC$_{50}$ using a standardized method [25,26].

2.3. Live Imaging

Images of untreated and treated (with resveratrol and pterostilbene) cells were taken every 10 min for 24 h to generate video files using a Zeiss Axio Observer Z1 microscope.

2.4. Clonogenic Assay

Two hundred thousand cells were plated on 6-well plates and allowed to grow for 24 h prior to treatment with pterostilbene (50 μM) and resveratrol (50 μM) for 24 h. After 24 h, cells were trypsinized to single cell suspensions. After cell counting, 150 viable cells from each treatment set were plated in one well from a 6-well plate and allowed to grow in complete DMEM/F-12 medium for 15 days. After said period of time, cells were washed once with $1\times$ PBS then fixed and stained with 0.5% crystal violet in 6% glutaraldehyde for 30 min. The cells were briefly rinsed with tap water and allowed to air dry. Images of each well was taken and colonies were counted using ImageJ (NIH, Bethesda, Rockville, MD, USA). The plating efficiency and survival factor was calculated as determined previously [27].

2.5. Scratch Assay

Twelve thousand cells were grown on 96-well plates until a confluent monolayer was formed. A scratch was made with a sterile p200 tip in each well through the center of the culture. The debris was washed off with serum-free media and a marking was made on the bottom of the plate to take images at the same location. Cells were then treated with different concentrations (5 μM and 20 μM) of resveratrol or pterostilbene and brightfield images were taken after 48 h to allow closure of the control scratch. The images were analyzed using ImageJ and the area of closure was measured according to previous published methods [28].

2.6. Flow Cytometry

Two hundred and fifty thousand cells were cultured on 6-well plates and subsequently treated with resveratrol or pterostilbene (5 μM, 10 μM, and 15 μM) for 18 h. Cells were trypsinized, centrifuged, and washed with 0.1% Fetal Calf Serum (FCS) in $1\times$ PBS solution and resuspended in 70% ethanol at -20 °C, which was added dropwise while shaking the samples vigorously. Fixed samples were kept at 4 °C for 1 h followed by washing twice in $1\times$ PBS. Prior to flow cytometry, cells were incubated with RNase (500 μg/mL) for 30 min at 37 °C and then stained with propidium iodide (PI; 70 μM) for 30 mins. Cells were analyzed for DNA content by measuring PI fluorescence using an Accuri C6 flow cytometer (BD).

2.7. Western Blot Analysis

Two hundred and fifty thousand cells were cultured on 6-well plates and subsequently treated with resveratrol (10 μM, 50 μM) or pterostilbene (10 μM, 50 μM) for a period of 22 h. Extraction of proteins from cultured cells was performed using M-PER Mammalian protein extraction reagent (Thermo Fisher, Waltham, MA, USA) with protease and phosphatase inhibitors. The total amount of protein in each well was quantified using the Lowry method. To resolve the proteins, 25 μg of protein was subjected to sodium dodecyl sulfate-polyacrylamide gel electrophoresis using a 10% acrylamide separating gel and then transferred to nitrocellulose membrane for 1 h. The membrane was blocked at room temperature for 1 h with 5% nonfat dry milk in Tris Tween Buffered Saline (TTBS). The nitrocellulose membrane was then incubated overnight with a p53 antibody (sc-6243) followed by incubation at room temperature for 1 h with anti-rabbit IgG conjugated with horseradish peroxidase. SuperSignal West Pico chemiluminescence substrate (Pierce) was used for detection following the manufacturer's instructions. The membranes were scanned using APHA INNOTECH Fluorchem SP imaging system. Analysis of blots was done using ImageJ software.

2.8. Immunocytochemistry

Seven thousand HeLa cells were plated on 8-well chamber slides and allowed to grow for 48 h. Cells were then treated with different concentrations of resveratrol (5–50 μM) or pterostilbene (5–50 μM) for 22 h (for study of E6, p53 and cleaved caspase-3) and 18 h (for study of Phospho histone H3). All drug treatments were performed in serum-free DMEM/F-12 containing 1% supplement (ITS; insulin, transferrin, selenium; Gibco BRL, Grand Island, NY, USA). After treatment, cells were fixed in 4% paraformaldehyde at room temperature, rinsed with 1× PBS, and then permeabilized and blocked with 10% horse serum, 2% bovine serum albumin, and 0.5% Triton X-100 in PBS for 1 h. The cells were then incubated overnight with primary antibodies in blocking buffer. Subsequent to primary antibody treatment, the cells were washed and then incubated with the respective Fluorescein isothiocyanate (FITC) conjugated secondary antibodies for 3 h, followed by incubation with 4′,6-diamidino-2-phenylindole (DAPI) (10 μg/mL) and three washes with 1× PBS. The slides were then mounted with coverslips and cell images were acquired using a Zeiss Axio Observer Z1 microscope and an AxioVision 4.6.3-AP1. Images of different, randomly chosen fields were acquired with identical exposure times from each well for quantification. ImageJ was used to measure the fluorescence intensity and cell counting. The fluorescence intensities of E6 and P53 antibodies were normalized to DAPI intensity (blue).

Antibodies Used: E6 antibody (sc-460, Santa Cruz Biotechnology, Dallas, TX, USA), p53 antibody (sc-6243), cleaved caspase-3 antibody (D175, 9661, CST), Phospho Histone H3 (Ser 10) antibody (06–570, Millipore, Burlington, MA, USA).

2.9. Statistical Analysis

Statistical analyses were performed using Microsoft Excel® 2013 (Microsoft Corporation, Redmond, WA, USA) and GraphPad Prism® 5 (GraphPad Software, Inc., La Jolla, CA, USA). Means and standard deviations were calculated for each group. One-way ANOVA with Tukey test was used to compare three or more datasets and determine the significance between the groups. ANOVA is a test of variance and post hoc Tukey test used is for the determination of significance between groups [29,30]. $p < 0.05$ was considered as significant.

3. Results

3.1. Pterostilbene Is More Potent in Eliminating HPV+ HeLa Cells Compared to Resveratrol

In order to study the comparative cytotoxicity of pterostilbene and resveratrol on HeLa tumor cells, brightfield images (Figure 1A) and WST-1 cell viability assays (Figure 1B) were performed 24 h post-treatment. The brightfield images taken after 24 h of treatment (Figure 1A) showed that pterostilbene (40 μM) eliminates significantly more cells than resveratrol at the same concentration. Live imaging of cells treated with 60 μM of the two compounds show significantly more death and characteristic apoptotic blebbing in pterostilbene-treated cells when compared to untreated or resveratrol-treated cells (Supplementary Videos S1–S3). The WST-1 analysis revealed that although both pterostilbene and resveratrol eliminated HeLa cells significantly and in a dose-dependent manner, pterostilbene displayed a 1.97-fold lower IC_{50} when compared to resveratrol (42.3 μM vs. 83.5 μM; $p < 0.05$; Figure 1B). Additionally, both compounds, at 50 μM, significantly inhibited the clonogenicity of post-treated cells in a 15-day clonogenic assay (Figure 1C). Pterostilbene significantly reduced clonogenic survival by 87.5% compared to the control ($p < 0.05$), while resveratrol inhibited it by 63% ($p < 0.05$) (Figure 1C). Moreover, the difference between the survival percentages of the two treatment groups is significant ($p < 0.05$).

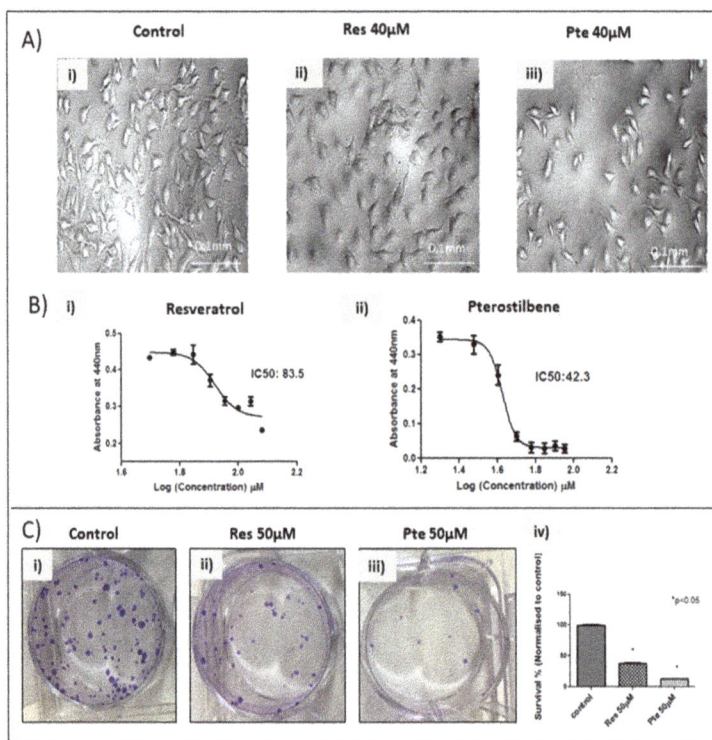

Figure 1. Pterostilbene is more potent in eliminating HeLa cervical cancer cells as compared to resveratrol: (**A**) Brightfield analysis of HeLa cells untreated (Ai) or treated for 24 h with 40 μM of resveratrol (Res; Aii) or 40 μM of pterostilbene (Pte; Aiii). Evidence of cell elimination was only seen robustly in cells treated with pterostilbene at 40 μM. (**B**) Analysis of IC_{50} values, generated by a Water Soluble Tetrazolium salt-1 (WST-1) assay after 24 h of exposure to resveratrol or pterostilbene indicates that pterostilbene ($IC_{50} = 42.3$ μM) is a more potent cytotoxic agent than resveratrol ($IC_{50} = 83.5$ μM; Bii). The graphs represent data from three independent experiments (mean ± S.E.M. (Standard error mean)). (**C**) Clonogenic assays performed to compare the relative effect of the two polyphenols on the clonogenicity of HeLa cells untreated (Ci) or treated with 50 μM of either resveratrol (Cii) or pterostilbene (Ciii). Results are from 15-days post-treatment and indicate that pterostilbene is more efficient in curbing the clonogenicity compared to resveratrol (Civ). Bar graph represents data from three independent experiments (mean ± S.E.M.; * $p < 0.05$; Civ).

3.2. Inhibition of Cell Migration of HeLa Cells Treated with Pterostilbene and Resveratrol

To determine the comparative efficacy of resveratrol and pterostilbene in inhibiting HeLa cell migration, two different sub-lethal concentrations of each compound were used in a 48-h scratch assay (Figure 2). Based on the WST-1 results and brightfield images (unpublished), we found that cells treated with a concentration below 25 μM showed no signs of cellular toxicity. To avoid any cytotoxicity, we used lower concentrations of 5 μM and 20 μM. At sub-lethal concentrations of 5 μM and 20 μM, both resveratrol and pterostilbene significantly inhibited HeLa cell migration relative to untreated cells ($p < 0.05$; Figure 2). Pterostilbene was more effective in inhibiting HeLa cell migration at 20 μM when compared to resveratrol; however, this result was not significant and no differences were seen between the two compounds at 5 μM (Figure 2). In an effort to analyze the effects of resveratrol and pterostilbene on cell migration, we normalized the amount of migration into the scratch (wound) by untreated cells, to 100%. Relative to this control, resveratrol-treated cells migrated only 71.2% (5 μM) and 63.7% (20 μM), while cells treated with pterostilbene migrated only 69.5% (5 μM) and 49.2% (20 μM) (Figure 2).

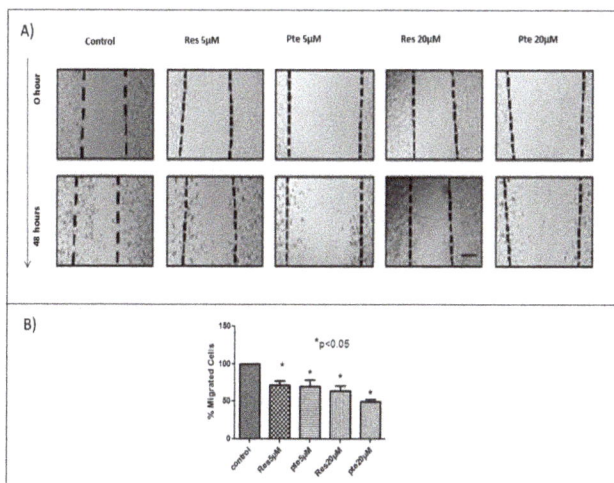

Figure 2. Resveratrol and pterostilbene inhibit cell migration: (**A**) HeLa cells were monitored for cell migration into a scratched "wound". Cells were either untreated or treated with sub-lethal concentrations (5 μM and 20 μM) of resveratrol (Res) or pterostilbene (Pte). The extent of migration into the scratched area was calculated after 48 h and revealed that both resveratrol and pterostilbene significantly inhibit cell migration, although pterostilbene had greater anti-migratory effect. (**B**) The graphs represents data from triplicate sample experiments normalized to the control (mean % migrated cells ± S.E.M.; * $p < 0.05$). Scale bar: 0.05 μm.

3.3. Cell Cycle Arrest at S-Phase in HeLa Cells Treated with Low Concentrations of Resveratrol and Pterostilbene

In order to compare the effect of sub-lethal doses of either resveratrol or pterostilbene on the cell cycle of HeLa cells, treatment was carried out with three different concentrations (5 μM, 10 μM, and 15 μM) of the two compounds for 18 h prior to flow cytometric analysis (Figure 3A). Flow cytometry analysis showed that the cells treated with either compound exhibited a significant decrease in the number of cells in the G2-M phase with respect to the control cells ($p < 0.05$) (Figure 3A,B, Table 1), indicating an S-phase cell cycle arrest. This effect corresponded with an increase in the number of cells arrested at the S-phase. Pterostilbene was significantly more potent than resveratrol in inhibiting cell cycle progression, showing effects at concentrations as low as

5 μM ($p < 0.05$) (Figure 3A,B, Table 1). At this concentration, pterostilbene had these percentages of cells in each phase: G1 = 53.4 ± 1.4, S = 34 ± 1.4, G2 =12.5 ± 0.2, while resveratrol had values of G1 = 64.8 ± 2.0, S = 16.3 ± 1.0, G2 = 18.3 ± 2.3. At a higher concentration (15 μM) both compounds significantly inhibited cells from entering into G2-M by arresting them in the S-phase, and difference between the extent of the arrest at this phase induced by the two compounds was significant ($p < 0.05$) (Figure 3A,B, Table 1).

To confirm the cell cycle data, which indicated that both compounds are potent inhibitors of cells entering into G2-M, we investigated the status of the M-phase mitotic marker phospho-histone-H3 by immunocytochemistry (Figure 3C,D). At concentrations of 10 μM, both compounds significantly suppressed the amount of cells positive for the mitotic marker phospho-histone-H3, when compared to the untreated cells control. Although resveratrol significantly suppressed the abundance of phospho-histone-H3 (mitotic cells) at 5 μM, when compared to the control cells, pterostilbene at this concentration was significantly more potent than resveratrol (Figure 3D). Relative to the control, which was set at 100%, cells treated with 5 μM pterostilbene exhibited only 13.8% mitotic cells positive for the marker, which was significantly lower than the resveratrol-treated sample at this concentration, which had 60% mitotic cells (Figure 3D; $p < 0.05$).

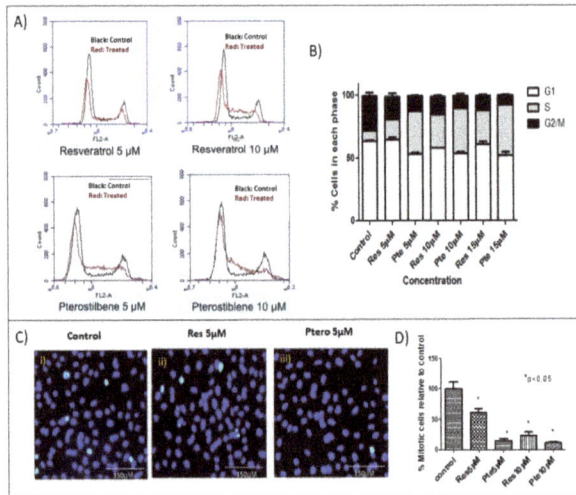

Figure 3. S-phase arrest in HeLa cells treated with low concentrations of resveratrol and pterostilbene: (**A**) Flow-cytometric evaluation of HeLa cells untreated or treated with sub-lethal doses of resveratrol (Res) and pterostilbene (Pte) for 18 h. Treated cells exhibited S-phase arrest and a subsequent decrease in the number of cells in G2/M. Pterostilbene was a more potent compound than resveratrol, showing a capacity to arrest cells at the S-phase at concentrations as low as 5 μM. (**B**) Graphical representation of the dose-dependent cell cycle effects induced by resveratrol and pterostilbene at three different concentrations (5 μM, 10 μM, and 15 μM). (**B**) The graph represents data from triplicate sample experiments normalized to the control (mean % cells in each phase ± S.E.M.) (**C**) Immunofluorescent images of HeLa cells probed for the M-phase marker phospho-histone-H3 (serine10). HeLa cells were untreated or treated with 5 μM and 10 μM of resveratrol or pterostilbene. Immunofluorescent images display a decrease of histone-H3 in cells treated with both the compounds, the effects at 5 μM of pterostilbene is much greater than those of resveratrol (at 5 μM). (**D**) Graphical representation of the percent of mitotic cells calculated from immunofluorescent images reveal that resveratrol and to a greater extent pterostilbene are effective in decreasing the number of mitotic HeLa cells. The graph represents data from experiments obtained from triplicate samples normalized to the control (mean % mitotic cells ± S.E.M.;* $p < 0.05$).

Table 1. Table showing the percentage of cells in each phase of the cell cycle (% ± S.E.M.) after treatment with different concentrations of resveratrol (Res) and pterostilbene (Pte).

	G1 ± S.E.M.	S ± S.E.M.	G2 ± S.E.M.
Control	64.1 ± 0.4	8.00 ± 2.5	27.7 ± 2.4
Res 5 μM	64.8 ± 2.0	16.3 ± 1.0	18.3 ± 2.3 ^
Pte 5 μM	53.4 ± 1.4 [+]	34.0 ± 1.4 *	12.5 ± 0.2 ^
Res 10 μM	58.5 ± 0.2	26.5 ± 0.2 *	14.4 ± 1.0 ^
Pte 10 μM	54.3 ± 0.8 [+]	35.6 ± 2.4 *	10.1 ± 1.5 ^
Res 15 μM	61.3 ± 1.9	27.1 ± 0.8 *,#	11.5 ± 1.2 ^
Pte 15 μM	52.3 ± 2.0 [+]	40.1 ± 3.4 *,#	7.7 ± 0.5 ^

[+] $p < 0.05$ relative to G1 control, * $p < 0.05$ relative to S control, ^ $p < 0.05$ relative to G2 control, # $p < 0.05$ relative to each other.

3.4. Downregulation of Viral Oncoprotein E6 and Upregulation of Active-Caspase-3 in HeLa Cells Treated with Pterostilbene and Resveratrol

In order to investigate how resveratrol and pterostilbene were affecting HeLa cell survival and cell cycle progression, we treated cells with either of the two compounds at sub-lethal (10 μM) and higher (50 μM) concentrations prior to analysis by immunostaining for E6, active caspase-3, and p53 (Figure 4A–C). At 10 μM, both resveratrol and pterostilbene failed to significantly affect levels of E6 and active caspase-3 levels relative to the control (Figure 4A,B). However, at 50 μM both compounds significantly suppressed E6 levels and elevated cleaved caspase-3 levels in treated cells relative to the untreated cells (Figure 3A–C). At this concentration (50 μM), pterostilbene was significantly more potent than resveratrol at suppressing E6 levels (resveratrol = 0.77 ± 0.11: 23% decrease vs. pterostilbene = 0.57 ± 0.06: 43% decrease; $p < 0.05$) and simultaneously elevating active caspase-3. It should be noted that we were unable to detect any noticeable differences in the sub-cellular localization of E6 in treated cells (Figure 4A).

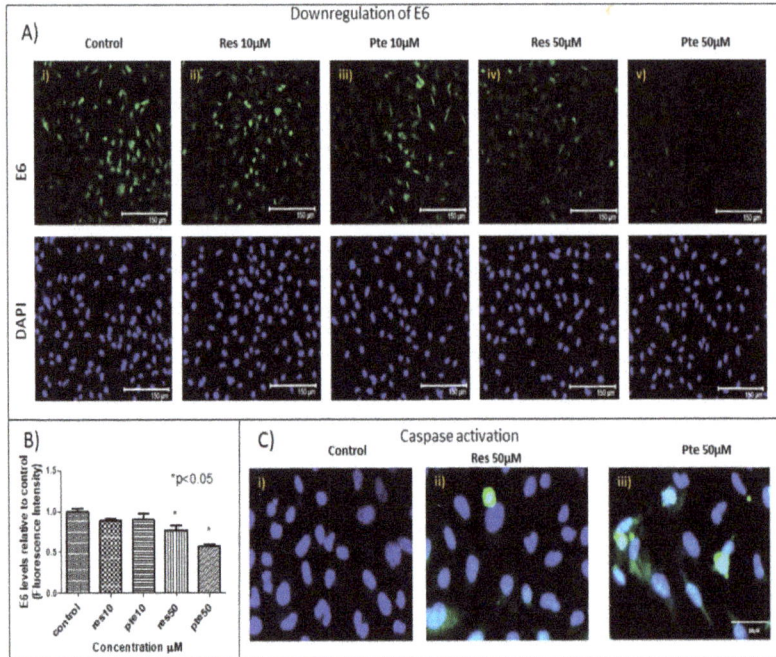

Figure 4. Downregulation of viral oncoprotein E6 and upregulation of active-caspase-3 in HeLa cells treated with resveratrol or pterostilbene: (**A**) HeLa cells immunostained for E6 levels (green) and counterstained with the nuclear dye 4′,6-diamidino-2-phenylindole (DAPI) (blue) after treatment with resveratrol (Res) and pterostilbene (Pte; 10 μM and 50 μM). Loss of E6 proteins are visually evident in cells treated with 50 μM of either resveratrol or pterostilbene. (**B**) Cell image analysis of the E6 fluorescent data revealed a significant 43% decrease of E6 protein levels in HeLa cells treated with pterostilbene at 50 μM and a 23% decrease of E6 levels in cells treated with resveratrol, both relative to the control. The graph represents data from experiments obtained from three independent experiments normalized to the control (mean % normalized to DAPI ± S.E.M.; * $p < 0.05$). (**C**) Immunofluorescent images probing for active-caspase-3 (green) shows a corresponding enhanced activation of this mediator of apoptosis by both resveratrol and pterostilbene.

3.5. Upregulation of Tumor Suppressor Protein p53 in HeLa Cells Treated with Pterostilbene and Resveratrol

Concomitant with E6 suppression, 50 μM pterostilbene treatment for 22 h caused an upregulation of p53 in HeLa cells (Figure 5A,B). When compared to the control, pterostilbene treatment elicited a 2-fold increase in p53 levels (staining normalized to DAPI; Figure 5B; $p < 0.05$). In comparison to the control, HeLa cells treated with 50 μM of resveratrol also caused an upregulation of p53 (1.75-fold increase; Figure 5A,B; $p < 0.05$) at 22 h.

Total protein levels of p53 were also analyzed by Western blot in cells treated with either resveratrol (10 μM and 50 μM) or pterostilbene (10 μM and 50 μM) for 22 h (Figure 5C,D). Both compounds elevated p53 levels at 50 μM; however, significance was only noted in cells treated with pterostilbene at this concentration (Figure 5C,D). Although cells treated with pterostilbene at 10 μM tended to have elevated p53 protein levels relative to both the control cells and cells treated with 10 μM of resveratrol, these differences were not significant based on an ANOVA test (Figure 5C,D).

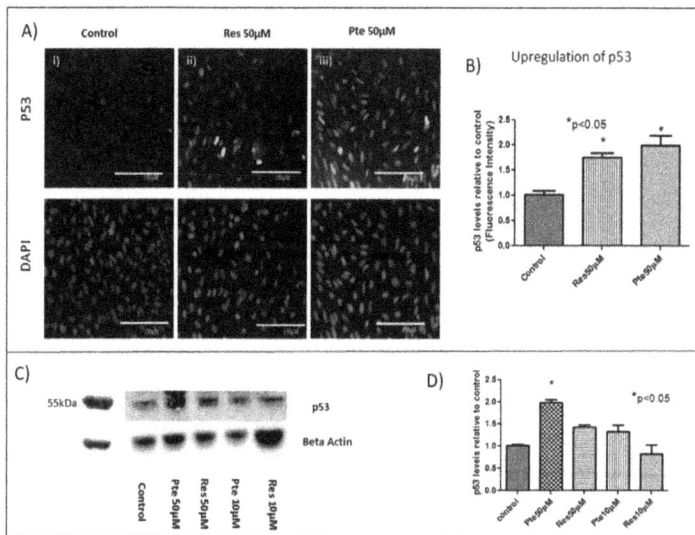

Figure 5. Upregulation of the tumor suppressor protein p53 in HeLa cells treated with resveratrol and pterostilbene: (**A**) Immunoflourescent images of p53 protein (green) untreated or after treatment with 50 μM of either resveratrol (Res) or pterostilbene (Pte) for 22 h. Levels of p53 are elevated in cells treated with either polyphenol. (**B**) Image analysis of p53 immunofluorescence indicates that pterostilbene treatment at 50 μM elicited a significant 2-fold increase in p53, while resveratrol exposure at similar concentrations induced a significant 1.75 increase in p53. The graph represents data from experiments obtained from three independent experiments normalized to the control (mean % normalized to DAPI ± S.E.M. * $p < 0.05$). (**C**) Western blot analysis also revealed that the elevation of p53 protein levels is evident in HeLa cells treated with 50 μM of resveratrol and pterostilbene; however, significant differences relative to the control were only reached with HeLa cells treated pterostilbene at 50 μM. (**D**) The graph represents data from experiments obtained from three independent experiments normalized to the control (mean % normalized to beta-actin ± S.E.M.; * $p < 0.05$).

4. Discussion and Conclusions

In the current study, for the first time to our knowledge, we have compared the antitumor potency of resveratrol and pterostilbene on E6+ cervical cancer cells in vitro. We demonstrated that pterostilbene was significantly more potent than resveratrol in eliminating and in abrogating the clonogenicity of these cervical cancer cells (Figure 1). To assess and study the effects of the two compounds, we used a wide range of concentrations. Sub IC$_{50}$ concentrations ranging from 5–20 μM were used to understand the action of these polyphenols at a low concentration. The results show that at these concentrations the polyphenols can inhibit cell division and migration. To further understand the cytotoxic mechanisms, it was imperative for us to look at supra IC$_{50}$ concentrations. We used 50 μM to understand the mechanism of action. The clonogenic assay using this high concentration elucidates the long-term effect of these polyphenols on surviving cells even after the removal of treatment. While sub-IC$_{50}$ values of both compounds inhibited the migration of E6+ cervical cancer cells, a higher sub-lethal concentration of resveratrol (20 μM) was needed to exert any significant inhibitory effect. Nonetheless, pterostilbene caused a more significant degree of inhibition to cell migration, attesting its superior antitumor potency (Figure 2). It is a notion held by cancer researchers that sub-IC$_{50}$ concentrations of chemotherapeutic drugs are ineffective in curtailing tumor malignancy. However, surprisingly, our data shows that even at a low sub-lethal concentration (5 μM), pterostilbene is more effective than resveratrol as an antiproliferative agent against cervical cancer cells by triggering cell cycle arrest at the S-phase (Figure 3). In addition to being effective at sub-IC_{50} concentrations, the supra-IC_{50} concentration of pterostilbene (50 µM) was also superior to resveratrol (at 50 µM) in suppressing E6 while upregulating p53 and active-caspase-3 expression, thus causing a greater degree of apoptosis-mediated cell elimination. This observed suppression of E6 and upregulation of p53 is of paramount importance because HPV infection and cancer progression in cervical cells relies on the expression of the viral E6 oncoprotein which targets p53 for degradation by the ubiquitination [24,31]. Thus, untreated cervical cancer cells continue to proliferate in the absence of p53, unable to respond to cell stress and DNA damage. Our data indicates that resveratrol and pterostilbene may restore an adequate p53 response and ultimately act as anticancer plant compounds.

A comparative study between resveratrol and pterostilbene on colon cancer cells had shown pterostilbene to be a more potent anticancer agent compared to resveratrol [15]. Our first approach to understand the comparative efficacy of resveratrol and pterostilbene in HeLa cells was a cytotoxicity analysis, in addition to ascertaining the inhibitory concentration (IC_{50}) (Figure 1 and Videos S1–S3). The results clearly indicated that pterostilbene could eliminate HeLa cells much faster and at a significantly lower concentration compared to resveratrol. We also further analyzed the cytotoxic potential of these polyphenols on a second cell line, E6-positive murine TC1 cells, and found a similar trend in IC_{50} results for resveratrol and pterostilbene, where pterostilbene is 2-fold more cytotoxic than resveratrol [32]. Since cancer cells are known to have enhanced clonogenecity [27,33], our study aimed to see the survival capability of the cells treated with supra-IC_{50} concentrations of either resveratrol or pterostilbene. Clonogenic studies show the long term-term effects of these polyphenols on cervical cancer cells after treatment for 24 h and then allowing the surviving cells to grow in normal growth medium for 15 days. Both compounds at supra-IC_{50} concentrations showed a dramatic decrease in the clonogenic capacity of the surviving cells. These results suggest that resveratrol and pterostilbene may suppress new tumor growth often seen in high-grade metastatic cervical cancer.

The migration of cancer cells is a very important factor responsible for the metastasizing of cancers [34]. Inhibition of migration can play a major role in checking the progression of cancer metastasis. Our study found that sub-cytotoxic doses of both compounds exhibit anti-migratory roles. These findings are supported by previous studies, which have shown that resveratrol shows anti-migratory activity by suppressing phorbol 12-myristate 13-acetate (PMA)-induced migration in cervical cancer cells [35]. Studies in hepatocellular carcinoma indicate that pterostilbene suppresses migration by downregulating MMP-9 expression [36]. These mechanisms might possibly be responsible for inhibiting migration in HeLa cells and remain to be determined in later studies.

Previous cell cycle arrest studies of resveratrol on HeLa cells showed that all the cells were arrested at the S-phase and none remained in the G2/M-phase [37,38]. Pterostilbene shows cell cycle arrest in several cancer studies [39]; however, to the best of our knowledge, no such study on cervical cancer has been carried out. Our current study showed that pterostilbene shows markedly better efficacy than resveratrol in arresting the cell cycle at the S-phase. To further analyze the effects of the two compounds on cell cycle arrest, we looked at phospho-histone H3 as a marker for mitosis [40]. Our observations strengthen and confirm the results obtained from flow cytometric analysis indicating that although both compounds are able to arrest mitosis, pterostilbene has enhanced capacity to arrest cancer cell growth.

Although we initially used sub-lethal concentrations of the two compounds on HeLa cells to decipher their antitumor mechanisms in the context of cell cycle arrest, it was imperative for us to delineate the possible mechanism of elimination of HeLa cells by these compounds at higher concentrations. Pterostilbene is known to be effective on cervical cancer cells by Endoplasmic reticulum (ER)-mediated stress development as well as by targeting the Nrf-2 pathway [41]. In HPV+ cancer cells, the oncoprotein E6 degrades the tumor-suppressor protein p53 by targeting it for proteasomal ubiquitination, which has been shown to augment the tumorigenic characteristics of cancer cells [24,42]. In contrast, inhibition of E6 expression in the cancer cells would be expected to allow p53 protein to trigger apoptosis and cell cycle arrest. Our findings support this latter statement, with resveratrol and pterostilbene activating caspase-3 while simultaneously downregulating E6 and upregulating p53. Our findings are partly supported by previous studies indicating that resveratrol treatment on cervical cancer cell lines upregulates p53 [43]. Our findings are the first to show a direct upregulation of p53 in HeLa cells by another polyphenol, namely, pterostilbene. Importantly previous studies have shown that p53 and simultaneous caspase-3 activation might be the key for triggering apoptosis in HeLa cells [44]. Our experiments support this finding and ascertain that resveratrol and pterostilbene act as robust agents capable of regulating the p53-dependent apoptotic pathway. The p53 protein, which is usually very low in HeLa cells, was upregulated by resveratrol and pterostilbene, leading us to hypothesize that reactivation of p53 in treated HeLa cells is a possible mechanism of action of these compounds.

Cervical cancer is a major concern in developing countries due to lack of affordable prophylaxis and treatment. As present modes of treatment like surgery, chemotherapy, or radiation involve high systemic toxicity, there is an urgent need to find affordable alternative therapies. Diet-based polyphenols like resveratrol and pterostilbene are therefore potential candidates for the effective therapy of cervical cancer with significantly low toxicity. We found pterostilbene to be a more potent anticancer agent than resveratrol in HeLa cells. This difference may be a function of pterostilbene being capable of upregulating p53 and downregulating E6 significantly more than resveratrol. As pterostilbene is non-toxic to normal cells [20], it has the potential to be a robust, cost-effective anti-E6+ tumor drug. Others have found that that pterostilbene possess greater bioavailability and stability [45] than resveratrol in vivo (80% vs. 20%). Resveratrol has been shown to be non-toxic to several cells lines like glial cells and neurons, even after a treatment dose of 100 µM for 48 h [46]. Other studies on normal fibroblasts also state the non-toxicity of resveratrol at our observed potent anticancer concentrations [47]. Additionally, pterostilbene shows no toxicity at these concentrations in normal skin fibroblasts and myoblasts [48]. According to clinical studies, the safe dosage for resveratrol and pterostilbene is 5 g/day [49] and 250 mg/day [20], respectively. Our initial in vivo studies in the laboratory using a non-toxic dosage of both resveratrol and pterostilbene has shown promising results in inhibiting tumor growth in a model of cervical cancer [32]. Taken together, our findings support the further evaluation of pterostilbene as a possible therapy against cervical cancer.

Here, we show that pterostilbene potently suppresses HPV E6 expression (Figure 4) and efficiently eliminates HPV+ cells in culture by p53-mediated apoptosis (Figures 1 and 5) while suppressing cell proliferation (Figure 3) and migration (Figure 2). We find that pterostilbene is a more promising agent against cervical cancer when compared to resveratrol. Based on such properties, the use of pterostilbene presents a relatively economical but highly hopeful therapeutic approach to treat HPV infections and cervical cancers. Our future studies will include signaling studies using HPV+ murine tumor models to confirm these observations in vivo.

Supplementary Materials: The following are available online at www.mdpi.com/2072-6643/10/02/243/s1, Video S1: Pterostilbene induces enhanced cell death compared to resveratrol: Time lapse video of cells untreated; Video S2: Pterostilbene induces enhanced cell death compared to resveratrol: Time lapse video of cells treated with 60 µM resveratrol; Video S3: Pterostilbene induces enhanced cell death compared to resveratrol: Time lapse video of cells treated with 60 µM pterostilbene obtained for 24 h showing elevated blebbing and cell death in pterostilbene treatment.

Acknowledgments: Kaushiki Chatterjee was supported by a teaching assistantship from the College of Staten Island (CUNY) and a doctoral scholarship from Northwell Health. We are grateful to Sumit Mukherjee for providing technical assistance and research input for this manuscript.

Author Contributions: Kaushiki Chatterjee and Jimmie E. Fata conceived and designed the experiments. Kaushiki Chatterjee, Dina AlSharif, Christina Mazza, Palwasha Syar, and Mohamed Al Sharif carried out the experiments and analyzed the data. All the authors contributed to the research and shaping of the article.

Conflicts of Interest: The authors declare no conflict of interest.

References

1. Safaeian, M.; Solomon, D.; Castle, P.E. Cervical cancer prevention—Cervical screening: Science in evolution. *Obstet. Gynecol. Clin. N. Am.* **2007**, *34*, 739–760. [CrossRef] [PubMed]
2. Ferlay, J.; Soerjomataram, I.; Dikshit, R.; Eser, S.; Mathers, C.; Rebelo, M.; Parkin, D.M.; Forman, D.; Bray, F. Cancer incidence and mortality worldwide: Sources, methods and major patterns in GLOBOCAN 2012. *Int. J. Cancer* **2015**, *136*, E359–E386. [CrossRef] [PubMed]
3. Burd, E.M. Human papillomavirus and cervical cancer. *Clin. Microbiol. Rev.* **2003**, *16*, 1–17. [CrossRef] [PubMed]
4. Parkin, D.M.; Bray, F. Chapter 2: The burden of HPV-related cancers. *Vaccine* **2006**, *24*. [CrossRef] [PubMed]
5. Palefsky, J.M. Human papillomavirus-related disease in men: Not just a women's issue. *J. Adolesc. Health* **2010**, *46*, S12–S19. [CrossRef] [PubMed]
6. Serrano, B.; Brotons, M.; Bosch, F.X.; Bruni, L. Epidemiology and burden of HPV-related disease. *Best Pract. Res. Clin. Obstet. Gynaecol.* **2017**. [CrossRef] [PubMed]
7. Wigle, J.; Coast, E.; Watson-Jones, D. Human papillomavirus (HPV) vaccine implementation in low and middle-income countries (LMICs): Health system experiences and prospects. *Vaccine* **2013**, *31*, 3811–3817. [CrossRef] [PubMed]
8. Stanley, M. Potential mechanisms for HPV vaccine-induced long-term protection. *Gynecol. Oncol.* **2017**, *118*, S2–S7. [CrossRef] [PubMed]
9. Kitagawa, R.; Katsumata, N.; Shibata, T.; Kamura, T.; Kasamatsu, T.; Nakanishi, T.; Nishimura, S.; Ushijima, K.; Takano, M.; Satoh, T.; et al. Paclitaxel Plus Carboplatin Versus Paclitaxel Plus Cisplatin in Metastatic or Recurrent Cervical Cancer: The Open-Label Randomized Phase III Trial JCOG0505. *J. Clin. Oncol.* **2015**, *33*, 2129–2135. [CrossRef] [PubMed]
10. Astolfi, L.; Ghiselli, S.; Guaran, V.; Chicca, M.; Simoni, E.; Olivetto, E.; Lelli, G.; Martini, A. Correlation of adverse effects of cisplatin administration in patients affected by solid tumours: A retrospective evaluation. *Oncol. Rep.* **2013**, *29*, 1285–1292. [CrossRef] [PubMed]
11. Stoner, G.D.; Mukhtar, H. Polyphenols as cancer chemopreventive agents. *J. Cell. Biochem.* **1995**, *59*, 169–180. [CrossRef]
12. Mukherjee, S.; Ranjan Debata, P.; Hussaini, R.; Chatterjee, K.; NE Baidoo, J.; Sampat, S.; Navarra, J.P.; Fata, J.; Severinova, E.; Banerjee, P.; et al. Unique synergistic formulation of curcumin, epicatechin gallate and resveratrol, tricurin, suppresses HPV E6, eliminates HPV+ cancer cells, and inhibits tumor progression. *Oncotarget* **2017**, *8*, 60904–60916. [CrossRef] [PubMed]
13. Wang, D.-G.; Liu, W.-Y.; Chen, G.-T. A simple method for the isolation and purification of resveratrol from Polygonum cuspidatum. *J. Pharm. Anal.* **2013**, *3*, 241–247. [CrossRef] [PubMed]
14. Mukherjee, S.; Dudley, J.I.; Das, D.K. Dose-dependency of resveratrol in providing health benefits. *Dose Response* **2010**, *8*, 478–500. [CrossRef] [PubMed]
15. Nutakul, W.; Sobers, H.S.; Qiu, P.; Dong, P.; Decker, E.A.; McClements, D.J.; Xiao, H. Inhibitory effects of resveratrol and pterostilbene on human colon cancer cells: A side-by-side comparison. *J. Agric. Food Chem.* **2011**, *59*, 10964–10970. [CrossRef] [PubMed]
16. Francioso, A.; Mastromarino, P.; Masci, A.; d'Erme, M.; Mosca, L. Chemistry, stability and bioavailability of resveratrol. *Med. Chem.* **2014**, *10*, 237–245. [CrossRef] [PubMed]
17. Fulda, S. Resveratrol and derivatives for the prevention and treatment of cancer. *Drug Discov. Today* **2010**, *15*, 757–765. [CrossRef] [PubMed]
18. Langcake, P.; Cornford, C.A.; Pryce, R.J. Identification of pterostilbene as a phytoalexin from Vitis vinifera leaves. *Phytochemistry* **1979**, *18*, 1025–1027. [CrossRef]
19. McCormack, D.; McFadden, D. Pterostilbene and cancer: Current review. *J. Surg. Res.* **2012**, *173*. [CrossRef] [PubMed]
20. Riche, D.M.; McEwen, C.L.; Riche, K.D.; Sherman, J.J.; Wofford, M.R.; Deschamp, D.; Griswold, M. Analysis of safety from a human clinical trial with pterostilbene. *J. Toxicol.* **2013**, *2013*, 463595. [CrossRef] [PubMed]
21. Estrela, J.M.; Ortega, A.; Mena, S.; Rodriguez, M.L.; Asensi, M. Pterostilbene: Biomedical applications. *Crit. Rev. Clin. Lab. Sci. 50* **2013**, *50*, 65–78. [CrossRef] [PubMed]

22. Paul, S.; Rimando, A.M.; Lee, H.J.; Ji, Y.; Reddy, B.S.; Suh, N. Anti-inflammatory Action of Pterostilbene Is Mediated through the p38 Mitogen-Activated Protein Kinase Pathway in Colon Cancer Cells. *Cancer Prev. Res.* **2009**, *2*, 650–657. [CrossRef] [PubMed]

23. Kumar, S.; Jena, L.; Sahoo, M.; Kakde, M.; Daf, S.; Varma, A.K.; Hoory, T.; Monie, A.; Gravitt, P.; Wu, T.; et al. *In Silico* Docking to Explicate Interface between Plant-Originated Inhibitors and E6 Oncogenic Protein of Highly Threatening Human Papillomavirus 18. *Genom. Inform.* **2015**, *13*, 60. [CrossRef] [PubMed]

24. Scheffner, M.; Huibregtse, J.M.; Vierstra, R.D.; Howley, P.M. The HPV-16 E6 and E6-AP complex functions as a ubiquitin-protein ligase in the ubiquitination of p53. *Cell* **2017**, *75*, 495–505. [CrossRef]

25. Chung, E.; Prelli, F.; Dealler, S.; Lee, W.S.; Chang, Y.-T.; Wisniewski, T. Styryl-based and tricyclic compounds as potential anti-prion agents. *PLoS ONE* **2011**, *6*, e24844. [CrossRef] [PubMed]

26. Kusaczuk, M.; Krętowski, R.; Stypułkowska, A.; Cechowska-Pasko, M. Molecular and cellular effects of a novel hydroxamate-based HDAC inhibitor—belinostat—in glioblastoma cell lines: A preliminary report. *Invest. New Drugs* **2016**, *34*, 552–564. [CrossRef] [PubMed]

27. Munshi, A.; Hobbs, M.; Meyn, R.E. Clonogenic Cell Survival Assay. In *Chemosensitivity*; Humana Press: Totowa, NJ, USA, 2005; Volume 110, pp. 021–028.

28. Liang, C.-C.; Park, A.Y.; Guan, J.-L. In vitro scratch assay: A convenient and inexpensive method for analysis of cell migration in vitro. *Nat. Protoc.* **2007**, *2*, 329–333. [CrossRef] [PubMed]

29. Aumailley, L.; Warren, A.; Garand, C.; Dubois, M.J.; Paquet, E.R.; Le Couteur, D.G.; Marette, A.; Cogger, V.C.; Lebel, M. Vitamin C modulates the metabolic and cytokine profiles, alleviates hepatic endoplasmic reticulum stress, and increases the life span of Gulo-/- mice. *Aging (Albany NY)* **2016**, *8*, 458–483. [CrossRef] [PubMed]

30. Correa-Costa, M.; Braga, T.T.; Semedo, P.; Hayashida, C.Y.; Bechara, L.R.G.; Elias, R.M.; Barreto, C.R.; Silva-Cunha, C.; Hyane, M.I.; Gonçalves, G.M.; et al. Pivotal role of Toll-like receptors 2 and 4, its adaptor molecule MyD88, and inflammasome complex in experimental tubule-interstitial nephritis. *PLoS ONE* **2011**, *6*, e29004. [CrossRef] [PubMed]

31. DeFilippis, R.A.; Goodwin, E.C.; Wu, L.; DiMaio, D. Endogenous human papillomavirus E6 and E7 proteins differentially regulate proliferation, senescence, and apoptosis in HeLa cervical carcinoma cells. *J. Virol.* **2003**, *77*, 1551–1563. [CrossRef] [PubMed]

32. Chatterjee, K.; Mukherjee, S.; Vanmanen, J.; Banerjee, P.; Fata, J.E. CUNY Graduate Center, College of Staten Island. Unpublished work. 2018.

33. Pajonk, F.; Pajonk, K.; McBride, W.H. Inhibition of NF-κB, Clonogenicity, and Radiosensitivity of Human Cancer Cells. *JNCI J. Natl. Cancer Inst.* **1999**, *91*, 1956–1960. [CrossRef] [PubMed]

34. Yamaguchi, H.; Wyckoff, J.; Condeelis, J. Cell migration in tumors. *Curr. Opin. Cell Biol.* **2005**, *17*, 559–564. [CrossRef] [PubMed]

35. Kim, Y.S.; Sull, J.W.; Sung, H.J. Suppressing effect of resveratrol on the migration and invasion of human metastatic lung and cervical cancer cells. *Mol. Biol. Rep.* **2012**, *39*, 8709–8716. [CrossRef] [PubMed]

36. Pan, M.-H.; Chiou, Y.-S.; Chen, W.-J.; Wang, J.-M.; Badmaev, V.; Ho, C.-T. Pterostilbene inhibited tumor invasion via suppressing multiple signal transduction pathways in human hepatocellular carcinoma cells. *Carcinogenesis* **2009**, *30*, 1234–1242. [CrossRef] [PubMed]

37. Kramer, M.P.; Wesierska-Gadek, J. Monitoring of long-term effects of resveratrol on cell cycle progression of human HeLa cells after administration of a single dose. *Ann. N. Y. Acad. Sci.* **2009**, *1171*, 257–263. [CrossRef] [PubMed]

38. Zoberi, I.; Bradbury, C.M.; Curry, H.A.; Bisht, K.S.; Goswami, P.C.; Roti Roti, J.L.; Gius, D. Radiosensitizing and anti-proliferative effects of resveratrol in two human cervical tumor cell lines. *Cancer Lett.* **2002**, *175*, 165–173. [CrossRef]

39. Pan, M.-H.; Chang, Y.-H.; Badmaev, V.; Nagabhushanam, K.; Ho, C.-T. Pterostilbene Induces Apoptosis and Cell Cycle Arrest in Human Gastric Carcinoma Cells. *J. Agric. Food Chem.* **2007**, *55*, 7777–7785. [CrossRef] [PubMed]

40. Veras, E.; Malpica, A.; Deavers, M.T.; Silva, E.G. Mitosis-specific Marker Phospho-histone H3 in the Assessment of Mitotic Index in Uterine Smooth Muscle Tumors: A Pilot Study. *Int. J. Gynecol. Pathol.* **2009**, *28*, 316–321. [CrossRef] [PubMed]

41. Zhang, B.; Wang, X.-Q.; Chen, H.-Y.; Liu, B.-H. Involvement of the Nrf2 Pathway in the Regulation of Pterostilbene-Induced Apoptosis in HeLa Cells via ER Stress. *J. Pharmacol. Sci.* **2014**, *126*, 216–229. [CrossRef] [PubMed]

42. Yim, E.-K.; Park, J.-S. The role of HPV E6 and E7 oncoproteins in HPV-associated cervical carcinogenesis. *Cancer Res. Treat.* **2005**, *37*, 319–324. [CrossRef] [PubMed]

43. Athar, M.; Back, J.H.; Kopelovich, L.; Bickers, D.R.; Kim, A.L. Multiple molecular targets of resveratrol: Anti-carcinogenic mechanisms. *Arch. Biochem. Biophys.* **2009**, *486*, 95–102. [CrossRef] [PubMed]

44. Liu, Y.; McKalip, A.; Herman, B. Human papillomavirus type 16 E6 and HPV-16 E6/E7 sensitize human keratinocytes to apoptosis induced by chemotherapeutic agents: Roles of p53 and caspase activation. *J. Cell. Biochem.* **2000**, *78*, 334–349. [CrossRef]

45. Kapetanovic, I.M.; Muzzio, M.; Huang, Z.; Thompson, T.N.; McCormick, D.L. Pharmacokinetics, oral bioavailability, and metabolic profile of resveratrol and its dimethylether analog, pterostilbene, in rats. *Cancer Chemother. Pharmacol.* **2011**, *68*, 593–601. [CrossRef] [PubMed]

46. Shu, X.-H.; Li, H.; Sun, X.-X.; Wang, Q.; Sun, Z.; Wu, M.-L.; Chen, X.-Y.; Li, C.; Kong, Q.-Y.; Liu, J. Metabolic patterns and biotransformation activities of resveratrol in human glioblastoma cells: Relevance with therapeutic efficacies. *PLoS ONE* **2011**, *6*, e27484. [CrossRef] [PubMed]

47. Gosslau, A.; Chen, M.; Ho, C.-T.; Chen, K.Y. A methoxy derivative of resveratrol analogue selectively induced activation of the mitochondrial apoptotic pathway in transformed fibroblasts. *Br. J. Cancer* **2005**, *92*, 513–521. [CrossRef] [PubMed]

48. Dewi, N.I.; Yagasaki, K.; Miura, Y. Anti-proliferative effect of pterostilbene on rat hepatoma cells in culture. *Cytotechnology* **2015**, *67*, 671–680. [CrossRef] [PubMed]

49. Patel, K.R.; Scott, E.; Brown, V.A.; Gescher, A.J.; Steward, W.P.; Brown, K. Clinical trials of resveratrol. *Ann. N. Y. Acad. Sci.* **2011**, *1215*, 161–169. [CrossRef] [PubMed]

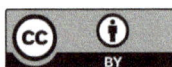

nutrients

MDPI

Review

Chinese Medicines in the Treatment of Prostate Cancer: From Formulas to Extracts and Compounds

Xueni Wang [1], Gang Fang [2,*] and Yuzhou Pang [1,2]

1   Guangxi Zhuang Yao Medicine Center of Engineering and Technology, Guangxi University of Chinese Medicine, 13 Wuhe Road, Qingxiu District, Nanning 530200, China; 000831@gxtcmu.edu.cn (X.W.); 000387@gxtcmu.edu.cn (Y.P.)
2   Laboratory of Zhuang Medicine Prescriptions Basis and Application Research, Guangxi University of Chinese Medicine, 179 Mingxiudong Road, Xixiangtang District, Nanning 530001, China
*   Correspondence: 000573@gxtcmu.edu.cn; Tel.: +86-77-1313-4025

Received: 18 January 2018; Accepted: 26 February 2018; Published: 28 February 2018

Abstract: In order to fully understand the progresses and achievements in Chinese medicines for the treatment of prostate cancer, we summarize all the available reports on formulas, extracts, and compounds of Chinese medicines against prostate cancer. A number of clinical trials verified that traditional Chinese formulas had some unique advantages in the treatment of prostate cancer. Many Chinese medicine extracts could protect against prostate cancer, and many compounds isolated from Chinese traditional medicines showed a clear anti-prostate cancer effect. However, Chinese medicines are facing many problems regarding their multicomponent nature, complicated mechanisms of action, and high doses required for therapy. Herein, we review the functions of Chinese medicines in prostate cancer and focus on their mechanisms. The review will deepen the understanding of Chinese medicines potential in the anti-prostate cancer field. In addition, we put forward a question concerning the current research on Chinese medicines: in order to better illustrate that Chinese medicines can be used in the clinical treatment of prostate cancer, should our research focus on formulas, extracts, or compounds?

Keywords: prostate cancer; Chinese medicines; formulas; extracts; compounds

---

1. Introduction

Prostate cancer (PCa) is a common cancer in elderly men. The incidence of PCa is different in different countries, and the general mortality rate of prostate cancer reaches 1–2% [1]. The mechanisms of PCa progression have been explored, and key progresses have been made in the treatment of PCa. Personalized therapies based on nanomedicines, Chinese medicines, and genetic factors, have become one of the study hotspots of PCa treatment [2]. However, why are the complex Chinese medicines increasingly concerned?

Because of their low toxicity, non-apparent side effects, and obvious curative effects in tumor treatment, Chinese medicines have been accepted by doctors, experts, and patients [3]. Chinese medicines can inhibit tumor growth and metastasis, prolong patients' life span, and improve patients' life quality [4]. Some patients, who were found to have cancers in the late stage, could not undergo surgery, radiotherapy, and chemotherapy, and finally accepted Chinese medicines treatment, which restrained the tumor progression, improved their quality of life, and obviously extended their survival [4]. Herbal medicines are the traditional medicine resources in China, with unique advantages. Medicinal plant resources are widely distributed in China. More than 50% of anticancer drugs approved by the U.S. Food and Drug Administration (FDA) are extracted from terrestrial plants [5], indicating that herbal medicines are important in the development of anticancer drugs.

Traditional Chinese medicine formulas are widely used in clinical cancer treatment in Chinese hospitals [6]. Many Chinese herbal extracts have been proved to inhibit the development of prostate cancer. More and more compounds isolated from Chinese medicine herbs were found to inhibit the development of prostate cancer via different pathways. A number of clinical trials have shown that traditional Chinese medicines play a definite role in the protection against prostate cancer and will be used in clinical treatment of prostate cancer in the future. Chinese medicines have a great potential in PCa treatment.

Pharmacological research on the antitumor efficacy of Chinese herbal extracts and formulas is developing promptly, and the application of Chinese medicine compounds in clinical oncology has been widely accepted. Soiqnet et al. established arsenic trioxide as an effective therapy for patients with relapsed acute promyelocytic leukemia and recorded high rates of 5-year disease-free survival and 5-year overall survival after a long-term follow-up of newly diagnosed patients with acute promyelocytic leukemia treated with a single-agent therapy based on arsenic trioxide [6,7]. The combination of Chinese medicines and other treatment methods has been widely used in China and has achieved a good therapeutic efficacy [8–11]. Although studies on Chinese medicines in anticancer therapy have demonstrated some achievements, there is still a long way for the wide application of Chinese medicines in the treatment of prostate cancer. This work intends to summarize the recent progresses in the use of Chinese medicines for PCa treatment and points out possible future breakthroughs.

2. Chinese Medicine Formulas in the Treatment of Prostate Cancer

PC-SPES is a Chinese medicine formula containing eight herbal medicines. It was launched into the market as a health care product in 1996 by Botanic Lab [12]. The New England Journal of Medicine first reported the biological activity and the clinical effect of PC-SPES in 1998 [13]. A series of reports showed that PC-SPES can significantly reduce serum testosterone and prostate-specific antigen in patients with prostate cancer in a time- and dose-dependent manner [14–17]. However, in 2001, patients taking PC-SPES showed diffuse intravascular coagulation and bleeding tendency [18,19]. In 2002, some batches of PC-SPES were found to contain diethylstilbestrol, warfarin, and indomethacin, which made the efficacy and side effects of PC-SPES controversial [20]. Considering the stability and safety of Chinese herbal remedies, National Center for Complementary and Alternative Medicine (NCCAM) suspended research on PC-SPES and its related compounds and withdrew it from the USA market in February 2000 [21].

From 2010 to 2012, Lin et al. reported a series of clinical data on prostate cancer treated with Chinese medicines. Firstly, they found that traditional Chinese medicine (TCM) treatment was only a complementary treatment rather than an alternative treatment. Then, they found that TCM treatment showed an increasing trend in popularity among prostate cancer patients in Taiwan. Later, they confirmed that TCM treatment was popular among prostate cancer patients in Taiwan [22–25].

A retrospective nationwide cohort study of prostate cancer patients was conducted based on data from 1998 to 2003 from the Taiwan National Health Insurance Research Database. Patients were classified as TCM users or nonusers and monitored from the day of prostate cancer diagnosis to death or to the end of 2012. The correlation between death risk and TCM use was determined with cox-proportional-hazards models and Kaplan–Meier curves. The correlation analysis results showed TCM users had a decreased mortality. A lower death risk was observed in patients with longer-term TCM use, especially in those who used TCM for at least 200 days. TCM users with metastatic prostate cancer had a significantly lower hazard ratio than non-TCM users [26].

PC-SPES's entry into the US market has convinced that this Chinese medicine formula has a definite efficacy on prostate cancer, although PC-SPES was withdrawn from the US market after 4 years. Chinese medicine researchers realize that it is a key issue to ensure Chinese medicines' stability and safety. Many scientists in China today are devoted to the quality control of Chinese medicines.

A leading cause of the prostate cancer treatment failure is chemoresistance, which often involves multiple mechanisms. Chinese medicines usually contain multiple components, which can potentially target many mechanisms simultaneously and may offer an advantage over single compounds. The characteristic of Chinese medicines can be used as a strategy to avoid chemoresistance.

Chinese medicines have been applied for a long time. The mechanisms of Chinese medicines should be further explored with advanced scientific and technological methods to control the stability and safety of Chinese medicines for human health.

3. Chinese Medicine Extracts Inhibit Prostate Cancer

Traditional plant-derived products play a significant role in the development of potential medicinal agents. *Ganoderma lucidum* (Leyss. ex Fr.) Karst. is a type of mushroom and has been used as a home remedy for the general promotion of health and longevity in traditional Chinese medicines [27]. Spores and unpurified fruiting bodies of *G. lucidum* (0.5–2.5 mg/mL) could inhibit the invasion of breast MDA-MB-231 and prostate PC-3 cancer cells by downregulating the expression of NF-kappaB, urokinase plasminogen activator (uPA), and uPA receptor [28]. Meanwhile, *G. lucidum* (0.125–0.5 mg/mL) could induce apoptosis, inhibit cell proliferation, and suppress the migration of highly invasive PC-3 human prostate cancer cells [29]. Furthermore, *G. lucidum* (0.125–0.5 mg/mL) was reported to inhibit prostate cancer-dependent angiogenesis by modulating MAPK and Akt signaling in PC-3 cells [30]. These results indicated that *G. lucidum* had a potential therapeutic efficacy for the treatment of prostate cancer.

Litchi chinensis Sonn. (Litchi) is a subtropical fruit tree growing in south China. Litchi seed extracts were found to possess diverse pharmacological effects including significantly inhibiting cell viability and clonogenic growth of prostate cancer PC-3, DU145, RM-1, and C4-2B cells in a dose-dependent manner (31.25–250 µg/mL) and inducing cell apoptosis and cell cycle G1/S phase arrest by inactivating protein kinase B (Akt or PKB) signaling pathway [31]. In addition, the extracts significantly decreased cell migration and invasion via a phenotypic inversion of epithelial–mesenchymal transition [31]. Remarkably, the extracts significantly decreased the size of PC3 xenograft nude mice, showing no toxicity [31]. These findings suggested that Litchi seed extracts might be used to develop a safe alternative therapy for prostate cancer patients.

Saussurea lappa Clarke has been applied in the treatment of inflammation, abdominal pain, tenesmus, nausea, and cancer in China [32,33]. Hexane extracts of *S. lappa* inhibited the basal and Epidermal Growth Factor (EGF)-induced migration of prostate cancer DU145 and TRAMP-C2 cells in a dose-dependent manner (1–4 µg/mL), whereas they did not influence the viability of these cancer cells. In addition, the extracts reduced matrix metalloproteinase (MMP)-9 and tissue inhibitor of metalloproteinase (TIMP)-1 secretion, but increased TIMP-2 levels in the absence or presence of EGF [34]. The results indicated that hexane extracts of *S. lappa* might be used as anti-metastatic agents for the treatment of prostate cancer.

Scutellaria baicalensis Georgi is a widely used Chinese herbal medicine in anti-inflammatory and anti-cancer therapy [35–37]. *S. baicalensis* (0.2–0.8 mg/mL) exerted dose- and time-dependent growth inhibition effects on both LNCaP and PC3 cell lines and also inhibited prostate-specific antigen production in LNCaP cells. Animal experiments of *S. baicalensis* showed a reduction of 50% in tumor volume after a 7-week treatment at a dose of 200 mg/kg/day [38]. These results imply that *S. baicalensis* possess anti-prostate cancer activity in vitro and in vivo.

Scutellaria barbata D. Don has been used to treat various cancers in China [39–41]. Wong et al.'s in vivo data showed that *S. barbata* (32 mg/day) delayed tumor development in a transgenic prostate adenocarcinoma mouse model ,and the complementary in vitro data indicated that *S. barbata* (1 mg/mL) might exert this function by upregulating the apoptotic pathway and downregulating the survival pathway in TRAMP-C1 and LNCaP prostate cancer cells [42]. According to these results, *S. barbata* might possess chemopreventive properties for cancer treatment.

Tripterygium wilfordii Hook F (12.5–50 µg/mL) combined with docetaxel could overcome the chemoresistance and suppress prostate tumor growth in docetaxel-resistant PC3 and DU145 prostate cancer cell lines by inhibiting P-glycoprotein activity and inducing a significant change in the expression of genes related to angiogenesis, cell cycle regulation, and differentiation [43]. This findings imply that *T. wilfordii* might be developed as a combined agent to prevent chemoresistance.

Wedelia chinensis (Osbeck) Merr. is a common ingredient in anti-inflammatory herbal medicines in China [44–46]. The anti-prostate cancer effect of *W. chinensis* extracts is ascribed to three active compounds: wedelolactone, luteolin, and apigenin, which inhibit the androgen receptor (AR) signaling pathway in LNCaP and 22Rv1 cells. Oral administration of *W. chinensis* extracts (4 or 40 mg/kg) impeded prostate cancer tumorigenesis [47].

On the basis of the above-mentioned results, we found that these Chinese medicines had anti-prostate cancer activity (Table 1). These results also suggested that many potential natural compounds with anti-prostate cancer activity might exist in Chinese herbal extracts.

Table 1. Chinese medicine extracts inhibit prostate cancer.

Scientific Name	Chinese Name	Plant Organs	Extraction Solvents
Ganoderma lucidum (Leyss. ex Fr.) Karst.	Ling Zhi	Spores and unpurified fruiting bodies	No solvent
Litchi chinensis Sonn.	Li Zhi	Seed	n-butyl alcohol
Saussurea lappa Clarke	Guang Mu Xiang	Root	n-Hexane
Scutellaria baicalensis Georgi	Huang Qin	Root	Water
Scutellaria barbata D. Don	Ban Zhi Lian	Whole plant	Water
Tripterygium wilfordii Hook F.	Lei Gong Teng	Root	EtOH
Wedelia chinensis (Osbeck) Merr.	Peng Qi Ju	Whole plant	EtOH

4. Compounds Isolated from Chinese Medicines Inhibit Prostate Cancer

4.1. Compounds Inhibiting the Growth of Prostate Cancer Cells

Andrographolide is a diterpenoid lactone derived from a traditional Chinese medicine plant *Andrographis paniculata* (Burm. f.) Nees. Chun et al. demonstrated that andrographolide (1–20 µM) could inhibit IL-6-induced signaling and induce signal transducer and activator of transcription 3 (STAT3) and the phosphorylation of extracellular signal-regulated kinases (ERK). Meanwhile, it could inhibit cell viability and induce apoptosis of PC3 and DU145 prostate cancer cell lines. Moreover, andrographolide suppressed tumor growth in a mouse xenograft model with castration-resistant DU145 cell-derived human prostate tumors. These findings imply that andrographolide could be developed as a therapeutic agent to treat prostate cancer [48].

Evodiamine is isolated from the Chinese herbal medicine *Evodia rutaecarpa* (Juss.) Benth. Recent results showed that evodiamine suppressed the growth of LNCaP cells in a dose-dependent manner (100 nM–100 µM) by arresting the cell cycle at the G2/M phase and inducing apoptosis [49].

Guttiferone F (10 µM and 20 µM) could induce apoptosis of LNCaP and PC3 prostate cancer cells under serum starvation via JNK activation and Ca^{2+} elevation, respectively. Furthermore, it exerted a significant growth inhibition on PC3 cells xenografts in vivo at a dose of 20 mg/kg [50].

Honokiol is a compound contained in the traditional Chinese herb *Magnolia officinalis* Rehd. et Wils. The viability of PC-3 and LNCaP human prostate cancer cells was decreased when the cells were treated with honokiol (20–60 µM). These results were confirmed to be correlated with G0/G1 phase cell cycle arrest [51]. Honokiol (5–20 µM) induced apoptosis in PCa cell lines by activating caspases 3/8/9 and cleaving poly-adenosine diphosphate ribose polymerase. In addition, honokiol (100 mg/kg) combined with docetaxel (5 mg/kg) showed growth-inhibitory, apoptotic, and antiangiogenic effects in C4-2B tumor xenografts [52]. Moreover, the exposure of PC-3, LNCaP, and Myc-CaP cells to 20–40 µM honokiol resulted in ROS-mediated cytoprotective autophagy [53].

Isorhapontigenin (ISO) is widely distributed in Chinese herbs, fruits, and vegetables [54–56]. Isorhapontigenin (ISO, 20–100 µM) induced cell growth inhibition and apoptosis of LNCaP and 22Rv1 by targeting EGFR and its downstream signal pathways and showed no obvious effects on normal prostate cells [57]. Moreover, the treatment with ISO decreased the protein level of AR by promoting the ubiquitination and degradation of AR proteins in proteasome and inhibiting the expression of AR gene [57]. In vivo, 50 mg/kg of ISO inhibited the growth of subcutaneously xenotransplanted tumors in nude mice by inducing PCa cell growth inhibition and apoptosis [57]. EGFR-related signal pathways are involved in ISO-induced cell growth inhibition and apoptosis in PCa cells, suggesting the application potential of ISO in prostate cancer treatment.

Peperotetraphin is a novel cyclobutane-type norlignan isolated from the whole plant of *Peperomia tetraphylla* [58]. Peperotetraphin (50–100 μM) inhibited the growth of PC-3 cells and induced cancer cells to undergo G1 phase arrest and apoptosis [59].

Quercetin is a natural polyphenolic compound widely distributed in Chinese herbal medicines [60]. A large body of evidence showed that quercetin could induce the apoptosis of prostate cancer cells via multiple possible signaling pathways [61–65]. Liu et al. reported that 50–200 μM quercetin might induce apoptosis by direct activation of the caspase cascade via the mitochondrial pathway and endoplasmic reticulum stress in PC-3 cells [66].

Tetrandrine is an alkaloid from the traditional Chinese medicine *Stephania tetrandra* S. Moore [67]. Tetrandrine (2.5–30 μM) inhibited the growth and cell cloning of PC-3 and DU145 cells [68]. In addition, tetrandrine induced apoptosis by inhibiting phosphoinositide 3-kinase–Akt signal pathway and by activating the caspase cascade [68].

Triptolide is one of the main active components of *Tripterygium wilfordii* Hook.f [69]. Tumor necrosis factor-related apoptosis-inducing ligand (TRAIL) is a promising cancer therapy agent [70]. Although a number of prostate cancer cells exhibited high resistance to TRAIL effect [71], 50–200 nM triptolide significantly sensitized LNCaP and PC-3M prostate cancer cells to TRAIL-mediated cellular apoptosis by upregulating the expression of death receptor 5 and inhibiting prostate cancer development [72].

Vitexicarpin is a polymethoxy flavone isolated from *Vitex rotundifolia* Linne fil. and has long been used as an anti-inflammatory herb in China [73]. Meng et al. revealed that vitexicarpin (10–50 μM) induced apoptosis by upregulating the proapoptotic protein Bax, downregulating the antiapoptotic protein Bcl-2, releasing cytochrome C from mitochondria, and decreasing mitochondrial membrane potential in PC3 cells [73].

These Chinese medicine compounds can inhibit the growth of prostate cancer cells mainly by inducing cell apoptosis, arresting the cell cycle at different phases, activating caspase cascade, and/or regulating the expression of apoptosis-related proteins. Moreover, AR signaling pathway and the cytoprotective effect mediated by ROS are also involved in the inhibition effect of Chinese Medicine compounds.

4.2. Compounds Inhibiting the Proliferation of Prostate Cancer Cells

Arsenic sulphide is a main component of realgar (As4S4), and 0.5–1 μM arsenic sulphide can repress the overexpression of miRNA-372 in DU145 and PC3 prostate cancer cell lines [74]. An in vivo study confirmed that repressing the overexpression of miR-372 by 2 mg/kg/day of As4S4 for 3 weeks could inhibit the proliferation and migration of prostate cancer cells [74].

Baicalin, isolated from the dried roots of *Scutellaria baicalensis* Georgi, is widely used in China for its anti-inflammatory, anti-pyretic, and anti-hypersensitivity properties [75]. Baicalin (150 μM) could inhibit the proliferation of DU145, PC-3, LNCaP, and CA-HPV-10 prostate cancer cells, and, particularly, of the androgen-independent DU145 cells. It was confirmed that this effect was associated with the induction of apoptosis, although the exact mechanisms are not clear [75].

Pang et al. indicated that celastrol could inhibit prostate cancer development and angiogenesis and that its effects were correlated with the extent of inhibition of AKT/mTOR/P70S6K signaling [76]. Celastrol (0.03–3 μM) could suppress PC-3 cell proliferation by downregulating IL-6 gene expression through the NF-kappaB-dependent pathway [77]. In addition, Yang et al. first reported that celastrol was a natural proteasome inhibitor with a great potential for prostate cancer prevention and treatment [78].

Gypensapogenin H is a novel dammarane-type triterpene from *Gynostemma pentaphyllum* (Thunb.) Makino [79]. Zhang et al. found that 5–60 μM Gypensapogenin H induced apoptosis in DU145 and 22RV-1 human prostate cancer cells by decreasing survival, inhibiting proliferation, and inducing cell cycle arrest in G1 phase [80].

Scoparone, a natural compound isolated from *Artemisia capillaris* Thunb. has anti-allergic effects in a mast cell-mediated allergy model [81]. Kim et al. indicated that scoparone could suppress the transcription of STAT3 and decrease phosphorylation and nuclear accumulation of STAT3 [82]. Scoparone treatment suppressed anchorage-independent growth in soft agar at the concentration of 50–200 μM, and tumor growth of DU145 xenografts in nude mice at the concentration of 30 mg/kg every 2–3 days for 18 days [82]. In addition, computational modeling suggested that scoparone might bind to the SH2 domain of STAT3 [82]. According to these findings, scoparone exerted an anti-prostate cancer effect by inhibiting STAT3 activity.

Triptolide could inhibit the proliferation of RM-1 cells in mice by decreasing the expression of Bcl-2 and increasing the expression of caspase 3 at a dose of 10 and 20 ng/mL [83].

These compounds inhibited the proliferation of prostate cancer cells by repressing the overexpression of miRNA-372, inhibiting inflammation pathways such as the NF-kappaB-dependent pathway, inducing apoptosis, acting as a poroteasome inhibitor, and inhibiting STAT3 activity.

4.3. Compounds Inhibiting Metastasis of Prostate Cancer Cells

Metastasis development is still a huge challenge in prostate cancer treatment. Most of the treatment failures of prostate cancer are generally ascribed to the formation of bone metastases [84,85].

Pretreatment with 2–8 μM celastrol significantly slowed down PC3 cell migration [86]. After celastrol administration, the number of cells penetrating a gel layer in a classical invasion assay was significantly decreased, and their bone invasive ability was significantly undermined. Pretreatment with celastrol inhibited the tumorigenicity of PC-3 cells, and almost no bone invasion occurred in an in vivo mouse model [86]. Celastrol could target the VEGFR-2 signaling pathway and inhibit the formation of blood vessel [86].

Curcumin is a well-known natural compound of curcuminoids. Yang et al. found that curcumin could suppress prostate cancer by reducing the function of the PSA promoter and inhibiting PSA and AR protein expression in LNCaP cells [87]. Meanwhile, 10 μM curcumin was demonstrated to inhibit prostate cancer by upregulating miR-143 and FOXD3 and downregulating PGK1 expression in DU145 and PC3 cells [88]. Furthermore, 10–50 μM curcumin could inhibit the metastasis and survival of DU145 and PC3 prostate cancer cells via the Notch-1 signaling pathway [89].

Hu et al. found three novel cyclotides from the leaves and root of *Hedyotis Diffusa* Willd, termed Diffusa cyclotide 1 to 3 (DC1–3). DC3 was found to show potent cytotoxicity against PC3, DU145, and LNCaP prostate cancer cell lines [90]. Furthermore, 0.05 μM DC3 inhibited cell migration and invasion of LNCap cells and significantly inhibited tumor development in a prostate xenograft model [90].

D-pinitol inhibited the invasion and migration of PC3 and DU145 prostate cancer cells at the noncytotoxic concentration of 3–30 μM [91]. D-pinitol metastatic activity was mediated by the downregulation of αvβ3 integrin activity through focal adhesion kinase (FAK), c-Src, and NF-κB pathways [91].

Dihydroisotanshinone I, a bioactive compound in *Salvia miltiorrhiza* Bunge. could inhibit the migration of androgen-dependent (22Rv1 cells) and androgen-independent (PC3 and DU145 cells) prostate cancer cells at the concentration of 5 μM–10 μM [92]. Dihydroisotanshinone I inhibited the migration of these prostate cancer cells by interrupting the cross-talk between macrophages and prostate cancer cells through the repression of the CCL2–STAT3 axis [92].

Shikonin is an active naphthoquinone from the Chinese medicine *Lithospermum erythrorhizon* Sieb. et Zucc. Shikonin potently suppressed PC-3 and DU145 cell metastasis in a dose-dependent manner (0.5–2 μM) and inhibited the migration and invasion of the two aggressive prostate cancer cell lines by reducing MMP-2/-9 expression via AKT/mTOR and ROS/ERK1/2 pathways [93].

Transwell invasion assays showed that 2.5–30 µM tetrandrine significantly weakened the invasion capacity of DU145 and PC-3 cells; in addition, this compound exhibited a strong inhibitory effect on the proliferation of these prostate cancer cells [68]. However, the exact molecular mechanisms are still unknown.

Some studies indicated that the tested compounds could inhibit metastasis of prostate cancer cells, but the specific molecular mechanisms are not yet known. Some other findings showed that the tested compounds exerted the inhibitory effect on prostate cancer cell metastasis mainly by inhibiting the VEGFR-2 signaling pathway, regulating the Notch-1 signaling pathway, downregulating FAK, c-Src, and NF-κB pathways, repressing the CCL2–STAT3 axis, and suppressing MMP-2/-9 expression via AKT–mTOR and ROS–ERK1/2 pathways.

4.4. Summary

Among the above summarized compounds, Ten compounds showed inhibition of the growth of prostate cancer cells. Six compounds were confirmed to inhibit the proliferation of prostate cells and seven compounds inhibited metastasis of prostate cancer cells. Tetrandrine and celastrol were the only two compounds which could inhibit both growth/proliferation and metastasis of prostate cancer cells. Triptolide suppressed the growth or proliferation of prostate cancer cells was verified in two different studies. Table 2 lists the compounds which can inhibit the growth or proliferation, and metastasis of prostate cancer cells through similar or different targets. These findings suggest that there are numerous natural small molecules which are potentially active against prostate cancer in Chinese medicines. The discovery of these compounds will help to study the anti-prostate cancer activity of Chinese medicines.

Table 2. Compounds isolated from Chinese medicines inhibiting prostate cancer.

General Name	Chemical Structure	Compound Classification	Inhibit prostate Cancer		
			Gro.	Pro.	Met.
Andrographolide		Diterpenoid lactone	+		
Evodiamine		Alkaloid	+		
Guttiferone F		Prenylated benzophenone derivative	+		
Honokiol		Aromatic phenol	+		

Table 2. *Cont.*

General Name	Chemical Structure	Compound Classification	Inhibit prostate Cancer		
			Gro.	Pro.	Met.
Isorhapontigenin		phytopolyphenol	+		
Peperotetraphin		Norlignan	+		
Quercetin		Flavone	+		
Tetrandrine		Alkaloid	+		+
Triptolide		Heterocycle	+	+	
Vitexicarpin		Flavone	+		
Arsenic sulphide		Metal chalcogenide			+
Baicalin		Flavone glycoside			+

Table 2. *Cont.*

General Name	Chemical Structure	Compound Classification	Inhibit prostate Cancer		
			Gro.	Pro.	Met.
Celastrol		Pentacyclic triterpenoid		+	+
Gypensapogenin H		Triterpene		+	
Scoparone		coumarin		+	
Curcumin		Diphenyl heptyl hydrocarbon			+
dihydroisotanshinone I		Phenanthraquinone			+
D-pinitol		Alcohol			+
Shikonin		Anthraquinone			+

Note: "Gro" = Growth, "Pro" = Proliferation, "Met" = Metastasis, "+" = Has effect on it.

5. Perspectives and Outlook

In the past years, PCa has been widely studied in China. More and more extracts, formulas, and compounds from traditional Chinese medicines have been found to have anti-prostate cancer activity. Most of these Chinese herbal extracts with anti-prostate cancer activity also show anti-inflammatory activities. Most of the Chinese medicine formulas with anticancer effects have the functions of promoting positive blood flow, removing blood stasis, alleviating fever, and detoxifying. The main compounds present in Chinese medicines with anti-prostate cancer activity are polyphenols, alkaloids, and terpenoids. As shown in Table 3, the extracts of *G. lucidum*, Litchi, *S. lappa* and *T. wilfordii* are active in the androgen-independent prostate cancer cells, and *S. barbata* suppresses androgen-dependent prostate cancer cells growth. In addition, the extracts of *S. baicalensis* and *W. chinensis* inhibit both androgen-dependent and androgen-independent prostate cancer cells. Moreover, 8 of the 19 compounds involved in this review, including Guttiferone F, Honokiol, Quercetin, Triptolide, Baicalin, Gypensapogenin H, Curcumin, and dihydroisotanshinone I, inhibit both androgen-dependent and androgen-independent prostate cancer cells. These extracts and/or compounds may be potential anti-prostate cancer agents present in Chinese medicines and deserve further study. The extracts and compounds of Chinese medicines mainly produce the anti-prostate effect in the following ways. Firstly, Chinese medicines induce apoptosis, inhibit cell proliferation, and suppress the migration of invasive human prostate cancer cells. Secondly, Chinese medicines inhibit prostate cancer-dependent angiogenesis and impede prostate cancer tumorigenesis. Thirdly, Chinese medicines induce apoptosis and downregulate survival pathways in prostate cancer cells. Fourthly, Chinese medicines act as anti-metastatic agents. Fifthly, Chinese medicines suppress prostate tumor growth and overcome cell chemoresistance. Chinese herb extracts are a mixture of many compounds at low concentrations, and the effects of the extracts derive from the interactions of all their components. Theompounds isolated from Chinese herbs here discussed perform well in inhibiting the growth, proliferation, and metastasis of prostate cancer cells, and most of them act as selective androgen receptor modulators to exert anti-prostate cancer activity.

Table 3. Activity of extracts and compounds isolated from Chinese medicines against prostate cancer cells in vitro.

Cell Type	Androgen-Dependent Human Prostate Cancer Cell Lines		Androgen-Independent Human Prostate Cancer Cell Lines				HPV-18-Transfected Human Prostate Cancer Cell Line	Mouse Transgenic Prostate Cancer Cell Lines		Mouse Prostate Cancer Cell Lines	
Name	LNCaP	22Rv1	PC3	PC-3M	DU145	C4-2B	CA-HPV-10	TRAMP-C1	TRAMP-C2	RM-1	Myc-CaP
Ganoderma lucidum (Leyss. ex Fr.) Karst.			+								
Litchi chinensis Sonn.			+		+	+				+	
Saussurea lappa Clarke				+					+		
Scutellaria baicalensis Georgi	+		+								
Scutellaria barbata D. Don	+							+			
Tripterygium wilfordii Hook F.			+	+							
Wedelia chinensis (Osbeck) Merr.	+	+	+								
Andrographolide			+	+							
Evodiamine	+										
Guttiferone F	+		+								
Honokiol	+		+								+
Isorhapontigenin	+	+									
Peperotetraphin			+								
Quercetin	+		+		+						
Tetrandrine			+		+						
Triptolide	+				+					+	
Vitexicarpin			+								
Arsenic sulphide			+		+						
Baicalin	+		+		+		+				
Celastrol			+								
Gypensapogenin H		+			+						
Scoparone					+						
Curcumin	+		+		+						
dihydroisotanshinone I		+	+		+						
D-pinitol			+		+						
Shikonin			+		+						

Note: "+" = has inhibitory effect on prostate cancer cell lines.

In this review, we collected formulas, extracts, and compounds of Chinese medicines with anti-prostate cancer activity and classified their mechanisms of action. We hope these findings can guide and enlighten researchers to explore the use of Chinese medicines in the treatment of prostate cancer.

Chinese researchers have carried out a large number of anti-prostate cancer studies on Chinese medicines under the guidance of the theory of traditional Chinese medicine. Meanwhile, the commonly used research ideas and methods that they have applied are consistent with those used in research for western drugs. The difference is that formulas, extracts, and compounds characteristic of traditional Chinese medicines are natural products. However, traditional Chinese medicines are often not a single Chinese herb extract, but a mixture of many Chinese herbs. Therefore, it is important to note that a Chinese medicine formula is an entirety. Although traditional Chinese medicines have been used for a long time, their mechanism have not been fully elucidated. Therefore, researchers often explored the mechanism of a single compound as a breakthrough point, and then gradually clarified the multi-target and multilevel function of multicomponent Chinese medicines. Chinese scientists and clinicians now are facing unprecedented opportunities and challenges to develop Chinese medicines. In the near future, a research cooperation network for the study of Chinese medicines as anti-prostate cancer agents will be established to impel the use of Chinese medicines in the treatment of prostate cancer.

6. Conclusions

This study has reviewed the progresses of Chinese medicines in the field of anti-prostate cancer treatment. Since prostate cancer treatment with Chinese medicines is not popular in the world at present, the available data on their adverse or toxic effects are not sufficient. We did not specifically address the adverse or toxic effects of the formulas, extracts, and compounds discussed in this review. The safety and stability of Chinese medicines have been widely examined, and scientists realize that this is a vacancy to be eliminated. Another point requiring study is the administration dose of Chinese medicines. The human dose of each Chinese medicine involved in a formula was stipulated by the Chinese Pharmacopoeia to ensure safety. The human doses of extracts and compounds should be verified through a series of pharmacological, pharmacokinetic, and toxicological studies. In our research on the bioactivity of Chinese medicines, we found that the administered doses of some extracts or compounds were high. High doses might be decreased by improving the extraction processes or by modifying the structures of the active compounds. There is still a long way to go to discover new anti-prostate cancer agents from Chinese medicines.

Acknowledgments: We thank Yang Yang of Tianjin University of Traditional Chinese Medicine for her advice on manuscript writing.

Author Contributions: G.F. and Y.P. designed the study. X.W. was involved in literature search and manuscript writing.

Conflicts of Interest: The authors declare that there are no conflicts of interest.

Funding: This work was supported by the Guangxi Colleges and Universities Key Laboratory of Zhuang Medicine Prescriptions Basis and Application Research. No.: Gui Jiao Ke Yan (2016) 6.

References

1. Attard, G.; Parker, C.; Eeles, R.A.; Eeles, R.A.; Schröder, F.; Tomlins, S.A.; Tannock, I.; Drake, C.G.; de Bono, J.S. Prostate cancer. *Lancet* **2015**, *387*, 70–82. [CrossRef]
2. Ren, S.C.; Chen, R.; Sun, Y.H. Prostate cancer research in China. *Asian J. Androl.* **2013**, *15*, 350–353. [CrossRef] [PubMed]
3. Ling, C.Q.; Yue, X.Q.; Ling, C. Three advantages of using traditional Chinese medicines to prevent and treat tumor. *J. Integr. Med.* **2014**, *12*, 331–335. [CrossRef]
4. Lin, L.Z.; Zhou, D.H.; Zheng, X.T. Effect of traditional Chinese medicines in improving quality of life of patients with non-small cell lung cancer in late stage. *Chin. J. Integr. Tradit. West. Med.* **2006**, *26*, 389–393.

5. Kim, J.; Park, E.J. Cytotoxic anticancer candidates from natural resources. *Curr. Med. Chem. Anticancer Agents* **2002**, *2*, 485–537. [CrossRef] [PubMed]

6. Soignet, S.L.; Frankel, S.R.; Douer, D.; Tallman, M.S.; Kantarjian, H.; Calleja, E.; Stone, R.M.; Kalaycio, M.; Scheinberg, D.A.; Steinherz, P.; et al. United States multicenter study of arsenic trioxide in relapsed acute promyelocytic leukemia. *J. Clin. Oncol.* **2001**, *19*, 3852–3860. [CrossRef] [PubMed]

7. Ghavamzadeh, A.; Alimoghaddam, K.; Rostami, S.; Ghaffari, S.H.; Jahani, M.; Iravani, M.; Mousavi, S.A.; Bahar, B.; Jalili, M. Phase II study of single-agent arsenic trioxide for the front-line therapy of acute promyelocytic leukemia. *J. Clin. Oncol.* **2011**, *29*, 2753–2757. [CrossRef] [PubMed]

8. Jiang, C.M.; Pang, M.R.; Gong, L.Y. Clinical observation on effect of chemotherapy combined with Chinese medicines in treating advanced tumor patients and on immunologic parameters. *Chin. J. Integr. Tradit. West. Med.* **2001**, *21*, 885–887.

9. Yan, G.Y.; Xu, Z.Y.; Deng, H.B.; Wan, Z.Y.; Zhang, L.; Zhu, J.Y. Effects of chemotherapy combined with Chinese herbal medicine Kangliu Zengxiao decoction on tumor markers of patients with advanced non-small-cell lung cancer: A randomized, controlled trial. *J. Chin. Integr. Med.* **2011**, *9*, 525–530. [CrossRef]

10. Tang, Z.Y. Combination of traditional Chinese medicines and western medicine in the treatment of liver cancer. *J. Clin. Hepatol.* **2011**, *27*, 449–450.

11. Shen, F.L.; Jin, J.G.; Cao, F.J. Clinical observation of combination of Chinese medicines combined with chemoradiotherapy in treatment of patients with stage-III non-small-cell lung cancer. *Med. J. West China* **2014**, *26*, 445–449.

12. Kosty, M.P. PC-SPES: Hope or hype? *J. Clin. Oncol.* **2004**, *22*, 3657–3659. [CrossRef] [PubMed]

13. DiPaola, R.S.; Zhang, H.; Lambert, G.H.; Meeker, R.; Licitra, E.; Rafi, M.M.; Zhu, B.T.; Spaulding, H.; Goodin, S.; Toledano, M.B.; et al. Clinical and biologic activity of an estrogenic herbal combination (PC-SPES) in prostate cancer. *N. Engl. J. Med.* **1998**, *339*, 785–791. [CrossRef] [PubMed]

14. Halicka, H.; Ardelt, B.; Juan, G.; Mittelman, A.; Chen, S.; Traganos, F.; Darzynkiewicz, Z. Apoptosis and cell cycle effects induced by extracts of the Chinese herbal preparation PC SPES. *Int. J. Oncol.* **1997**, *11*, 437–448. [CrossRef] [PubMed]

15. Tiwari, R.K.; Geliebter, J.; Garikapaty, V.P.; Yedavelli, S.P.; Chen, S.; Mittelman, A. Anti-tumor effects of PC-SPES, an herbal formulation in prostate cancer. *Int. J. Oncol.* **1999**, *14*, 713–719. [CrossRef] [PubMed]

16. De la Taille, A.; Buttyan, R.; Hayek, O.; Bagiella, E.; Shabsigh, A.; Burchardt, M.; Burchardt, T.; Chopin, D.K.; Katz, A.E. Herbal therapy PC-SPES: In vitro effects and evaluation of its efficacy in 69 patients with prostate cancer. *J. Urol.* **2000**, *164*, 1229–1234. [CrossRef]

17. Kubota, T.; Hisatake, J.; Hisatake, Y.; Said, J.W.; Chen, S.S.; Holden, S.; Taguchi, H.; Koeffler, H.P. PC-SPES: A unique inhibitor of proliferation of prostate cancer cells in vitro and in vivo. *Prostate* **2000**, *42*, 163–171. [CrossRef]

18. Lock, M.; Loblaw, D.A.; Choo, R.; Imrie, K. Disseminated intravascular coagulation and PC-SPES: A case report and literature review. *Can. J. Urol.* **2001**, *8*, 1326–1329. [PubMed]

19. Weinrobe, M.C.; Montgomery, B. Acquired bleeding diathesis in a patient taking PC-SPES. *N. Engl. J. Med.* **2001**, *345*, 1213–1214. [CrossRef] [PubMed]

20. Sovak, M.; Seligson, A.L.; Konas, M.; Hajduch, M.; Dolezal, M.; Machala, M.; Nagourney, R. Herbal composition PC-SPES for management of prostate cancer: Identification of active principles. *J. Natl. Cancer Inst.* **2002**, *94*, 1275–1281. [CrossRef] [PubMed]

21. Olaku, O.; White, J.D. Herbal therapy use by cancer patients: A literature review on case reports. *Eur. J. Cancer* **2011**, *47*, 508–514. [CrossRef] [PubMed]

22. Lin, Y.H.; Chen, K.K.; Chiu, J.H. Prevalence, patterns, and costs of Chinese medicines use among prostate cancer patients: A population-based study in Taiwan. *Integr. Cancer Ther.* **2010**, *9*, 16–23. [CrossRef] [PubMed]

23. Lin, Y.H.; Chen, K.K.; Chiu, J.H. Trends in Chinese medicines use among prostate cancer patients under national health insurance in Taiwan: 1996–2008. *Integr. Cancer Ther.* **2011**, *10*, 317–327. [CrossRef] [PubMed]

24. Lin, Y.H.; Chen, K.K.; Chiu, J.H. Use of Chinese medicines among prostate cancer patients in Taiwan: A retrospective longitudinal cohort study. *Int. J. Urol.* **2011**, *18*, 383–386. [CrossRef] [PubMed]

25. Lin, Y.H.; Chen, K.K.; Chiu, J.H. Coprescription of Chinese Herbal Medicine and Western Medications among Prostate Cancer Patients: A Population-Based Study in Taiwan. *Evid. Based Complement. Altern. Med.* **2012**, *2012*, 147015. [CrossRef] [PubMed]

26. Liu, J.M.; Lin, P.H.; Hsu, R.J.; Chang, Y.H.; Cheng, K.C.; Pang, S.T.; Lin, S.K. Complementary traditional Chinese medicines therapy improves survival in patients with metastatic prostate cancer. *Medicine* **2016**, *95*, 1–7.

27. Unlu, A.; Nayir, E.; Kirca, O.; Ozdogan, M. Ganoderma Lucidum (*Reishi Mushroom*) and cancer. *J. BUON* **2016**, *21*, 792–798. [PubMed]

28. Sliva, D.; Labarrere, C.; Slivova, V.; Sedlak, M.; Lloyd, F.P., Jr.; Ho, N.W. Ganoderma lucidum suppresses motility of highly invasive breast and prostate cancer cells. *Biochem. Biophys. Res. Commun.* **2002**, *298*, 603–612. [CrossRef]

29. Jiang, J.; Slivova, V.; Valachovicova, T.; Sedlak, M.; Lloyd, F.P., Jr.; Ho, N.W. Ganoderma lucidum inhibits proliferation and induces apoptosis in human prostate cancer cells PC-3. *Int. J. Oncol.* **2004**, *24*, 1093–1099. [CrossRef] [PubMed]

30. Stanley, G.; Harvey, K.; Slivova, V.; Jiang, J.; Sliva, D. Ganoderma lucidum suppresses angiogenesis through the inhibition of secretion of VEGF and TGF-β1 from prostate cancer cells. *Biochem. Biophys. Res. Commun.* **2005**, *330*, 46–52. [CrossRef] [PubMed]

31. Guo, H.; Luo, H.; Yuan, H.; Xia, Y.; Shu, P.; Huang, X.; Lu, Y.; Liu, X.; Keller, E.T.; Sun, D.; et al. Litchi seed extracts diminish prostate cancer progression via induction of apoptosis and attenuation of EMT through Akt/GSK-3β signaling. *Sci. Rep.* **2017**, *7*, 41656. [CrossRef] [PubMed]

32. Sunkara, Y.; Robinson, A.; Suresh, B.K.; Naidu, V.G.M.; Vishnuvardhan, M.V.P.S.; Suresh, B.K.; Ramakrishna, S.; Madhavendra, S.S.; Rao, J.M. Anti-inflammatory and cytotoxic activity of chloroform extract of roots of *Saussurea lappa* Clarke. *J. Pharm. Res.* **2010**, *3*, 1775–1778.

33. Kretschmer, N.; Blunder, M.; Kunert, O.; Kahl, S.; Efferth, T.; Boechzelt, H.; Hao, X.J.; Bauer, R. Activity-Guided Isolation of AntiTumor Compounds from *Saussurea lappa* Clarke. *Sci. Pharm.* **2009**, *77*, 246. [CrossRef]

34. Kim, E.J.; Hong, J.E.; Lim, S.S.; Kwon, G.T.; Kim, J.; Kim, J.S.; Lee, K.W.; Park, J.H. The hexane extract of *Saussurea lappa* and its active principle, dehydrocostus lactone, inhibit prostate cancer cell migration. *J. Med. Food* **2012**, *15*, 24–32. [CrossRef] [PubMed]

35. Zhang, D.Y.; Wu, J.; Ye, F.; Xue, L.; Jiang, S.; Yi, J.; Zhang, W.; Wei, H.; Sung, M.; Wang, W.; et al. Inhibition of cancer cell proliferation and prostaglandin E2 synthesis by *Scutellaria baicalensis*. *Cancer Res.* **2003**, *63*, 4037–4043. [PubMed]

36. Kim, E.H.; Shim, B.; Kang, S.; Jeong, G.; Lee, J.S.; Yu, Y.B.; Chun, M. Anti-inflammatory effects of *Scutellaria baicalensis* extract via suppression of immune modulators and MAP kinase signaling molecules. *J. Ethnopharmacol.* **2009**, *126*, 320–331. [CrossRef] [PubMed]

37. Yoon, S.B.; Lee, Y.J.; Park, S.K.; Kim, H.C.; Bae, H.; Kim, H.M.; Ko, S.G.; Choi, H.Y.; Oh, M.S.; Park, W. Anti-inflammatory effects of *Scutellaria baicalensis* water extract on LPS-activated RAW 264.7 macrophages. *J. Ethnopharmacol.* **2009**, *125*, 286–290. [CrossRef] [PubMed]

38. Ye, F.; Jiang, S.; Volshonok, H.; Wu, J.; Zhang, D.Y. Molecular mechanism of anti-prostate cancer activity of *Scutellaria baicalensis* extract. *Nutr. Cancer* **2007**, *57*, 100–110. [CrossRef] [PubMed]

39. Zhang, L.; Ren, B.; Zhang, J.; Liu, L.; Liu, J.; Jiang, G.; Li, M.; Ding, Y.; Li, W. Anti-tumor effect of *Scutellaria barbata* D. Don extracts on ovarian cancer and its phytochemicals characterisation. *J. Ethnopharmacol.* **2017**, *206*, 184–192. [CrossRef] [PubMed]

40. Yang, X.; Yang, Y.; Tang, S.; Tang, H.; Yang, G.; Xu, Q.; Wu, J. Anti-tumor effect of polysaccharides from *Scutellaria barbata* D. Don on the 95-D xenograft model via inhibition of the C-met pathway. *J. Pharmacol. Sci.* **2014**, *125*, 255–263. [CrossRef] [PubMed]

41. Yin, X.; Zhou, J.; Jie, C.; Xing, D.; Zhang, Y. Anticancer activity and mechanism of *Scutellaria barbata* extract on human lung cancer cell line A549. *Life Sci.* **2004**, *75*, 2233–2244. [CrossRef] [PubMed]

42. Wong, B.Y.; Nguyen, D.L.; Lin, T.; Wong, H.H.; Cavalcante, A.; Greenberg, N.M.; Hausted, R.P.; Zheng, J. Chinese medicinal herb *Scutellaria barbata* modulates apoptosis and cell survival in murine and human prostate cancer cells and tumor development in TRAMP mice. *Eur. J. Cancer Prev.* **2009**, *18*, 331–341. [CrossRef] [PubMed]

43. Wang, Z.; Ravula, R.; Shi, L.; Song, Y.; Yeung, S.; Liu, M.; Lau, B.; Hao, J.; Wang, J.; Lam, C.W.; et al. Overcoming chemoresistance in prostate cancer with Chinese medicines *Tripterygium wilfordii* via multiple mechanisms. *Oncotarget* **2016**, *7*, 61246–61261. [CrossRef] [PubMed]

44. Sureshkumar, S.; Sivakumar, T.; Chandrasekar, M.J.N.; Suresh, B. Investigating the Anti-Inflammatory and Analgesic Activity of Leaves of *Wedelia chinensis* (Osbeck) Merr. In Standard Experimental Animal models. *Iran. J. Pharm. Res.* **2006**, *5*, 123–129.

45. Manjamalai, A.; Shukoor, S.A.; Haridas, A.; Berlin, G. Evaluation of antifungal and anti-inflammatory effect on methanolic extract of *Wedelia chinensis* leaves. *Int. J. Pharm. Biomed. Res.* **2011**, *2*, 446–454.

46. Manjamalai, A.; Jiflin, G.J.; Grace, V.M.B. Study on the effect of essential oil of *Wedelia chinensis* (Osbeck) against microbes and inflammation. *Asian J. Pharm. Clin. Res.* **2012**, *5*, 155–164.

47. Tsai, C.H.; Lin, F.M.; Yang, Y.C.; Lee, M.T.; Cha, T.L.; Wu, G.J.; Hsieh, S.C.; Hsiao, P.W. Herbal extract of *Wedelia chinensis* attenuates androgen receptor activity and orthotopic growth of prostate cancer in nude mice. *Clin. Cancer Res.* **2009**, *15*, 5435–5444. [CrossRef] [PubMed]

48. Chun, J.Y.; Tummala, R.; Nadiminty, N.; Lou, W.; Liu, C.; Yang, J.; Evans, C.P.; Zhou, Q.; Gao, A.C. Andrographolide, an herbal medicine, inhibits interleukin-6 expression and suppresses prostate cancer cell growth. *Genes Cancer* **2010**, *1*, 868–876. [CrossRef] [PubMed]

49. Kan, S.F.; Huang, W.J.; Lin, L.C.; Wang, P.S. Inhibitory effects of evodiamine on the growth of human prostate cancer cell line LNCaP. *Int. J. Cancer* **2004**, *110*, 641–651. [CrossRef] [PubMed]

50. Li, X.; Lao, Y.; Zhang, H.; Wang, X.; Tan, H.; Lin, Z.; Xu, H. The natural compound Guttiferone F sensitizes prostate cancer to starvation induced apoptosis via calcium and JNK elevation. *BMC Cancer* **2015**, *15*, 254. [CrossRef] [PubMed]

51. Hahm, E.R.; Singh, S.V. Honokiol causes G0-G1 phase cell cycle arrest in human prostate cancer cells in association with suppression of retinoblastoma protein level/phosphorylation and inhibition of E2F1 transcriptional activity. *Mol. Cancer Ther.* **2007**, *6*, 2686–2695. [CrossRef] [PubMed]

52. Shigemura, K.; Arbiser, J.L.; Sun, S.Y.; Zayzafoon, M.; Johnstone, P.A.; Fujisawa, M.; Gotoh, A.; Weksler, B.; Zhau, H.E.; Chung, L.W. Honokiol, a natural plant product, inhibits the bone metastatic growth of human prostate cancer cells. *Cancer* **2007**, *109*, 1279–1289. [CrossRef] [PubMed]

53. Hahm, E.R.; Sakao, K.; Singh, S.V. Honokiol activates reactive oxygen species-mediated cytoprotective autophagy in human prostate cancer cells. *Prostate* **2014**, *74*, 1209–1221. [CrossRef] [PubMed]

54. Fang, Y.; Yu, Y.; Hou, Q.; Zheng, X.; Zhang, M.; Zhang, D.; Li, J.; Wu, X.R.; Huang, C. The Chinese Herb Isolate Isorhapontigenin Induces Apoptosis in Human Cancer Cells by Down-regulating Overexpression of Antiapoptotic Protein XIAP. *J. Biol. Chem.* **2012**, *287*, 35234–35243. [CrossRef] [PubMed]

55. Fernández-Marín, M.I.; Guerrero, R.F.; García-Parrilla, M.C.; Puertas, B.; Richard, T.; Rodriguez-Werner, M.A.; Winterhalter, P.; Monti, J.P.; Cantos-Villar, E. Isorhapontigenin: A novel bioactive stilbene from wine grapes. *Food Chem.* **2012**, *135*, 1353–1359. [CrossRef] [PubMed]

56. Fang, Y.N.; Liu, G.T. Effect of isorhapontigenin on respiratory burst of rat neutrophils. *Phytomedicine* **2002**, *9*, 734–738. [CrossRef] [PubMed]

57. Zhu, C.; Zhu, Q.; Wu, Z.; Yin, Y.; Kang, D.; Lu, S.; Liu, P. Isorhapontigenin induced cell growth inhibition and apoptosis by targeting EGFR-related pathways in prostate cancer. *J. Cell. Physiol.* **2018**, *233*, 1104–1119. [CrossRef] [PubMed]

58. Li, Y.Z.; Huang, J.; Gong, Z.; Tian, X.Q. A Novel Norlignan and a Novel Phenylpropanoid from *Peperomia tetraphylla. Helv. Chim. Acta* **2010**, *90*, 2222–2226. [CrossRef]

59. Li, Y.; He, N.; Zhai, C. Peperotetraphin inhibits the proliferation of human prostate cancer cells via induction of cell cycle arrest and apoptosis. *Med. Oncol.* **2015**, *32*, 468. [CrossRef] [PubMed]

60. Boots, A.W. Health effects of quercetin: From mechanism to nutraceutical. *Eur. J. Pharmacol.* **2006**, *585*, 325–337. [CrossRef] [PubMed]

61. Lee, D.H.; Szczepanski, M.; Yong, J.L. Role of Bax in quercetin-induced apoptosis in human prostate cancer cells. *Biochem. Pharm.* **2008**, *75*, 2345–2355. [CrossRef] [PubMed]

62. Jung, Y.H.; Heo, J.; Lee, Y.J.; Kwon, T.K.; Kim, Y.H. Quercetin enhances TRAIL-induced apoptosis in prostate cancer cells via increased protein stability of death receptor 5. *Life Sci.* **2010**, *86*, 351–357. [CrossRef] [PubMed]

63. Aalinkeel, R.; Bindukumar, B.; Reynolds, J.L.; Sykes, D.E.; Mahajan, S.D.; Chadha, K.C.; Schwartz, S.A. The Dietary Bioflavonoid, Quercetin, Selectively Induces Apoptosis of Prostate Cancer Cells by Down-Regulating the Expression of Heat Shock Protein 90. *Prostate* **2008**, *68*, 1773–1789. [CrossRef] [PubMed]

64. Vijayababu, M.R.; Kanagaraj, P.; Arunkumar, A.; Ilangovan, R.; Dharmarajan, A.; Arunakaran, J. Quercetin induces p53-independent apoptosis in human prostate cancer cells by modulating Bcl-2-related proteins: A possible mediation by IGFBP-3. *Oncol. Res.* **2006**, *16*, 67–74. [CrossRef] [PubMed]

65. Wang, G.; Song, L.; Wang, H.; Xing, N. Quercetin synergizes with 2-methoxyestradiol inhibiting cell growth and inducing apoptosis in human prostate cancer cells. *Oncol. Rep.* **2013**, *30*, 357–363. [CrossRef] [PubMed]

66. Liu, K.C.; Yen, C.Y.; Wu, R.S.; Yang, J.S.; Lu, H.F.; Lu, K.W.; Lo, C.; Chen, H.Y.; Tang, N.Y.; Wu, C.C.; et al. The roles of endoplasmic reticulum stress and mitochondrial apoptotic signaling pathway in quercetin-mediated cell death of human prostate cancer PC-3 cells. *Environ. Toxicol.* **2014**, *29*, 428–439. [CrossRef] [PubMed]

67. Xu, W.; Debeb, B.G.; Lacerda, L.; Li, J.; Woodward, W.A. Tetrandrine, a Compound Common in Chinese Traditional Medicine, Preferentially Kills Breast Cancer Tumor Initiating Cells (TICs) In Vitro. *Cancers* **2011**, *3*, 2274–2285. [CrossRef] [PubMed]

68. Liu, W.; Kou, B.; Ma, Z.K.; Tang, X.S.; Lv, C.; Ye, M.; Chen, J.Q.; Li, L.; Wang, X.Y.; He, D.L. Tetrandrine suppresses proliferation, induces apoptosis, and inhibits migration and invasion in human prostate cancer cells. *Asian J. Androl.* **2015**, *17*, 850–853. [PubMed]

69. Chen, B.J. Triptolide, a novel immunosuppressive and anti-inflammatory agent purified from a Chinese herb *Tripterygium wilfordii* Hook F. *Leuk. Lymphoma* **2001**, *42*, 253–265. [CrossRef] [PubMed]

70. Fulda, S. Tumor-necrosis-factor-related apoptosis-inducing ligand (TRAIL). *Adv. Exp. Med. Biol.* **2014**, *818*, 167–180. [PubMed]

71. Thakkar, H. Constitutively active Akt is an important regulator of TRAIL sensitivity in prostate cancer. *Oncogene* **2001**, *20*, 6073–6083.

72. Xiaowen, H.; Yi, S. Triptolide sensitizes TRAIL-induced apoptosis in prostate cancer cells via p53-mediated DR5 up-regulation. *Mol. Boil. Rep.* **2012**, *39*, 8763–8770. [CrossRef] [PubMed]

73. Meng, F.M.; Yang, J.B.; Yang, C.H.; Jiang, Y.; Zhou, Y.F.; Yu, B.; Yang, H. Vitexicarpin induces apoptosis in human prostate carcinoma PC-3 cells through G2/M phase arrest. *Asian Pac. J. Cancer Prev.* **2012**, *13*, 6369–6374. [CrossRef] [PubMed]

74. Cao, H.; Feng, Y.; Chen, L. Repression of MicroRNA-372 by Arsenic Sulphide Inhibits Prostate Cancer Cell Proliferation and Migration through Regulation of large tumour suppressor kinase 2. *Basic Clin. Pharmacol. Toxicol.* **2017**, *120*, 256–263. [CrossRef] [PubMed]

75. Chan, F.L.; Choi, H.L.; Chen, Z.Y.; Chan, P.S.; Huang, Y. Induction of apoptosis in prostate cancer cell lines by a flavonoid, baicalin. *Cancer Lett.* **2000**, *160*, 219–228. [CrossRef]

76. Pang, X.; Yi, Z.; Zhang, J.; Lu, B.; Sung, B.; Qu, W.; Aggarwal, B.B.; Liu, M. Celastrol suppresses angiogenesis-mediated tumor growth through inhibition of AKT/mammalian target of rapamycin pathway. *Cancer Res.* **2010**, *70*, 1951–1959. [CrossRef] [PubMed]

77. Chiang, K.C.; Tsui, K.H.; Chung, L.C.; Yeh, C.; Chen, W.; Chang, P.; Juang, H. Celastrol blocks interleukin-6 gene expression via downregulation of NF-κB in prostate carcinoma cells. *PLoS ONE* **2014**, *9*, e93151. [CrossRef] [PubMed]

78. Yang, H.; Chen, D.; Cui, Q.C.; Yuan, X.; Dou, Q.P. Celastrol, a triterpene extracted from the Chinese "Thunder of God Vine", is a potent proteasome inhibitor and suppresses human prostate cancer growth in nude mice. *Cancer Res* **2006**, *66*, 4758–4765. [CrossRef] [PubMed]

79. Zhang, X.S.; Cao, J.Q.; Zhao, C.; Wang, X.D.; Wu, X.J.; Zhao, Y.Q. Novel dammarane-type triterpenes isolated from hydrolyzate of total Gynostemma pentaphyllum saponins. *Bioorg. Med. Chem. Lett.* **2015**, *25*, 3095–3099. [CrossRef] [PubMed]

80. Zhang, X.S.; Zhao, C.; Tang, W.Z.; Wu, X.J.; Zhao, Y.Q. Gypensapogenin H, a novel dammarane-type triterpene induces cell cycle arrest and apoptosis on prostate cancer cells. *Steroids* **2015**, *104*, 276–283. [CrossRef] [PubMed]

81. Choi, Y.H.; Yan, G.H. Anti-allergic effects of scoparone on mast cell-mediated allergy model. *Phytomedicine* **2009**, *16*, 1089–1094. [CrossRef] [PubMed]

82. Kim, J.-K.; Kim, J.-Y.; Kim, H.-J.; Park, K.-G.; Harris, R.A.; Cho, W.J.; Lee, J.-T.; Lee, I.-K. Scoparone exerts anti-tumor activity against DU145 prostate cancer cells via inhibition of STAT3 activity. *PLoS ONE* **2013**, *8*, e80391. [CrossRef] [PubMed]

83. Zhang, R.; Zhang, P.Y.; Guo, J.; Yang, D.; Wang, W.J.; Zheng, M.H.; Ma, Y.C. Effects of triptolide on prostate carcinoma in mouse RM-1 cells. *Natl. J. Androl.* **2007**, *13*, 237–241.

84. Cher, M.L. Mechanisms governing bone metastasis in prostate cancer. *Curr. Opin. Urol.* **2001**, *11*, 483–488. [CrossRef] [PubMed]

85. Msaouel, P.; Pissimissis, N.; Halapas, A.; Koutsilieris, M. Mechanisms of bone metastasis in prostate cancer: Clinical implications. Best practice & research. *Clin. Endocrinol. Metab.* **2008**, *22*, 341–355.

86. Kuchta, K.; Xiang, Y.; Huang, S.; Tang, Y.; Peng, X.; Wang, X.; Zhu, Y.; Li, J.; Xu, J.; Lin, Z.; et al. Celastrol, an active constituent of the TCM plant Tripterygium wilfordii Hook.f., inhibits prostate cancer bone metastasis. *Prostate Cancer Prostatic Dis.* **2017**, *20*, 156–164. [CrossRef] [PubMed]

87. Yang, L.; Zhang, L.Y.; Chen, W.W.; Kong, F.; Zhang, P.J.; Hu, X.Y.; Zhang, J.Y.; Cui, F.A. Inhibition of the expression of prostate specific antigen by curcumin. *Acta Pharm. Sin.* **2005**, *40*, 800–803.

88. Cao, H.; Yu, H.; Feng, Y.; Chen, L.; Liang, F. Curcumin inhibits prostate cancer by targeting PGK1 in the FOXD3/miR-143 axis. *Cancer Chemother. Pharmacol.* **2017**, *79*, 985–994. [CrossRef] [PubMed]

89. Yang, J.; Wang, C.; Zhang, Z.; Chen, X.; Jia, Y.; Wang, B.; Kong, T. Curcumin inhibits the survival and metastasis of prostate cancer cells via the Notch-1 signaling pathway. *APMIS* **2017**, *125*, 134–140. [CrossRef] [PubMed]

90. Hu, E.; Wang, D.; Chen, J.; Tao, X. Novel cyclotides from Hedyotis diffusa induce apoptosis and inhibit proliferation and migration of prostate cancer cells. *Int. J. Clin. Exp. Med.* **2015**, *8*, 4059–4065. [PubMed]

91. Lin, T.H.; Tan, T.W.; Tsai, T.H.; Chen, C.C.; Hsieh, T.F.; Lee, S.S.; Liu, H.H.; Chen, W.C.; Tang, C.H. D-pinitol inhibits prostate cancer metastasis through inhibition of $\alpha V\beta 3$ integrin by modulating FAK, c-Src and NF-kappaB pathways. *Int. J. Mol. Sci.* **2013**, *14*, 9790–9802. [CrossRef] [PubMed]

92. Wu, C.Y.; Yang, Y.H.; Lin, Y.Y.; Kuan, F.C.; Lin, Y.S.; Lin, W.Y.; Tsai, M.Y.; Yang, J.J.; Cheng, Y.C.; Shu, L.H.; et al. Anti-cancer effect of danshen and dihydroisotanshinone I on prostate cancer: Targeting the crosstalk between macrophages and cancer cells via inhibition of the STAT3/CCL2 signaling pathway. *Oncotarget* **2017**, *8*, 40246–40263. [CrossRef] [PubMed]

93. Chen, Y.; Zheng, L.; Liu, J.; Zhou, Z.; Cao, X.; Lv, X.; Chen, F. Shikonin inhibits prostate cancer cells metastasis by reducing matrix metalloproteinase-2/-9 expression via AKT/mTOR and ROS/ERK1/2 pathways. *Int. Immunopharm.* **2014**, *21*, 447–455. [CrossRef] [PubMed]

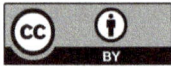

nutrients

MDPI

Article

Deciphering the Molecular Mechanism Underlying the Inhibitory Efficacy of Taiwanese Local Pomegranate Peels against Urinary Bladder Urothelial Carcinoma

Ching-Ping Chang [1], Yu-Yi Chan [2], Chien-Feng Li [2,3], Lan-Hsiang Chien [1], Song-Tay Lee [2] and Ting-Feng Wu [2,*]

[1] Department of Medical Research, Chi Mei Medical Center, Tainan 710, Taiwan;
    jessica.cpchang@gmail.com (C.-P.C.); m96h0207@stust.edu.tw (L.-H.C.)
[2] Department of Biotechnology, Southern Taiwan University of Science and Technology, Tainan 710, Taiwan;
    yuyichan@stust.edu.tw (Y.-Y.C.); angelo.p@yahoo.com.tw (C.-F.L.); songtlee@stust.edu.tw (S.-T.L.)
[3] Department of Pathology, Chi Mei Medical Center, Tainan 710, Taiwan
*   Correspondence: wutingfe@stust.edu.tw; Tel.: +886-6-253-3131 (ext. 8394)

Received: 3 April 2018; Accepted: 24 April 2018; Published: 27 April 2018

Abstract: Pomegranate (*Punica granatum* L.) fruit has been demonstrated to have the inhibitory activities to various tumors. In this study, we try to uncover the molecular mechanism underlying the inhibitory capability of Taiwanese local pomegranate fruit to urinary bladder urothelial carcinoma. The results collected from the 3-(4,5-dimethylthiazol-2-yl)-2,5-diphenyltetrazolium bromide assay indicated that the ethanol extract of pomegranate peel exhibited better inhibitory activity to human urinary bladder urothelial carcinoma T24 and J82 cells than that of pulp. Furthermore, the ethylacetate layer of peel ethanol extract was observed to have the best inhibitory activity against urinary bladder urothelial carcinoma cells. One of the eight fractions (PEPE2 fraction) collected from the ethylacetate layer with Diaion HP-20 column chromatography demonstrated the highest inhibitory activity in urinary bladder urothelial carcinoma cells. The results of the flow cytometry and apoptotic pathway studies suggested that the inhibitory activity of PEPE2 fraction were attributed to the UBUC cell apoptosis. To confirm the above results, our results of xenograft-induced bladder tumor in nude mice showed that the oral consumption of the ethylacetate layer (2, 5, 10 and 100 mg/kg) could decrease the volume and weight of T24 tumors and caused the apoptosis in the xenografted tumors, which was observed by terminal deoxynucleotidyl transferase-mediated deoxyuridine triphosphate nick end-labeling assay. This study provided the likelihood that the traditionally non-edible pomegranate peel waste is re-utilized to make an affordable and promising chemopreventive product to prevent UBUC incidence or recurrence.

Keywords: apoptosis; T24 cells; death receptor pathway; mitochondrial pathway; endoplasmic reticulum stress; pomegranate peel; urinary bladder urothelial carcinoma

1. Introduction

Bladder cancer is the most common tumor of the urinary system in the world and ranked the 9th in male cancer incidence in Taiwan in 2014 [1,2]. Urothelial carcinoma is the most encountered lesion among various bladder tumor types, which contributes to more than 90% of the bladder cancer cases in developed countries [1]. According to WHO classification (2004), urinary bladder urothelial carcinoma (UBUC) cells can be classified into the low or high grades. Most of the UBUCs are papillary/non-invasive or superficially invasive types and can be treated by curettage. However, local recurrence can be observed in some UBUCs even followed by lethal distal spreading [3]. In terms of disease management, it may be beneficial that a chemopreventive product for bladder cancer can be used by cancer patients or high-risk persons to avoid tumor recurrence or incidence.

Pomegranate (*Punica granatum* L.) is an edible fruit collected from a deciduous tree species. Today, it is widely grown in Mediterranean countries, Northern India, Northern/Southern America, Europe, and even in Taiwan, mainly as gardening trees. The pomegranate fruit is observed to have a reddish peel and white to deep red seeds. Pomegranate pericarp (peel) is a rich resource of phenolics, flavonoids, ellagitannins (predominantly punicalagin), and proanthocyanins compounds [4]. Pomegranate seeds are edible and have strong anti-oxidant activities attributed to the high amount of hydrolyzable tannins and anthocyanins [4]. Pomegranate juice (PJ) squeezed from seed pulp is rich in phenolics and flavonoids, mainly anthocyanins [4].

Many studies exploring the chemopreventive capability of pomegranate have indicated that the pomegranate fruit demonstrates inhibitory activities to various tumors. Pomegranate fruit extract (PFE) prepared from the edible portions (seed coats and pulp juice) of the pomegranate fruit with 70% acetone was proved to display the apoptotic impacts on human lung cancer A549 cells but have minimal effects on normal bronchial epithelial cells [5]. PFE treatment also induces g_0/G_1 arrest and inhibits not only NF-κB activities but also various MAP kinase pathways [5]. PFE administration also ameliorates tumor growth/progression/angiogenesis of B(a)P or NTCU induced primary lung tumors in A/J mice by dwindled activation of NF-κB, MAP kinase pathways, and mammalian target of rapamycin (mTOR) signaling [6]. In addition to the effects on lung cancer, PFE may be a promising chemopreventive/chemotherapeutic agent against human prostate cancer as well. Malik et al. [7] found that apoptosis is evoked in PFE-treated highly aggressive PC3 cells, resulting in a decrease in Bcl-2 along with an increase in Bax. Their studies showed that PFE treatment impairs various cell cycle cyclins and p21 as well as p27. Additionally, the oral administration of 0.1% or 0.2% PFE in drinking water (equivalent to the ingredients present in 250 or 500 mL of pomegranate juice) to TRAMP mice can obviously inhibit prostate carcinogenesis by inhibiting IGF-1/Akt/mTOR pathways [8]. Retting et al. [9] reported that the treatment of polyphenols/ellagitannin-abundant extract (PE) purified from pomegranate fruit peels can restrict LAPC4 androgen-independent xenograft via the inhibition of the NF-κB signaling pathway. The clinical trial in patients with increasing prostate-specific antigens (PSA) after surgery or radiotherapy demonstrated that daily oral consumption of 8 ounces of pomegranate juice (PJ) significantly extends the PSA doubling time (PSADT) from 15 to 54 months in men with prostate cancer (PCa) [10]. However, a randomized, double-blind, placebo-controlled clinical study also showed that PFE treatment does not significantly extend the PSADT in PCa patients with rising PSA after primary therapy, compared to the placebo-treated group [11]. Our previous documented results demonstrated that Taiwanese local pomegranate juice (PJ) could evoke cell apoptosis via the intrinsic mitochondrial pathway and the extrinsic death receptor signaling in PCa cells. It also can de-regulate the expression levels of genes linked to cytoskeletal functions, anti-apoptosis, metabolism, NF-B signaling in PJ-treated PCa cells [12]. Based on the above-documented findings, pomegranates may be a promising chemopreventive or chemotherapeutic source against UBUC carcinogenesis and recurrence.

In this study, we found that the ethanol extract isolated from pomegranate peels (PEP) exhibited a better inhibitory activity comparatively to UBUC cells than that of pulps. Fractionation of PEP with increasing polarity showed that the EtOAc fraction of PEP had the best anti-cancer efficacy. Treatment of 1 of 8 column-fractionation parts of the EtOAc fraction, PEPE6, could evoke UBUC cell apoptosis. Oral administration of the EtOAc fraction of PEP to UBUC xenografted nude mice caused a significant reduction in tumor growth and evoked cell apoptosis. Taken together, our results implied that the ingredients present in pomegranate peels demonstrated the inhibitory activity of UBUC cells.

2. Materials and Methods

2.1. Materials

The following antibodies were used for western immunoblotting: Actin (1:5000, Millipore, Billerica, MA, USA), Bip (1:1000, BD Biosciences, San Jose, CA, USA), Caspase-3 (1:250, Gene Tex, Irvine, CA, USA), Caspase-8 (1:250, BD Biosciences, San Jose, CA, USA), Caspase-9 (1:1000, BD Biosciences, San Jose, CA, USA), Caspase-12 (1:1000, Gene Tex, Irvine, CA, USA), DR4 (1:1000, Gene Tex, Irvine, CA, USA), DR5 (1:2000, Gene Tex, Irvine, CA, USA), VCP (1:1000, Abnova, Taipei, Taiwan, ROC), Anti-rabbit IgG (1:10,000, GE Healthcare, Mickleton, NJ, USA), and Anti-mouse IgG (1:10,000, GE Healthcare, Mickleton, NJ, USA). Annexin V conjugated with FITC was bought from the Strong Biotech Corporation in Tainan, Taiwan. Chemiluminescence ECL detection system was purchased from GE Healthcare Bio-Sciences AB in Uppsala, Sweden. Dulbecco's Modified Eagle Medium, McCoy's5A, and fetal bovine serum were purchased from GIBCO, Grand Island in NY, USA. MTT was bought from Merck in Darmstadt, Germany. Propidium iodide was purchased from Sigma, Saint Louis in MO, USA. PVDF membrane was bought from Stratagene, La Jolla in CA, USA. TUNEL reaction mixture was purchased from Rochel in Mannheim, Germany.

2.2. Collection and Identification of Plant Materials

The fruits of the *P. granatum* were field collected from a farmland (22°41′59.3267″ N, 120°30′45.1836″ E) located in Jiuru, a suburban township in the Pingtung county in southern Taiwan from August to September 2012. The plant specimens were identified by Dr. Gwo-Ing Liao from National Chen-Kung University, Taiwan and were pressed/dried for voucher specimens (Nan-Kai Lin, STUSTG308-001 to STUSTG308-003) deposited in the herbarium of Taiwan Forestry Research Institute (TFRI), Taiwan.

2.3. Preparation of the Ethanol Extracts from Pulps and Peels of Pomegranates

Fresh pomegranate pulps (452 g) and peels (392 g) were extracted respectively with 95% ethanol, three times, at a ratio of 1:3 at room temperature for 24 h. The filtrates were evaporated under reduced pressure to yield the dark brown syrups from pulp (PEG, 51 g) and peel (PEP, 74 g) extracts respectively. PEP was suspended in water (300 mL) and then partitioned with ethyl acetate (EtOAc) (4 × 300 mL) and *n*-butanol (4 × 300 mL) successively to yield individual layers of extracts of EtOAc (4.5 g), *n*-butanol (29.8 g) and water (28.7 g), respectively. The above three layers were examined for their anticancer bioactivities. Among these three layers, the EtOAc layer exhibited the most potent effectiveness (Figure 1). Hence, the EtOAc layer (4.5 g) was subjected directly to Diaion HP-20 column chromatography, eluted with water containing increasing proportions of ethanol to render eight fractions labeled PEPE1 (0.1256 g), PEPE2 (0.1064 g), PEPE3 (1.712 g), PEPE4 (1.4595 g), PEPE5 (0.3758 g), PEPE6 (0.1384 g), PEPE7 (0.1731 g), and PEPE8 (0.1567 g). The eight fractions were then evaluated for their anticancer bioactivities.

2.4. Cell Lines

Human UBUC T24 cells, identified as high grade and invasive, were purchased from the Bioresource Collection and Research Center, Hsinchu, Taiwan and cultured at 37 °C in McCoy's5A supplemented with 10% (*v/v*) fetal bovine serum. Human UBUC J82 cells recognized as high grade were provided by Dr. Chien-Feng Li from Department of Pathology, Chi-Mei Medical Center, Tainan, Taiwan and maintained at 37 °C in Dulbecco's Modified Eagle Medium supplemented with 10% (*v/v*) fetal bovine serum. Human papillomavirus E7 immortalized uroepithelial cell was kindly provided by Professor Hsiao-Sheng Liu from the department of microbiology and immunology, college of medicine, National Cheng Kung University, Tainan, Taiwan and maintained as described previously [13].

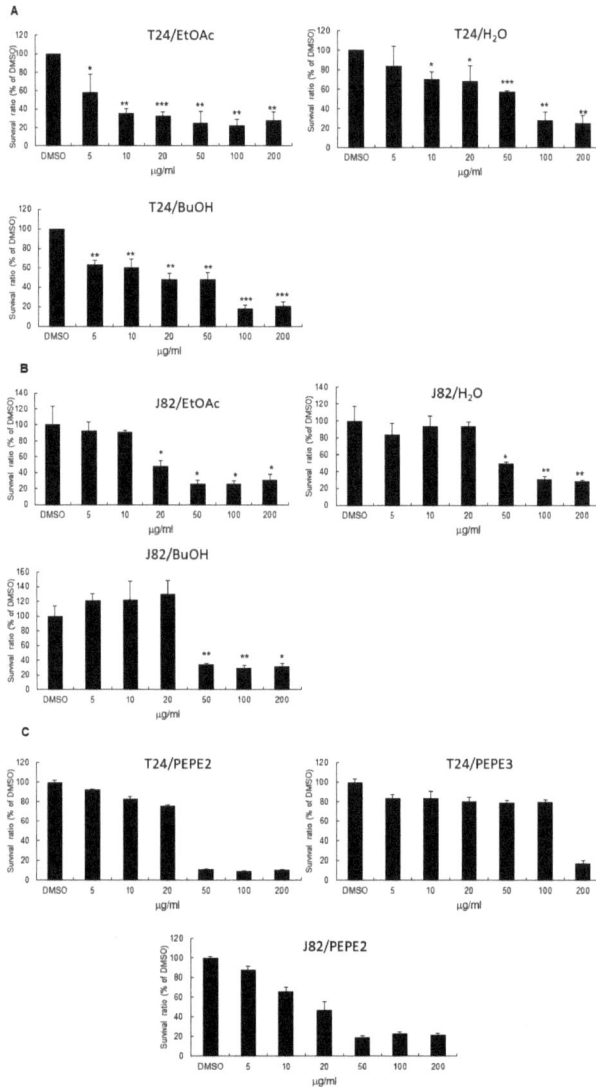

Figure 1. The inhibitory activities of Taiwanese local pomegranate fruit. The ethylacetate, butanol, and water layers extracted from pomegranate peel extract (PEP) were tested for the inhibitory efficacy to T24 (**A**) or J82 (**B**) cells using MTT assay as described in Materials and Methods. PEPE2 and PEPE3 (**C**) were also investigated for the inhibitory effectiveness to T24 or J82 cells. 0.1% (v/v) Dimethyl sulfoxide (DMSO)-treated urinary bladder urothelial carcinoma (UBUC) cells were regarded as the solvent control. Each MTT result was the typical data of at least three independent experiments. * $p \leq 0.05$, ** $p \leq 0.01$, *** $p \leq 0.001$.

2.5. 3-(4,5-Dimethylthiazol-2-yl)-2,5-diphenyltetrazolium Bromide (MTT) Assay

As indicated in Figure 1, 5, 10, 20, 50, and 100 µg/mL of ethanol extracts of pomegranate peels were added to a 96-well plate seeded with 5000 human T24 cells, 6000 human J82 cells, or 3000 human E7 cells per well. The same concentrations and protocol were also conducted with pulp ethanol extracts and further with EtOAc, BuOH and H_2O layers from peel ethanol extracts and PEP2/PEP3 column fractions. After incubation for the time period shown in Figure 1, 20 μL of MTT solution (5 mg/mL PBS) was added to each well and the plate was incubated at 37 °C for 4 h. After medium removal, 200 μL of dimethyl sulfoxide (DMSO) was added to each well and the plate was gently shaken for 5 min. The absorbance was measured at 540 nm. Quadruplicate wells were applied to each concentration for a specific time period. 0.1% (*v*/*v*) DMSO (vehicle)-treated UBUC cells were recognized as the control.

2.6. Cell Cycle Analysis of PEPE2-Treated UBUC Cells

1×10^6 T24 or 7×10^5 J82 cells were first seeded on a 10-cm plate. After overnight incubation, 50 μg/mL and 20 μg/mL of PEPE2 was added to respectively T24 and J82 cells seeded on each 10-cm plate and the cells were harvested at the appropriate time duration. The collected cells of each plate were suspended in 500 μL of ice-cold 70% ethanol at 4 °C overnight. After treatment, the cells were washed with 1 mL ice-cold PBS and re-suspended in 100 μL PBS. Afterward, the cells were incubated in 300 μL propidium iodide (PI) solution (3 μL RNase and 20 μg PI per mL) in the dark at 37 °C for 30 min. The stained cells were analyzed by FACSCalibur flow cytometer (Becton Dickinson, Franklin Lakes, NJ, USA). 0.1% (*v*/*v*) DMSO-treated UBUC cells were regarded as the control and analyzed as described above.

2.7. Annexin V/PI Analyses of PEPE2-Treated UBUC Cells

T24 and J82 cells were treated as indicated in the annexin V/PI analyses. The collected cells of each plate were washed with 1 mL ice-cold PBS and re-suspended in 100 μL binding buffer. Then 2 μL of annexin V conjugated with FITC and 2 μL of PI solution were administrated to the re-suspended cells and incubated in the dark on ice for 15 min. After incubation, the cells were measured using a FACSCalibur flow cytometer (Becton Dickinson). A percentage of 0.1% (*v*/*v*) DMSO-treated UBUC cells were deemed as the control and analyzed as described above.

2.8. Western Immunoblotting

After treatment, as described in the results, T24 or J82 cells were harvested and lysed in the lysis buffer (10 mMTris (pH 8.0), 0.32 M sucrose, 1% (*v*/*v*) Triton X-100, 5 mM EDTA, 2 mM DTT, and 1 mM PMSF). After determining its protein concentration using Bio-Rad DC protein assay kit, equal volume of 2× sample buffer (0.1 M Tris (pH 6.8), 2% (*w*/*v*) SDS, 0.2% (*v*/*v*) β-mercaptoethanol, 10% (*v*/*v*) glycerol, and 0.0016% (*w*/*v*) bromophenol blue) was mixed with the protein lysate. The protein lysates were separated by SDS-PAGE at 100 V for the suitable time and further transferred onto a PVDF membrane. After blocking for 1 h in 3% (*w*/*v*) bovine serum albumin at room temperature, the membranes were hybridized for 2 h at room temperature with primary antibodies. Then the membranes were washed and hybridized with correspondent secondary antibodies for 1 h at room temperature. The secondary antibodies binding on the membrane were detected by a chemiluminescence ECL detection system using Fujifilm LAS-4000 Luminescent Image Analyzer (Fujifilm Corporation, Tokyo, Japan). The intensity of each protein band of interest was quantified by PDQUEST Quantity One software (Bio-Rad Laboratory, Hercules, CA, USA) and normalized with actin protein expression level. The acquired data were analyzed with Student's *t*-Test (STATISTICA, StatSoft, Tulsa, OK, USA). The 0.1% (*v*/*v*) of DMSO-treated UBUC cells were deemed as the control and analyzed as described above.

2.9. Xenografted Tumors of T24 Cells in Nude Mice

Relevant animal studies were performed in accordance with the guide for Laboratory Animal Facilities and Care as promulgated by the Council of Agriculture, Executive Yuan, Taiwan. The protocol was approved by the Animal Research Committee (permit number: MED-100-05; project code: NSC 101-2632-B-218-001-MY3) of Southern Taiwan University of Science and Technology. Male nude mice (BALB/cAnN-Foxn1, 9 weeks old) were purchased from the animal center of the National Science Council in Taiwan. The animals were nurtured at 23–25 °C and 30–70% humidity with 12-h light/12-h darkness cycle. The mice intake rodent Lab Diet 5001 (Lab Supply, Fort Worth, TX, USA) and sterile water ad libitium. The mice were quarantined for 7 days before the experiment. The mice were subcutaneously (s.c.) inoculated on the right lower abdomen with 100 µL T24 cell/matrigel mixture prepared by blending 1×10^7 of T24 cells with an equal volume of the gel. All efforts were made to minimize the suffering of the mice. Dried EtOAc extract was suspended thoroughly in water and then the suspension was used for oral gavage (o.g.). The mice were separated into 4 subgroups. The xenografted mice were fed o.g. with water ($n = 11$), 2 mg/kg ($n = 8$), 5 mg/kg ($n = 10$), 10 mg/kg ($n = 10$), and 100 mg/kg ($n = 6$) of EtOAc extract. For the extract-treated groups, after implanted with T24 cells, the mice were fed with EtOAc extract suspension by o.g. in the next day and then administrated with the suspension once a day until the endpoint. At the endpoint, each mouse was euthanized by intraperitoneal (i.p.) injecting with 0.5 mL of 500 mg/mL urethane and the tumor, as well as liver, was collected. growth of the xenografted tumors was measured by vernier calipers at 3-day intervals. The tumor volume was calculated as $V =$ length $\times$ width^2/2 as described previously [14]. For Statistical Analysis, the results are expressed as the mean $\pm$ standard error (SE) of at least 3 independent experiments. Statistical significance was determined by Student's *t*-test and one-way ANOVA using the SigmaPlot program for Windows, version 12.0 (Systat Software Inc., San Jose, CA, USA).

2.10. Terminal Deoxynucleotidyl Transferase-Mediated Deoxyuridine Triphosphate Nick End-Labeling Assay (TUNEL)

Histologic specimens were prepared in the way as described for preparation of the subcutaneous xenografts. Animal specimens were fixed in 10%-buffered formalin solution and embedded in paraffin. For morphological analysis, the hematoxylin-eosin (H&E) staining and microscopic examination were performed on the 3-µm-thick sections of the paraffin-embedded tumor blocks. Slides were either stained with H&E according to the aforementioned specifications or exposed to TUNEL assay. The sections were treated with xylene and then with ethanol. After paraffin removal and dehydration, the sections were washed with PBS and incubated with 3% (v/v) H_2O_2 solution for 20 min. Then the specimens were treated with 5 µg/mL proteinase k at room temperature for 2 min. After enzyme incubation, the specimens were washed with 0.1 M PBS (pH 7.4) and incubated with a TUNEL reaction mixture at 37 °C for 1 h. Then the treated sections were washed with distilled water and hybridized with a horse-radish peroxidase-conjugated fluorescent antibody at room temperature for 30 min. Lastly the sections were washed with distilled water. The TUNEL-positive cells were evaluated in at least 6 fields per section ($\times 200$ magnification) by two persons under a blinding condition.

2.11. Statistical Analyses

Student's *t*-test (STATISTICA Ver 10.0 MR1, StatSoft, Tulsa, OK, USA) were used for the statistical analyses of MTT assay, flow cytometry, and western immunoblotting. Student's *t*-test and one-way ANOVA of the SigmaPlot program for Windows, version 12.0 (Systat Software Inc., San Jose, CA, USA) were exploited for the statistical significance of animal studies.

3. Results

3.1. Pomegranate Fruits Exhibited the Inhibitory Impacts on UBUC Cell Proliferation

In this investigation, the pulps and peels of fresh pomegranate fruits were extracted with ethanol, respectively, to give pulp extract (PEG) and peel extract (PEP). The results of MTT assays showed that PEP exhibited better suppressive ability than that of PEG toward UBUC cells (Figure S1A,B). Therefore, PEP was partitioned successively between H_2O/EtOAc and between H_2O/*n*-BuOH, respectively, to yield three layers of EtOAc, *n*-BuOH, and H_2O. The results of the MTT assays demonstrated that IC_{50} of EtOAc, butanol, and water layers from PEP were 5, 10, and 50 µg/mL, respectively, against the T24 cells while for the J82 cells IC_{50} of these three layers were 20, 50, and 50 µg/mL (Figure 1A,B).

Taken together, the EtOAc layer had the best inhibitory activity against the UBUC cell lines. The HPLC profile of EtOAc layer was shown in Supplementary Figure S2A.

Furthermore, the EtOAc layer was fractionated into 8 fractions by Diaion HP-20 column chromatography as described in Materials and Methods. We first examined the toxicity of each column fraction to normal-like urothelial E7 cell and found that IC_{50} of PEPE2 and PEPE3 were >200 µg/mL, respectively, (Figure S1C) and the other PEP fractions would harm E7 cell (data not shown). Findings in Figure 1C demonstrated that the PEPE2 fraction showed the best inhibitory effects on human T24 and J82 cells and the least harmful impacts on normal-like human E7 urothelial cells. The HPLC map of PEPE2 was shown in Supplementary Figure S2B.

3.2. PEPE2-Evoked Retardation of Human UBUC Cell Proliferation Attributed to Cell Apoptosis

To discover which mechanism was engaged in the inhibition of human UBUC cell proliferation, the cell cycle analyses conducted following incubation of T24 cells with 50 µg/mL PEPE2 showed that the PEPE2 treatment induced 20.9% on average of T24 cells in the sub-G_1 phase at 72-h as compared to 2.45% on the average DMSO-treated cells (Figure 2A), whereas treatment with 20 µg/mL PEPE2 evoked 41.78% on average of J82 cells in the subG1 phase at 72-h as compared to 4.17% on average of DMSO-treated cells (Figure 2B). Furthermore, the annexin V/PI analysis indicated that 50 µg/mL of PEPE2 incubation for 72 h enhanced the early apoptotic T24 cells significantly from 2.9 to 46.2% on average as compared to the vehicle-treated cells (Figure 2C) while 20 µg/mL PEPE2 treatment for 72 h augmented the early/late J82 apoptotic cells prominently from 6.4 to 66.3% on average as compared to the DMSO-treated cells (Figure 2D), suggesting that the PEPE2 treatment could induce apoptosis in the T24 and J82 cells and J82 cells that were more susceptible to PEPE2 than that of T24 cells.

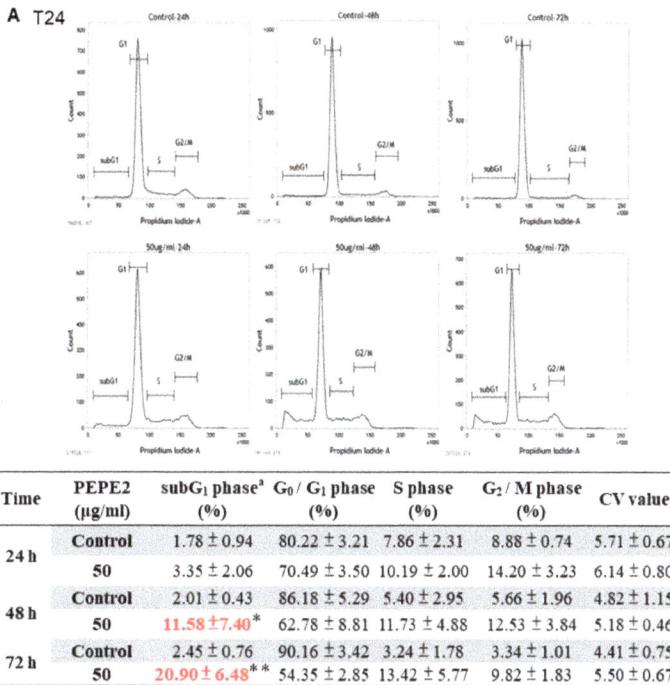

Time	PEPE2 (µg/ml)	subG$_1$ phase[a] (%)	G$_0$/G$_1$ phase (%)	S phase (%)	G$_2$/M phase (%)	CV value
24 h	Control	1.78 ± 0.94	80.22 ± 3.21	7.86 ± 2.31	8.88 ± 0.74	5.71 ± 0.67
	50	3.35 ± 2.06	70.49 ± 3.50	10.19 ± 2.00	14.20 ± 3.23	6.14 ± 0.80
48 h	Control	2.01 ± 0.43	86.18 ± 5.29	5.40 ± 2.95	5.66 ± 1.96	4.82 ± 1.15
	50	11.58 ± 7.40*	62.78 ± 8.81	11.73 ± 4.88	12.53 ± 3.84	5.18 ± 0.46
72 h	Control	2.45 ± 0.76	90.16 ± 3.42	3.24 ± 1.78	3.34 ± 1.01	4.41 ± 0.75
	50	20.90 ± 6.48**	54.35 ± 2.85	13.42 ± 5.77	9.82 ± 1.83	5.50 ± 0.67

[a]The results of three independent experiments

Figure 2. *Cont.*

B J82

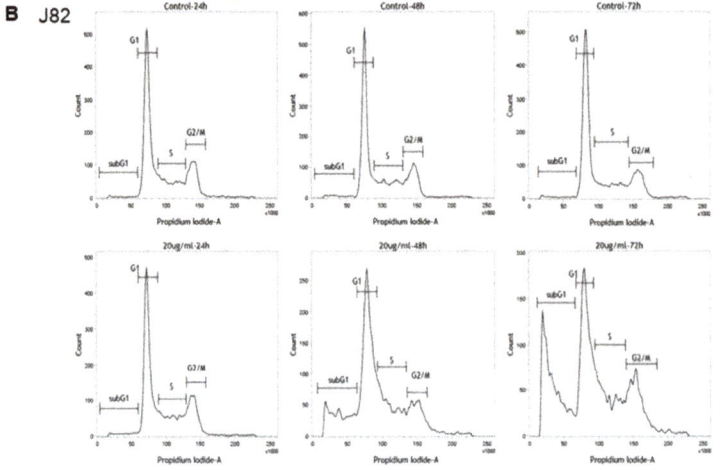

Time	PEPE2 (μg/ml)	subG₁ phase[a] (%)	G₀/G₁ phase (%)	S phase (%)	G₂/M phase (%)	CV value
24 h	**Control**	1.87± 0.52	55.20 ± 4.16	20.57 ± 2.84	18.95 ± 1.77	5.70 ± 0.57
	20	2.39 ± 0.81	54.80 ± 4.96	23.14 ± 3.70	15.91 ± 3.30	6.15 ± 0.54
48 h	**Control**	3.04 ± 0.86	50.54 ± 1.21	22.78 ± 2.09	19.96 ± 1.68	5.19± 0.24
	20	16.59 ±4.30***	44.24 ± 4.28	21.35 ± 3.95	12.62± 0.83	8.12± 0.87
72 h	**Control**	4.17 ± 0.60	51.75 ± 1.48	21.05 ± 0.66	19.53 ± 1.43	5.14 ± 0.20
	20	47.18 ± 14.67**	27.31 ± 4.74	14.20 ± 4.82	8.98± 5.83	9.42 ± 2.68

[a]The results of three independent experiments

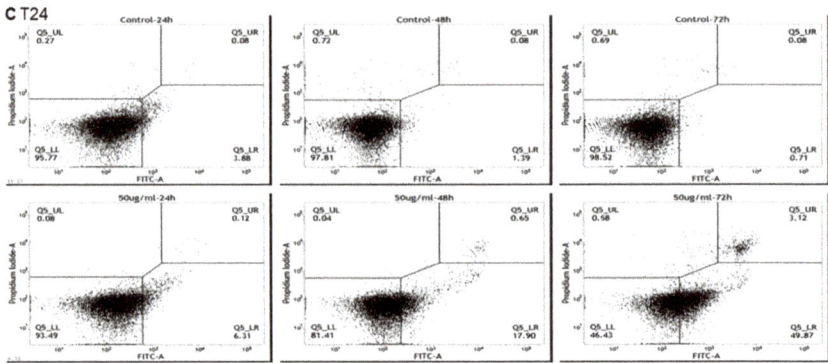

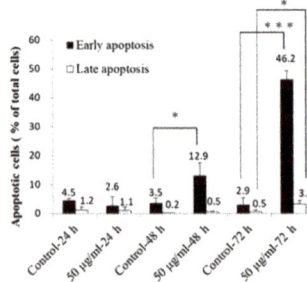

C T24

Figure 2. *Cont.*

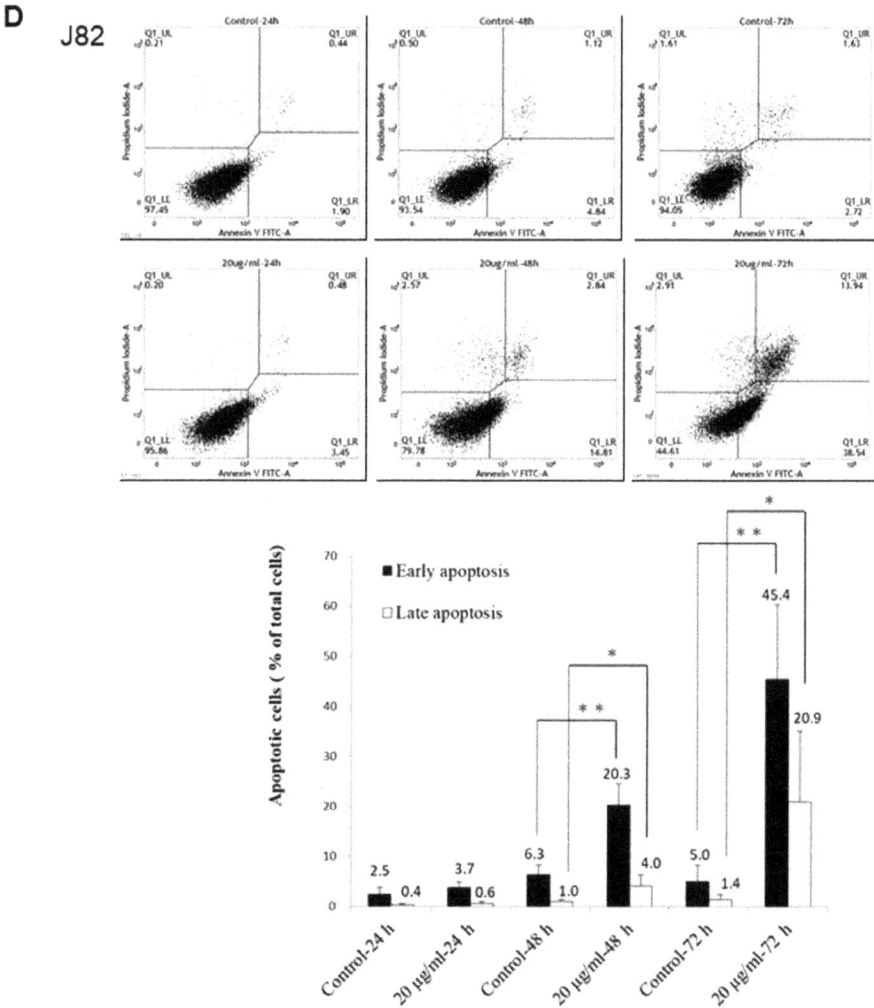

Figure 2. The propidium iodide (PI) and PI/annexin V analyses of UBUC cells treated with PEPE2. The results of PI analyses were represented in (**A**) the T24 cells and (**B**) the J82 cells. The data of the PI/annexin V measurement were shown in (**C**) T24 cells and (**D**) J82 cells. Each flow cytometry figure was the typical result of three independent experiments. The diagram under the PI/annexin V panel was the results of the three independent experiments. The cell cycles and apoptosis detection of the T24 or J82 cells treated with PEPE2 were measured with PI and PI/annexin V analyses, respectively, using flow cytometry as described in the supplementary document. The 0.1% (v/v) DMSO-treated UBUC cells were implemented as the vehicle control. * $p \leq 0.05$, ** $p \leq 0.01$, *** $p \leq 0.001$.

3.3. Molecular Mechanism of the Apoptotic Pathway Induced in PEPE2-Treated UBUC Cells

The previous results showed that the PEPE2 treatment could induce bladder cancer cell apoptosis. However, the cytometric analysis cannot decipher whether PEPE2 resulted in the apoptosis by death receptor signaling, the mitochondrial damage pathway, or ER stress. Caspase-3 is a key player in mitochondrial damage, death receptor signaling, and ER stress. Meanwhile, Caspase-3 can be activated by caspase-8 in death receptor signaling, by caspase-9 in mitochondrial damage, and by caspase-12 in endothelium reticulum (ER) stress [15]. In order to search for the molecular mechanism by which PEPE2 evoked the apoptosis, the processing and activation of caspase-3 was measured in drug-treated UBUC cells. The results in Figure 3A showed that the activated caspase-3 (21 and 17 kDa) amount was increased in PEPE2-treated T24 cells in a time-dependent response, implicating that caspase-3 was activated while the apoptosis might be initiated in PEPE2-incubated T24 cells. The data in Figure 3B and Figure S3A also demonstrated that the expressions of DR4 as well as DR5 and activated caspase-8 were augmented, implicating that the death receptor pathway was evoked in PEPE2-treated T24 and J82 cells. In PEPE2-incubated T24 and J82 cells, the apoptosis-activator Bax level was increased while the anti-apoptotic Bcl-2 amount was decreased and thus, the pro-caspase-9 level dwindled, implying that the mitochondrial pathway was related to cancer cell apoptosis (Figures 3C and S3B). Our studies also showed that the amount of Bip and VCP (ER stress markers) was increased in PEPE2-treated T24 and J82 cells and thus, pro-caspase-12 was activated (Figures 3D and S3C), implying that the ER stress was also associated with UBUC cell apoptosis.

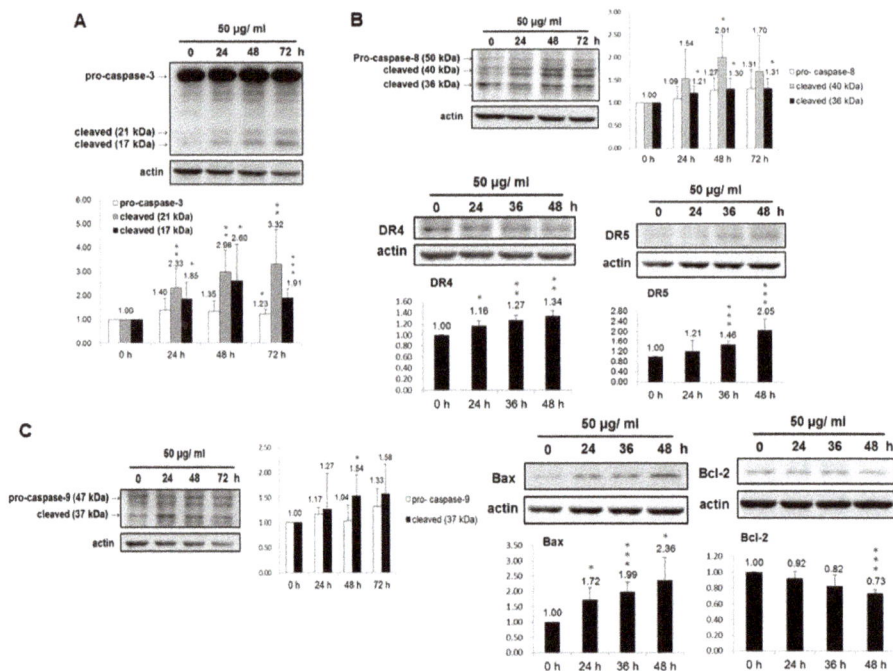

Figure 3. *Cont.*

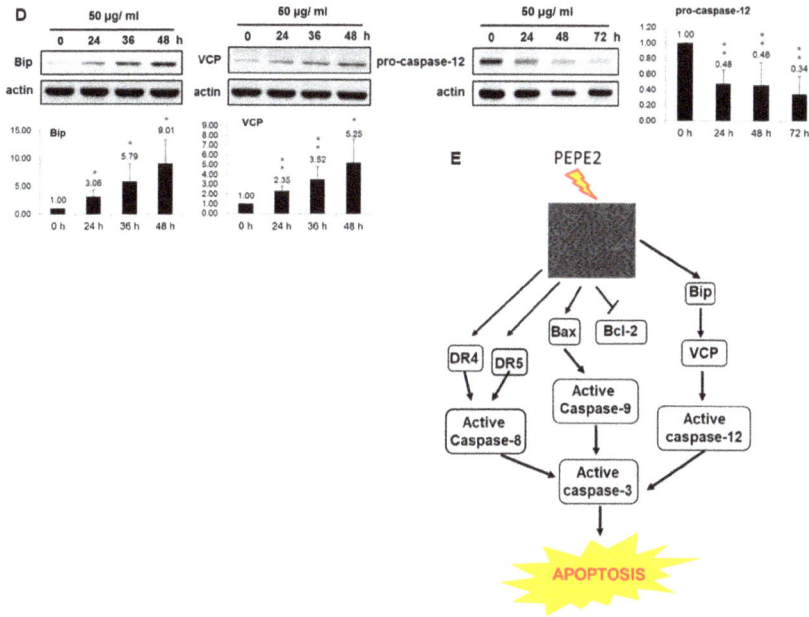

Figure 3. The molecular mechanisms of apoptotic pathway evoked in PEPE2-incubated UBUC cells. T24 and J82 cells were treated with 50 and 20 µg/mL PEPE2 respectively. Then the protein levels of (**A**) pro-/cleaved caspase-3; (**B**) pro-/cleaved caspase-8, DR4 and DR5; (**C**) pro-/cleaved caspase-9, Bax and Bcl-2 and (**D**) Bip, VCP and pro- caspase-12 in PEPE2-treated T24 cells were measured using western immunoblotting as described in the supporting information. The 0.1% (v/v) DMSO-treated UBUC cells were used as the solvent control; (**E**) The proposed molecular apoptotic pathway provoked in the PEPE2-treated UBUC cells. The immunoblot in each figure was the representative result of at least three independent experiments. The diagram (ratio (mean ± standard deviation (S.D.)) under each immunoblot indicated the ratio of the normalized protein intensity (observed protein/actin) of PEPE2-treated cells at the indicated time interval, divided by that at the 0-h time point. * $p \leq 0.05$, ** $p \leq 0.01$, *** $p \leq 0.001$.

3.4. The EtOAc Layer of PEP Could Reduce Xenografted Tumor growth in Nude Mice

In order to further confirm the UBUC-cell-line-associated inhibitory activity of pomegranate fruits, xenografted tumors induced by implanting T24 cells into nude mice as described in Materials and Methods were exploited to investigate the inhibitory effectiveness of the EtOAc layer of PEP on tumor growth in vivo. The results in Figure 4A demonstrated that the oral consumption of the EtOAc layer affected slightly the body weight of mice. The effects were more obvious in mice fed with 100 mg/kg EtOAc layer. As indicated in Figure 4B,C, the volume and weight of T24 tumors of the EtOAc layer-treated group (2, 5, 10, and 100 mg/kg) grew at a slower rate than those of the untreated tumors. On week 10, the tumor volumes of the control group had increased significantly to 600 mM^3 on average, which is the endpoint of the animal protocol, whereas the tumor volumes of 5 and 10 mg/kg of EtOAc layer-fed animals had only reached 200 mM^3 on average, respectively. The tumor weight of the control group increased to 456.5 mg on average while those of 5, 10, and 100 mg/kg EtOAc layer-fed mice decreased dramatically to 94.6, 94.9, and 39.4 mg, on average. The inhibitory effects on the tumor volume/weight were much higher than the body weight, suggesting that the decreased tumor volume/weight did not attribute to the body weight loss. Although EtOAc administration might impact the body weight, hematoxylin/eosin (H/E) staining of liver specimens showed that

EtOAc layer demonstrated no lesion to the liver. The H/E stainings of the liver specimens were presented in Supplementary Figure S4.

To observe the impacts of the EtOAc layer on the xenografted tumors, T24 xenografted tumors, treated with H_2O (vehicle), 2 mg/kg, 5 mg/kg, or 10 mg/kg of the EtOAc layer, were dissected from nude mice for histological examination. The hematoxylin/eosin (H/E) staining of H_2O-treated tumors revealed large neoplastic areas while the 5 and 10 mg/kg treated counterparts showed less neoplastic areas comparatively (Figure 4B). Furthermore, the TUNEL assay was performed to evaluate if apoptosis was induced in treated xenografted tumors. The results in Figure 4C demonstrated that the amount of TUNEL-positive T24 cells had increased obviously in tumors treated with the EtOAc layer (2, 5, 10, and 100 mg/kg) after 10 weeks as compared to that of the control groups, suggesting that the apoptosis was evoked in treated xenografted tumors. The above results indicated that the apoptosis could be induced in UBUC in vivo, which was in line with the findings observed in UBUC cells.

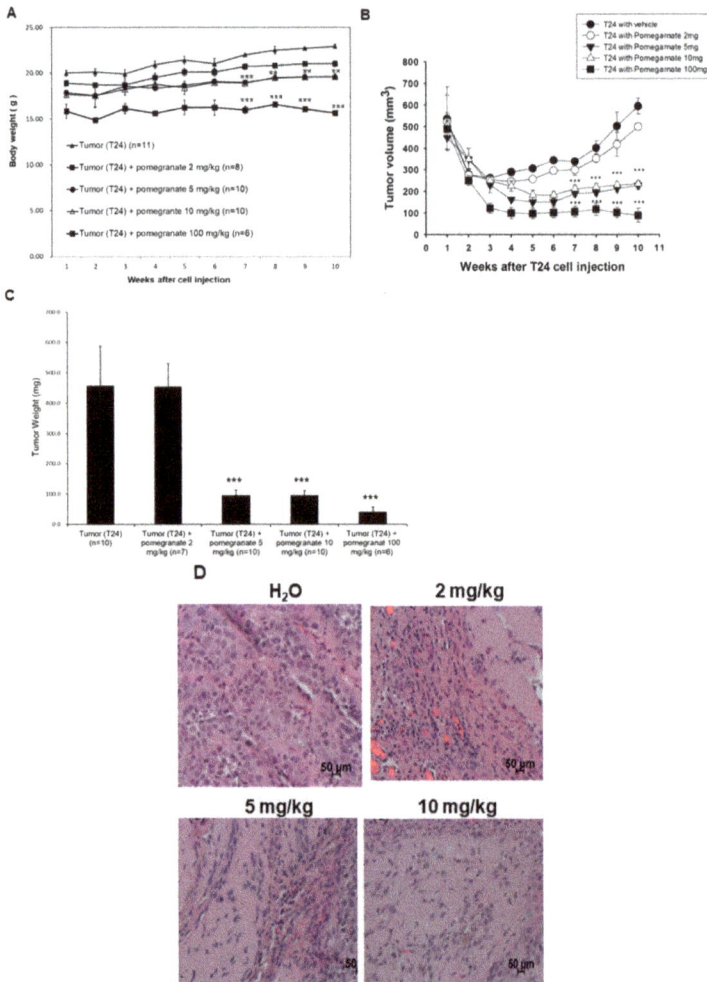

Figure 4. *Cont.*

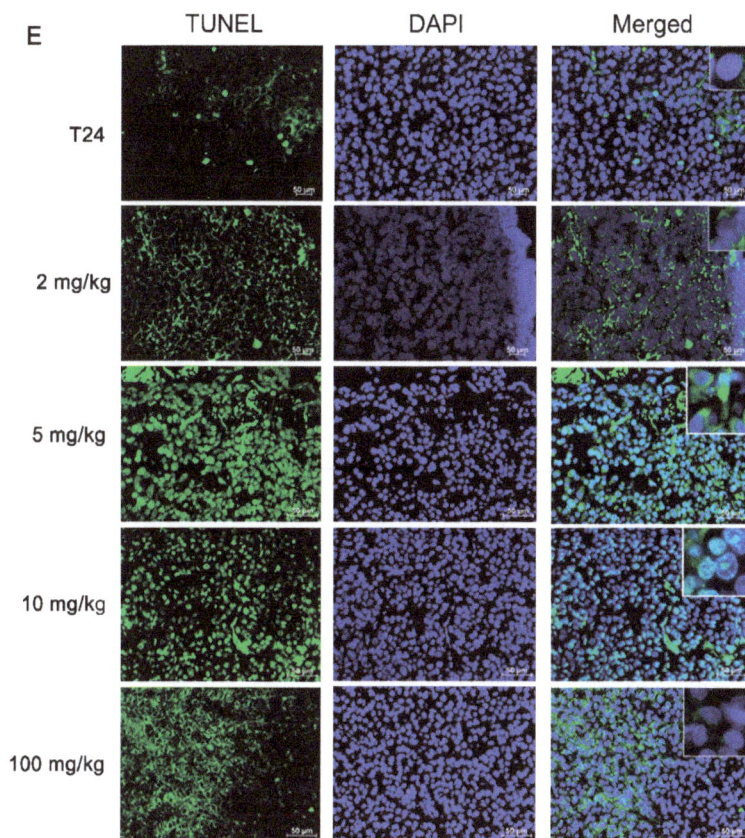

Figure 4. The inhibition of the xenografted UBUC growth in nude mice by the treatment of the EtOAc layer. T24 cells were injected s.c. into nude mice and were o.g. administrated with water (control), 2, 5, 10, or 100 mg/kg EtOAc layer as described in Materials and Methods. (**A**) The body weights of the extract-treated mice. *** $p < 0.001$, ** $p < 0.005$; (**B**) The effects of the EtOAc layer on tumor growth in the xenografted nude mice. The volumes of tumors from the extract-fed mice were compared to those of the water-fed mice. *** $p < 0.001$; (**C**) The tumor weight. The tumor weight was measured at the 10th week. *** $p < 0.001$; (**D**) The typical H/E images (400×) of tumor specimens dissected from xenografted nude mice; (**E**) The representative terminal deoxynucleotidyl transferase-mediated deoxyuridine triphosphate nick end-labeling (TUNEL) images (400×) of tumor lesions from xenografted nude mice. H&E and TUNEL assays were performed as described in Material and Methods.

4. Discussion

In this study, we found that the ethanol extract isolated from pomegranate peels exhibited a better inhibitory activity comparatively T24 and J82 cells than that of pulps. Fractionation of PEP with increasing polarity showed that the EtOAc layer of PEP had the best anti-cancer efficacy. Among 8 collecting parts of PEP fractionated with the Diaion HP-20 column chromatography, the PEPE2 fraction demonstrated the best inhibitory activity on UBUC cells along with the least influence on normal-like urothelial E7 cells. Annexin V/PI and western immunoblotting analyses demonstrated that PEPE2 treatment evoked UBUC cell apoptosis through stimulation of the death receptor pathway, the mitochondrial pathway, and ER stress. The suggested apoptotic pathway evoked by PEPE2 was shown in Figure 3E. The mitochondrial pathway starts with the increased permeabilization of the mitochondrial outer membrane, causing the rupturing of the outer membrane. The outer membrane rupturing the release of cytochrome c, apoptosis-inducing factor (AIF), endonuclease g, and Smac/DIABLO (second mitochondria-derived activator of caspases/direct IAP-associated binding protein with low pI) [16–18]. Cytochrome c along with apoptosis protease activating factor (APAF-1) and pro-caspase 9 form an apoptosome which activates caspase 9. Caspase 9, in turn, activates the effector caspases which orchestrates the progression of apoptosis [19]. AIF and endonuclease g participate in DNA fragmentation and subsequent chromosomal condensation, which is typical phenomena of apoptosis [17,18]. Smac/DIABLO can antagonize IAP (inhibitor of apoptosis protein) to promote caspase activation [20]. In addition to our proposed apoptotic mechanism, pomegranate peels might impair the release of cytochrome c, apoptosis-inducing factor (AIF), endonuclease g and Smac/DIABLO to interfere with the activation effector caspases. Taken together, our results implied that the components present in pomegranate peels demonstrated the inhibitory activity against UBUC cells and owned much better intervention capability than those of the pulps. The anti-cancer efficacy of PEP was further confirmed in the xenografted mice. It was observed that oral administration of the EtOAc layer of PEP to nude mice implanted with T24 cells caused a significant reduction in tumor growth. Besides, the TUNEL-positive cells were extensively observed in EtOAc layer-treated T24 tumors, suggesting cell apoptosis was evoked in extract-treated tumors.

Most of the chemopreventive/chemotherapeutic cancer studies of pomegranate fruits focus on the juice or various extracts prepared from the juice [1]. Very few documented findings emphasize the medicinal value of the pomegranate peels. The studies carried out by Zahin et al. (2014) showed that A549 and H1299 lung cancer cell lines demonstrate the comparable susceptibility to punicalagin and ellagic acid, the main ingredients of pomegranate peels [21]. In addition, treatment of the methanol extract of pomegranate pericarps (PME) results in the significant dose-responsive inhibition on cell proliferation in MCF7 cell lines that are positive for estrogen receptors (ER) while showing no impacts on that of ER^- MDAMB-231 cells. PME also reduces the expression of estrogen-responsive genes such as ERα, pS2, and PR in MCF7 cells. Examination on the PME estrogenicity indicated that there are no obvious differences in the uterus weight and the proliferation of uterine endometrium between PME- and vehicle-treated 17 β-estradiol-evoked ovariectomized mice, implying that PME is a selective estrogen receptor modulator [22]. Consistent with the above findings, Dikmen et al. (2011) also observed that the administration of pomegranate fruit peels (PPE) inhibits MCF7 cell proliferation and induces cancer cell apoptosis [23].

In addition to the above cancer cells, Asmaa et al. (2015) reported that the treatment of 80% ethanol extract of pomegranate peels (PGPE) mainly evokes g_2/M cell cycle arrest to inhibit chronic myeloid leukemia K562 cells [24]. The compounds present in pomegranate peels possess inhibitory activities against prostate cancer. The effects of pomegranate peel extract (PoPx) on prostate cancer cell lines examined by Deng et al. (2017) demonstrated that PoPx incubation can induce apoptosis by the loss of mitochondrial transmembrane potential (Δym), the increased reactive oxygen species (ROS) as well as the augmented Bax/Bcl-2. Furthermore, they reported that PoPx treatment can retard migration/invasion likely through the down-regulation of matrix metallopeptidase (MMP) 2/MMP9 and the up-regulation of Metallopeptidase Inhibitor 2 (TIMP2) [25]. gou et al. (2016) indicated that ellagic acid purified from pomegranate peels provokes Hela cell apoptosis by increasing the IGFBP7 expression level [26]. Song et al. (2016) found that treatment of polyphenol of pomegranate peels can induce HepG2 cells apoptosis by increasing cytochrome c amount, p53 expression level, Bax/Bcl-2 and caspase-3/9 activities. It can also arrest HepG2 cell at S-phase [27]. Most of the above-mentioned literature with regard to pomegranate peels focuses on the investigations of single cancer cell line. However, in this study, two cancer cell lines and animal studies were implemented for examination.

Besides anti-cancer activities, the pomegranate peel is demonstrated to have activities for other ailments. Due to its abundant phenolics and flavonoids, the pomegranate peel is indicated to possess high anti-oxidant activities [28]. Morzelle et al. demonstrated that the administration of pomegranate

Nutrients **2018**, *10*, 543

peel extract (PPE) decreases amyloid plaque density, augments the expression of neurotrophin BDNF, and reduces TNF-α production in mice infused with amyloid-β peptide. Their results imply that treatment of PPE provides neuroprotective effectiveness to the neurodegeneration provoked by infusion with amyloid-β peptide in mice [29]. PPE is also shown to alleviate the hepatic pathology, body weight, liver enzymes, and retard lipogenesis. It can enhance the cellular redox status in the liver tissues of rats with a non-alcoholic fatty liver disease to reduce oxidative damage [30]. Pomegranate peel extract is also showed to reduce significantly fasting blood glucose in type 2 diabetic mice, suggesting that it might be recommended for the management of type 2 diabetes [31]. Although a variety of studies related to the therapeutic effects of pomegranate peel have been reported, there are no clinical trial results.

Most of the UBUCs are papillary/non-invasive, or papillary/superficially invasive lesions. The lesions are normally treated by curettage but the local recurrence is often observed in papillary UBUCs, even followed by lethal distal spreading. The results of our studies implicated that the pomegranate peel extract may be a potential chemopreventive product for lowering the possibility of UBUC recurrence. Pomegranate peels cover the whole fruits and are handy to be separated from the fruit bodies, thus, it is easier to obtain than pulps. Furthermore, our results provide the likelihood that the traditionally non-edible pomegranate peel waste is re-utilized to make an affordable and promising chemopreventive product.

Supplementary Materials: The following are available online at http://www.mdpi.com/2072-6643/10/5/543/s1. Supplementary document: legends for supplementary figure, Figure S1: The inhibitory activities of peel and pulp of pomegranate fruit. T24 (**A**) or J82 (**B**) cells were used to examine the inhibitory activities. PEP2 and PEP3 fractions from the EtOAc layer were examined for the toxicity to normal-like E7 cells (**C**), Figure S2: The HPLC profiles of EtOAc layer of PEP and PEPE2. (**A**) The HPLC profile of EtOAc layer of PEP. (**B**) The profile of PEPE2, Figure S3: The molecular mechanisms of apoptotic pathway evoked in PEPE2-incubated UBUC J82 cells. (**A**) pro-/cleaved caspase-8, DR4 and DR5, (**B**) pro-/cleaved caspase-9, Bax and Bcl-2, (**C**) Bip, VCP and pro-caspase-12 in PEPE2-incubated J82 cells. The immunoblot in each figure was the representative result of at least three independent experiments. The diagram (ratio (mean $\pm$ SD)) under each immunoblot indicated the ratio of normalized protein intensity (observed protein/actin) of PEPE2-treated cells at indicated time interval divided by that at 0-h time point. * $p \leq 0.05$, ** $p \leq 0.01$, *** $p \leq 0.001$, Figure S4: liver specimens collected at 10th week from non-fed- and EtOAc layer-fed xenografted mice.

Author Contributions: C.-P.C. designed the xenografted animal studies and performed the TUNEL assay. Y.-Y.C. carried out all the preparation of various extracts, C.-F.L. conducted TUNEL assay and evaluated the results, L.-H.C. performed MTT assay and apoptotic pathway studies. S.-T.L. performed apoptotic pathway studies. T.-F.W. managed and design the whole study and performed the apoptotic pathway studies.

Acknowledgments: The authors would like to thank the ministry of Science and Technology of Taiwan to provide the grants MOST 105-2320-B-218-001-MY3 and MOST 101-2632-B-218-001-MY3 to support this research.

Conflicts of Interest: The authors declare no conflict of interest.

References

1. Siegel, R.L.; Miller, K.D.; Jemal, A. Cancer Statistics, 2017. *CA Cancer J. Clin.* **2017**, *6*, 7–30. [CrossRef] [PubMed]

2. Health Promotion Administration, Ministry of Health and Welfare, Taiwan, Cancer Registry Annual Report. 2014. Available online: https://www.hpa.gov.tw/File/Attach/7330/File_6792.pdf (accessed on 13 March 2018).

3. Zieger, K.; Wolf, H.; Olsen, P.-R.; Hojgaard, K. Long-term follow-up of noninvasive bladder tumours (stage Ta): Recurrence and progression. *BJU Int.* **2000**, *85*, 824–828. [CrossRef] [PubMed]

4. Sharma, P.; McClees, S.F.; Afaq, F. Pomegranate for prevention and treatment of Cancer: An update. *Molecules* **2017**, *22*, 177. [CrossRef] [PubMed]

5. Khan, N.; Hadi, N.; Afaq, F.; Syed, D.-N.; Kweon, M.H.; Mukhtar, H. Pomegranate fruit extract inhibits prosurvival pathways in human A549 lung carcinoma cells and tumor growth in athymic nude mice. *Carcinogenesis* **2007**, *28*, 163–173. [CrossRef] [PubMed]

6. Khan, N.; Afaq, F.; Kweon, M.H.; Kim, K.; Mukhtar, H. Oral consumption of pomegranate fruit extract inhibits growth and progression of primary lung tumors in mice. *Cancer Res.* **2007**, *67*, 3475–3482. [CrossRef] [PubMed]

7. Malik, A.; Afaq, F.; Sarfaraz, S.; Adhami, V.M.; Syed, D.N.; Mukhtar, H. Pomegranate fruit juice for chemoprevention and chemotherapy of prostate cancer. *Proc. Natl. Acad. Sci. USA* **2005**, *102*, 14813–14818. [CrossRef] [PubMed]

8. Adhami, V.M.; Siddiqui, I.A.; Syed, D.N.; Lall, R.K.; Mukhtar, H. Oral infusion of pomegranate fruit extract inhibits prostate carcinogenesis in the TRAMP model. *Carcinogenesis* **2012**, *33*, 644–651. [CrossRef] [PubMed]

9. Rettig, M.B.; Heber, D.; An, J.; Seeram, N.P.; Rao, J.Y.; Liu, H.; Klatte, T.; Belldegrun, A.; Moro, A.; Henning, S.M.; et al. Pomegranate extract inhibits androgen-independent prostate cancer growth through a nuclear factor-kappa B-dependent mechanism. *Mol. Cancer Ther.* **2008**, *7*, 2662–2671. [CrossRef] [PubMed]

10. Pantuck, A.J.; Leppert, J.T.; Zomorodian, N.; Aronson, W.; Hong, J.; Barnard, R.J.; Seeram, N.; Liker, H.; Wang, H.; Elashoff, R.; et al. Phase II study of pomegranate juice for men with rising prostate-specific antigen following surgery or radiation for prostate cancer. *Clin. Cancer Res.* **2006**, *12*, 4018–4026. [CrossRef] [PubMed]

11. Pantuck, A.J.; Pettaway, C.A.; Dreicer, R.; Corman, J.; Katz, A.; Ho, A.; Aronson, W.; Clark, W.; Simmons, G.; Heber, D. A randomized, double-blind, placebo-controlled study of the effects of pomegranate extract on rising PSA levels in men following primary therapy for prostate cancer. *Prostate Cancer Prostatic Dis.* **2015**, *18*, 242–248. [CrossRef] [PubMed]

12. Lee, S.T.; Wu, Y.L.; Chien, L.H.; Chen, S.T.; Tzeng, Y.K.; Wu, T.F. Proteomic exploration of the impacts of pomegranate fruit juice on the global gene expression of prostate cancer cell. *Proteomics* **2012**, *12*, 3251–3262. [CrossRef] [PubMed]

13. Chen, S.H.; Wang, Y.W.; Hsu, J.L.; Chang, H.Y.; Wang, C.Y.; Shen, P.T.; Chiang, C.W.; Chuang, J.J.; Tsai, H.W.; Gu, P.W.; et al. Nucleophosmin in the pathogenesis of arsenic-related bladder carcinogenesis revealed by quantitative proteomics. *Toxicol. Appl. Pharmacol.* **2010**, *242*, 126–135. [CrossRef] [PubMed]

14. Naito, S.; von Eschenbach, A.C.; giavazzi, r.; Fidler, I.J. growth and metastasis of tumor cells isolated from a human renal cell carcinoma implanted into different organs of nude mice. *Cancer Res.* **1986**, *46*, 4109–4115. [PubMed]

15. Kurokawa, M.; Kornbluth, S. Caspases and kinases in a death grip. *Cell* **2009**, *138*, 838–854. [CrossRef] [PubMed]

16. Yang, J.C.; Cortopassi, G.A. Induction of the mitochondrial permeability transition causes release of the apoptogenic factor cytochrome c. *Free Radic. Biol. Med.* **1998**, *24*, 624–631. [CrossRef]

17. Li, L.Y.; Luo, X.; Wang, X. Endonuclease g is an apoptotic DNase when released from mitochondria. *Nature* **2001**, *412*, 95–99. [CrossRef] [PubMed]

18. Susin, S.A.; Lorenzo, H.K.; Zamzami, N.; Marzo, I.; Snow, B.E.; Brothers, G.M.; Mangion, J.; Jacotot, E.; Costantini, P.; Loeffler, M.; et al. Molecular characterisation of mitochondrial apoptosis-inducing factor. *Nature* **1999**, *397*, 441–446. [CrossRef] [PubMed]

19. Zou, H.; Yuchen, L.; Xuesing, L.; Wang, X. An APAF-1-cytochrome c multimeric complex is a functional apoptosome that activates procaspase 9. *J. Biol. Chem.* **1999**, *274*, 11549–11556. [CrossRef] [PubMed]

20. Du, C.; Fang, M.; Li, Y.; Li, L.; Wang, X. Smac, a mitochondrial protein that promotes cytochrome c-dependent caspase activation by eliminating IAP inhibition. *Cell* **2000**, *102*, 33–42. [CrossRef]

21. Zahin, M.; Ahmad, I.; gupta, R.C.; Aqil, F. Punicalagin and ellagic acid demonstrate antimutagenic activity and inhibition of benzo[a]pyrene induced DNA adducts. *BioMed Res. Int.* **2014**, *2014*, 467465. [CrossRef] [PubMed]

22. Sreeja, S.; Santhosh Kumar, T.R.; Lakshmi, B.S.; Sreeja, S. Pomegranate extract demonstrates a selective estrogen receptor modulator profile in human tumor cell lines and in vivo models of estrogen deprivation. *J. Nutr. Biochem.* **2012**, *23*, 725–732. [CrossRef] [PubMed]

23. Dikmen, M.; Ozturk, N.; Ozturk, Y. The antioxidant potency of *Punica granatum* L. fruit peel reduces cell proliferation and induces apoptosis on breast cancer. *J. Med. Food* **2011**, *14*, 1638–1646. [CrossRef] [PubMed]

24. Asmaa, M.J.; Ali, A.J.; Farid, J.M.; Azman, S. growth inhibitory effects of crude pomegranate peel extract on chronic myeloid leukemia, K562 cells. *Int. J. Appl. Basic Med. Res.* **2015**, *5*, 100–105. [CrossRef] [PubMed]

Nutrients **2018**, *10*, 543

25. Deng, Y.; Li, Y.; Yang, F.; Zeng, A.; Yang, S.; Luo, Y.; Zhang, Y.; Xie, Y.; Ye, T.; Xia, Y.; et al. The extract from *Punica granatum* (pomegranate) peel induces apoptosis and impairs metastasis in prostate cancer cells. *Biomed. Pharmacother.* **2017**, *93*, 976–984. [CrossRef] [PubMed]

26. Guo, H.; Zhang, D.; Fu, Q. Inhibition of cervical cancer by promoting IGFBP7 expression using ellagic acid from pomegranate peel. *Med. Sci. Monit.* **2016**, *22*, 4881–4886. [CrossRef] [PubMed]

27. Song, B.; Li, J.; Li, J. Pomegranate peel extract polyphenols induced apoptosis in human hepatoma cells by mitochondrial pathway. *Food Chem. Toxicol.* **2016**, *93*, 158–166. [CrossRef] [PubMed]

28. Derakhshan, Z.; Ferrante, M.; Tadi, M.; Ansari, F.; Heydari, A.; Hosseini, M.S.; Conti, G.O.; Sadrabad, E.K. Antioxidant activity and total phenolic content of ethanolic extract of pomegranate peels, juice and seeds. *Food Chem. Toxicol.* **2018**, *114*, 108–111. [CrossRef] [PubMed]

29. Morzelle, M.C.; Salgado, J.M.; Telles, M.; Mourelle, D.; Bachiega, P.; Buck, H.S.; Viel, TA. Neuroprotective Effects of Pomegranate Peel Extract after Chronic Infusion with Amyloid-β Peptide in Mice. *PLoS ONE* **2016**, *11*, e0166123. [CrossRef] [PubMed]

30. Al-Shaaibi, S.N.; Waly, M.I.; Al-Subhi, L.; Tageldin, M.H.; Al-Balushi, N.M.; Rahman, M.S. Ameliorative Effects of Pomegranate Peel Extract against Dietary-Induced Nonalcoholic Fatty Liver in Rats. *Prev. Nutr. Food Sci.* **2016**, *21*, 14–23. [CrossRef] [PubMed]

31. Banihani, S.; Swedan, S.; Alguraan, Z. Pomegranate and type 2 diabetes. *Nutr. Res.* **2013**, *33*, 341–348. [CrossRef] [PubMed]

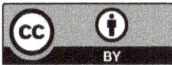

![nutrients logo] *nutrients*

MDPI

Article

Frondoside A Enhances the Anti-Cancer Effects of Oxaliplatin and 5-Fluorouracil on Colon Cancer Cells

Samir Attoub [1,2,*], **Kholoud Arafat** [1], **Tamam Khalaf** [1], **Shahrazad Sulaiman** [1] and **Rabah Iratni** [3]

1 Department of Pharmacology & Therapeutics, College of Medicine & Health Sciences, United Arab Emirates University, Al-Ain P.O. Box 17666, UAE; kholoud.arafat@uaeu.ac.ae (K.A.); tamam.es.khalaf@gmail.com (T.K.); sharazadjeffy@uaeu.ac.ae (S.S.)
2 Institut National de la Santé et de la Recherche Médicale (INSERM), 75571 Paris Cedex 12, France
3 Department of Biology, College of Science, United Arab Emirates University, Al-Ain P.O. Box 15551, UAE; R_iratni@uaeu.ac.ae
* Correspondence: samir.attoub@uaeu.ac.ae; Tel.: +971-371-37219

Received: 28 February 2018; Accepted: 27 April 2018; Published: 1 May 2018

Abstract: Over recent years, we have demonstrated that Frondoside A, a triterpenoid glycoside isolated from an Atlantic sea cucumber, has potent in vitro and in vivo anti-cancer effects against human pancreatic, breast, and lung cancer. We have also demonstrated that Frondoside A is able to potentiate and/or synergize the anti-cancer effects of major classical cytotoxic agents, namely, gemcitabine, paclitaxel, and cisplatin, in the treatment of pancreatic, breast, and lung cancer, respectively. This study evaluates the impact of Frondoside A alone and in combination with the standard cytotoxic drugs oxaliplatin and 5-fluorouracil (5-FU) in the treatment of colon cancer using three human colon cancer cell lines, namely, HT-29, HCT-116, and HCT8/S11. We demonstrate that Frondoside A, oxaliplatin, and 5-FU cause a concentration- and time-dependent reduction in the number of HT-29 colon cancer cells. A concentration of 2.5 µM of Frondoside A led to almost 100% inhibition of cell numbers at 72 h. A similar effect was only observed with a much higher concentration (100 µM) of oxaliplatin or 5-FU. The reduction in cell numbers by Frondoside A, oxaliplatin, and 5-FU was also confirmed in two other colon cancer cell lines, namely, HCT8/S11 and HCT-116, treated for 48 h. The combinations of low concentrations of these drugs for 48 h in vitro clearly demonstrated that Frondoside A enhances the inhibition of cell numbers induced by oxaliplatin or 5-FU. Similarly, such a combination also efficiently inhibited colony growth in vitro. Interestingly, we found that the inhibition of ERK1/2 phosphorylation was significantly enhanced when Frondoside A was used in combination treatments. Moreover, we show that Frondoside A and 5-FU, when used alone, induce a concentration-dependent induction of apoptosis and that their pro-apoptotic effect is dramatically enhanced when used in combination. We further demonstrate that apoptosis induction upon the treatment of colon cancer cells was at least in part a result of the inhibition of phosphorylation of the survival kinase AKT, leading to caspase-3 activation, poly (ADP-ribose) polymerase (PARP) inactivation, and consequently DNA damage, as suggested by the increase in the level of γH2AX. In light of these findings, we strongly suggest that Frondoside A may have a role in colon cancer therapy when used in combination with the standard cytotoxic drugs oxaliplatin and 5-FU.

Keywords: colon cancer; Frondoside A; oxaliplatin; 5-fluorouracil; cell proliferation; apoptosis

1. Introduction

Colorectal cancer is the third leading cause of cancer death in the world and represents a serious threat to human health [1]. Without treatment, patients with inoperable or metastatic colorectal cancer have a median life expectancy of about 8 months. The standard cytotoxic drugs for the treatment of metastatic colorectal cancer are 5-fluorouracil (5-FU) (combined with folinic acid), oxaliplatin, and irinotecan. These chemotherapeutic agents currently in use for colon cancer remain unsatisfactory because of their associated collateral toxicity and resistance. In the last decade, the survival rate of patients with metastatic colorectal cancer has improved with the application of targeted drugs such as Bevacizumab. Despite these advances, patients still die, and a cure remains elusive [2].

Patients, oncologists, and scientists have for decades expressed interest in using natural compound remedies because of the overall disappointing results and side effects of the current cytotoxic drugs and targeted therapies. Recent studies have demonstrated that low concentrations of Frondoside A, a triterpenoid glycoside isolated from the Atlantic cucumber *Cucumaria frondosa*, induces apoptosis in human pancreatic, leukemic, breast, lung, and prostate cancer cells, leading to the inhibition of their tumor xenograft growth in vivo [3–7]. Investigators have also demonstrated that Frondoside A was able to synergize or to potentiate the anti-cancer effects of major classical cytotoxic agents, namely, gemcitabine, paclitaxel, and cisplatin, in the treatment of pancreatic [8], breast [5], and lung [6] cancer xenografts, respectively.

We know from clinical trials that single-agent treatments rarely result in clinical benefits to cancer patients and that combination therapy is necessary for the effective treatment of tumors. This study investigates the potential anti-cancer effects of Frondoside A alone and in combination with the standard cytotoxic drugs oxaliplatin and 5-FU (FOLFOX protocol) in the treatment of colon cancer.

2. Materials and Methods

2.1. Cell Culture and Reagents

The human colon cancer cell lines HT-29, HCT-116, and HCT8/S11 were maintained in DMEM (Hyclone, Cramlington, UK) supplemented with antibiotics (penicillin: 50 U/mL; streptomycin: 50 μg/mL) (Hyclone, Cramlington, UK) and with 10% fetal bovine serum (FBS; Biowest, Nouaille, France). In all experiments, the cell viability was higher than 99% using trypan blue dye exclusion. Frondoside A, oxaliplatin, and 5-FU were purchased from Sigma-Aldrich (Sigma-Aldrich, Saint Louis, MO, USA). Antibodies to phospho-AKT, phospho-p44/42 MAPK (ERK1/2), cleaved caspase-3 (Asp175), and cleaved poly (ADP-ribose) polymerase (PARP) were obtained from Cell Signaling Technology (Cell Signaling, Beverly, MA, USA). The AKT antibody was obtained from Abcam (Abcam, Cambridge, UK). The antibody to phospho-histone H2AX was obtained from Millipore (Millipore, Hayward, CA, USA). Antibodies to ERK2 and β-actin were obtained from Santa Cruz Biotechnology, Inc. (Santa Cruz, CA, USA).

2.2. Impact of Frondoside A, Oxaliplatin, 5-Fluorouracil, and Their Combinations on Colon Cancer Cell Numbers

Cells were seeded at a density of 50,000 cells per well into 6-well plates. After 24 h, the cells were treated for another 24, 48, and 72 h with increasing concentrations of Frondoside A (0.1–5 μM), oxaliplatin (1–100 μM), or 5-FU (1–100 μM) in triplicate. Control cultures were treated with 0.1% DMSO (the drug vehicle). In the second set of experiments, cells were treated with a combination of Frondoside A and oxaliplatin or Frondoside A and 5-FU. The effects of these combinations on the cell numbers were determined at the indicated times using the Scepter 2.0 Handheld Automated Cell Counter (Millipore, Hayward, CA, USA). Data were presented as the proportional cell numbers (%) by comparing the drug-treated cells with the DMSO-treated cells, the cell numbers of which were assumed to be 100%.

2.3. Impact of the Treatments on Colony Growth in Matrigel Matrix

A layer of 150 μL of matrigel was poured into the wells of a 24-well cell culture dish and allowed to set at 37 °C for 30 min. A second layer (300 μL) composed of 150 μL of matrigel dissolved in 150 μL of growth media containing 1.5×10^3 cells was placed on top of the first layer and allowed to set in the humidified incubator at 37 °C for 30 min. Growth medium (0.5 mL) was added on top of the second layer, and the cells were incubated in a humidified incubator at 37 °C for 14 days and then treated for another 7 days with Frondoside A, oxaliplatin, 5-FU, or the combinations. Control cells were exposed to 0.1% DMSO. The medium was changed twice a week. At the end of the experiment, colonies were stained for 1 h with 2% Giemsa stain and incubated with PBS overnight to remove excess Giemsa stain. The colonies were photographed and scored, and the percentages of colonies larger than 100 μm were determined. Data presented compare the drug-treated colonies with the DMSO-treated colonies. Colonies larger than 100 μm were expressed as a percentage of the total counted colonies and were then compared to the DMSO-treated controls.

2.4. Quantification of Apoptosis by Annexin V Labeling

Apoptosis was examined using the Annexin V Dead Cell kit (Millipore, Hayward, CA, USA) according to the manufacturer's instructions. Briefly, HT-29 cells were treated with or without each compound individually or in combination for 48 h. Detached and adherent cells were collected and incubated with Annexin V and 7-AAD, a dead cell marker, for 20 min at room temperature in the dark. The early and late apoptotic cells were counted with the Muse Cell Analyzer (Millipore, Hayward, CA, USA). Experiments were carried out in triplicate and were repeated three times.

2.5. Impact of Frondoside A, Oxaliplatin, 5-Fluorouracil, and Their Combinations on Pro-Apoptotic and Anti-Proliferation Proteins' Expression and Phosphorylation Levels

Cells were seeded in 100 mm dishes at 2×10^6 cells per dish for 24 h and were then treated with Frondoside A (0.5 μM), oxaliplatin (10 μM), 5-FU (10 μM), a combination of Frondoside A and oxaliplatin, or Frondoside A and 5-FU, for another 24 h. Control cultures were treated with 0.1% DMSO (the drug vehicle). In a second set of experiments, cells were treated with increasing concentrations of Frondoside A (0.5–2.5 μM) for 2 h. Total cellular proteins were isolated using a RIPA buffer (25 mM Tris.HCl, pH 7.6; 1% Nonidet P-40; 1% sodium deoxycholate; 0.1% SDS; 0.5% protease inhibitor cocktail; 1% PMSF; 1% phosphatase inhibitor cocktail) from the DMSO- and drug-treated cells. The whole cell lysates were recovered by centrifugation at 14,000 rpm for 20 min at 4 °C to remove insoluble material, and the protein concentrations of the lysates were determined using a BCA protein assay kit (Thermo Fisher Scientific, Waltham, MA, USA). Proteins (30 μg) were separated by SDS-PAGE gel to determine the expression and the phosphorylation levels of different pro-apoptotic and anti-proliferation proteins (AKT, p-AKT, activated caspase-3, cleaved PARP, p-H2AX, ERK-2, p-ERK, and β-actin). After electrophoresis, the proteins were transferred onto a nitrocellulose membrane, blocked for 1 h at room temperature with 5% non-fat milk in TBST (TBS and 0.05% Tween 20), and then probed with specific primary antibodies and β-actin (1:1000) overnight at 4 °C. The blots were washed, exposed to secondary antibodies, and visualized using the ECL system (Thermo Fisher Scientific, Waltham, MA, USA). Membrane stripping was performed by incubating the membrane in Restore Western blot stripping buffer (Thermo Fisher Scientific, Waltham, MA, USA) according to the manufacturer's instructions. Densitometry analysis was performed using an HP Deskjet F4180 Scanner (HP Development Company, Palo Alto, CA, USA) with ImageJ software.

2.6. Statistics

Results are expressed as means $\pm$ S.E.M. of the indicated data. The difference between the experimental and control values was assessed by ANOVA followed by Dunnett's post hoc multiple comparison test (*** $p < 0.001$, ** $p < 0.01$, and * $p < 0.05$ indicate a significant difference).

3. Results and Discussion

3.1. Effect of Frondoside A, Oxaliplatin and 5-Fluorouracil on Cell Numbers

As shown in Figure 1, Frondoside A (0.1–5 μM), oxaliplatin (1–100 μM), and 5-FU (1–100 μM) caused a concentration- and time-dependent decrease in HT-29 cell numbers over 24, 48, and 72 h (Figure 1A–C). The concentration-dependent effects of Frondoside A, oxaliplatin, and 5-FU were also confirmed on two other colon cancer cell lines, namely, HCT-116 and HCT8/S11 (Figure 1D–F). At 48 h, the IC_{50} concentration of Frondoside A was 0.5 μM in HT-29 cells and approximately 0.75 μM in both HCT-116 and HCT8/S11 cells (Table 1). On the other hand, the IC_{50} concentrations of oxaliplatin and 5-FU were found to be much higher than for Frondoside A (Table 1). Because previous work has reported the anti-tumor activity of oxaliplatin and 5-FU in HT-29 colon cancer cells [9], we therefore decided to pursue the rest of this study on HT-29 cells.

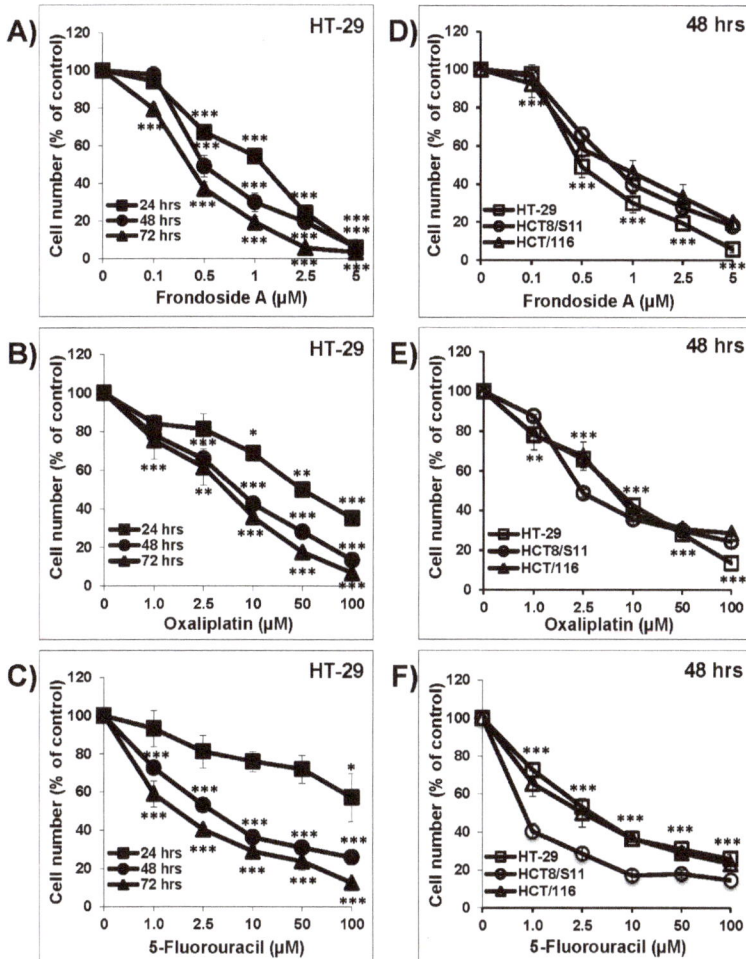

Figure 1. Frondoside A inhibition of colon cancer cell numbers compared to oxaliplatin and 5-fluorouracil. Exponentially growing HT-29 cells were treated with vehicle (0.1% DMSO) and the indicated concentrations of Frondoside A (**A**), oxaliplatin (**B**), and 5-fluorouracil (**C**) for 24 to 72 h. The effects of the three drugs were confirmed at 48 h in two additional colon cancer cell lines, namely, HCT8/S11 and HCT-116 (**D–F**). Cell count was determined as described in Materials and Methods. All experiments were repeated at least three times. Shapes represent means; bars represent S.E.M. * Significantly different at $p < 0.05$. ** Significantly different at $p < 0.01$. *** Significantly different at $p < 0.001$.

Table 1. IC_{50} (µM) of Frondoside A compared to oxaliplatin and 5-fluorouracil at 48 h of treatment.

	IC_{50} (µM)		
	Frondoside A	**Oxaliplatin**	**5-Fluorouracil**
HT-29	0.5	5	2.6
HCT-116	0.75	5	2.5
HCT8/S11	0.75	2.5	0.9

3.2. Frondoside A Enhanced the Anti-Tumor Activity of Oxaliplatin and 5-Fluorouracil on HT-29 in Cell Count and Colony Growth Assays

The treatment of HT-29 cells for 48 h using the IC_{50} concentration of Frondoside A (0.5 µM) significantly enhanced the growth inhibitory effects of increasing concentrations of oxaliplatin (1–10 µM) (Figure 2A) and 5-FU (0.5–2.5 µM) (Figure 2B). We next examined the impact of these combinations on the growth of already formed HT-29 colonies. First, HT-29 cells were allowed to grow and form visible colonies in the absence of any treatment. After two weeks of growth, the colonies were treated for one more week with DMSO as the control, Frondoside A (0.5 µM), oxaliplatin (10 µM), 5-FU (10 µM), or a combination. Although the number of colonies obtained in each treatment seemed unchanged, we noticed, however, that the sizes of the colonies were significantly reduced. Indeed, while large colonies represented approximately 70% of the total number of colonies in the control, they represented only 25% and 35% of the total number of colonies exposed to both oxaliplatin (Figure 3A) and 5-FU (Figure 3B) alone. Although Frondoside A did not lead to significant colony growth inhibition when compared to oxaliplatin or 5-FU alone, when used in combination, Frondoside A significantly enhanced the inhibition of colony growth mediated by oxaliplatin (Figure 3A) or 5-FU (Figure 3B). We speculate that the effect of these drugs alone and in combination on the size of the colony growth may be due to cell death and/or inhibition of cellular proliferation.

It is well documented that the MAPK signaling pathway is mainly involved in regulating cellular proliferation and that a blockade of this pathway suppresses the growth of colon tumors [10]. ERK1 and ERK2, the final effectors of the MAPK pathway, activated through phosphorylation, lead to the activation of a variety of substrates responsible for the induction of cell proliferation. Hence, we decided to investigate the activation of ERK1/2 in response to Frondoside A alone and in combination with oxaliplatin and 5-FU. Interestingly, although we observed a marked inhibition of ERK1/2 phosphorylation with single treatments, a combination of the drugs enhanced this inhibition (Figure 3C,D).

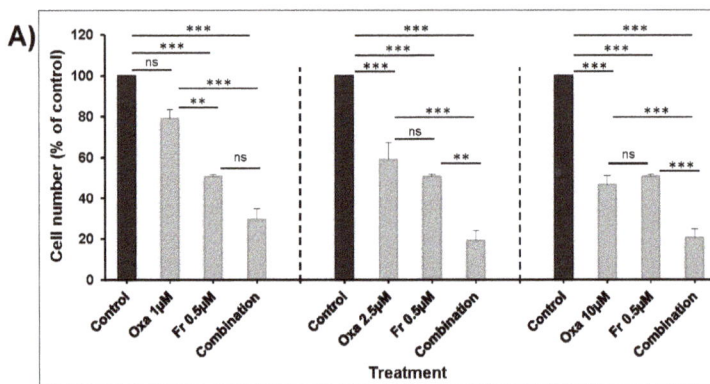

Figure 2. *Cont.*

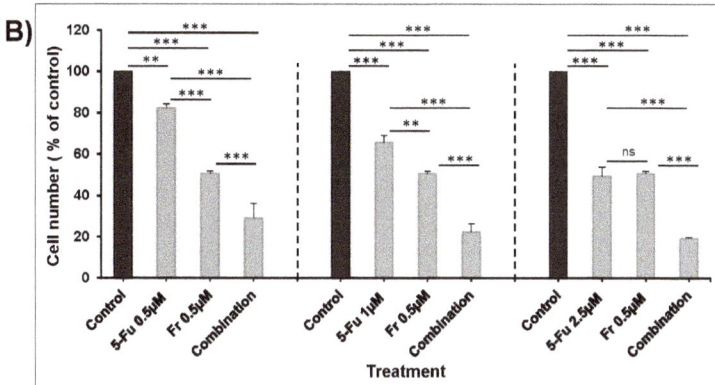

Figure 2. Frondoside A enhances the inhibition of HT-29 cell numbers by (**A**) oxaliplatin (1–10 µM), and (**B**) 5-fluorouracil (0.5–2.5 µM). Cells were treated for 48 h, and all experiments were repeated at least three times. Columns are means; bars are S.E.M. ** Significantly different at $p < 0.01$. *** Significantly different at $p < 0.001$. ns (not significant).

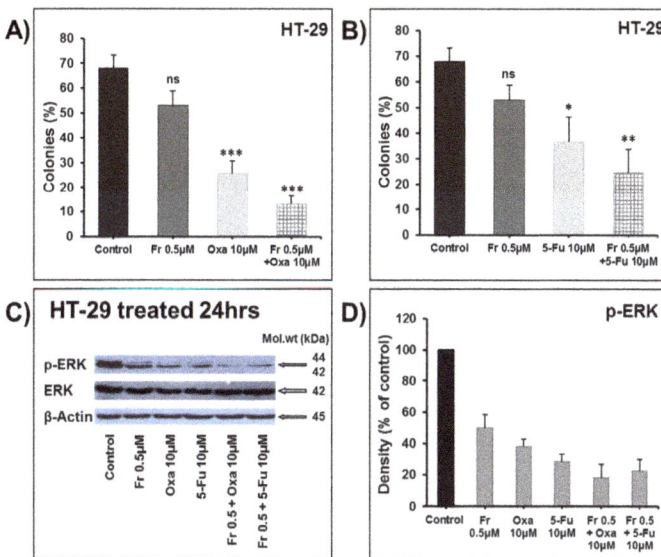

Figure 3. Frondoside A enhances the inhibition of colonies' growth by (**A**) oxaliplatin (10 µM), and (**B**) 5-fluorouracil (10 µM). Data are presented as histograms of the mean percentage of large colonies' growth ± S.E.M. (**C**) The inhibition of ERK phosphorylation by oxaliplatin and 5-fluorouracil was enhanced by Frondoside A in HT-29 colon cancer cells. (**D**) Densitometry analysis of p-ERK from three different experiments. β-actin was used as an internal loading control of the protein levels, and the normalized p-ERK bands' densities are expressed as percentage change in comparison to control samples considered equal to 100%. * Significantly different at $p < 0.05$. ** Significantly different at $p < 0.01$. *** Significantly different at $p < 0.001$. ns (not significant).

3.3. Combination of Frondoside A with 5-Fluorouracil or Oxaliplatin Enhances Apoptotic Cell Death in HT-29 Colon Cancer Cells

Next, we investigated whether the enhanced decrease in HT-29 cell numbers when Frondoside A was used in combination with 5-FU or oxaliplatin was the result of increased apoptotic cell death. Toward this aim, HT-29 colon cancer cells were incubated with Frondoside A (0.5 μM) alone or in combination with increasing concentrations of oxaliplatin (1–10 μM) or 5-FU (0.5–10 μM), and apoptosis was examined after 48 h using Annexin V staining. As shown in Figure 4, a combination of Frondoside A and oxaliplatin caused no increase in the level of apoptosis in comparison with either drug alone. On the other hand, and very interestingly, we found that a combination of Frondoside A and 5-FU led to an increased number of apoptotic cells. Indeed, the population of apoptotic cells rose from 21% for Frondoside A (0.5 μM) and 23% for 5-FU (10 μM) when used alone to 66% when used in combination, suggesting a possible synergism between Frondoside A and 5-FU at these concentrations (Figure 5).

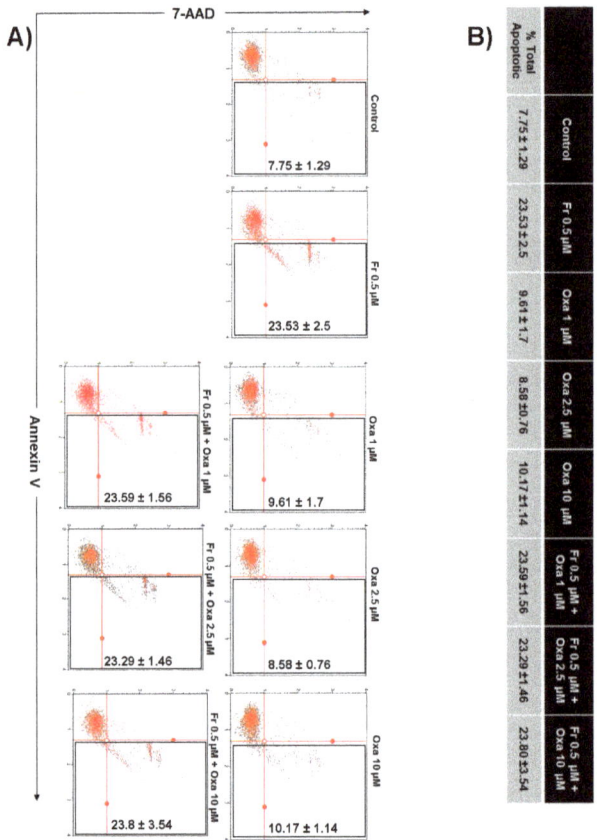

Figure 4. Impact of Frondoside A on apoptotic cell death induced by oxaliplatin in HT-29 colon cancer cells. (**A**,**B**) Annexin V binding was carried out using Annexin V Dead Cell kit. HT-29 cells were treated with or without Frondoside A (0.5 μM) and indicated concentrations of oxaliplatin (1, 2.5, and 10 μM) individually and in combination for 48 h. Detached and adherent cells were collected and stained with Annexin V and 7-AAD, and then the events for early and late apoptotic cells were counted with the Muse Cell Analyzer as described in Materials and Methods. Data represent the mean ± S.E.M. of at least three independent experiments. Fr represents Frondoside A and Oxa represents oxaliplatin.

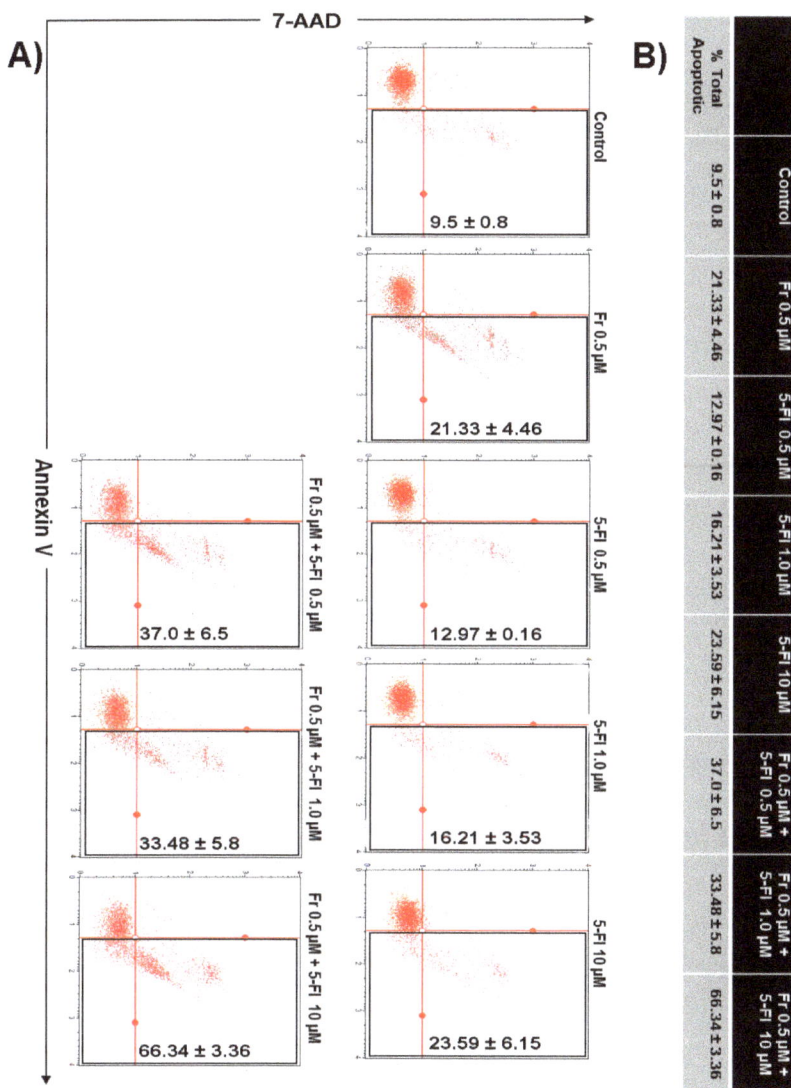

Figure 5. Frondoside A enhances apoptotic cell death induced by 5-fluorouracil in HT-29 colon cancer cells. (**A,B**) Annexin V binding was carried out using Annexin V Dead Cell kit. HT-29 cells were treated with or without Frondoside A (0.5 μM) and indicated concentrations of 5-fluorouracil (0.5, 1, and 10 μM) individually and in combination for 48 h. Detached and adherent cells were collected and stained with Annexin V and 7-AAD, and then the events for early and late apoptotic cells were counted with the Muse Cell Analyzer as described in Materials and Methods. Data represent the mean ± S.E.M. of at least three independent experiments. Fr represents Frondoside A and 5-FU represents 5-fluorouracil.

3.4. Effects of Frondoside A, Oxaliplatin, and 5-Fluorouracil alone or in Combination on Survival and Apoptotic Pathways and on the DNA Damage

A marked inhibition of AKT phosphorylation was noted with all three drugs when used alone; however, no further decrease in the level of phosphorylation was observed when the drugs were used in combination (Figure 6A). As expected, neither of the treatments carried out affected the level of total AKT proteins (Figure 6A). It has been reported that downregulation of AKT phosphorylation induces caspase-3-dependent apoptosis [11,12]. In line with these reports, oxaliplatin was shown to induce dephosphorylation of AKT, leading to the accumulation of cleaved caspase-3 [13]. We and others have previously reported that Frondoside A induced caspase-3 cleavage in pancreatic, breast, lung, and prostate cancer cells [3,5–7]. In this context, apoptosis induced by Frondoside A alone and in combination with oxaliplatin and 5-FU was further assessed by measuring caspase-3 activation and consequently PARP cleavage and inactivation. Cells treated with Frondoside A (0.5 μM), oxaliplatin (10 μM), and 5-FU (10 μM) for 24 h induced the activation of the executioner caspase-3, a key step to induce apoptosis. This activation was further slightly enhanced when Frondoside A was used in combination with either oxaliplatin or 5-FU (Figure 6A). Caspase-3 activation leads to the cleavage and consequently the inactivation of the downstream PARP, a nuclear protein involved in DNA repair and apoptosis. Similarly, downstream PARP cleavage was also observed in the single and combined treatments of HT-29 cells. This is supported by previous reports demonstrating that Frondoside A, oxaliplatin, and 5-FU induce PARP cleavage [3,7,14].

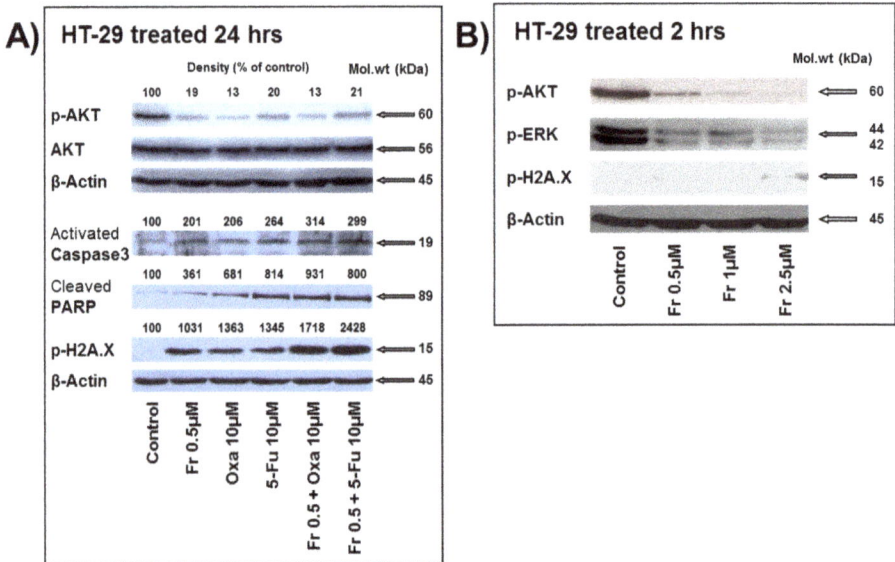

Figure 6. Western blot analysis of: (**A**) the effects of Frondoside A, oxaliplatin, 5-fluorouracil, and their combinations on the phosphorylation of the survival kinase AKT and on caspase-3 activation, Poly (ADP-ribose) polymerase (PARP) inactivation and H2AX phosphorylation. HT-29 cells were treated for 24 h with the indicated concentrations of Frondoside A, oxaliplatin, 5-fluorouracil, and their combinations. Densitometry analysis is from three different experiments. β-actin was used as an internal loading control of the protein levels, and the normalized bands' densities are expressed as percentage change in comparison to control samples considered equal to 100%. (**B**) The levels of p-AKT, p-ERK, and p-H2AX after 2 h of treatment with Frondoside A (0.5–2.5 μM).

PARP inhibition using PARP inhibitors is known to increase the levels of DNA-damage-associated phosphorylation of H2AX [15]. Phosphorylated H2AX histone (γH2AX) is a marker of DNA double-strand breaks. 5-FU was previously reported to induce DNA damage in colon cancer cells [16]. To check whether the induction of cell death by Frondoside A, oxaliplatin, and 5-FU is associated with DNA damage, HT-29 cells were exposed to the drugs either alone or in combination, and the total proteins were evaluated for γH2AX expression. We found that cells treated with the three drugs alone underwent DNA damage. Interestingly, when the drugs were used in combination, this further increased the level of DNA damage in the treated cells (Figure 6A). To determine whether Frondoside A mediates its effect through DNA damage, the inhibition of ERK1/2, AKT signaling pathways, or a combination, we performed an experiment to measure the levels of DNA damage, p-AKT, and p-ERK1/2 after 2 h of treatment with Frondoside A (0.5–2.5 μM). Figure 6B clearly demonstrates that the concentration of 0.5 μM of Frondoside A used in this study had no effect on the DNA damage, while it strongly reduced the levels of phosphorylated AKT and ERK. DNA damage occurred at a minimal level only at a very high concentration of Frondoside A. Hence, this result strongly suggests that the inhibition of ERK and AKT signaling is an early event that occurs in response to Frondoside A treatment and that DNA damage is a late event that might result from excessive DNA damage as a consequence of active apoptosis. Taken together, our results strongly suggest that Frondoside A, when used in combination, enhances the anti-proliferative and the pro-apoptotic effects of oxaliplatin and 5-FU.

4. Conclusions

To the best of our knowledge, the present study identifies for the first time that Frondoside A treatment significantly inhibits proliferation and induces apoptosis in colon cancer cells. The combinations of Frondoside A with the DNA-damaging agent oxaliplatin or with the thymidylate synthase inhibitor 5-FU were significantly more effective in inhibiting HT-29 cell proliferation and triggering apoptosis, leading to the inhibition of the HT-29 colonies' growth, than either cytotoxic agent alone.

Our data suggests that the inactivation of the proliferation (ERK) and pro-survival (AKT) pathways along with caspase-3 activation, PARP cleavage, and consequently DNA damage account, at least partly, for the anti-cancer effect of Frondoside A. Moreover, combination therapy either with oxaliplatin or 5-FU enhanced these effects and further clarified the capacity of Frondoside A to enhance the apoptosis induced mainly by 5-FU. The data also suggests that the inhibition of ERK1/2 phosphorylation with single treatments and its enhanced inhibition under the combination conditions suggests a potential impact of the treatments on colon cancer cell proliferation.

The dual inhibitory effect of our treatments on the PI3K–AKT and the Raf–MEK–ERK pathways is in line with the previously reported interactions between these two pathways [17]. Here, we demonstrate that the inhibition of AKT and ERK phosphorylation is crucial for the anti-tumor activity of Frondoside A. These results are in agreement with previous reports showing that Frondoside A inhibited AKT and ERK1/2 activation in TPA-stimulated breast cancer cells [18] and ERK1/2 activation in PGE2-stimulated breast cancer cells [19].

The current findings are in line with a study by Janakiran et al. demonstrating that Frondanol A5, a *Cucumaria frondosa* extract that contains several agents, including monosulphated triterpenoid glycoside Frondoside A, the disulphated glycoside Frondoside B, the trisulphated glycoside Frondoside C, 12-methyltetradecanoic acid, eicosapentaenoic acid, fucosylated chondroitin sulfate, and canthaxanthin/astaxanthin, inhibits HCT-116 colon cancer cell growth by inducing a G2 arrest followed by the induction of apoptosis [20].

This study provides sufficient rationale to carry out in vivo studies to confirm the relevance of the combination therapy. We believe that Frondoside A in combination with the standard cytotoxic drugs oxaliplatin and 5-FU currently used in colon cancer treatment may improve colon cancer therapy.

Author Contributions: S.A. conceived and designed the experiments; K.A., T.K., S.S., and R.I. performed the experiments; S.A. and R.I. analyzed the data; S.A. and R.I. wrote the paper.

Acknowledgments: This work was supported by the CMHS Grant (31M146), was partly supported by the Terry Fox UAE Grant (21M081) to S.A., and was partly supported by the ZCHS Research Grant (31R086) to R.I. The funders had no role in the study design, the data collection and analysis, the decision to publish, or the preparation of the manuscript.

Conflicts of Interest: The authors declare no conflict of interest. The authors have no other relevant affiliations or financial involvement with any organization or entity with a financial interest in or financial conflict with the subject matter or materials discussed in the manuscript apart from those disclosed.

References

1. Torre, L.A.; Bray, F.; Siegel, R.L.; Ferlay, J.; Lortet-Tieulent, J.; Jemal, A. Global cancer statistics, 2012. *CA Cancer J. Clin.* **2015**, *65*, 87–108. [CrossRef] [PubMed]

2. Chemotherapy of Metastatic Colorectal Cancer. Available online: https://www.ncbi.nlm.nih.gov/pubmed/21180382 (accessed on 19 October 2010).

3. Li, X.; Roginsky, A.B.; Ding, X.Z.; Woodward, C.; Collin, P.; Newman, R.A.; Bell, R.H., Jr.; Adrian, T.E. Review of the apoptosis pathways in pancreatic cancer and the anti-apoptotic effects of the novel sea cucumber compound, Frondoside A. *Ann. N. Y. Acad. Sci.* **2008**, *1138*, 181–198. [CrossRef] [PubMed]

4. Jin, J.O.; Shastina, V.V.; Shin, S.W.; Xu, Q.; Park, J.I.; Rasskazov, V.A.; Avilov, S.A.; Fedorov, S.N.; Stonik, V.A.; Kwak, J.Y. Differential effects of triterpene glycosides, frondoside A and cucumarioside A2-2 isolated from sea cucumbers on caspase activation and apoptosis of human leukemia cells. *FEBS Lett.* **2009**, *583*, 697–702. [CrossRef] [PubMed]

5. Al Marzouqi, N.; Iratni, R.; Nemmar, A.; Arafat, K.; Al Sultan, M.A.; Yasin, J.; Collin, P.; Mester, J.; Adrian, T.E.; Attoub, S. Frondoside A inhibits human breast cancer cell survival, migration, invasion and the growth of breast tumor xenografts. *Eur. J. Pharmacol.* **2011**, *668*, 25–34. [CrossRef] [PubMed]

6. Attoub, S.; Arafat, K.; Gelaude, A.; Al Sultan, M.A.; Bracke, M.; Collin, P.; Takahashi, T.; Adrian, T.E.; De Wever, O. Frondoside a suppressive effects on lung cancer survival, tumor growth, angiogenesis, invasion, and metastasis. *PLoS ONE* **2013**, *8*, e53087. [CrossRef] [PubMed]

7. Dyshlovoy, S.A.; Menchinskaya, E.S.; Venz, S.; Rast, S.; Amann, K.; Hauschild, J.; Otte, K.; Kalinin, V.I.; Silchenko, A.S.; Avilov, S.A.; et al. The marine triterpene glycoside frondoside A exhibits activity in vitro and in vivo in prostate cancer. *Int. J. Cancer* **2016**, *138*, 2450–2465. [CrossRef] [PubMed]

8. Al Shemaili, J.; Mensah-Brown, E.; Parekh, K.; Thomas, S.A.; Attoub, S.; Hellman, B.; Nyberg, F.; Adem, A.; Collin, P.; Adrian, T.E. Frondoside A enhances the antiproliferative effects of gemcitabine in pancreatic cancer. *Eur. J. Cancer* **2014**, *50*, 1391–1398. [CrossRef] [PubMed]

9. Raymond, E.; Buquet-Fagot, C.; Djelloul, S.; Mester, J.; Cvitkovic, E.; Allain, P.; Louvet, C.; Gespach, C. Antitumor activity of oxaliplatin in combination with 5-fluorouracil and the thymidylate synthase inhibitor AG337 in human colon, breast and ovarian cancers. *Anticancer Drugs* **1997**, *8*, 876–885. [CrossRef] [PubMed]

10. Sebolt-Leopold, J.S.; Dudley, D.T.; Herrera, R.; Van Becelaere, K.; Wiland, A.; Gowan, R.C.; Tecle, H.; Barrett, S.D.; Bridges, A.; Przybranowski, S.; et al. Blockade of the MAP kinase pathway suppresses growth of colon tumors in vivo. *Nat. Med.* **1999**, *5*, 810–816. [CrossRef] [PubMed]

11. Moon, D.O.; Park, S.Y.; Choi, Y.H.; Kim, N.D.; Lee, C.; Kim, G.Y. Melittin induces Bcl-2 and caspase-3-dependent apoptosis through downregulation of Akt phosphorylation in human leukemic U937 cells. *Toxicon* **2008**, *51*, 112–120. [CrossRef] [PubMed]

12. Weng, H.Y.; Hsu, M.J.; Chen, C.C.; Chen, B.C.; Hong, C.Y.; Teng, C.M.; Pan, S.L.; Chiu, W.T.; Lin, C.H. Denbinobin induces human glioblastoma multiforme cell apoptosis through the IKKα-Akt-FKHR signaling cascade. *Eur. J. Pharmacol.* **2013**, *698*, 103–109. [CrossRef] [PubMed]

13. Shiragami, R.; Murata, S.; Kosugi, C.; Tezuka, T.; Yamazaki, M.; Hirano, A.; Yoshimura, Y.; Suzuki, M.; Shuto, K.; Koda, K. Enhanced antitumor activity of cerulenin combined with oxaliplatin in human colon cancer cells. *Int. J. Oncol.* **2013**, *43*, 431–438. [CrossRef] [PubMed]

14. Flis, S.; Gnyszka, A.; Misiewicz-Krzeminska, I.; Spławiński, J. Decytabine enhances cytotoxicity induced by oxaliplatin and 5-fluorouracil in the colorectal cancer cell line Colo-205. *Cancer Cell Int.* **2009**, *9*, 10. [CrossRef] [PubMed]

15. Dale Rein, I.; Solberg Landsverk, K.; Micci, F.; Patzke, S.; Stokke, T. Replication-induced DNA damage after PARP inhibition causes G2 delay, and cell line-dependent apoptosis, necrosis and multinucleation. *Cell Cycle* **2015**, *14*, 3248–3260. [CrossRef] [PubMed]

16. Matuo, R.; Sousa, F.G.; Escargueil, A.E.; Grivicich, I.; Garcia-Santos, D.; Chies, J.A.; Saffi, J.; Larsen, A.K.; Henriques, J.A. 5-Fluorouracil and its active metabolite FdUMP cause DNA damage in human SW620 colon adenocarcinoma cell line. *J. Appl. Toxicol.* **2009**, *29*, 308–316. [CrossRef] [PubMed]

17. McCubrey, J.A.; Steelman, L.S.; Franklin, R.A.; Abrams, S.L.; Chappell, W.H.; Wong, E.W.T.; Lehmann, B.; Terrian, D.M.; Basecke, J.; Stivala, F.; et al. Targeting the RAF/MEK/ERK, PI3K/AKT and p53 pathways in hematopoietic drug resistance. *Adv. Enzym. Regul.* **2007**, *47*, 64–103. [CrossRef] [PubMed]

18. Park, S.Y.; Kim, Y.H.; Kim, Y.; Lee, S.J. Frondoside A has an anti-invasive effect by inhibiting TPA-induced MMP-9 activation via NF-kappaB and AP-1 signaling in human breast cancer cells. *Int. J. Oncol.* **2012**, *41*, 933–940. [CrossRef] [PubMed]

19. Ma, X.; Kundu, N.; Collin, P.D.; Goloubeva, O.; Fulton, A.M. Frondoside A inhibits breast cancer metastasis and antagonizes prostaglandin E receptors EP4 and EP2. *Breast Cancer Res. Treat.* **2012**, *132*, 1001–1008. [CrossRef] [PubMed]

20. Janakiram, N.B.; Mohammed, A.; Zhang, Y.; Choi, C.I.; Woodward, C.; Collin, P.; Steele, V.E.; Rao, C.V. Chemopreventive Effects of Frondanol A5, a Cucumaria frondosa Extract, against Rat Colon Carcinogenesis and Inhibition of Human Colon Cancer Cell Growth. *Cancer Prev. Res.* **2010**, *3*, 82–91. [CrossRef] [PubMed]

nutrients

MDPI

Review

Pro-Apoptotic and Anti-Cancer Properties of Diosgenin: A Comprehensive and Critical Review

Gautam Sethi [1,2,3,*,†], Muthu K. Shanmugam [3,†], Sudha Warrier [4], Myriam Merarchi [3], Frank Arfuso [5], Alan Prem Kumar [3] and Anupam Bishayee [6,*]

1   Department for Management of Science and Technology Development, Ton Duc Thang University, Ho Chi Minh City 700000, Vietnam
2   Faculty of Pharmacy, Ton Duc Thang University, Ho Chi Minh City 700000, Vietnam
3   Department of Pharmacology, Yong Loo Lin School of Medicine, National University of Singapore, Singapore 117600, Singapore; phcsmk@nus.edu.sg (M.K.S.); myriammerarchi@hotmail.fr (M.M.); phcapk@nus.edu.sg (A.P.K.)
4   Division of Cancer Stem Cells and Cardiovascular Regeneration, Manipal Institute of Regenerative Medicine, Manipal University, Bangalore 560065, India; sudha.warrier@manipal.edu
5   Stem Cell and Cancer Biology Laboratory, School of Biomedical Sciences, Curtin Health Innovation Research Institute, Curtin University, Perth, WA 6102, Australia; frank.arfuso@curtin.edu.au
6   Department of Pharmaceutical Sciences, College of Pharmacy, Larkin University, 18301 N. Miami Avenue, Miami, FL 33169, USA
*   Correspondence: gautam.sethi@tdt.edu.vn or phcgs@nus.edu.sg (G.S.); abishayee@ULarkin.org or abishayee@gmail.com (A.B.)
†   These authors contributed equally to this work.

Received: 17 March 2018; Accepted: 16 May 2018; Published: 19 May 2018

Abstract: Novel and alternative options are being adopted to combat the initiation and progression of human cancers. One of the approaches is the use of molecules isolated from traditional medicinal herbs, edible dietary plants and seeds that play a pivotal role in the prevention/treatment of cancer, either alone or in combination with existing chemotherapeutic agents. Compounds that modulate these oncogenic processes are potential candidates for cancer therapy and may eventually make it to clinical applications. Diosgenin is a naturally occurring steroidal sapogenin and is one of the major bioactive compounds found in dietary fenugreek (*Trigonella foenum-graecum*) seeds. In addition to being a lactation aid, diosgenin has been shown to be hypocholesterolemic, gastro- and hepato-protective, anti-oxidant, anti-inflammatory, anti-diabetic, and anti-cancer. Diosgenin has a unique structural similarity to estrogen. Several preclinical studies have reported on the pro-apoptotic and anti-cancer properties of diosgenin against a variety of cancers, both in in vitro and in vivo. Diosgenin has also been reported to reverse multi-drug resistance in cancer cells and sensitize cancer cells to standard chemotherapy. Remarkably, diosgenin has also been reported to be used by pharmaceutical companies to synthesize steroidal drugs. Several novel diosgenin analogs and nano-formulations have been synthesized with improved anti-cancer efficacy and pharmacokinetic profile. In this review we discuss in detail the multifaceted anti-cancer properties of diosgenin that have found application in pharmaceutical, functional food, and cosmetic industries; and the various intracellular molecular targets modulated by diosgenin that abrogate the oncogenic process.

Keywords: diosgenin; steroidal sapogenins; anti-cancer; apoptosis; oncogenic; metastasis

---

1. Introduction

Cancer is a complex and heterogeneous disease that afflicts men and women worldwide; it is expected to increase due to human lifestyle changes and a rapidly aging population [1]. Hanahan and Weinberg's proposed hallmarks of cancer are widely accepted towards understanding the biology of cancer cells, through a multi-stage and progressive process [2–6]. These hallmarks include sustained proliferation of cells, constitutive activation of pro-survival transcription factors, deregulated cellular functions, evading cell death signals and growth suppressors, an increased pro-inflammatory tumor microenvironment, camouflaging against immune cell destruction, promoting angiogenesis, activating cell movement from the primary site and metastasis, enabling replicative immortality, and finally, severe genome instability [2,3,5–10]. In addition, several deregulated cellular signaling networks underlying the above hallmarks have been extensively investigated in pre-clinical and clinical drug development [3,4,11–18]. In spite of detailed information of these semi-synthetic and synthetic anti-cancer agents, they only provide limited therapeutic advantages to patients due to highly toxic unwanted side effects and the development of chemoresistance [19–21]. Emerging approaches should include the identification of novel drug targets that are very effective in inhibiting the growth of cancer cells, while exhibiting fewer adverse effects. Natural products are a good source of compounds with novel chemical structures that are effective and less toxic [18,22–27]. High throughput technologies should be exploited for the screening of a large library of compounds for their anti-cancer activities [28–30]. The mainstream of United States Food and Drug Administration (US FDA)-approved compounds divulge that natural products and their derivatives occupy one-third of all novel drugs [22–24,31]. These natural compounds, in general, show multi-targeted effects and can modulate several oncogenic transcription factors that block the tumor microenvironment targets that usually sustain tumor growth [22,27,32]. These compounds can also be classified as cytotoxic or cytostatic compounds [30]. Therefore, many secondary metabolites and pure molecules isolated from herbs, spices, dietary fruits and vegetables, and even marine sources have been explored [33–35].

Several novel bioactive molecules have been found in various edible cereals, pulses, roots, and in several parts of medicinal plants. Fenugreek (*Trigonella foenum-graecum*) belongs to the family Leguminosae and is considered a traditional medicinal herb that is commonly used in India, China, Thailand, and South-East Asian countries; it is also cultivated in the Mediterranean region and Northern Africa [36–41]. Fenugreek seeds, shoots and leaves are used in Indian curry preparation as a condiment. Bibliometric data indicates that fenugreek extract has several pharmacological properties, such as being hypocholesterolemic, a lactation aid, antibacterial, a gastric stimulant, anti-anorexic, antidiabetic, galactogogic, hepatoprotective, and anti-cancer both in in vitro and in vivo studies [40–43]. Fenugreek seed extract contains several bioactive molecules in various classes of compounds, such as saponins, flavonoids, coumarins, and alkaloids that target several molecules involved in inflammation and cancer cell proliferation, invasion, migration, angiogenesis, and metastasis [40]. Sapogenins are a class of compounds that widely occur in natural products in their glycoside form and promote general healthy living. Among these compounds, steroidal sapogenins (otherwise known as spirostans) are the most potent bioactive compounds isolated from natural product sources [44,45]. Steroidal sapogenins exhibit ubiquitous pharmacological properties and the majority of them demonstrate anti-cancer activity in vitro and in pre-clinical animal models. Several clinical trials have been conducted with fenugreek seed extract, they are either completed or ongoing; however, diosgenin anti-cancer trials are yet to start [36,41]. Diosgenin is the most abundant steroidal sapogenin in fenugreek seeds. Fujii and Matsukawa isolated and identified diosgenin from *Dioscorea tokoro* Makino in 1935 [41,46] (Figure 1). Diosgenin is a phytosteroidal saponin and a major bioactive compound found in the seeds of *T. foenum-graecum*, commonly known as fenugreek, and in the roots of wild yam (*Dioscorea villosa*) [36,40, 41,47,48]. Interestingly, diosgenin is also found in high levels in numerous plant species including *Costus speciosus*, *Smilax menispermoidea*, species of *Paris*, *Aletris* and *Trillum*, and in species of *Dioscorea* [41,49,50]. The steroidal saponin, diosgenin, is biosynthesized from cholesterol. Cholesterol is formed from lanosterol and catalysed by the cytochrome P450 system. Several other routes of synthesis have been identified, such as from squalene-2,3-oxide in two ways: From cycloartenol through the formation of sitosterol [51] and from lanosterol via cholesterol [52]. Several studies have demonstrated the diverse biological activities of diosgenin, such as hypolipidemic, anti-inflammatory, anti-proliferative, hypoglycemic activity, and as a potent anti-oxidant [44]. In addition, diosgenin inhibited cancer cell proliferation and induced apoptosis in a variety of cancer cell lines including colorectal, hepatocellular, breast, osteosarcoma, and leukemia [53–55]. The primary mechanism of action of diosgenin is through the modulation of multiple cell signaling pathways that play prominent roles in cell-cycle regulation, differentiation, and apoptosis [56]. Remarkably, pharmaceutical companies use diosgenin as a principal precursor compound for the manufacturing of several steroidal drugs [48]. Diosgenin is also an attractive molecule with multifaceted properties that has found application in pharmaceutical, functional food, and cosmetic industries. In this review we provide an in-depth evaluation of literature on diosgenin and its pharmacodynamics and pharmacokinetics, and discuss several of its novel derivatives and nanoformulations that increase its bioavailability and therapeutic efficacy. Diosgenin, over the years, has provided abundant data on the prevention and treatment of various inflammation-driven diseases, including cancers [36] (Figure 2).

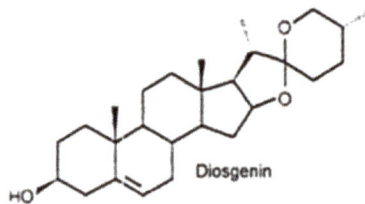

Figure 1. Chemical structure of diosgenin.

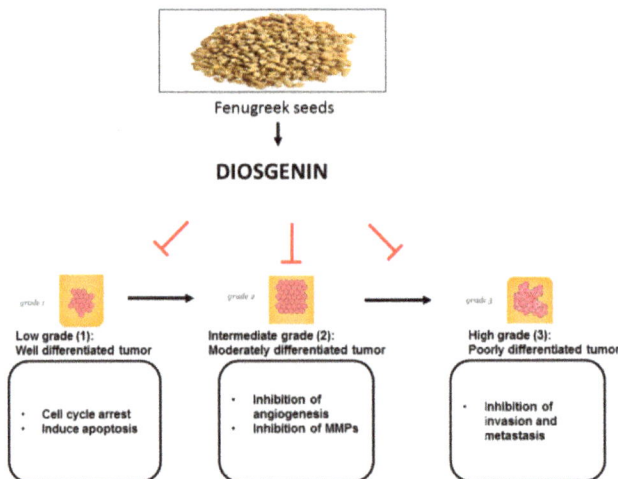

Figure 2. Tumor stage-specific inhibition of molecular targets by diosgenin.

2. Fenugreek Seed Bioactive Compounds

Fenugreek contains several chemical constituents, such as alkaloids, steroidal sapogenins, saponins, flavonoids, lipids, amino acids, and carbohydrates. Diosgenin is a major bioactive steroidal sapogenin in the fenugreek seed, which is reported to have chemopreventive and therapeutic effects against inflammation and chronic inflammation-driven cancers in preclinical in vitro and in vivo models of cancer [36,57]. Table 1 illustrates the major constituents of fenugreek seeds and leaves.

Table 1. Main phytochemical constituents of fenugreek (*T. foenum-graecum*).

Class of Compounds	Phytochemical Constituents	Reference
Steroidal sapogenins	Diosgenin, Yamogenin, Smilagenin, Sarsasapogenin, Tigogenin, Neotigogenin, Gitogenin, Yuccagenin, Saponaretin	[40]
Flavonoids	Quercetin, Rutin, Vitexin, Isovitexin	[40]
Saponins	Graecunins, Fenugrin B, Fenugreekine, Trigofoenosides A–G	[40]
Alkaloids	Trimethylamine, Neurin, Trigonelline, Choline, Gentianine, Carpaine, and Betain	[40]
Fibers	Gum, Neutral detergent fiber	[40]
Lipids	Lipids, Triacylglycerols, Diacylglycerols, Monoacylglycerols, Phosphatidylcholine, Phosphatidylethanolamine, Phosphatidylinositol, Free fatty acids	[40]
Others	Coumarin, Amino acids, Vitamins, Minerals. 28% Mucilage; 22% Proteins; 5% of a stronger swelling, Bitter fixed oil	[40]

3. In Vitro Anti-Cancer Effects of Diosgenin

Diosgenin, the major steroidal sapogenin in the fenugreek seed, has been shown to potently suppress constitutively-activated pro-inflammatory and pro-survival signaling pathways in a variety of cancer cells, and induced apoptosis [58]. Some of the earlier studies by Shishodia and Aggarwal [58] reported that diosgenin abrogated TNF-α-induced NF-κB activation and suppressed osteoclastogenesis in RAW 264.7 macrophage cells [58]. In Her-2 positive breast cancer cells, diosgenin inhibited the expression of AKT, mTOR, JNK and their associated pro-survival signaling pathways, and induced apoptosis in these cells [53]. In another study by Li et al., they reported that diosgenin could inactivate the STAT3 signaling pathway in hepatocellular carcinoma (HCC) cells, by inhibiting intracellular signaling molecules such as c-SRC, JAK1, and JAK2 (Figure 3). Diosgenin also suppressed STAT3 transcriptional activity and the expression of its downstream gene products involved in proliferation, invasion and metastasis. In addition, diosgenin sensitized HCC cells to doxorubicin and paclitaxel, and synergistically augmented apoptosis, thereby suggesting that diosgenin is a potential bioactive compound for the treatment of HCC and other cancers [54]. Diosgenin inhibited proliferation, AKT and JNK in a dose- and time-dependent manner and induced caspase-dependent apoptosis in A431 and Hep2 skin squamous cell carcinoma cells [59]. HT-29 colon cancer cells have been reported to be resistant to TRAIL-induced apoptosis. Diosgenin was shown to sensitize the HT-29 colon cancer cell to TRAIL. In addition, it potently suppressed cell proliferation and induced apoptosis by suppressing the p38/MAPK signaling pathway and the overexpression of DR5 [60]. Furthermore, Romero-Hernandez et al. [61] demonstrated that diosgenin-derived thio(seleno)ureas and glycomimetics, bearing a 1,2,3-triazolyl tether on C-3, showed more potent anti-cancer activity against MDA-MB-231 and MCF-7 breast cancer cells, HepG2 hepatocellular carcinoma cells, and induced apoptosis, compared to its parent compound diosgenin [61]. In another study, diosgenin conjugated to methotrexate was found to be more potent in inhibiting the growth of transport-resistant breast cancer cells and dihydrofolate reductase (enzyme involved in DNA synthesis), compared to the parent diosgenin [62]. In chronic myeloid leukemia cells, diosgenin-induced autophagy inhibited the mTOR signaling pathway and induced apoptotic cell death [63]. Diosgenin induced cytotoxicity and significantly inhibited the growth and proliferation of MCF-7 breast cancer cells in a dose- and time-dependent manner. Diosgenin was also shown to inhibit *N*-nitroso-*N*-methylurea-induced breast cancer in rats [64].

Of several factors that contribute to the sustained growth and proliferation of tumors, one important factor is the abundant neovascularization or formation of new micro blood vessels at the tumor site, or within the tumor. This process is also known as tumor angiogenesis. Thus, the formation of new blood vessels in tumors actively supplies the essential nutrients and growth factors that allow tumors to acquire the ability to reject chemotherapeutic drugs and develop chemoresistance [27,65–68]. Diosgenin is also a potent inhibitor of cancer cell invasion, migration, and tumor-associated angiogenesis [27,69]. He et al., reported that diosgenin inhibited the invasion and migration of triple-negative breast cancer cells and was associated with the concomitant suppression of actin polymerization, phosphorylation of Vav2, and activation of Cdc42 oncoprotein expression. These proteins have been shown to be involved in the initiation of cancer cells' invasive and migratory potential [70]. Similarly, diosgenin was found to inhibit PC3 androgen-independent prostate cancer cell invasion and migration. The inhibitory effect was mediated by the downregulation of matrix metalloproteinase (MMP)-2 and MMP-9, the key enzymes in matrix degradation and stroma invasion. Furthermore, diosgenin also downregulated the tissue inhibitors of metalloproteinase (TIMP)-2, vascular endothelial growth factor (VEGF), extracellular regulated kinase (ERK), Janus kinase (JNK), phosphotidyl-inositol-3 kinase/protein kinase B (PI3K/AKT), and NF-κB transcriptional activity [56]. In addition, diosgenin was reported to inhibit the expression of E-cadherin, integrin 5a and 6b, invasion, migration, and angiogenesis in hypoxia-sensitive BGC-823 gastric cancer cells [71]. Diosgenin was reported to inhibit proliferation of ER-positive MCF-7 breast cancer cells by the upregulation of the p53 tumor suppressor gene and activation of caspase 3, while it downregulated BCL2 in ER negative MDA-MB-231 triple-negative breast cancer cells [72]. Diosgenin, either alone, or in combination with thymoquinone, inhibited A431 and Hep2 squamous cell carcinoma cell proliferation, increased the Bax/Bcl2 ratio, and induced caspase 3-mediated apoptosis [59] (Table 2). The potential effect of diosgenin on NF-κB and STAT3 signaling pathways in tumor cells, is shown in Figure 3.

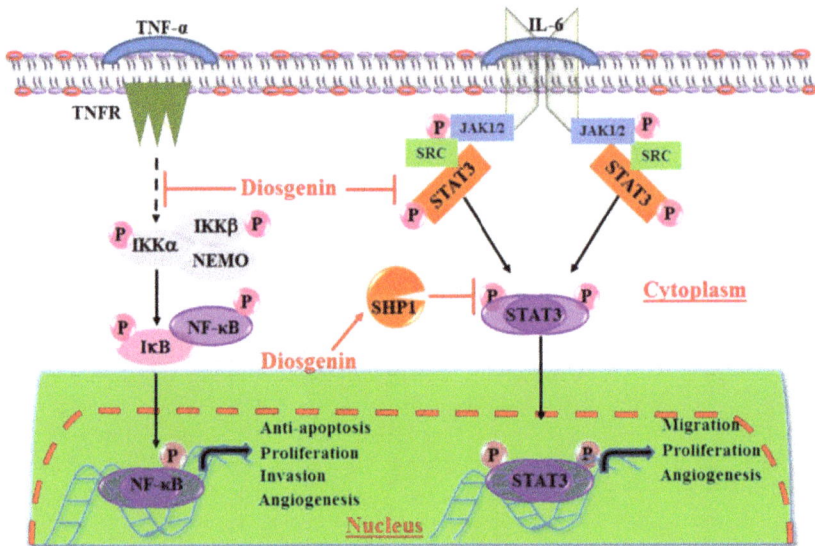

Figure 3. Role of diosgenin in NF-κB and STAT3 signaling pathways. Diosgenin abrogates TNF-α -induced activation of NF-κB and IL6-induced STAT3 signaling pathways in tumor cells. Diosgenin can hence prevent proliferation, invasion and angiogenesis; and induce apoptosis, a characteristic vastly looked for in cancer therapy.

Table 2. In vitro anti-cancer effects of diosgenin.

Cancer model	Cell Lines	Diosgenin Dose	Molecular Target	References
Breast carcinoma	Estrogen receptor positive and estrogen receptor negative human breast cancer MCF-7 and MDA 231 cells	20 μM and 30 μM	Inhibition of cell proliferation Induces apoptosis	[72]
	MDA-MB-231 breast cancer cells	20 μM, 40 μM, and 60 μM	Downregulation of Bcl2	[57]
	Her2 over-expressing breast cancer cells	5–20 μM	Modulation of Akt, mTOR, and JNK phosphorylation	[53]
	MCF-7 breast cancer cells	20 μM and 40 μM	Upregulation of p53 tumor suppressor gene	[73]
Hepatocellular carcinoma	C3A, HUH-7, and HepG2 cells	50 μM and 100 μM	Downregulation of STAT3 signaling pathway Upregulates SH-PTP2 expression Induces apoptosis Potentiates the apoptotic effects of doxorubicin and paclitaxel	[54]
Prostate carcinoma	PC3 cells	5 μM, 10 μM, and 20 μM	Downregulates NF-κB signaling pathway Inhibits matrix metalloproteinases Inhibits invasion and migration of cells	[56]
Osteosarcoma	1547 cells	40 μM, 80 μM, and 100 μM	Inhibits cell proliferation Induces apoptosis	[55]
	1547 cells	40 μM	Inhibits cell proliferation Induces apoptosis Upregulation of p53 tumor suppressor gene	[74]
	HEL cells, K562 cells	40 μM	Inhibits NF-κB signaling pathway	[75]
Human erythroleukemia	HEL cells	40 μM	Inhibits proliferation Induces apoptosis Upregulation of p21	[76]
Human Laryngocarcinoma Human Melanoma	HEp-2 cells M4Beu cells	40 μM	Inhibits cell proliferation Induces caspase-3 dependent apoptosis Upregulates p53 tumor suppressor gene	[77]
Human cancer cells	Human epithelial carcinoma cell line (A431), human NSCLC cell line (A549), human ovarian cancer cell line (A2780), Human erythroleukemia (K562) and Dukes' type C, colorectal adenocarcinoma (HCT-15)	10 mmol/L	Induces apoptosis via mitochondrial dependent pathway	[78]
	Multiple myeloma (U266), leukemia (U937), and breast cancer (MCF-7)	50 μM and 100 μM	Inhibits NF-κB signaling pathway	[58]

4. In Vivo Anti-Cancer Effects of Diosgenin

In addition to in vitro inhibition of cancer cell proliferation by dietary fenugreek seeds and its bioactive constituent diosgenin, several studies have provided evidence that diosgenin is a potent inhibitor of tumor growth in vivo in rodent models of cancer. In a rat colorectal tumor model, administration of diosgenin, given during the promotional stage, reduced azoxymethane (AOM)-induced colonic aberrant crypt foci formation [79]. Similarly, Malisetty et al., showed that diosgenin, at a dose of 15 mg/kg, significantly suppressed both the incidence and invasive potential of AOM-induced rat colon adenocarcinoma mass by 60% and colon tumor multiplicity (adenocarcinomas/rat) by 68% [80]. However, in the murine model of AOM/dextran sodium sulfate-induced colon aberrant crypt foci, diosgenin at doses of 20, 100 and 200 mg/kg b.w. in the diet did not reduce adenocarcinoma mass; nonetheless, a significant reduction in tumor multiplicity was observed with all three doses tested [81]. In another study, diosgenin (at a dose of 10 mg/kg b.w. administered intra-tumorally) significantly inhibited the growth of MCF-7 and MDA-MB-231 human breast cancer xenografts in mice [72]. In another study using inbred T739 mice, diosgenin was shown to significantly inhibit the growth of mouse LA795 lung adenocarcinoma tumors by 33.94% [82]. Diosgenin, at a dose of 80 mg/kg administered by oral gavage, was reported to inhibit the growth of oral tumors in a DMBA-induced hamster buccal pouch model [64]. Diosgenin, in combination with thymoquinone, exhibited significant tumor growth inhibition in a mice xenograft model [59]. Therefore, diosgenin modulates multiple targets and suppresses tumor growth in preclinical models of cancer. However, diosgenin's poor solubility in organic solvents and its lack of bioavailability greatly hinder its translational process as a therapeutic compound. Further clinical trials are required to evaluate its potential either as a preventive or therapeutic anti-cancer agent.

5. Semisynthetic Derivatives of Diosgenin That Exhibit Anti-Cancer Activity

Diosgenin is used in the pharmaceutical industry as the main precursor in the synthesis of steroids [83]. It has the ability to penetrate cell membranes and bind to specific receptors [84]. Steroidal sapogenins are bioactive molecules that have shown exceptional antiproliferative activity against several human cancer cells. By making specific changes in the steroidal structure of diosgenin, it can affect its biological activity. In a recent report, using diosgenin as the parent molecule, the authors synthesized two novel steroidal oxime compounds that showed significant antiproliferative activity on cervical cancer cells and human lymphocytes. These compounds induced apoptosis and activated caspase 3 [85]. In another study Mohammad et al., reported on the anti-proliferative activity of diosgenin and its semi-synthetic derivatives against breast (HBL-100), colon (HCT-116 and HT-19) and lung (A549) cancer cells. A structure-activity relationship study revealed that the potent anti-proliferative activity was mainly attributed to the analogs with the simple phenyl R moiety or electron-withdrawing ortho-substituted R moieties attached to the parent diosgenin [86]. In another study, diosgenin was used as a parent compound to synthesize 1α-hydroxysolasodine; it showed significant anti-cancer activity against prostate cancer (PC3), cervical carcinoma (HeLa), and hepatocellular carcinoma (HepG2) cells [87]. Twelve different analogs of diosgenin containing a long chain fatty acid/ester of diosgenin-7-ketoxime exhibited anti-cancer activity when tested against a panel of cancer cell lines. Compound 16 in this series exhibited potent anti-proliferative activity against DU145 prostate cancer cells, which was associated to the suppression of lipopolysaccharide-induced activation of TNF-α and IL6. The compound was also identified as safe, with a maximum tolerated dose of 300 mg/kg in Swiss albino mice [88]. In a recent article by Ghosh et al., they reported the synthesis of diosgenin functionalized iron oxide nanoparticles that exhibited anti-breast cancer activity by inhibiting proliferation and migration, and by inducing apoptosis [89].

6. Conclusions and Future Perspectives

Compounds derived either from medicinal or dietary plant sources embrace distinct advantages, such as novel bioactive structures, low toxicity, and being multi-targeted in abrogating oncogenic processes; thereby, they may form the source of improved therapeutic options. A vast body of pre-clinical experimental evidence suggests that diosgenin has great potential as an anti-cancer agent. In this review we have compiled and analyzed the role of diosgenin in modulating various oncogenic transcription factors and intracellular molecular targets that drive tumor initiation, progression and metastasis. It is well known that the majority of cancers are a consequence of chronic inflammation, infection, dysfunctional cell death mechanisms, and deregulation of cell cycle molecules. The ability of diosgenin to prevent carcinogenesis by acting as an anti-oxidant and anti-inflammatory agent, and its ability to induce apoptosis of cancer cells, suggests that it can be useful as an anti-carcinogenic agent. Due to the complexities in the cellular processes involved, several new studies need to be conducted to decipher the exact molecular targets that can be exploited to prevent cancer progression. Interestingly, there are 12 reported clinical trials on fenugreek seed extract on a variety of human ailments, as reported in www.clinicaltrials.gov. However, to date, there are no cancer-related clinical trials reported either on diosgenin or on fenugreek seed extract. Several novel synthetic diosgenin derivatives have been shown to improve its anti-cancer efficacy. Several nano-formulations and delivery systems of diosgenin are also shown to improve its bioavailability. In conclusion, several challenges such as developing novel delivery systems, pharmaceutical formulations, and semi-synthetic derivatives that are water soluble, need to be overcome to uncover diosgenin's benefits either as a chemopreventive or therapeutic agent.

Author Contributions: G.S. and M.K.S. wrote the paper, F.A., A.P.K., S.W., M.M. and A.B. critically analyzed and revised the manuscript.

Acknowledgments: A.P.K. was supported by grants from National Medical Research Council of Singapore, Medical Science Cluster, Yong Loo Lin School of Medicine, National University of Singapore and by the National Research Foundation Singapore and the Singapore Ministry of Education under its Research Centers of Excellence initiative to Cancer Science Institute of Singapore, National University of Singapore.

Conflicts of Interest: The authors declare no conflict of interest.

References

1. Siegel, R.L.; Miller, K.D.; Jemal, A. Cancer statistics, 2017. *CA Cancer J. Clin.* **2017**, *67*, 7–30. [CrossRef] [PubMed]
2. Hanahan, D.; Weinberg, R.A. The hallmarks of cancer. *Cell* **2000**, *100*, 57–70. [CrossRef]
3. Hanahan, D.; Weinberg, R.A. Hallmarks of cancer: The next generation. *Cell* **2011**, *144*, 646–674. [CrossRef] [PubMed]
4. Hanahan, D. Rethinking the war on cancer. *Lancet* **2014**, *383*, 558–563. [CrossRef]
5. Floor, S.L.; Dumont, J.E.; Maenhaut, C.; Raspe, E. Hallmarks of cancer: Of all cancer cells, all the time? *Trends Mol. Med.* **2012**, *18*, 509–515. [CrossRef] [PubMed]
6. Pietras, K.; Ostman, A. Hallmarks of cancer: Interactions with the tumor stroma. *Exp. Cell Res.* **2010**, *316*, 1324–1331. [CrossRef] [PubMed]
7. Massague, J.; Obenauf, A.C. Metastatic colonization by circulating tumour cells. *Nature* **2016**, *529*, 298–306. [CrossRef] [PubMed]
8. Chaffer, C.L.; Weinberg, R.A. How does multistep tumorigenesis really proceed? *Cancer Discov.* **2015**, *5*, 22–24. [CrossRef] [PubMed]
9. Iwatsuki, M.; Mimori, K.; Yokobori, T.; Ishi, H.; Beppu, T.; Nakamori, S.; Baba, H.; Mori, M. Epithelial-mesenchymal transition in cancer development and its clinical significance. *Cancer Sci.* **2010**, *101*, 293–299. [CrossRef] [PubMed]
10. Almendro, V.; Marusyk, A.; Polyak, K. Cellular heterogeneity and molecular evolution in cancer. *Annu. Rev. Pathol.* **2013**, *8*, 277–302. [CrossRef] [PubMed]
11. Steeg, P.S. Targeting metastasis. *Nat. Rev. Cancer* **2016**, *16*, 201–218. [CrossRef] [PubMed]

12. Wang, Z.; Dabrosin, C.; Yin, X.; Fuster, M.M.; Arreola, A.; Rathmell, W.K.; Generali, D.; Nagaraju, G.P.; El-Rayes, B.; Ribatti, D.; et al. Broad targeting of angiogenesis for cancer prevention and therapy. *Semin. Cancer Biol.* **2015**, *35*, S224–S243. [CrossRef] [PubMed]

13. Sethi, G.; Ahn, K.S.; Aggarwal, B.B. Targeting nuclear factor-kappa B activation pathway by thymoquinone: Role in suppression of antiapoptotic gene products and enhancement of apoptosis. *Mol. Cancer Res.* **2008**, *6*, 1059–1070. [CrossRef] [PubMed]

14. Tang, C.H.; Sethi, G.; Kuo, P.L. Novel medicines and strategies in cancer treatment and prevention. *BioMed Res. Int.* **2014**, *2014*, 474078. [CrossRef] [PubMed]

15. Ahn, K.S.; Sethi, G.; Aggarwal, B.B. Nuclear factor-kappa B: From clone to clinic. *Curr. Mol. Med.* **2007**, *7*, 619–637. [CrossRef] [PubMed]

16. Chai, E.Z.; Shanmugam, M.K.; Arfuso, F.; Dharmarajan, A.; Wang, C.; Kumar, A.P.; Samy, R.P.; Lim, L.H.; Wang, L.; Goh, B.C.; et al. Targeting transcription factor stat3 for cancer prevention and therapy. *Pharmacol. Ther.* **2016**, *162*, 86–97. [CrossRef] [PubMed]

17. Li, F.; Zhang, J.; Arfuso, F.; Chinnathambi, A.; Zayed, M.E.; Alharbi, S.A.; Kumar, A.P.; Ahn, K.S.; Sethi, G. NF-kappaB in cancer therapy. *Arch. Toxicol.* **2015**, *89*, 711–731. [CrossRef] [PubMed]

18. Shanmugam, M.K.; Kannaiyan, R.; Sethi, G. Targeting cell signaling and apoptotic pathways by dietary agents: Role in the prevention and treatment of cancer. *Nutr. Cancer* **2011**, *63*, 161–173. [CrossRef] [PubMed]

19. Deorukhkar, A.; Krishnan, S.; Sethi, G.; Aggarwal, B.B. Back to basics: How natural products can provide the basis for new therapeutics. *Expert Opin. Investig. Drugs* **2007**, *16*, 1753–1773. [CrossRef] [PubMed]

20. Kneller, R. The importance of new companies for drug discovery: Origins of a decade of new drugs. *Nat. Rev. Drug Discov.* **2010**, *9*, 867–882. [CrossRef] [PubMed]

21. Bishayee, A.; Sethi, G. Bioactive natural products in cancer prevention and therapy: Progress and promise. *Semin. Cancer Biol.* **2016**, *40–41*, 1–3. [CrossRef] [PubMed]

22. Newman, D.J.; Cragg, G.M. Natural products as sources of new drugs from 1981 to 2014. *J. Nat. Prod.* **2016**, *79*, 629–661. [CrossRef] [PubMed]

23. Newman, D.J. Developing natural product drugs: Supply problems and how they have been overcome. *Pharmacol. Ther.* **2016**, *162*, 1–9. [CrossRef] [PubMed]

24. Newman, D.J. Bioactive cyclic molecules and drug design. *Expert Opin. Drug Discov.* **2018**, *13*, 379–385. [CrossRef] [PubMed]

25. Shanmugam, M.K.; Lee, J.H.; Chai, E.Z.; Kanchi, M.M.; Kar, S.; Arfuso, F.; Dharmarajan, A.; Kumar, A.P.; Ramar, P.S.; Looi, C.Y.; et al. Cancer prevention and therapy through the modulation of transcription factors by bioactive natural compounds. *Semin. Cancer Biol.* **2016**, *40–41*, 35–47. [CrossRef] [PubMed]

26. Shanmugam, M.K.; Nguyen, A.H.; Kumar, A.P.; Tan, B.K.; Sethi, G. Targeted inhibition of tumor proliferation, survival, and metastasis by pentacyclic triterpenoids: Potential role in prevention and therapy of cancer. *Cancer Lett.* **2012**, *320*, 158–170. [CrossRef] [PubMed]

27. Shanmugam, M.K.; Warrier, S.; Kumar, A.P.; Sethi, G.; Arfuso, F. Potential role of natural compounds as anti-angiogenic agents in cancer. *Curr. Vasc. Pharmacol.* **2017**, *15*, 503–519. [CrossRef] [PubMed]

28. Mishra, K.P.; Ganju, L.; Sairam, M.; Banerjee, P.K.; Sawhney, R.C. A review of high throughput technology for the screening of natural products. *Biomed. Pharmacother.* **2008**, *62*, 94–98. [CrossRef] [PubMed]

29. Cragg, G.M.; Grothaus, P.G.; Newman, D.J. Impact of natural products on developing new anti-cancer agents. *Chem. Rev.* **2009**, *109*, 3012–3043. [CrossRef] [PubMed]

30. Harvey, A.L.; Edrada-Ebel, R.; Quinn, R.J. The re-emergence of natural products for drug discovery in the genomics era. *Nat. Rev. Drug Discov.* **2015**, *14*, 111–129. [CrossRef] [PubMed]

31. Newman, D.J. Natural products as leads to potential drugs: An old process or the new hope for drug discovery? *J. Med. Chem.* **2008**, *51*, 2589–2599. [CrossRef] [PubMed]

32. Chai, E.Z.; Siveen, K.S.; Shanmugam, M.K.; Arfuso, F.; Sethi, G. Analysis of the intricate relationship between chronic inflammation and cancer. *Biochem. J.* **2015**, *468*, 1–15. [CrossRef] [PubMed]

33. Sung, B.; Prasad, S.; Yadav, V.R.; Aggarwal, B.B. Cancer cell signaling pathways targeted by spice-derived nutraceuticals. *Nutr. Cancer* **2012**, *64*, 173–197. [CrossRef] [PubMed]

34. Newman, D.J.; Cragg, G.M. Current status of marine-derived compounds as warheads in anti-tumor drug candidates. *Mar. Drugs* **2017**, *15*, 99. [CrossRef] [PubMed]

35. Newman, D.J.; Cragg, G.M. Drugs and drug candidates from marine sources: An assessment of the current "state of play". *Planta Med.* **2016**, *82*, 775–789. [CrossRef] [PubMed]

36. El Bairi, K.; Ouzir, M.; Agnieszka, N.; Khalki, L. Anticancer potential of trigonella foenum graecum: Cellular and molecular targets. *Biomed. Pharmacother.* **2017**, *90*, 479–491. [CrossRef] [PubMed]

37. Shabbeer, S.; Sobolewski, M.; Anchoori, R.K.; Kachhap, S.; Hidalgo, M.; Jimeno, A.; Davidson, N.; Carducci, M.A.; Khan, S.R. Fenugreek: A naturally occurring edible spice as an anticancer agent. *Cancer Biol. Ther.* **2009**, *8*, 272–278. [CrossRef] [PubMed]

38. Aggarwal, B.B.; Kunnumakkara, A.B.; Harikumar, K.B.; Tharakan, S.T.; Sung, B.; Anand, P. Potential of spice-derived phytochemicals for cancer prevention. *Planta Med.* **2008**, *74*, 1560–1569. [CrossRef] [PubMed]

39. Kenny, O.; Smyth, T.J.; Hewage, C.M.; Brunton, N.P. Antioxidant properties and quantitative UPLC-MS analysis of phenolic compounds from extracts of Fenugreek (*Trigonella foenum-graecum*) seeds and bitter melon (*Momordica charantia*) fruit. *Food Chem.* **2013**, *141*, 4295–4302. [CrossRef] [PubMed]

40. Wani, S.A.; Kumar, P. Fenugreek: A review on its nutraceutical properties and utilization in various food products. *J. Saudi Soc. Agric. Sci.* **2018**, *17*, 97–106. [CrossRef]

41. Kim, J.K.; Park, S.U. An update on the biological and pharmacological activities of diosgenin. *EXCLI J.* **2018**, *17*, 24–28. [PubMed]

42. Bahmani, M.; Shirzad, H.; Mirhosseini, M.; Mesripour, A.; Rafieian-Kopaei, M. A review on ethnobotanical and therapeutic uses of Fenugreek (*Trigonella foenum-graceum* L.). *J. Evid. Based Complement. Altern. Med.* **2016**, *21*, 53–62. [CrossRef] [PubMed]

43. Srinivasan, K. Fenugreek (*Trigonella foenum-graecum*): A review of health beneficial physiological effects. *Food Rev. Int.* **2006**, *22*, 203–224. [CrossRef]

44. Jesus, M.; Martins, A.P.; Gallardo, E.; Silvestre, S. Diosgenin: Recent highlights on pharmacology and analytical methodology. *J. Anal. Methods Chem.* **2016**, *2016*, 4156293. [CrossRef] [PubMed]

45. Yang, S.F.; Weng, C.J.; Sethi, G.; Hu, D.N. Natural bioactives and phytochemicals serve in cancer treatment and prevention. *Evid. Based Complement. Altern. Med.* **2013**, *2013*, 698190. [CrossRef] [PubMed]

46. Djerassi, C.; Rosenkranz, G.; Pataki, J.; Kaufmann, S. Steroids, xxvii. Synthesis of allopregnane-3beta, 11beta, 17alpha-, 20beta, 21-pentol from cortisone and diosgenin. *J. Biol. Chem.* **1952**, *194*, 115–118. [PubMed]

47. Patel, K.; Gadewar, M.; Tahilyani, V.; Patel, D.K. A review on pharmacological and analytical aspects of diosmetin: A concise report. *Chin. J. Integr. Med.* **2013**, *19*, 792–800. [CrossRef] [PubMed]

48. Chen, Y.; Tang, Y.M.; Yu, S.L.; Han, Y.W.; Kou, J.P.; Liu, B.L.; Yu, B.Y. Advances in the pharmacological activities and mechanisms of diosgenin. *Chin. J. Nat. Med.* **2015**, *13*, 578–587. [CrossRef]

49. Tang, Y.; Yi, T.; Chen, H.; Zhao, Z.; Liang, Z.; Chen, H. Quantitative comparison of multiple components in dioscorea nipponica and d. Panthaica by ultra-high performance liquid chromatography coupled with quadrupole time-of-flight mass spectrometry. *Phytochem. Anal.* **2013**, *24*, 413–422. [CrossRef] [PubMed]

50. Tang, Y.N.; Pang, Y.X.; He, X.C.; Zhang, Y.Z.; Zhang, J.Y.; Zhao, Z.Z.; Yi, T.; Chen, H.B. UPLC-QTOF-MS identification of metabolites in rat biosamples after oral administration of dioscorea saponins: A comparative study. *J. Ethnopharmacol.* **2015**, *165*, 127–140. [CrossRef] [PubMed]

51. Ciura, J.; Szeliga, M.; Grzesik, M.; Tyrka, M. Next-generation sequencing of representational difference analysis products for identification of genes involved in diosgenin biosynthesis in Fenugreek (*Trigonella foenum-graecum*). *Planta* **2017**, *245*, 977–991. [CrossRef] [PubMed]

52. Vaidya, K.; Ghosh, A.; Kumar, V.; Chaudhary, S.; Srivastava, N.; Katudia, K.; Tiwari, T.; Chikara, S.K. De novo transcriptome sequencing in *Trigonella foenum-graecum* L. to identify genes involved in the biosynthesis of diosgenin. *Plant. Genome* **2013**, *6*, 1–11. [CrossRef]

53. Chiang, C.T.; Way, T.D.; Tsai, S.J.; Lin, J.K. Diosgenin, a naturally occurring steroid, suppresses fatty acid synthase expression in HER2-overexpressing breast cancer cells through modulating Akt, mTOR and JNK phosphorylation. *FEBS Lett.* **2007**, *581*, 5735–5742. [CrossRef] [PubMed]

54. Li, F.; Fernandez, P.P.; Rajendran, P.; Hui, K.M.; Sethi, G. Diosgenin, a steroidal saponin, inhibits STAT3 signaling pathway leading to suppression of proliferation and chemosensitization of human hepatocellular carcinoma cells. *Cancer Lett.* **2010**, *292*, 197–207. [CrossRef] [PubMed]

55. Moalic, S.; Liagre, B.; Corbiere, C.; Bianchi, A.; Dauca, M.; Bordji, K.; Beneytout, J.L. A plant steroid, diosgenin, induces apoptosis, cell cycle arrest and cox activity in osteosarcoma cells. *FEBS Lett.* **2001**, *506*, 225–230. [CrossRef]

56. Chen, P.S.; Shih, Y.W.; Huang, H.C.; Cheng, H.W. Diosgenin, a steroidal saponin, inhibits migration and invasion of human prostate cancer pc-3 cells by reducing matrix metalloproteinases expression. *PLoS ONE* **2011**, *6*, e20164. [CrossRef] [PubMed]

57. Raju, J.; Rao, C.V. Diosgenin, a steroid saponin constituent of yams and fenugreek: Emerging evidence for applications. In *Bioactive Compounds Medicine in Phytomedicine*; Rasooli, I., Ed.; InTech.: London, UK, 2012; pp. 125–142.

58. Shishodia, S.; Aggarwal, B.B. Diosgenin inhibits osteoclastogenesis, invasion, and proliferation through the downregulation of Akt, I kappa B kinase activation and NF-kappa B-regulated gene expression. *Oncogene* **2006**, *25*, 1463–1473. [CrossRef] [PubMed]

59. Das, S.; Dey, K.K.; Dey, G.; Pal, I.; Majumder, A.; MaitiChoudhury, S.; kundu, S.C.; Mandal, M. Antineoplastic and apoptotic potential of traditional medicines thymoquinone and diosgenin in squamous cell carcinoma. *PLoS ONE* **2012**, *7*, e46641. [CrossRef] [PubMed]

60. Lepage, C.; Leger, D.Y.; Bertrand, J.; Martin, F.; Beneytout, J.L.; Liagre, B. Diosgenin induces death receptor-5 through activation of p38 pathway and promotes trail-induced apoptosis in colon cancer cells. *Cancer Lett.* **2011**, *301*, 193–202. [CrossRef] [PubMed]

61. Romero-Hernandez, L.L.; Merino-Montiel, P.; Montiel-Smith, S.; Meza-Reyes, S.; Vega-Baez, J.L.; Abasolo, I.; Schwartz, S., Jr.; Lopez, O.; Fernandez-Bolanos, J.G. Diosgenin-based thio(seleno)ureas and triazolyl glycoconjugates as hybrid drugs. Antioxidant and antiproliferative profile. *Eur. J. Med. Chem.* **2015**, *99*, 67–81. [CrossRef] [PubMed]

62. Cai, B.; Liao, A.; Lee, K.K.; Ban, J.S.; Yang, H.S.; Im, Y.J.; Chun, C. Design, synthesis of methotrexate-diosgenin conjugates and biological evaluation of their effect on methotrexate transport-resistant cells. *Steroids* **2016**, *116*, 45–51. [CrossRef] [PubMed]

63. Jiang, S.; Fan, J.; Wang, Q.; Ju, D.; Feng, M.; Li, J.; Guan, Z.B.; An, D.; Wang, X.; Ye, L. Diosgenin induces ros-dependent autophagy and cytotoxicity via mtor signaling pathway in chronic myeloid leukemia cells. *Phytomedicine* **2016**, *23*, 243–252. [CrossRef] [PubMed]

64. Jagadeesan, J.; Langeswaran, K.; Gowthamkumar, S.; Balasubramanian, M.P. Diosgenin exhibits beneficial efficiency on human mammary carcinoma cell line MCF-7 and against N-nitroso-N-methylurea (NMU) induced experimental mammary carcinoma. *Biomed. Prev. Nutr.* **2013**, *3*, 381–388. [CrossRef]

65. Albini, A.; Tosetti, F.; Li, V.W.; Noonan, D.M.; Li, W.W. Cancer prevention by targeting angiogenesis. *Nat. Rev. Clin. Oncol.* **2012**, *9*, 498–509. [CrossRef] [PubMed]

66. Folkman, J. Tumor angiogenesis: Therapeutic implications. *N. Engl. J. Med.* **1971**, *285*, 1182–1186. [PubMed]

67. Folkman, J. Role of angiogenesis in tumor growth and metastasis. *Semin. Oncol.* **2002**, *29*, 15–18. [CrossRef] [PubMed]

68. Folkman, J. Angiogenesis: An organizing principle for drug discovery? *Nat. Rev. Drug Discov.* **2007**, *6*, 273–286. [CrossRef] [PubMed]

69. Selim, S.; Al Jaouni, S. Anti-inflammatory, antioxidant and antiangiogenic activities of diosgenin isolated from traditional medicinal plant, costus speciosus (Koen ex.Retz.) Sm. *Nat. Prod. Res.* **2016**, *30*, 1830–1833. [CrossRef] [PubMed]

70. He, Z.; Chen, H.; Li, G.; Zhu, H.; Gao, Y.; Zhang, L.; Sun, J. Diosgenin inhibits the migration of human breast cancer MDA-MB-231 cells by suppressing VAV2 activity. *Phytomedicine* **2014**, *21*, 871–876. [CrossRef] [PubMed]

71. Mao, Z.J.; Tang, Q.J.; Zhang, C.A.; Qin, Z.F.; Pang, B.; Wei, P.K.; Liu, B.; Chou, Y.N. Anti-proliferation and anti-invasion effects of diosgenin on gastric cancer BGC-823 cells with HIF-1alpha shrnas. *Int. J. Mol. Sci.* **2012**, *13*, 6521–6533. [CrossRef] [PubMed]

72. Srinivasan, S.; Koduru, S.; Kumar, R.; Venguswamy, G.; Kyprianou, N.; Damodaran, C. Diosgenin targets AKT-mediated prosurvival signaling in human breast cancer cells. *Int. J. Cancer* **2009**, *125*, 961–967. [CrossRef] [PubMed]

73. Sowmyalakshmi, S.; Ranga, R.; Gairola, C.G.; Chendil, D. Effect of diosgenin (Fenugreek) on breast cancer cells. *Proc. Am. Assoc. Cancer Res.* **2005**, *46*, 1382.

74. Corbiere, C.; Liagre, B.; Bianchi, A.; Bordji, K.; Dauca, M.; Netter, P.; Beneytout, J.L. Different contribution of apoptosis to the antiproliferative effects of diosgenin and other plant steroids, hecogenin and tigogenin, on human 1547 osteosarcoma cells. *Int. J. Oncol.* **2003**, *22*, 899–905. [CrossRef] [PubMed]

75. Liagre, B.; Bertrand, J.; Leger, D.Y.; Beneytout, J.L. Diosgenin, a plant steroid, induces apoptosis in COX-2 deficient K562 cells with activation of the p38 map kinase signalling and inhibition of NF-kappaB binding. *Int. J. Mol. Med.* **2005**, *16*, 1095–1101. [CrossRef] [PubMed]

Nutrients **2018**, *10*, 645

76. Leger, D.Y.; Liagre, B.; Corbiere, C.; Cook-Moreau, J.; Beneytout, J.L. Diosgenin induces cell cycle arrest and apoptosis in hel cells with increase in intracellular calcium level, activation of CPLA2 and COX-2 overexpression. *Int. J. Oncol.* **2004**, *25*, 555–562. [CrossRef] [PubMed]

77. Corbiere, C.; Liagre, B.; Terro, F.; Beneytout, J.L. Induction of antiproliferative effect by diosgenin through activation of p53, release of apoptosis-inducing factor (AIF) and modulation of caspase-3 activity in different human cancer cells. *Cell. Res.* **2004**, *14*, 188–196. [CrossRef] [PubMed]

78. Wang, S.L.; Cai, B.; Cui, C.B.; Liu, H.W.; Wu, C.F.; Yao, X.S. Diosgenin-3-O-alpha-L-rhamnopyranosyl-(1→4)-beta-d-glucopyranoside obtained as a new anticancer agent from dioscorea futschauensis induces apoptosis on human colon carcinoma HCT-15 cells via mitochondria-controlled apoptotic pathway. *J. Asian Nat. Prod. Res.* **2004**, *6*, 115–125. [CrossRef] [PubMed]

79. Raju, J.; Patlolla, J.M.; Swamy, M.V.; Rao, C.V. Diosgenin, a steroid saponin of *Trigonella foenum graecum* (Fenugreek), inhibits azoxymethane-induced aberrant crypt foci formation in F344 rats and induces apoptosis in HT-29 human colon cancer cells. *Cancer Epidemiol. Biomarkers Prev.* **2004**, *13*, 1392–1398. [PubMed]

80. Malisetty, V.S.; Patlolla, J.M.R.; Raju, J.; Marcus, L.A.; Choi, C.L.; Rao, C.V. Chemoprevention of colon cancer by diosgenin, a steroidal saponin constituent of fenugreek. *Proc. Am. Assoc. Cancer Res.* **2005**, *46*, 2473.

81. Miyoshi, N.; Nagasawa, T.; Mabuchi, R.; Yasui, Y.; Wakabayashi, K.; Tanaka, T.; Ohshima, H. Chemoprevention of azoxymethane/dextran sodium sulfate-induced mouse colon carcinogenesis by freeze-dried yam sanyaku and its constituent diosgenin. *Cancer Prev. Res. (Phila.)* **2011**, *4*, 924–934. [CrossRef] [PubMed]

82. Yan, L.L.; Zhang, Y.J.; Gao, W.Y.; Man, S.L.; Wang, Y. In vitro and in vivo anticancer activity of steroid saponins of paris polyphylla var. Yunnanensis. *Exp. Oncol.* **2009**, *31*, 27–32. [PubMed]

83. Marker, R.E.; Sterols, C.V. The preparation of testosterone and related compounds from sarsasapogenin and diosgenin. *J. Am. Chem. Soc.* **1940**, *62*, 2543–2547. [CrossRef]

84. Tietze, L.F.; Bell, H.P.; Chandrasekhar, S. Natural product hybrids as new leads for drug discovery. *Angew. Chem. Int. Ed.* **2003**, *42*, 3996–4028. [CrossRef] [PubMed]

85. Sanchez-Sanchez, L.; Hernandez-Linares, M.G.; Escobar, M.L.; Lopez-Munoz, H.; Zenteno, E.; Fernandez-Herrera, M.A.; Guerrero-Luna, G.; Carrasco-Carballo, A.; Sandoval-Ramirez, J. Antiproliferative, cytotoxic, and apoptotic activity of steroidal oximes in cervicouterine cell lines. *Molecules* **2016**, *21*, 1533. [CrossRef] [PubMed]

86. Masood Ur, R.; Mohammad, Y.; Fazili, K.M.; Bhat, K.A.; Ara, T. Synthesis and biological evaluation of novel 3-O-tethered triazoles of diosgenin as potent antiproliferative agents. *Steroids* **2017**, *118*, 1–8. [CrossRef] [PubMed]

87. Liu, C.; Xie, F.; Zhao, G.D.; Wang, D.F.; Lou, H.X.; Liu, Z.P. Synthetic studies towards 1alpha-hydroxysolasodine from diosgenin and the unexpected tetrahydrofuran ring opening in the birch reduction process. *Steroids* **2015**, *104*, 214–219. [CrossRef] [PubMed]

88. Hamid, A.A.; Kaushal, T.; Ashraf, R.; Singh, A.; Chand Gupta, A.; Prakash, O.; Sarkar, J.; Chanda, D.; Bawankule, D.U.; Khan, F.; et al. (22beta,25R)-3beta-hydroxy-spirost-5-en-7-iminoxy-heptanoic acid exhibits anti-prostate cancer activity through caspase pathway. *Steroids* **2017**, *119*, 43–52. [CrossRef] [PubMed]

89. Ghosh, S.; More, P.; Derle, A.; Kitture, R.; Kale, T.; Gorain, M.; Avasthi, A.; Markad, P.; Kundu, G.C.; Kale, S.; et al. Diosgenin functionalized iron oxide nanoparticles as novel nanomaterial against breast cancer. *J. Nanosci. Nanotechnol.* **2015**, *15*, 9464–9472. [CrossRef] [PubMed]

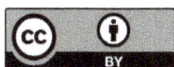

nutrients

MDPI

Article

α-Chaconine and α-Solanine Inhibit RL95-2 Endometrium Cancer Cell Proliferation by Reducing Expression of Akt (Ser473) and ERα (Ser167)

Ayşe Kübra Karaboğa Arslan * and Mükerrem Betül Yerer *

Department of Pharmacology, Faculty of Pharmacy, Erciyes University, Kayseri 38039, Turkey
* Correspondence: aysekubrakaraboga@gmail.com (A.K.K.A.); eczbetul@yahoo.com (M.B.Y.);
  Tel.: +90-352-207-66-66 (ext. 28277) (A.K.K.A.); +90-352-206-77-77 (ext. 28275) (M.B.Y.)

Received: 18 April 2018; Accepted: 23 May 2018; Published: 25 May 2018

Abstract: The aim of this study is to investigate the potential inhibitory effect of α-chaconine and α-solanine on RL95-2 estrogen receptor (ER) positive human endometrial cancer cell line and to identify the effect of these glycoalkaloids on the Akt signaling and ERα. The cell proliferation profiles and the cytotoxicity studies were performed by Real-Time Cell Analyzer (xCELLigence) and compared with Sulphorhodamine B (SRB) assay. The effects of α-chaconine (2.5, 5, 10 µM), α-solanine (20, 30, 50 µM), API-1 (25 µM) and MPP (20 µM) effects on Akt (Ser473) and ERα (Ser167) expressions evaluated by Western blot and qPCR method. Their IC_{50} values were as α-chaconine (4.72 µM) < MPP (20.01 µM) < α-solanine (26.27 µM) < API-1 (56.67 µM). 10 µM α-chaconine and 20, 30 and 50 µM α-solanine were effective in decreasing p-Akt(Ser473)/Akt ratio compared to positive control API-1. When the p-ERα/ERα ratios were evaluated, it was observed that α-chaconine (2.5, 5, 10 µM) and α-solanine (50 µM) were as effective as the specific ERα inhibitor MPP in reducing the ratio of p-ERα/ERα compared to the control group. In conclusion, it has been shown that the proliferation of α-chaconine and α-solanine in human endometrial carcinoma cells reduces the expression and activity of the Akt and ERα signaling pathway.

Keywords: α-chaconine; α-solanine; *Solanum tuberosum* L.; API-1; MPP dihydrochloride; RL95-2; endometrium cancer; steroidal glycoalkaloids; Akt; ERα

---

1. Introduction

Glycoalkaloids, a class of nitrogen-containing steroidal glycosides, are biologically active secondary plant metabolites, usually found in plants of the genus Solanum. These plants include many agricultural plants, especially the plants from Solanaceae family such as *Solanum tuberosum* L. (potato), *Solanum lycopersicum* (tomato) and *Solanum melongena* (eggplant) [1]. *S. tuberosum* L. (potato) contains significant amount of glycoalkaloids α-chaconine and α-solanine, which are trisaccharide steroidal glycoalkaloids [2].

S. tuberosum glycoalkaloids are naturally produced and the main glycoalkaloids are α-chaconine and α-solanine, which make up 95% of the total glycoalkaloid content. The molecules of both substances contain the same steroid scaffold (aglycone), but differ in the trisaccharide moiety [1]. Steroidal glycoalkaloids are produced from the cytosolic terpenoid (mevalonate) biosynthetic pathway. Cholesterol is produced starting from acetyl-CoA. Cholesterol is modified by various glycoalkaloid metabolism enzymes via hydroxylation, oxidation and transamination, and thus solanidine (Figure 1a) is synthesized in *S. tuberosum*. Aglycone solanidine is glycosylated by solanidine glycosyltransferase enzymes to produce α-solanine and α-chaconine [3,4]. α-Chaconine and α-solanine are derived from the compound solanidine and include a carbohydrate side-chain; the side-chain is composed of glucose and two rhamnose molecules and glucose, rhamnose and galactose molecules, respectively [5].

The glycoalkaloids are found at all parts of the potato plant. The highest glycoalkaloid level is in flowers and sprouts while the lowest glycoalkaloid level is in potato tubers. Glycoalkaloids are concentrated in the skins and the prolonged exposure of the tubers to the light promotes the formation of glycoalkaloids on the surface of the tuber [1]. Steroidal alkaloids and their glycosides are known to possess a variety of biological activities including anti-tumor [6], anti-fungal [7], anti-inflammatory [8], teratogenic [9], anti-viral [10], antimicrobial [11], antiestrogenic [12,13], antiandrogenic [14] and anti-cancer activities [15]. There are some studies related to the evaluation of α-chaconine and α-solanine which are naturally occurring toxic steroidal glycoalkaloids in potato sprouts effects on different cancer cells such as lymphoma and lung [16], prostate [17], cervical [18], stomach [19], melanoma [20], pancreatic [21], breast [22] and colorectal [23].

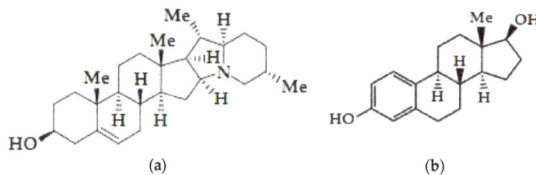

Figure 1. Structural similarities of the potato aglycone solanidine to the estradiol: (**a**) The molecular structure of solanidine; (**b**) The molecular structure of estradiol.

Endometrial cancer is the fifth most common gynecological malignancy in the world in 2012, but its incidence varies between regions [24,25]. In 2012, 320,000 new cases of endometrial cancer were diagnosed worldwide. The number of new cases is expected to increase by about 70% over the next 20 years [26]. Approximately 30% of patients diagnosed with endometrial cancer are under 54 years of age, with 20% between 45–54 years of age and approximately 9% under the age of 44. For this reason, it is necessary to carefully select women with fertility-protective approaches in managing endometrial cancer [27]. Because early detection and treatment modalities have not had a major influence on mortality and fertility, searching out and developing novel approaches for treatment of endometrial cancer is very important.

Akt, a serine-threonine protein kinase, central signaling molecule in the PI3K pathway and plays an important role in controlling the balance between cell survival and apoptosis [28]. Alterations in the Akt pathway have been identified in a variety of human cancer types, including endometrial cancer. Akt is activated by phosphorylation, on account of this Akt phosphorylation is a marker for the activation of this enzyme. The serine/threonine kinase Akt pathway integrates both extracellular and intracellular oncogenic signals, and therefore presents a promising new target for molecular therapeutics [29]. The central negative regulator of the Akt signaling cascade is the tumor suppressor gene PTEN. Mutations in PTEN result in notably increased Akt activity. PTEN mutations occur in 50% of endometrial carcinomas. Patients with increased Akt phosphorylation as a result of loss of PTEN expression have a poor prognosis. Consequently, targeting the Akt pathway may be an appropriate strategy in addressing endometrial cancer [30]. Selective inhibition of Akt represents a potential approach for the treatment of endometrium cancer. Akt/protein kinase B inhibitor, 4-amino-5,8-tetrahydro-5-oxo-8-(β-D-ribofuranosyl)pyrido[2,3-d]pyrimidine-6-carboxamide (API-1) is a novel, small molecule and potent selective inhibitor of Akt signaling that binds to the pleckstrin homology (PH) domain of Akt. It blocks its membrane translocation, which cause inhibition of Akt-regulated cell growth and cell survival *in vitro* and *in vivo* [31,32].

ERα plays a role in mediating the activity of estrogen [33]. The biological effects of 17β-estradiol (E2) (Figure 1b) are mainly mediated by ERα and estrogen receptor β (ERβ) receptors and ERα is primarily expressed in the uterus. E2 stimulates the growth of cancer cells as well as many type of cells [34]. Oncogenic transformation of cells in the uterus can initiate to the development of cancerous lesions and these lesions take advantage of E2 signaling pathways for growth [35]. Methyl-piperidino-pyrazole (MPP) is a highly selective ERα antagonist [36].

Although α-chaconine and α-solanine as being steroidal glycoalkaloid exhibit anti-carcinogenic potential against several cancer cell lines, its effect on endometrium cancer is still unclear. The aim of this study is to investigate the potential inhibitory effect of α-chaconine and α-solanine to clarify the potential of inhibiting proliferation, and to explain the effect of these glycoalkaloids on the Akt signaling and estrogen receptor α (ERα) in RL95-2, which is estrogen receptor (ER) positive human endometrial cancer cell line.

2. Materials and Methods

2.1. Materials

α-Chaconine (Cat No: A9544) was purchased from Applichem (Darmstadt, Germany), whereas α-solanine (Cat No: S3757) was Sigma (St. Louis, MO, USA). Chemical inhibitors API-1 (Cat No: 3897) and 1,3-Bis(4-hydroxyphenyl)-4-mtehyl-5-[4-(2-piperidiylethoxy) phenol]-1H-pyrazole dihydrochloride (MPP dihydrochloride) (Cat No: 1991) were purchased from Tocris bioscience (Bristol, UK). Stock solutions of α-chaconine, α-solanine and the chemical inhibitors were prepared in dimethyl sulfoxide (DMSO). DMSO (Cat No: A3672) and phosphate-buffered saline (PBS) (Cat No: A9177) were purchased from Applichem. Dulbecco's modified eagle's medium with F-12 nutrient mixture (DMEM: F-12) (Cat No: 01-170-1A) and penicillin/streptomycin solution (Cat No: 03-031-1C) were obtained from Biological Industries (Cromwell, CT, USA). Fetal bovine serum (FBS) (Cat No: S0115) obtained from Biochrom (Cambridge, UK). Insulin (Cat No: I9278), RNAzol (Cat No: R4533, Sigma) and trypsin-EDTA (T3924) were purchased from Sigma. Sulforhodamine B (SRB) sodium salt (Cat No: sc-253615A) and radio immuneprecipitation assay (RIPA) buffer (Cat No: sc-24948) were purchased from Santa Cruz Biotechnology (Heidelberg, Germany). Akt (Cat No: 9272), phospo-Akt (Ser473) (Cat No: 9271) and β-actin (Cat No: 4967) antibodies, estrogen receptor α (D8H8) rabbit mAb (Cat No: 8644), phospho-estrogen receptor α (Ser167) (D1A3) rabbit mAb (Cat No: 5587) and HRP-linked secondary antibody (Cat No: 7074) and BCA kit (Cat No: 7780) were purchased from Cell Signaling Technology, Inc (Leiden, The Netherlands). Reagents for electrophoresis and Western blotting were obtained from Sigma. Polyvinylidene difluoride (PVDF) membrane obtained from (Cat No: 162-0177) Bio-Rad (Dubai, United Arab Emirates). Chemiluminescence solution (ECL) (Cat No: 34080) obtained from Thermo Scientific (Paisley, UK). FastStart Essential DNA Probes Master (06 402 682 001), Transcriptor High Fidelity cDNA Synthesis Kit (05 081 955 001), RealTime ready human β-actin, Akt and ER-α catalog assays (05 532 957 001), E-plate (05 232 368 001), Cedex Smart Slides (05 650 801 001) were purchased from Roche (Roche, Laval, QC, Canada).

2.2. Cancer Cell Line and Culture

Human endometrial cancer cell lines RL95-2 was purchased from the American Type Cell Collection (Cat No: CRL-1671™ ATCC, Manassas, VA, USA). The cell line was grown in DMEM:F-12 that was supplemented with 10% (v/v) FBS, 1% penicillin/streptomycin and 0.005 mg/mL insulin. The cells were cultivated in 75 cm² culture flasks at 37 °C in humidify atmosphere of 95% air and 5% CO_2. When the cells had approximately reached 80% confluence, trypsin containing 0.25% EDTA was used to remove them from the flasks for subculture or for the corresponding experimental treatments. An inverted microscope was used to observe the changes in cell morphology. α-Chaconine, α-solanine, API-1 and MPP dihydrochloride were dissolved in DMSO and the final DMSO concentration in the medium was less than 0.1%.

2.3. Cell Growth and Proliferation Assay Using xCELLigence Real-Time Cell Analysis (RTCA)

The essence of the real-time growth profile is based on measuring the change in the adhesive properties of the cells as they are attached to the microelectrode-coated surface of special e-plates of xCELLigence system. Impedance measurement gives time quantitative information about the current state of cells such as cell number, viability, morphology and movement. Measurement is possible without using any label or chemicals. By eliminating the need for label or dye, it is possible to maximize the acquired data physiologically. The device's software allows real-time monitoring of the experiment and real-time data visualization and analysis functions [37,38].

RL95-2 cells were resuspended in the culture medium and then seeded, to e-plate of xCELLigence RTCA SP system (ACEA Biosciences Inc., San Diego, CA, USA). In this experiment, different number of cells varying from 1.250 to 40.000 were used to obtain growth profile of RL95-2 cell line. xCELLigence system calculates the impedances parameter called "Cell Index (CI)". CI values of RL95-2 were used to examine cell profile depending on proliferation and viability during 96 h. All experiments were performed at least three times.

2.4. Cytotoxicity Assay Using xCELLigence RTCA

According to SRB assay results, novel concentrations were determined in order to evaluate its effects on cell growth and proliferation of α-chaconine (1–10 μM), α-solanine (10–30 μM), API-1 (10–25 μM) and MPP dihydrochloride (5–50 μM). In brief, RL95-2 cells were seeded at a density of 20.000 cells per well of a 96-well E-plate (Catalog No. 05232368001; ACEA Biosciences, Inc., San Diego, CA, USA). The compounds added to cells at their growth phase. The assay was monitored during 96 h. Effects of α-chaconine, α-solanine, API-1 and MPP dihydrochloride on cell growth curve was assessed with the RTCA system xCELLigence. After obtaining cell profile data, another RTCA assay was performed by using 20.000 cells/100 μL per well to monitor the cytotoxicity of α-chaconine, α-solanine, API-1 and MPP dihydrochloride. Proliferation, spreading and cell attachment kinetics were monitored every 15 min. IC_{50} values were defined as the inhibition of the cell line by the compounds at 24 h. The RTCA software performs a curve-fitting of selected "sigmoidal dose–response equation" to the experimental data points and calculates logarithmic half maximum effect of concentration (log [IC_{50}]) values at a given time point based on log of concentration producing 50% reduction of CI value relative to solvent control CI value (100%), expresses as log IC_{50} [37,38]. All experiments were performed at least three times and the results were given as the mean ± Standart Deviation (SD) of independent experiments.

2.5. Determination of Cell Viability via Sulphorhodamine B Assay

The effect of α-chaconine, α-solanine, API-1 and MPP dihydrochloride on RL95-2 cell viability were determined by the method of SRB assay [39,40]. The compounds were dissolved in DMSO to a stock concentration of 50 mM. 20.000 cells/wells seeded and after 24 h incubation cells treated with different final concentrations of α-chaconine (1 nM-100 μM), α-solanine (1 nM-100 μM), API-1 (1–100 μM) and MPP dihydrochloride (1–100 μM) for 24 h, followed by fixing the cells in 10% (*v/v*) of trichloroacetic acid (TCA) for 1 h at 4 °C. After washing 5 times, cells were exposed to 0.5% (*w/v*) SRB solution for 30 min in a dark place and subsequently washed with 1% (*v/v*) acetic acid. After drying, 10 mM (pH 10.5) Tris base solution was used to dissolve the SRB-stained cells using a plate-shaker (PST-60 HL plus Biosan) and color intensity was measured at 510 nm in a microplate reader (Biotek Synergy HT). Data are represented as a percentage of control cells. The measurement of the "half maximal inhibitory concentration" (IC_{50}) values was calculated with the Microsoft Excel program. All experiments were performed at least three times and the results were given as the mean ± SD of independent experiments.

2.6. Protein Extraction and Western Blot Analysis

1×10^6 cells were seeded in 6 well plate to be left overnight and incubated with α-chaconine (2.5; 5; 10 μM), α-solanine (20; 30; 50 μM), API-1 (25 μM) and MPP dihydrochloride (20 μM) for 24 h. The cells were scraped using a cell scraper and centrifuged at 10.000 rpm for 10 min, after which the sample was rinsed again with PBS. Proteins were isolated with RIPA buffer. After cell lysates sonication, total protein contents were determined by using a BCA kit. A 10% separating and 5% stacking gel was prepared freshly on western blotting day. Electrophoresis was carried out at a voltage of 70 V, which was then raised to 100 V after the specimens had reached the separation gel. PVDF membrane was activated in 100% methanol for 10 s. The transfer was performed at 100 V for 1 h and 20 min in cold conditions. 5% non-fat dry milk in tris buffered saline with tween (TBST) was used for blockage for 1 h. Membranes were washed with TBST three times for 10 min. 1:1000 dilution of primary rabbit antibodies in TBST were applied to membrane and incubated overnight at 4 °C. The membranes were subsequently washed with TBST and incubated with a 1:2000 dilution of secondary antibody for 2 h at room temperature. After washing the membrane three times for 10 min in TBST, the proteins were visualized using ECL. Blue sensitive X-ray film was used for detection in a dark room. A Developer, water and fixer were used for photographic process. The band intensity was analyzed using Image J (ImageJ 1.48, ABD). β-actin was used for normalization. All experiments were performed three times and the results were given as the mean ± SD of independent experiments.

2.7. RNA Isolation and Quantitative Real-Time Polymerase Chain Reaction (qRT-PCR)

RL95-2 cells were seeded at a density of 1×10^6 cells per well of a 6-well plate and cells were harvested for RNA isolation 24 h after the treatment with α-chaconine (2.5; 5; 10 μM), α-solanine (20; 30; 50 μM), API-1 (25 μM) and MPP dihydrochloride (20 μM). Total RNA was isolated using RNAzol in accordance with the manufacturer's instructions. The RNA concentration and purity were determined by measurement of absorbance at 260 and 280 nm using a NanoDrop (DeNovix) and 1000 ng of each total RNA sample was used for cDNA synthesis with the Transcriptor High Fidelity cDNA Synthesis Kit (Roche, Quebec, Canada) according to the manufacturer's specifications. qRT-PCR was performed using the FastStart Essential DNA Probes Master (Roche, Quebec, Canada) with primers. The qRT-PCR primer sequences were as follows: *ACTB* 5′-TCCTCCCTGGAGAAGAGCTA-3′ (forward) and 5′-CGTGGATGCCACAGGACT-3′ (reverse); *AKT1*, 5′-GCAGCACGTGTACGAGAAGA-3′ (forward) and 5′-GGTGTCAGTCTCCGACGTG-3′ (reverse). *ESR1*, 5′-TTACTGACCAACCTGGCAGA-3′ (forward) and 5′-ATCATGGAGGGTCAAATCCA-3′ (reverse). Threshold cycle (C_T) values obtained from the instrument's software were used to calculate the fold change of the respective mRNAs. $\Delta\Delta C_T$ for each mRNA was calculated by subtracting the C_T value of the control from the experimental value. Fold change was calculated by the formula $2^{-\Delta\Delta CT}$. All experiments were performed at least three times and the results were given as the mean ± SD of independent experiments.

2.8. Statistical Analysis

All calculations from xCELLigence were obtained using the RTCA-integrated software of the xCELLigence system. Statistical analysis was performed GraphPad Prism Software Version 7.01 (La Jolla, CA, USA) using to compare differences in values between the control and experimental group. The results are expressed as the mean ± SD. Statistically significant values were compared using one-way ANOVA and Dunnett's post-hoc test, and p-values of less than 0.05 were considered statistically significant.

3. Results

3.1. Real Time Cell Growth Profile Curve

A cell number titration experiment is necessary to assess cell growth and proliferation and to decide the optimum cell number for further steps of the study. This approach not only helps to determine the appropriate seeding density but also the time for compound addition [37].

The dynamic cell proliferation of the RL95-2 cells was monitored for a period of 96 h, and the growth curves at different densities are shown in Figure 2. When we examined the growth profile of RL95-2 cells, it was seen that the CI values were low. The factors affecting the value of CI may include cell dimension, morphology and cell-substrate adhesion quality [37,41]. Lack of CI fluctuation in cell attachment and spreading stages was characteristic for RL95-2 cells. The growth curve after cell seeding showed a linear adhesion period that was followed by a continuous increase of CI for all tested densities. According to the growth profile of the cells, even after 96 h, it has been observed that the 20,000 cells/well did not reach the plateau and continued to proliferate at a constant rate. Densities of 10,000 cells/well and above were not considered suitable for further studies as their logarithmic phase lasted before than 20,000 cells/well. It was decided that the optimal cell number for the surface area of 0.20 cm^2/well was 20,000 cells/well. The density of 20,000 cells/well produced the most ideal growth curve for further experiments. Approximately 24-h after seeding was selected as the ideal time for compound addition.

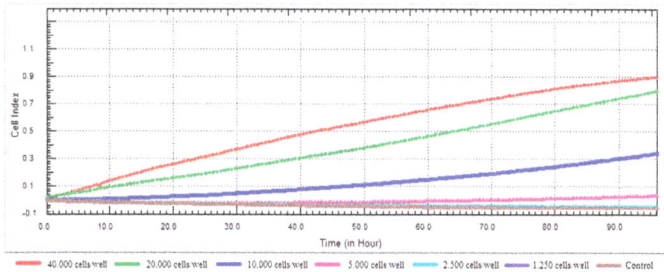

Figure 2. Dynamic monitoring of cell adhesion and proliferation using the xCELLigence system. RL95-2 cell at a density of 40,000; 20,000; 10,000; 5000; 2500; 1250 cells/well in E-Plates 96 were observed during 96 h.

3.2. Effects of the Compounds on the Cell Viability

This test is the first test elucidated the cytotoxic effect of API-1, MPP dihydrochloride, α-chaconine and α-solanine on RL95-2 endometrium cancer cells (Figures 3, 4, 5 and 6b). The cell viabilities in the presence of various concentrations of these compounds were analyzed by SRB assay. Seven different concentrations (1, 3, 5, 10, 25, 50 and 100 μM) of API-1, six different concentrations (1, 5, 10, 25, 50 and 100 μM) of MPP dihydrochloride, eight different concentrations (10 and 100 nM, 1, 5, 10, 25, 50 and 100 μM) of α-chaconine and α-solanine were selected to assess the effect of the compounds on cell viability over a wide range.

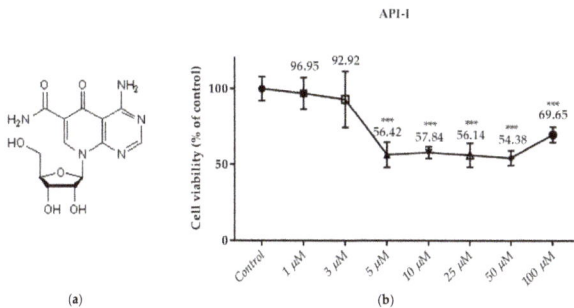

(a)   (b)

Figure 3. Dose dependent cytotoxic effects of API-1 was determined by SRB assay and shown for 24 h. (**a**) The molecular structure of API-1; (**b**) Effect of API-1 on viability of RL95-2 cell. Cells were treated with various concentrations of API-1 for 24 h. The absorbance was determined after 1 h-incubation of the cells with SRB. Cell viability is presented as the mean ± SD at least three independent experiments. *** $p < 0.001$ compared with the untreated control.

MPP dihydrochloride

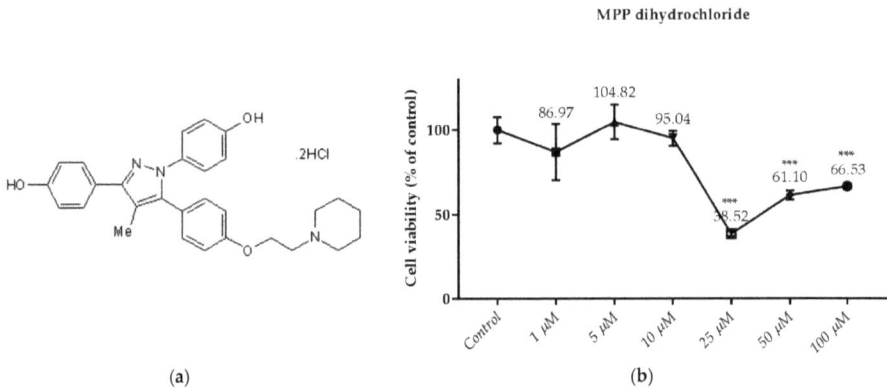

(a)

(b)

Figure 4. Dose dependent cytotoxic effects of MPP dihydrochloride was determined by SRB assay and shown for 24 h: (**a**) The molecular of MPP dihydrochloride; (**b**) Effect of MPP dihydrochloride on viability of RL95-2 cell. Cells were treated with various concentrations of MPP dihydrochloride for 24 h. The absorbance was determined after 1 h-incubation of the cells with SRB. Cell viability is presented as mean ± SD at least three independent experiments. *** $p < 0.001$ compared with the untreated control.

α-Chaconine

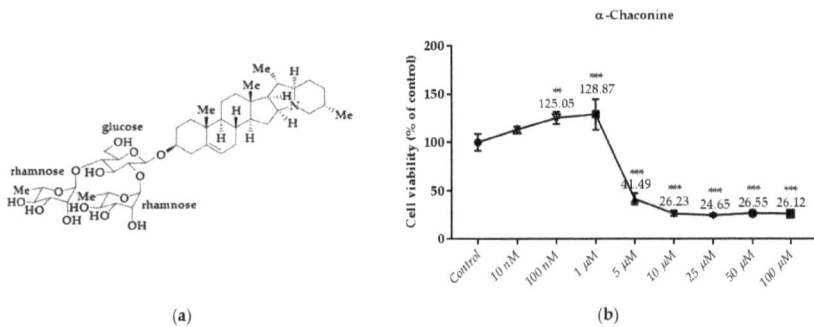

(a)

(b)

Figure 5. Dose dependent cytotoxic effects of α-chaconine was determined by SRB assay and shown for 24 h: (**a**) The molecular structure of α-chaconine; (**b**) Effect of α-chaconine on viability of RL95-2 cell. Cells were treated with various concentrations of α-chaconine for 24 h. Cell viability is presented as mean ± SD at least three independent experiments. ** $p < 0.01$ and *** $p < 0.001$ compared with the untreated control.

As shown in Figure 4b, the treatment of MPP dihydrochloride with 25; 50 and 100 μM for 24 h decreased cell viability significantly. However, cell viability was not significantly changed by MPP dihydrochloride at concentration below 25 μM.

At 1, 3, 5 and 10 μM concentrations there was no significant decrease compared to the control, whereas the cell viability did not change at higher than 5 μM. The next step was to work with a lower concentration of 25 μM, as it reduced viability at the same significance compared to the control at 25 and 50 μM concentration. In addition, the RTCA viability test results show a similar profile at concentrations of 10 and 25 μM, but supporting this, 25 μM concentration when evaluated together with the SRB assay results.

As shown in Figure 3b, the treatment of API-1 (5; 10; 25; 50 and 100 μM) for 24 h decreased cell viability significantly. However, cell viability was not significantly changed by API-1 at concentration below 5 μM.

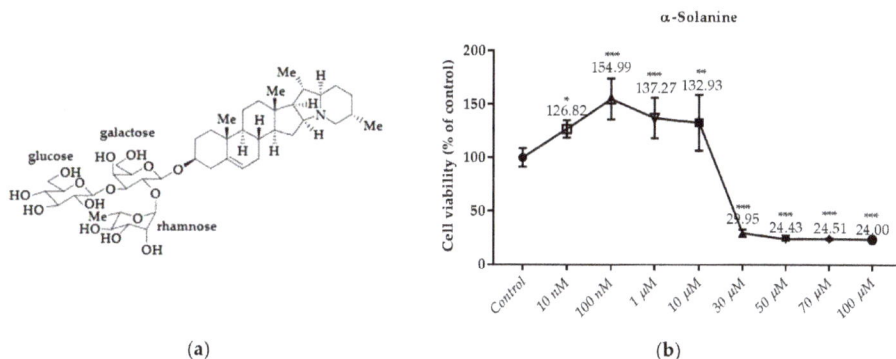

(a) (b)

Figure 6. Dose dependent cytotoxic effects of α-solanine was determined by SRB assay and shown for 24 h: (**a**) The molecular structure of α-solanine; (**b**) Effect of α-solanine on viability of RL95-2 cell. Cells were treated with various concentrations of α-solanine for 24 h. Cell viability is presented as mean ± SD at least three independent experiments. ** $p < 0.01$ and *** $p < 0.001$ compared with the untreated control.

As shown in Figure 5b, the treatment of α-chaconine with 5; 10; 25; 50 and 100 μM for 24 h decreased cell viability significantly. However, cell viability was not decreased by α-chaconine at concentrations below 5 μM.

α-Chaconine at concentrations of 5 μM and over were found to reduce viability in the same sense of significance compared to the control. However, at concentrations of 10 μM and higher it was considered cytotoxic since it reduced viability by more than 70% whereas α-chaconine decreased the viability by about 50% compared to the control at the concentration of 5 μM.

As shown in Figure 6b, the treatment of α-solanine with 30; 50; 70 and 100 μM for 24 h decreased cell viability significantly. However, cell viability did not decrease by α-solanine at concentration below 30 μM. It was found that the cytotoxicity produced by α-Solanine at 50 μM and higher concentrations did not increase due to the dose. A significant increase in α-solanine was observed at 10 μM compared to the control, and a decrease in viability was observed at 30 μM and over at the same concentrations.

3.3. Monitoring of Cytotoxicity in Real-Time Using xCELLigence System

To monitor and validate the reliability and accuracy of the SRB assay in evaluating the cytotoxic effects of the compounds, the cell viability was evaluated using the xCELLigence system in parallel with the studies above. As the cells interacted with these compounds, continuous CI alterations resulting from changes of cell number, morphology, and adhesion on the microelectrodes were measured by the RTCA SP instrument for approximately 72 h. A correlation was noted between results obtained from the impedance-based detection and those from SRB assay. As shown in Figures 3, 4, 5 and 6b, the concentration-response curves of the given time points marked with dashed lines in Figures 7–10 corresponded well with at the same dose of the xCELLigence system. The concentration-response curves and the viability of treated cells at the indicated time points are exhibited in Figures 7–10. Control groups without compound treatment indicated the normal cell growth in electronic microwells. As shown in Figure 7, the CI values of the treated cells decreased from 5 μM in a concentration-dependent manner after an initial rise, while the CI values of the control kept rising until the maximal value at about 72 h after the treatment. In order to compare the cytotoxic effects of the four compounds, their 50% inhibitory concentrations (IC_{50}) were calculated after 24-h exposure. The IC_{50} values of α-chaconine, α-solanine, API-1 and MPP dihydrochloride were 4.72, 26.27, 56.67 and 20.01 μM, respectively (Table 1).

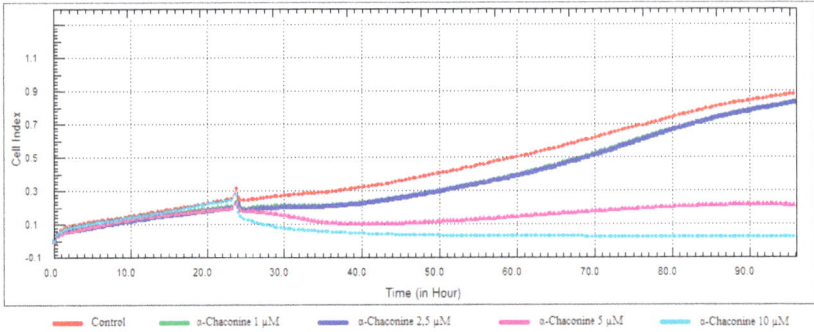

Figure 7. Dose and time-dependent cytotoxic effect and alteration of CI of α-chaconine determined by xCELLigence system: Effect of α-chaconine on proliferation of RL95-2 cell. Cells were treated with various concentrations of α-chaconine for 72 h. The CI was calculated from four repeated measurements.

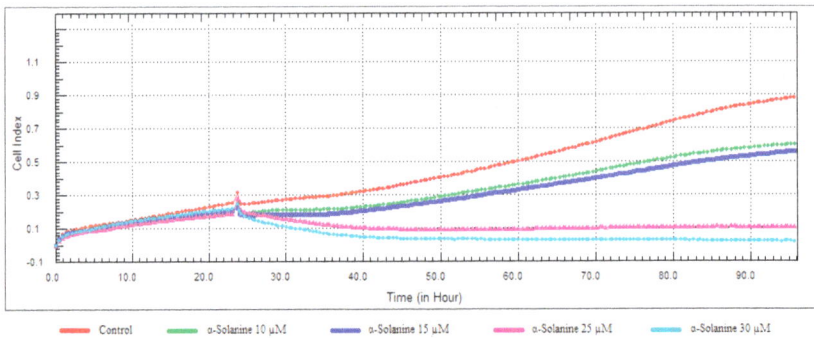

Figure 8. Dose and time-dependent cytotoxic effect and alteration of CI of α-solanine determined by xCELLigence system: Effect of α-solanine on proliferation of RL95-2 cell. Cells were treated with various concentrations of α-solanine for 72 h. The CI was calculated from four repeated measurements.

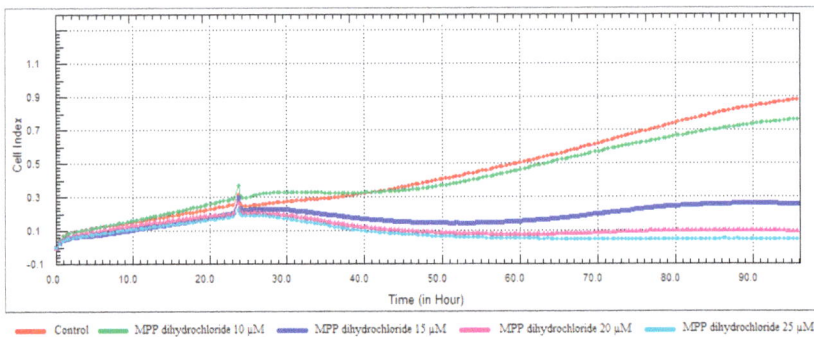

Figure 9. Dose and time-dependent cytotoxic effect and alteration of CI of MPP dihydrochloride determined by xCELLigence system: Effect of MPP dihydrochloride on proliferation of RL95-2 cell. Cells were treated with various concentrations of MPP dihydrochloride for 72 h. The CI was calculated from four repeated measurements.

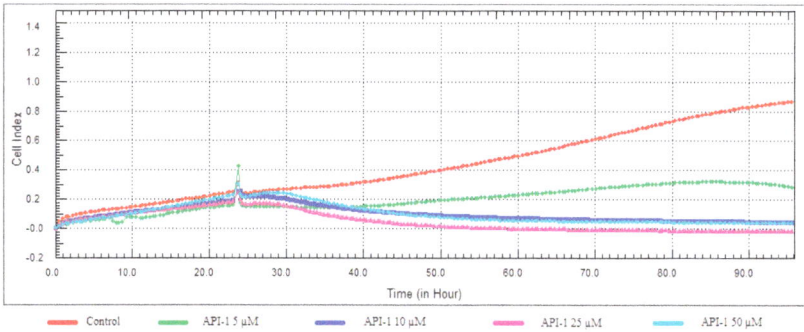

Figure 10. Dose and time-dependent cytotoxic effect and alteration of CI of API-1 determined by xCELLigence system: Effect of API-1 on proliferation of RL95-2 cell. Cells were treated with various concentrations of API-1 for 72 h. The CI was calculated from four repeated measurements.

Table 1. IC$_{50}$ values of RL95-2 cells for 24 h [1].

Compound	24 h
α-Chaconine	4.72 μM
α-Solanine	26.27 μM
API-1	56.67 μM
MPP dihydrochloride	20.01 μM

[1] The IC$_{50}$ of the four compounds were obtained based on the dose–response curves of CI during 24 h exposure in and calculated from repeated experiments (*n* = 4) with the real-time xCELLigence system.

α-Chaconine has an antiproliferative effect at concentrations of 1 and 2.5 μM; it was observed that cell viability decreased at concentrations of 5 and 10 μM in a dose-dependent manner (Figures 7 and 11). RTCA viability assay results showed similar profiles at 10 μM concentrations (Figure 5b), while 2.5 μM α-chaconine reduced viability by at least 70%. A decision was made to work with this concentration since the CI value was 50% change at 5 μM and was close to IC$_{50}$ (4.71 μM).

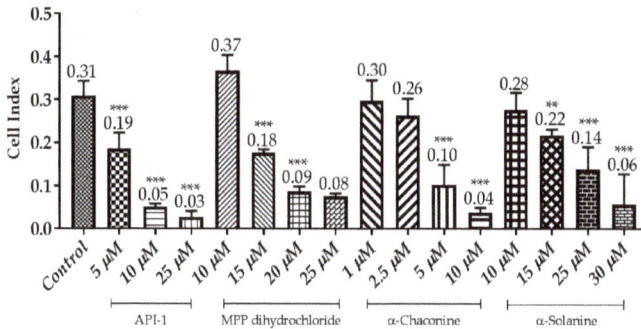

Figure 11. Correlation between cell index and the compounds effects using the xCELLigence system. Cells were treated with various concentrations of the compounds for 24 h. The CI was calculated from four repeated data and presented as mean ± SD. ** *p* < 0.01 and *** *p* < 0.001 compared with the untreated control.

It was observed that 10 and 15 μM concentrations of α-solanine had an antiproliferative effect and decreased cell viability at 25 and 30 μM concentrations (Figures 8 and 11). RTCA exhibited similar profiles to the control at concentrations of 10 and 15 μM according to the viability test results.

α-Solanine did not provide a 50% CI change at 25 μM concentration and was close to a value of 26.27, which was calculated as the IC_{50} value, therefore 30 μM concentration has been selected for further studies.

MPP dihydrochloride showed antiproliferative activity at a concentration of 10 μM, while cell viability decreased at concentrations of 15, 20 and 25 μM in a dose-dependent manner (Figures 9 and 11). According to RTCA and SRB results, IC_{50} value was calculated 20 μM for MPP dihydrochloride and this concentration was selected for further studies.

While 5 μM concentration of API-1 showed antiproliferative activity, cell viability was reduced at 10, 25 and 50 μM concentrations and the CI value at 25 μM concentration decreased to below 0.05 (Figures 10 and 11).

SRB and real-time xCELLigence measurements show that RL95-2 cells are more sensitive to α-chaconine then the other tested compounds (Table 1).

3.4. α-Chaconine, α-Solanine Inhibits Phosphorylation of Akt (Ser473) and ERα

Since Akt is crucial for cancer progression, being a critical mediator and required for metastasis, the effect of the glycoalkaloids were investigated on the activation of Akt.

Data demonstrated that API-1 reduced the phosphorylation of Akt (Figure 12a,c), while it did not alter the phosphorylation of ERα (Figure 12b,c). MPP dihydrochloride reduced the phosphorylation of ERα, while it did not alter the phosphorylation of Akt. The quantitative results showed that α-chaconine significantly suppressed the phosphorylation of Akt and ERα in a dose-dependent manner (Figure 12a–c). α-Solanine significantly suppressed the phosphorylation of Akt in a dose-depend manner except for 30 μM (Figure 12b,c).

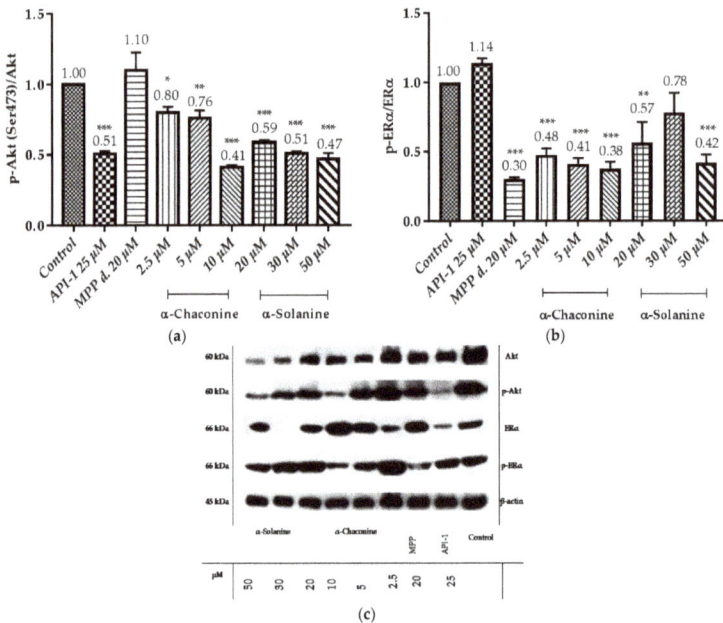

Figure 12. Western blot analysis of the expression of p-Akt, Akt, p-ERα and ERα proteins in the RL95-2 cell line: (**a**) In the bar graph the data represent the relative density of the bands p-Akt (Ser473)/Akt; (**b**) In the bar graph the data represent the relative density of the bands p-ERα/ERα; (**c**) RL95-2 cells were treated with the compounds. The relative intensity is presented as mean ± SD. three independent experiments. * $p < 0.1$, ** $p < 0.01$ and *** $p < 0.001$ compared with the untreated control.

3.5. Changes in the Expression of Akt and ERα Genes

Expression of genes associated with cancer progression was demonstrated by RT-qPCR (Figure 13a,b). It is demonstrated that α-chaconine and α-solanine suppressed the expression of Akt mRNA at concentration 5 μM and 30 μM, respectively as seen in Figure 13a. The results showed that API-1, α-chaconine and 30 μM α-solanine markedly suppressed the mRNA expression of ERα (Figure 13a,b).

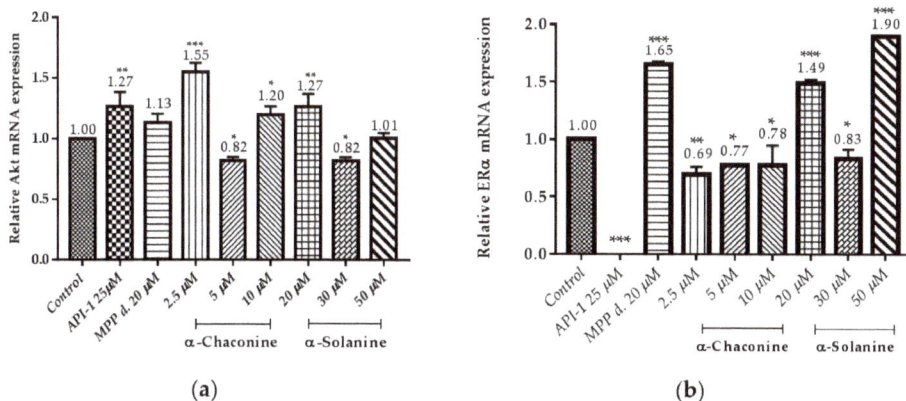

Figure 13. Effects of α-chaconine and α-solanine on suppressing the genes expression of: (a) Akt; (b) ERα in the RL95-2 cell line. The mRNA expressions were calculated from three repeated data and presented as mean ± SD. * $p < 0.1$, ** $p < 0.01$ *** $p < 0.001$ compared with the untreated control.

4. Discussion

The most basic steroidal trisaccharide glycoalkaloids are α-chaconine and α-solanine that are found in potato plants [16,20]. Solanidine, the aglycone of α-chaconine and α-solanine, shows structural similarities with diosgenin, the precursor of steroidal hormones. Solanidine is a nitrogen-containing equivalent of diosgenin (steroidal saponin) [42]. Although the potential toxicity of α-chaconine and α-solanine is well known, studies showing that they have beneficial effects such as anticholinesterase [43], anti-inflammatory [8], antibacterial [44], antiviral [10], antifungal [45], antimalarial [46] and anticancer [2] depending on dosage and use conditions are included in the literature.

α-Chaconine and α-solanine can cause toxicity in mouse and normal human liver cells in physiological functions [18,47]. Although the steroidal glycoalkaloids are toxic to normal cell membranes and lead to cell disruption [48], the compounds are thought to be possesses with the potential for therapeutic treatment against cancer cells. α-Chaconine exhibits anti-carcinogenic potential, including the ability to inhibit cell growth of various cancer cell lines in the human colon [49], lung [50,51], prostate [17], liver [18,52], cervical [18] cancer cells. Similarly, α-solanine exhibits anti-carcinogenic potentials, such as inhibiting cell growth of various cancer cell lines in human melanoma [20], prostate [2,52], pancreatic [21] and mice breast [22], lung [51] cancer cells. However, no information was available in the literature regarding whether it is effective in combatting endometrial cancer, and the effects on endometrial cancer were investigated for the first time in this study.

In endometrial cancer, inhibition of both extrinsic (Fas proteins) and intrinsic (Bcl-2 protein family) apoptotic pathways, alterations in PI3K/Akt activity and p53 mutation are known resistance mechanisms. Progressive and recurrent endometrial carcinomas continue to be a compelling tumor group with a high rate of multi-factor chemotherapy resistance. Chemotherapy resistance resulting from overexpression of drug flow efficacious proteins and mutations in β-tubulin isoforms in both primary and recurrent disease represent treatment difficulties. For this reason, the need for a less sensitive new agent for known resistance pathways arises [53]. The development of resistance to these drugs and the serious toxic effects of high doses lead researchers to search for different drug molecules.

When the effects of α-chaconine and α-solanine on cell viability is examined, most of the studies have been performed on various cell culture lines and confirm our findings [16,20,50,54]. The IC_{50} values of α-solanine in HepG2, human gastric carcinoma (SGC-7901) and human large intestine cancer (LS-174) cells were 14.47, >50 and >50 µg/mL, respectively, and HepG2 cells were more sensitive to α-solanine [55]. The IC_{50} value of α-solanine was found to be 34 µM in mouse mammary carcinoma cells (4T1) and 30 µM in human hepatocellular carcinoma cells (HuH-7) [22]. These findings agree with the IC_{50} value of our study of α-solanine. In our study, glycoalkaloids were not combined. However, it is shown that α-chaconine has a more acute toxicity in RL95-2 than α-solanine. According to our findings, α-chaconine increased cell viability at concentrations of 1 µM and lower at 10 µM and lower concentrations of α-solanine, similar to steroidal hormones [56] in the structure of solanidine, the aglycone of these glycoalkaloids, it was evaluated that they could be responsible for this effect.

Since α-chaconine and α-solanine have decreased both cell proliferation and apoptosis-inducing effects in different cancer types as mentioned above, we decided to investigate the effects of these compounds with API -1 and MPP in regulation of Akt and ERα signaling in estrogen-positive RL95-2 cells.

In this study, SRB cytotoxicity assay was chosen to give better linearity and signal-to-noise ratio than sensitive, simple, and formazan-based experiments when measuring the effect of α-chaconine and α-solanine on viability in RL95-2 cells [57].

Supporting the previous data with α-solanidine with MCF-7 cells, α-solanine significantly increased the viability relative to control group up to a concentration of 10 µM [56].

We showed that α-chaconine and α-solanine reveal similar effects at different concentrations and these differences might be their glycone group, although the aglycones are the same. It is also possible to discover more effective molecules by synthesizing chemical derivatives. The inhibition is related to a concentration—but not time—dependent manner. Both compounds might have an even stronger effect than API-1 and MPP dihydrochloride, although there was no significant difference between their IC_{50} values in this study. Their cytotoxic efficacy on RL95-2 cells was α-chaconine > MPP dihydrochloride > α-solanine > API-1. Thus, more studies should be conducted to investigate the activity of these compounds especially these steroidal glycoalkaloids. In this in vitro study, the activity of these glycoalkaloids and the potential structure–activity relationship was shown, and further in vivo investigation about the cellular mechanisms should be conducted in the future. As shown in Figures 5a and 6a, all the two steroidal glycoalkaloids have same aglycone but not glycone side chain. The cytotoxic effects of α-chaconine which contains chacotriose was significantly stronger than α-solanine with solatriose groups. Thus, the glycone groups besides aglycone ring might be an influencing factor for the cytotoxicity effects of potatoes steroidal glycoalkaloids on RL95-2 cells. There is another study in the literature where this effect is seen in different cell lines supporting our results [19].

When the effects of both glycoalkaloids on cell viability is examined, some of the studies have been performed on various cell culture lines and confirm our findings. From the results obtained, it can be concluded that α-chaconine can decrease phosphorylation of ERα as the same significance in positive control MPP dihydrochloride on RL95-2 cells whereas the specific Akt inhibitor API-1 did not show any effect on ERα phosphorylation. It has been shown for the first time that it may be related to the steroidal aglycone solanidine structure that they might have on the estrogen-dependent pathways on endometrium cancer cell line. This study showed for the first time the effect of α-chaconine on cell proliferation, ERα activity and expression in RL95-2 cells.

It has been shown that α-chaconine inhibits bovine aortic endothelial cell proliferation, migration and invasion. These effects have been shown to be mediated by JNK and PI3K/Akt signaling pathways and NF-κB activation by antiangiogenic activity [20]. α-Chaconine also showed anti-metastatic activity in human lung cancer cells A549. This effect has been shown to decrease MMP-2 and MMP-9 activities [50]. In another study, α-chaconine inhibited prostate cancer cells proliferation (LNCaP and PC-3) by increasing p27 levels and downregulating Cyclin D1, and apoptosis in these cells was associated with caspase-dependent and independent pathways. In addition, it has been shown that caspase-dependent apoptosis is induced via JNK activation in that study [17]. Beforehand α-solanine has been shown to inhibit metastasis, migration and invasion in human melanoma cells (A2058) by inhibiting JNK, PI3K, Akt phosphorylation and NF-κB activation and by decreasing MMP-2/9 activity/expression [20]. In another study, α-solanine down-regulated oncogenic microRNA-21 expression by decreasing MMP-2/9 expression via the ERK and PI3K/Akt signal pathway suppressed by human prostate cancer cell (PC-3) invasion and upregulated of tumor suppressor microRNA-138 [2]. α-Solanine has been shown to increase expression of radio-sensitivity and chemo-sensitivity by decreasing miR138 and focal adhesion kinase (FAK) expression in lung cancer cells (A549 and H1299) [58]. It has been reported in the literature that α-solanine acts as an antitumor agent in inhibition of Wnt/β-catenin, Akt/mTOR, Stat3 and NF-κB pathways in non-toxic concentrations in healthy cells and in pancreatic cancer cells (PANC-1) [21]. Another study has shown that α-solanine induces apoptosis by reducing the ratio of Bcl-2/Bax resulting in intracellular [Ca^{2+}]i, which can cause and alteration in the enzymatic activity of the caspase family in human hepatocarcinoma cells (HepG$_2$) [21]. In a study of the effects of α-solanine on the mitochondrial membrane potential and intracellular [Ca^{2+}]i in HepG2 cells, α-solanine resulted in lowering the membrane potential and reducing the Ca^{2+} concentration in the organs by facilitating the opening of the permeability transition (PT) channels in the mitochondria. This has been shown to increase the Ca^{2+} concentration in the cell and thus trigger the apoptosis mechanism [59]. Therefore, α-chaconine and α-solanine are thought to play an active role in the control of signal transduction pathways and signaling proteins and apoptosis-dependent or independent cell proliferative functions. However, so far, the mechanism of these steroidal glycoalkaloids actions and effects in endometrium cancer has not yet been elucidated. In this study it is found that α-chaconine may have led to an increase in cell viability related to an increase in mRNA overexpression of Akt compared with the control, but the level of growth factors in the environment is increased at the 2.5 μM concentration and should be investigated with different parameters in detail. The reason for preference for the investigation of Akt expressions of RL95-2 cells is the presence of active Akt in mutated PTEN human endometrial cancer cells [60]. In our study, it was found that API-1 25 μM strongly reduced p-Akt (Ser473) levels, resulting in RL95-2 cells sensitive to API-1. However, the relative p-Akt (Ser473) protein level results at a concentration of 10 μM α-solanine at 20, 30 and 50 μM α-chaconine were shown to be at the same level of significance as the 25 μM reduction of API-1. Thus, at these applied concentrations, α-chaconine and α-solanine were found to be as potent as API-1, the pure Akt inhibitor, inhibition of Akt phosphorylation. In our study, it was observed that 10 μM α-chaconine and 20, 30 and 50 μM α-solanine were effective in decreasing p-Akt (Ser473)/Akt ratio compared to control 25 μM API-1. At these concentrations, Akt was shown to act by reducing phosphorylation like API-1. This effect of α-chaconine and α-solanine was shown to be related to the dose and these findings were also confirmed in the RL95-2 cell of the α-chaconine A549 [50] and α-solanine [21] in the PANC-1 cells.

When the p-ERα/ERα ratios were evaluated, it was observed that α-chaconine (2.5, 5 and 10 μM), α-solanine (50 μM) and the specific ERα inhibitor was as effective as MPP dihydrochloride (20 μM) to reduce the ratio of p-ERα/ERα compared to the control group. At these concentrations, ERα, such as MPP dihydrochloride, was shown to be effective by reducing the phosphorylation. It has been shown for the first time that it may be effective in estrogen-dependent pathways and may be related to the steroidal aglycone solanidine structure. α-Chaconine showed this effect in a dose-dependent manner.

E2 stimulates the growth of many cancer cells. The mechanisms underpinning this effect include the blockade of MAPK/ERK and PI3K/Akt pathways that inhibit E2-induced DNA synthesis [34]. Estrogen-mediated signaling pathways are classified as genomic and non-genomic, depending on whether ER-dependence is transcriptionally regulated or not [61,62]. Taking into account the fact that RL95-2 cells are ER positive, we have investigated the effect of the compounds on the p-ERα/ERα expressions in these cells. In our study, p-ERα levels were increased α-chaconine (2.5, 5 μM) and α-solanine (20 μM) compared to the control group, and the increase in the concentration of α-chaconine 2.5 μM was found to be significant. This result is also consistent with the results of the RTCA and concludes that α-chaconine did not show cytotoxic effects up to 2.5 μM but may increase ERα phosphorylation through an estrogen receptor-dependent signaling pathway. However, contrary to protein expression, this decrease in mRNA level relative to control may be attributed to non-transcriptional activity of α-chaconine via non-genomic pathway using ERα interaction proteins and secondary messengers. This effect can also be caused by the estrogen-like effect of these steroidal compounds. The fact that RL95-2 cells are also ER positive confirms these results. The mRNA levels of Akt and ERα were decreased with α-chaconine and α-solanine at IC_{50} concentrations 5 and 30 μM respectively however these alterations were not concentration-dependent.

There are also limited data regarding the combination for these glycoalkaloids revealing that they have synergic toxic effects [63,64]. However, in our study the effects of the combination of these compounds has not been studied.

Furthermore, bioavailability of these compounds is not well-defined and there are a limited number of papers regarding the bioavailability of these glycoalkaloids [63,65,66]. Because of the steroidal structure and lipid solubility of the compounds they might probably go through pre-systemic elimination or enterohepatic cycle therefore the bioavailability of the compounds should be clarified with further in vivo studies.

Our study shows that α-chaconine and α-solanine have cytotoxic effects in RL95-2 cells, specifically affect cellular signaling pathways, and decrease phosphorylation of Akt and ERα. It is clear that there is a need for other scientific studies to be able to fully elucidate which mechanisms might be related to other effects. In addition, the scope of this study should be supported by expanded in vitro and in vivo studies. In this respect, α-chaconine and α-solanine are thought to be potential candidates for endometrial cancer therapy research.

5. Conclusions

In conclusion, we attributed the decrease in expression and activity of Akt and ERα by α-chaconine and α-solanine, and such suppressive effect might contribute to the inactivation of the PI3K/Akt and ERα signaling pathways in human endometrium cancer cells by both these steroidal glycoalkaloids. We demonstrated with a RL95-2 endometrial carcinoma cell line that α-chaconine and α-solanine alone seems to be as effective as both API-1 and MPP dihydrochloride. In ER positive cancers, active ER signaling is a pharmacological target so that ERα is a clinically important target for endometrial cancer. It is, therefore, necessary to carry out further research to explore novel candidates capable of both anti-estrogenic and cytotoxic potential. This should lead a strong insight into endometrial cancer therapy. In addition to this, steroidal glycoalkaloids which have anticancer potential to the estrogens, may also give further insight into endometrial cancer therapy. These findings reveal a new therapeutic potential for these glycoalkaloids on endometrial cancer therapy.

One of the main problems that should be taken into account while using such steroidal glycoalkaloids is the possible hormonal effects/interferences of these compounds on the physiological hormonal system. However, taking into account that conventional hormonal therapies are still being used for ERα positive endometrium cancer treatment, physicians should consider the benefit/risk ratio while treating these types of cancer, as this glycoalkaloids might be used to reduce the interference of these conventional hormonal therapies by lowering the doses with their synergistic effect which should be further investigated by in vivo studies.

On the other hand, it is possible to investigate whether pre- and combined estradiol administration to these glycoalkaloids leads to a change in Akt and ER expressions, and how it affects other endometrial cancer cell lines, Ishikawa and HEC-1A. When PI3K/Akt is thought to be one of the major signaling pathways in endometrial cancer, it is possible to investigate other signaling proteins associated with this pathway. It is also important to investigate whether the effects of these glycoalkaloids on cell migration are related to steroidal structural similarities.

Author Contributions: Conceptualization, A.K.K.A.; Methodology, A.K.K.A.; Formal Analysis, A.K.K.A. and M.B.Y.; Investigation, A.K.K.A.; Resources, M.B.Y.; Data Curation, A.K.K.A. and M.B.Y.; Writing-Original Draft Preparation, A.K.K.A. and M.B.Y.; Writing-Review & Editing, A.K.K.A. and M.B.Y.; Supervision, M.B.Y.; Project Administration, A.K.K.A. and M.B.Y.; Funding Acquisition, M.B.Y.

Acknowledgments: The present study was financially supported by Erciyes University Scientific Research Foundation (Project No: TDK-2014-5446).

Conflicts of Interest: The authors declare no conflict of interest.

References

1. Milner, S.E.; Brunton, N.P.; Jones, P.W.; O'Brien, N.M.; Collins, S.G.; Maguire, A.R. Bioactivities of glycoalkaloids and their aglycones from solanum species. *J. Agric. Food Chem.* **2011**, *59*, 3454–3484. [CrossRef] [PubMed]
2. Shen, K.H.; Liao, A.C.; Hung, J.H.; Lee, W.J.; Hu, K.C.; Lin, P.T.; Liao, R.F.; Chen, P.S. Alpha-solanine inhibits invasion of human prostate cancer cell by suppressing epithelial-mesenchymal transition and mmps expression. *Molecules* **2014**, *19*, 11896–11914. [CrossRef] [PubMed]
3. Cárdenas, P.; Sonawane, P.; Heinig, U.; Bocobza, S.; Burdman, S.; Aharoni, A. The bitter side of the nightshades: Genomics drives discovery in solanaceae steroidal alkaloid metabolism. *Phytochemistry* **2015**, *113*, 24–32. [CrossRef] [PubMed]
4. De Luca, A.; Maiello, M.R.; D'Alessio, A.; Pergameno, M.; Normanno, N. The RAS/RAF/MEK/ERK and the PI3K/AKT signalling pathways: Role in cancer pathogenesis and implications for therapeutic approaches. *Expert Opin. Ther. Targets* **2012**, *16*, S17–S27. [CrossRef] [PubMed]
5. Jiang, Q.W.; Chen, M.W.; Cheng, K.J.; Yu, P.Z.; Wei, X.; Shi, Z. Therapeutic potential of steroidal alkaloids in cancer and other diseases. *Med. Res. Rev.* **2016**, *36*, 119–143. [CrossRef] [PubMed]
6. Zhong, W.F.; Liu, S.P.; Pan, B.; Tang, Z.F.; Zhong, J.G.; Zhou, F.J. Solanine inhibits prostate cancer Du145 xenograft growth in nude mice by inducing cell cycle arrest in G1/S phase. *J. South. Med. Univ.* **2016**, *36*, 665–670.
7. Sánchez-Maldonado, A.F.; Schieber, A.; Gänzle, M.G. Antifungal activity of secondary plant metabolites from potatoes (*Solanum tuberosum* L.): Glycoalkaloids and phenolic acids show synergistic effects. *J. Appl. Microbiol.* **2016**, *120*, 955–965. [CrossRef] [PubMed]
8. Lee, K.G.; Lee, S.G.; Lee, H.H.; Lee, H.J.; Shin, J.S.; Kim, N.J.; An, H.J.; Nam, J.H.; Jang, D.S.; Lee, K.T. Alpha-chaconine isolated from a *Solanum tuberosum* L. cv Jayoung suppresses lipopolysaccharide-induced pro-inflammatory mediators via AP-1 inactivation in RAW 264.7 macrophages and protects mice from endotoxin shock. *Chem. Biol. Interact.* **2015**, *235*, 85–94. [CrossRef] [PubMed]
9. Wang, X.G. Teratogenic effect of potato glycoalkaloids. *Zhonghua Fu Chan Ke Za Zhi* **1993**, *28*, 73–75. [PubMed]
10. Thorne, H.V.; Clarke, G.F.; Skuce, R. The inactivation of herpes simplex virus by some solanaceae glycoalkaloids. *Antivir. Res.* **1985**, *5*, 335–343. [CrossRef]
11. Mitchell, G.; Lafrance, M.; Boulanger, S.; Séguin, D.L.; Guay, I.; Gattuso, M.; Marsault, É.; Bouarab, K.; Malouin, F. Tomatidine acts in synergy with aminoglycoside antibiotics against multiresistant staphylococcus aureus and prevents virulence gene expression. *J. Antimicrob. Chemother.* **2011**, *67*, 559–568. [CrossRef] [PubMed]
12. Chang, L.C.; Bhat, K.P.; Fong, H.H.; Pezzuto, J.M.; Kinghorn, A.D. Novel bioactive steroidal alkaloids from pachysandra procumbens. *Tetrahedron* **2000**, *56*, 3133–3138. [CrossRef]
13. Chang, L.C.; Bhat, K.P.; Pisha, E.; Kennelly, E.J.; Fong, H.H.; Pezzuto, J.M.; Kinghorn, A.D. Activity-guided isolation of steroidal alkaloid antiestrogen-binding site inhibitors from pachysandra procumbens. *J. Nat. Prod.* **1998**, *61*, 1257–1262. [CrossRef] [PubMed]
14. Gupta, R.; Dixit, V. Effects of short term treatment of solasodine on cauda epididymis in dogs. *Indian J. Exp. Biol.* **2002**, *40*, 169–173. [PubMed]
15. Zha, X.M.; Zhang, F.R.; Shan, J.Q.; Zhang, Y.H.; Liu, J.O.; Sun, H.B. Synthesis and evaluation of in vitro anticancer activity of novel solasodine derivatives. *Chin. Chem. Lett.* **2010**, *21*, 1087–1090. [CrossRef]

16. Lu, M.-K.; Chen, P.-H.; Shih, Y.-W.; Chang, Y.-T.; Huang, E.-T.; Liu, C.-R.; Chen, P.-S. Alpha-chaconine inhibits angiogenesis in vitro by reducing matrix metalloproteinase-2. *Biol. Pharm. Bull.* **2010**, *33*, 622–630. [CrossRef] [PubMed]

17. Reddivari, L.; Vanamala, J.; Safe, S.H.; Miller, J.C., Jr. The bioactive compounds α-chaconine and gallic acid in potato extracts decrease survival and induce apoptosis in LNCaP and PC3 prostate cancer cells. *Nutr. Cancer* **2010**, *62*, 601–610. [CrossRef] [PubMed]

18. Friedman, M.; Lee, K.R.; Kim, H.J.; Lee, I.S.; Kozukue, N. Anticarcinogenic effects of glycoalkaloids from potatoes against human cervical, liver, lymphoma, and stomach cancer cells. *J. Agric. Food Chem.* **2005**, *53*, 6162–6169. [CrossRef] [PubMed]

19. Nakamura, T.; Komori, C.; Lee, Y.-Y.; Hashimoto, F.; Yahara, S.; Nohara, T.; Ejima, A. Cytotoxic activities of solanum steroidal glycosides. *Biol. Pharm. Bull.* **1996**, *19*, 564–566. [CrossRef] [PubMed]

20. Lu, M.-K.; Shih, Y.-W.; Chang Chien, T.-T.; Fang, L.-H.; Huang, H.-C.; Chen, P.-S. Alpha-solanine inhibits human melanoma cell migration and invasion by reducing matrix metalloproteinase-2/9 activities. *Biol. Pharm. Bull.* **2010**, *33*, 1685–1691. [CrossRef] [PubMed]

21. Lv, C.; Kong, H.; Dong, G.; Liu, L.; Tong, K.; Sun, H.; Chen, B.; Zhang, C.; Zhou, M. Antitumor efficacy of α-solanine against pancreatic cancer in vitro and in vivo. *PLoS ONE* **2014**, *9*, e87868. [CrossRef] [PubMed]

22. Mohsenikia, M.; Alizadeh, A.M.; Khodayari, S.; Khodayari, H.; Karimi, A.; Zamani, M.; Azizian, S.; Mohagheghi, M.A. The protective and therapeutic effects of alpha-solanine on mice breast cancer. *Eur. J. Pharmacol.* **2013**, *718*, 1–9. [CrossRef] [PubMed]

23. Kenny, O.M.; Brunton, N.P.; Rai, D.K.; Collins, S.G.; Jones, P.W.; Maguire, A.R.; O'Brien, N.M. Cytotoxic and apoptotic potential of potato glycoalkaloids in a number of cancer cell lines. *J. Agric. Sci. Appl.* **2013**, *2*, 184–192. [CrossRef]

24. Morice, P.; Leary, A.; Creutzberg, C.; Abu-Rustum, N.; Darai, E. Endometrial cancer. *Lancet* **2016**, *387*, 1094–1108. [CrossRef]

25. Bansal, N.; Yendluri, V.; Wenham, R.M. The molecular biology of endometrial cancers and the implications for pathogenesis, classification, and targeted therapies. *Cancer Control J. Moffitt Cancer Cent.* **2009**, *16*, 8–13. [CrossRef] [PubMed]

26. Cancer 2017. Available online: http://www.who.int/mediacentre/factsheets/fs297/en/ (accessed on 20 August 2017).

27. Burke, W.M.; Orr, J.; Leitao, M.; Salom, E.; Gehrig, P.; Olawaiye, A.B.; Brewer, M.; Boruta, D.; Herzog, T.J.; Shahin, F.A. Endometrial cancer: A review and current management strategies: Part II. *Gynecol. Oncol.* **2014**, *134*, 393–402. [CrossRef] [PubMed]

28. Miyawaki, T.; Ofengeim, D.; Noh, K.-M.; Latuszek-Barrantes, A.; Hemmings, B.A.; Follenzi, A.; Zukin, R.S. The endogenous inhibitor of AKT, CTMP, is critical to ischemia-induced neuronal death. *Nat. Neurosci.* **2009**, *12*, 618–626. [CrossRef] [PubMed]

29. Cheng, J.Q.; Lindsley, C.W.; Cheng, G.Z.; Yang, H.; Nicosia, S.V. The AKT/PKB pathway: Molecular target for cancer drug discovery. *Oncogene* **2005**, *24*, 7482–7492. [CrossRef] [PubMed]

30. Engel, J.B.; Honig, A.; Schönhals, T.; Weidler, C.; Häusler, S.; Krockenberger, M.; Grunewald, T.G.; Dombrowski, Y.; Rieger, L.; Dietl, J.; et al. Perifosine inhibits growth of human experimental endometrial cancers by blockade of AKT phosphorylation. *Eur. J. Obstet. Gynecol. Reprod. Biol.* **2008**, *141*, 64–69. [CrossRef] [PubMed]

31. Saglam, A.S.; Alp, E.; Elmazoglu, Z.; Menevse, E.S. Effect of API-1 and FR180204 on cell proliferation and apoptosis in human DLD-1 and LoVo colorectal cancer cells. *Oncol. Lett.* **2016**, *12*, 2463–2474. [CrossRef] [PubMed]

32. Kim, D.; Sun, M.; He, L.; Zhou, Q.H.; Chen, J.; Sun, X.M.; Bepler, G.; Sebti, S.M.; Cheng, J.Q. A small molecule inhibits AKT through direct binding to AKT and preventing AKT membrane translocation. *J. Biol. Chem.* **2010**, *285*, 8383–8394. [CrossRef] [PubMed]

33. Zivadinovic, D.; Watson, C.S. Membrane estrogen receptor-α levels predict estrogen-induced ERK1/2 activation in MCF-7 cells. *Breast Cancer Res.* **2004**, *7*, R130. [CrossRef] [PubMed]

34. Marino, M.; Acconcia, F.; Ascenzi, P. Estrogen receptor signalling: Bases for drug actions. *Curr. Drug Targets Immune Endocr. Metab. Disord.* **2005**, *5*, 305–314. [CrossRef]

35. Vasquez, Y.M. Estrogen-regulated transcription: Mammary gland and uterus. *Steroids* **2018**, *133*, 82–86. [CrossRef] [PubMed]

36. Harrington, W.R.; Sheng, S.; Barnett, D.H.; Petz, L.N.; Katzenellenbogen, J.A.; Katzenellenbogen, B.S. Activities of estrogen receptor alpha- and beta-selective ligands at diverse estrogen responsive gene sites mediating transactivation or transrepression. *Mol. Cell. Endocrinol.* **2003**, *206*, 13–22. [CrossRef]

37. RTCA SP Instrument Operator's Manual. Available online: http://sydney.edu.au/medicine/bosch/facilities/molecular-biology/live-cell/RTCA%20SP%20Instrument'%20Operator'%20Manual'%20v4.pdf (accessed on 20 May 2017).

38. RTCA Software Manual Software Version 1.2. Available online: http://sydney.edu.au/medicine/bosch/facilities/molecular-biology/live-cell/RTCA%20SP%20Instrument'%20Operator'%20Manual'%20v4.pdf (accessed on 20 May 2017).

39. Vichai, V.; Kirtikara, K. Sulforhodamine B colorimetric assay for cytotoxicity screening. *Nat. Protoc.* **2006**, *1*, 1112–1116. [CrossRef] [PubMed]

40. Skehan, P.; Storeng, R.; Scudiero, D.; Monks, A.; McMahon, J.; Vistica, D.; Warren, J.T.; Bokesch, H.; Kenney, S.; Boyd, M.R. New colorimetric cytotoxicity assay for anticancer-drug screening. *J. Natl. Cancer Inst.* **1990**, *82*, 1107–1112. [CrossRef] [PubMed]

41. Xing, J.Z.; Zhu, L.; Jackson, J.A.; Gabos, S.; Sun, X.J.; Wang, X.B.; Xu, X. Dynamic monitoring of cytotoxicity on microelectronic sensors. *Chem. Res. Toxicol.* **2005**, *18*, 154–161. [CrossRef] [PubMed]

42. Kenny, O.M.; McCarthy, C.M.; Brunton, N.P.; Hossain, M.B.; Rai, D.K.; Collins, S.G.; Jones, P.W.; Maguire, A.R.; O'Brien, N.M. Anti-inflammatory properties of potato glycoalkaloids in stimulated jurkat and raw 264.7 mouse macrophages. *Life Sci.* **2013**, *92*, 775–782. [CrossRef] [PubMed]

43. Roddick, J.G. The acetylcholinesterase-inhibitory activity of steroidal glycoalkaloids and their aglycones. *Phytochemistry* **1989**, *28*, 2631–2634. [CrossRef]

44. Gubarev, M.I.; Enioutina, E.Y.; Taylor, J.L.; Visic, D.M.; Daynes, R.A. Plant-derived glycoalkaloids protect mice against lethal infection with salmonella typhimurium. *Phytother. Res.* **1998**, *12*, 79–88. [CrossRef]

45. Fewell, A.M.; Roddick, J.G. Interactive antifungal activity of the glycoalkaloids α-solanine and α-chaconine. *Phytochemistry* **1993**, *33*, 323–328. [CrossRef]

46. Chen, Y.; Li, S.; Sun, F.; Han, H.; Zhang, X.; Fan, Y.; Tai, G.; Zhou, Y. In vivo antimalarial activities of glycoalkaloids isolated from solanaceae plants. *Pharm. Biol.* **2010**, *48*, 1018–1024. [CrossRef] [PubMed]

47. Friedman, M. Analysis of biologically active compounds in potatoes (*Solanum tuberosum*), tomatoes (*Lycopersicon esculentum*), and jimson weed (*Datura stramonium*) seeds. *J. Chromatogr. A* **2004**, *1054*, 143–155. [CrossRef] [PubMed]

48. Keukens, E.A.; de Vrije, T.; van den Boom, C.; de Waard, P.; Plasman, H.H.; Thiel, F.; Chupin, V.; Jongen, W.M.; de Kruijff, B. Molecular basis of glycoalkaloid induced membrane disruption. *Biochim. Biophys. Acta* **1995**, *1240*, 216–228. [CrossRef]

49. Yang, S.A.; Paek, S.H.; Kozukue, N.; Lee, K.R.; Kim, J.A. Alpha-chaconine, a potato glycoalkaloid, induces apoptosis of HT-29 human colon cancer cells through caspase-3 activation and inhibition of ERK 1/2 phosphorylation. *Food Chem. Toxicol. Int. J. Publ. Br. Ind. Biol. Res. Assoc.* **2006**, *44*, 839–846. [CrossRef] [PubMed]

50. Shih, Y.W.; Chen, P.S.; Wu, C.H.; Jeng, Y.F.; Wang, C.J. Alpha-chaconine-reduced metastasis involves a PI3K/AKT signaling pathway with downregulation of NF-kappaB in human lung adenocarcinoma A549 cells. *J. Agric. Food Chem.* **2007**, *55*, 11035–11043. [CrossRef] [PubMed]

51. Öztürk, E.; Arslan, A.K.K.; Yerer, M.B. Continuously monitoring the cytotoxicity of api-1, α-chaconine and α-solanine on human lung carcinoma A549. *Multidiscip. Digit. Publ. Inst. Proc.* **2017**, *1*, 998. [CrossRef]

52. Lee, K.R.; Kozukue, N.; Han, J.S.; Park, J.H.; Chang, E.Y.; Baek, E.J.; Chang, J.S.; Friedman, M. Glycoalkaloids and metabolites inhibit the growth of human colon (HT29) and liver (HepG2) cancer cells. *J. Agric. Food Chem.* **2004**, *52*, 2832–2839. [CrossRef] [PubMed]

53. Zhang, J.; Shi, G. Inhibitory effect of solanine on prostate cancer cell line PC-3 in vitro. *Natl. J. Androl.* **2011**, *17*, 284–287.

54. Moxley, K.M.; McMeekin, D.S. Endometrial carcinoma: A review of chemotherapy, drug resistance, and the search for new agents. *Oncologist* **2010**, *15*, 1026–1033. [CrossRef] [PubMed]

55. Ji, Y.-B.; Gao, S.-Y. Antihepatocarcinoma effect of solanine and its mechanisms. *Chin. Herb. Med.* **2012**, *4*, 126–135.

56. Ji, Y.; Gao, S.; Ji, C.; Zou, X. Induction of apoptosis in HepG2 cells by solanine and Bcl-2 protein. *J. Ethnopharmacol.* **2008**, *115*, 194–202. [CrossRef] [PubMed]

57. Friedman, M.; Henika, P.R.; Mackey, B.E. Effect of feeding solanidine, solasodine and tomatidine to non-pregnant and pregnant mice. *Food Chem. Toxicol. Int. J. Publ. Br. Ind. Biol. Res. Assoc.* **2003**, *41*, 61–71. [CrossRef]

58. Keepers, Y.P.; Pizao, P.E.; Peters, G.J.; van Ark-Otte, J.; Winograd, B.; Pinedo, H.M. Comparison of the sulforhodamine B protein and tetrazolium (MTT) assays for in vitro chemosensitivity testing. *Eur. J. Cancer Clin. Oncol.* **1991**, *27*, 897–900. [CrossRef]

59. Zhang, F.; Yang, R.; Zhang, G.; Cheng, R.; Bai, Y.; Zhao, H.; Lu, X.; Li, H.; Chen, S.; Li, J. Anticancer function of α-solanine in lung adenocarcinoma cells by inducing microrna-138 expression. *Tumor Biol.* **2016**, *37*, 6437–6446. [CrossRef] [PubMed]

60. Gao, S.-Y.; Wang, Q.-J.; Ji, Y.-B. Effect of solanine on the membrane potential of mitochondria in HepG2 cells and [Ca^{2+}] i in the cells. *World J. Gastroenterol.* **2006**, *12*, 3359. [CrossRef] [PubMed]

61. Lilja, J.F.; Wu, D.; Reynolds, R.K.; Lin, J. Growth suppression activity of the PTEN tumor suppressor gene in human endometrial cancer cells. *Anticancer Res.* **2001**, *21*, 1969–1974. [PubMed]

62. Cui, J.; Shen, Y.; Li, R. Estrogen synthesis and signaling pathways during aging: From periphery to brain. *Trends Mol. Med.* **2013**, *19*, 197–209. [CrossRef] [PubMed]

63. Langkilde, S.; Mandimika, T.; Schrøder, M.; Meyer, O.; Slob, W.; Peijnenburg, A.; Poulsen, M. A 28-day repeat dose toxicity study of steroidal glycoalkaloids, α-solanine and α-chaconine in the Syrian Golden hamster. *Food Chem. Toxicol.* **2009**, *47*, 1099–1108. [CrossRef] [PubMed]

64. Rayburn, J.R.; Friedman, M.; Bantle, J.A. Synergistic interaction of glycoalkaloids α-chaconine and α-solanine on developmental toxicity in Xenopus embryos. *Food Chem. Toxicol.* **1995**, *33*, 1013–1019. [CrossRef]

65. Groen, K.; Pereboom-De Fauw, D.P.K.H.; Besamusca, P.; Beekhof, P.K.; Speijers, G.J.A.; Derks, H.J.G.M. Bioavailability and disposition of 'H-solanine in rat and hamster. *Xenobiotica* **1993**, *23*, 995–1005. [CrossRef] [PubMed]

66. Alozie, S.O.; Sharma, R.P.; Salunkhe, D.K. Physiological Disposition, Subcellular Distribution and Tissue Binding of A-Chaconine (3h). *J. Food Saf.* **1978**, *1*, 257–273. [CrossRef]

nutrients

MDPI

Review

Targeting Histone Deacetylases with Natural and Synthetic Agents: An Emerging Anticancer Strategy

Amit Kumar Singh [1], Anupam Bishayee [2] and Abhay K. Pandey [1,*]

[1] Department of Biochemistry, University of Allahabad, Allahabad 211 002, Uttar Pradesh, India; amitfbs21@gmail.com
[2] Department of Pharmaceutical Sciences, College of Pharmacy, Larkin University, Miami, FL 33169, USA; abishayee@ULarkin.org or abishayee@gmail.com
* Correspondence: akpandey23@rediffmail.com; Tel.: +91-983-952-1138

Received: 7 May 2018; Accepted: 4 June 2018; Published: 6 June 2018

Abstract: Cancer initiation and progression are the result of genetic and/or epigenetic alterations. Acetylation-mediated histone/non-histone protein modification plays an important role in the epigenetic regulation of gene expression. Histone modification is controlled by the balance between histone acetyltransferase and (HAT) and histone deacetylase (HDAC) enzymes. Imbalance between the activities of these two enzymes is associated with various forms of cancer. Histone deacetylase inhibitors (HDACi) regulate the activity of HDACs and are being used in cancer treatment either alone or in combination with other chemotherapeutic drugs/radiotherapy. The Food and Drug Administration (FDA) has already approved four compounds, namely vorinostat, romidepsin, belinostat, and panobinostat, as HDACi for the treatment of cancer. Several other HDACi of natural and synthetic origin are under clinical trial for the evaluation of efficiency and side-effects. Natural compounds of plant, fungus, and actinomycetes origin, such as phenolics, polyketides, tetrapeptide, terpenoids, alkaloids, and hydoxamic acid, have been reported to show potential HDAC-inhibitory activity. Several HDACi of natural and dietary origin are butein, protocatechuic aldehyde, kaempferol (grapes, green tea, tomatoes, potatoes, and onions), resveratrol (grapes, red wine, blueberries and peanuts), sinapinic acid (wine and vinegar), diallyl disulfide (garlic), and zerumbone (ginger). HDACi exhibit their antitumor effect by the activation of cell cycle arrest, induction of apoptosis and autophagy, angiogenesis inhibition, increased reactive oxygen species generation causing oxidative stress, and mitotic cell death in cancer cells. This review summarizes the HDACs classification, their aberrant expression in cancerous tissue, structures, sources, and the anticancer mechanisms of HDACi, as well as HDACi that are either FDA-approved or under clinical trials.

Keywords: cancer; histone deacetylases; histone deacetylase inhibitors; vorinostat; natural HDACi; apoptosis

1. Introduction

Cancer is the second leading cause of death worldwide and caused 8.8 million deaths in 2015. Globally, 1 out of 6 deaths is because of cancer. Low and middle-income countries are the hotspot of cancer deaths, accounting for approximately 70% of deaths. Lung cancer is the most common cause of cancer death worldwide. According to the National Center for Health Statistics about 1.73 million new cancer cases and 0.6 million cancer deaths are projected to occur in the United States in 2018 [1]. Cancer results from altered cell physiology leading to self-sufficient growth potential, loss of cell cycle control, extended angiogenesis, delay in replicative senescence, dysregulated apoptosis, invasion, and metastasis [2,3]. Progression of the disease is not only governed by genomic and genetic changes, such as translocation, amplification, deletion and point mutation, it also involves epigenetic changes; i.e., alteration in the pattern of gene expression without changing underlying DNA sequence.

Methylation of DNA, histone protein modifications and non-coding RNA-mediated gene silencing are the major epigenetic changes, reversible in nature [4].

Chromatin is a compact and highly ordered structure comprised of DNA and histone protein. Nucleosome, the basic unit of chromatin, is made up of 147 bp of DNA superhelix wrapped around histone core protein containing two copies each of H2A, H2B, H3 and H4. H1 is the linker histone. The core plays an important role in establishing interactions between the nucleosomes and within the nucleosome particle itself. N-terminals (histone tails) of core histones are flexible and unstructured while the rest of histone proteins are basically globular and highly ordered. Depending on the epigenetic changes in histone tail, chromatin undergoes various conformational changes responsible for upregulation or downregulation of respective genes [5,6]. The common posttranslational modifications occurring in histones are acetylation, methylation, phosphorylation, sumoylation, ubiquitinylation, and ADP ribosylation.

Acetylation of a lysine residue of histone was discovered by Vincent Allfrey and colleagues in 1964 and based on the finding it has been proposed that acetylation of ε-amino group of lysine residues could play a role in gene expression [7,8]. Acetylation and deacetylation of N-terminal ε-amino group of lysine residues are regulated by two enzymes, namely histone acetyltransferase (HAT) and histone deacetylase (HDAC) (Figure 1). Acetylation neutralizes the positive charge and decreases the affinity between the histone and DNA helix responsible for relaxation of conformation and greater accessibility to transcription machinery [4,9]. Therefore, acetylation is generally associated with gene activation, however, deacetylation catalyzed by HDAC induces chromatin condensation and downregulation of gene expression. N-terminal acetylation of lysine residue also occurs in non-histone proteins, such as cytoplasmic proteins, transcription factors responsible for alteration in gene expression and other cellular processes [10].

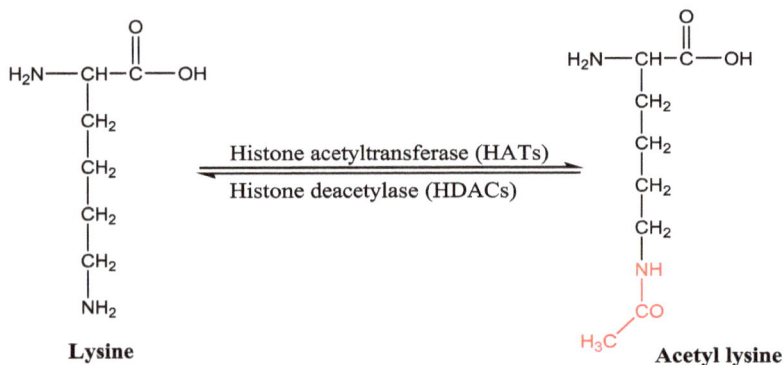

Figure 1. Histone acetylation at the N-terminus lysine by histone acetyltransferases (HATs) and deacetylation by histone deacetylases (HDACs).

Imbalance in the activities of enzymes HATs and HDACs is responsible for the development and progression of wide variety of cancers [2]. Histone deacetylase inhibitors (HDACi) increase the level of acetylated lysine residues of core histone which in turn restarts the expression of silenced regulatory genes in the cancerous cell and therefore, HDACi are now emerging as anticancer agents [11].

Epidemiological studies have suggested that vegetables, fruits, whole grains, microorganism-derived bioactive components, and fatty acids provide protection against some forms of cancer and other diseases without detectable side effects [12–14]. Many dietary compounds that have been identified as having HDAC-inhibitory activities implicated in therapeutic potential in the context of a whole food [11,15]. In the present review an effort has been made to highlight the role of HDACs in the tumor initiation and progression and their inhibitors from natural (dietary and non-dietary) as well as synthetic sources in the management of cancer either alone or in combination with other chemotherapeutic drugs/radiotherapy.

2. Classification of HDACs

In humans, 18 HDACs have been identified so far and are divided into two families and four classes based on their sequence homology to *Saccharomyces cerevisiae* HDACs (Figure 2) [16]. One of the family group members are zinc-dependent, they require Zn^{++} as a cofactor for their deacetylase activity and include HDAC 1 to HDAC 11. HDACs 1, 2, 3 and 8 are grouped into class 1 having a sequence similarity with yeast reduced potassium dependency-3 (Rpd3) and class II HDACs are subdivided into class IIA and Class IIB that include HDACs 4, 5, 6, 7, 9 and 10 which are reported to have sequence homology with yeast histone deacetylase-1 (hda-1) while HDAC 11 of class IV share sequence similarity with both classes of yeast deacetylase Rpd3 and hda-1.

Another group of the family requires nicotinamide adenine dinucleotide (NAD^+) as a cofactor for deacetylase activity classified as class III, has sequence similarity to yeast deacetylase silent information regulator-2 (Sir2) and includes seven members from sirtuins (SIRTs) 1 to 7. Sirtuins are known to regulate several cellular processes; e.g., survival, aging, stress response, and various metabolic processes. The members of class I and IV are located in the nucleus while class IIA is mainly located into the cytoplasm and class IIB is found shuttling between the nucleus and cytoplasm. Cellular localization of class III HDACs are nucleus, cytoplasm, and mitochondria [11,17]. Nomenclature of class I, II and IV HDACs are based on their chronological order of discovery; for example, both HDAC 1 and 2 were discovered in 1996 while HDAC 2 was discovered a few months after HDAC 1 [18,19]. Later on, HDAC 3 was discovered in the subsequent years [20]. While HDACs 4, 5, and 6 were first reported in 1999, the HDAC 7 was discovered in early 2000 and so on [21,22]. Table 1 summarizes the HDACs classification, number of amino acids, cellular and chromosomal locations, biological functions, relevant histone/non-histone target proteins, and their expression pattern [6,23,24].

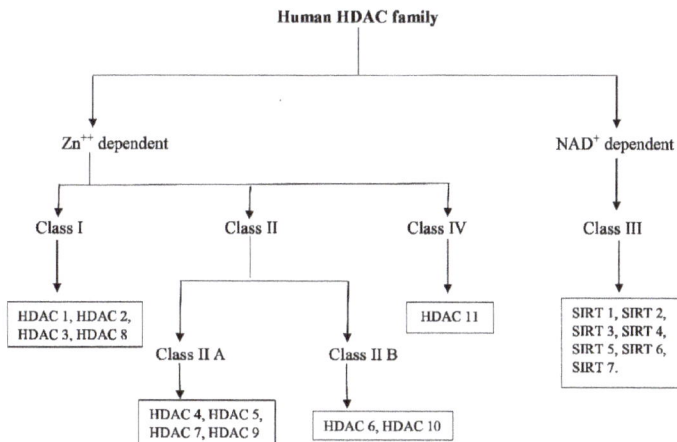

Figure 2. Classification of HDAC family.

Table 1. Histone deacetylase (HDAC) enzymes classification, number of amino acids, localization, function, protein targets and expression pattern.

Class	HDACs	Number of Amino Acid	Cellular Location	Chromosomal Location	Biological Function	Histone/Non-Histone Protein Target	Pattern of Expression of Gene
I	HDAC 1	483	Nucleus	1p35.2-p35.1	Proliferation and survival of cells	Histones, pRb, SHP, BRCA1, MECP2, ATM, MEF2, MyoD, p53, NF-κB, AR, DNMT1	Ubiquitous expression
	HDAC 2	488		6q21	Proliferation of cell and insulin resistance	Histones, BRCA1, NF-κB, MECP, GATA 2, pRb	
	HDAC 3	428		5q31.3	Proliferation and survival of cells	Histones, HDAC (4, 5, 7, 9), GATA 1, NF-κB, pRb	
	HDAC 8	377		Xq13.1	Proliferation of cell	HSP70	
IIA	HDAC 4	1084	Nucleus/Cytoplasm	2q37.3	Regulation of cytoskeleton dynamics and cell mobility	Histones, HDAC 3, 14-3-3, CaM, MEF 2	Tissue restricted expression
	HDAC 5	1122		17q21.31	Helps in endothelial cell function, gluconeogenesis, cardiac myocyte growth and function		
	HDAC 7	912		12q13.11	Helps in endothelial cell function and glyconeogenesis.		
	HDAC 9	1069		7p21.1	Helps in thymocyte differentiation, homologous recombination, cardiac cell function		
IIB	HDAC 6	1215	Cytoplasm	Xp11.23	Regulation of cytoskeleton dynamics and cell mobility	HDAC 11, SHP, HSP 90, α tubulin	Tissue restricted expression
	HDAC 10	669		2q13.33	Regulation of autophagy, homologous recombination.	LcoR, PP1	
III	SIRT 1	747	Nucleus/Cytoplasm	10q21.3	Autoimmunity, aging, redox balance, and cell survival	Histones, NF-κB, p53, p300	Variable expression
	SIRT 2	389	Nucleus	19q13.2	Survival, migration, and invasion of cell	Histone H4, PPAR-Y, p53, p300, α-tubulin, FOXO	

Table 1. *Cont.*

Class	HDACs	Number of Amino Acid	Cellular Location	Chromosomal Location	Biological Function	Histone/Non-Histone Protein Target	Pattern of Expression of Gene
	SIRT 3	399	Mitochondria	11p15.5	Regulate ATP production and metabolism, cell signaling, apoptosis, urea cycle	Complex I of ETC, PGC-1α, p53, Ku70, Acetyl-CoA Synthetase, FOXO	
	SIRT 4	314		12q24.31	Energy metabolism, Urea cycle, cell signaling	Glutamate dehydrogenase	
	SIRT 5	310		6p23	Regulate ATP production and metabolism, cell signaling, apoptosis, urea cycle	Carbamoyl phosphate synthetase I, Cytochrome c	
	SIRT 6	355	Nucleus	19p13.3	Regulate metabolism	Histone H3, TNF-α	
	SIRT 7	400		17q25.3	Apoptosis	p53, RNA polymerase I	
IV	HDAC 11	347	Nucleus	3p25.1	DNA replication, Immunomodulation	HDAC 6	Ubiquitous in nature

AR, androgen receptor; ATM, ataxia-telangiectasia-mutated; BRCA, breast cancer; CaM, calmodulin; CoA, co-enzyme A; DNMT, DNA methyltransferase; FOXO, forkhead box O; GATA, GATA binding protein; HIF, hypoxia-inducible factor; HSP, heat shock protein; LcoR, ligand-dependent receptor co-repressor; MECP, methyl-CpG-binding domain protein; MEF, myocyte enhancer factor; NF-κB, nuclear factor-kappa B; PGC, peroxisome proliferator-activated receptor gamma coactivator; PP1, protein phosphatase; PPAR, peroxisome proliferator-activated receptor; pRb, retinoblastoma protein; SHP, Src homology region 2-domain-containing phosphatase; SIRT, sirtuin; TNF, tumor necrosis factor.

3. Cellular Targets of Histone/Non-Histone Protein Acetylation

The acetylation or deacetylation status of histone proteins and transcription factors modulate the gene expression pattern. Hyperacetylation of lysine residues of histone proteins promotes the relaxed state of chromatin and activates gene expression [25]. Besides this, acetylation of transcription factors affects their cellular localization. For example, signal transducer and activator of transcription 1 (STAT 1) and nuclear factor-κB (NF-κB) are internalized into the nucleus from cytosol after the acetylation of specific lysine residues where they activate transcription of respective genes. The activity of other transcription factors, such as p53 and FOXO, is also positively regulated by the acetylation process. Acetylation process also affects the stability of proteins, i.e., acetylation of p53, p73, and mothers against decapentaplegic homolog 7 (SMAD 7) prevents their ubiquitinylation and degradation. Interestingly, cell mobility is also affected by the acetylation pattern of α-tubulin and cortactin. It has been reported that HDAC 6 and SIRT2 cause deacetylation of α-tubulin, which promotes microtubule depolymerization and therefore increases microtubule dynamics and cell mobility. Acetylation also affects the activity of retinoblastoma protein (pRB) by blocking its cyclin E-cdk2 dependent phosphorylation so acetylation-dependent hypophosphorylation causes cell cycle arrest [26,27].

4. HDAC Mutations in Cancer

Mutations of HDACs have also been observed. HDAC2 mutation in human epithelial cancer resulted in microsatellite instability. Interestingly, a truncating mutation of HDAC2 in human cancers confers resistance to HDACi. These findings suggest that the HDAC2 mutational status of patients should be assessed before therapies using HDACi [28]. HDAC3 are associated with DNA damage control response. Inactivation of HDAC3 causes genomic instability. HDAC4 acts s transcriptional repressor and its mutations have been identified at significant frequency in breast and colorectal cancers. SIRT 2 acts as a tumor suppressor and mutation in its catalytic domain eliminates its enzymatic activity, which compromises the mitotic checkpoint, contributing to genomic instability and tumorigenesis. HDAC9 and 10 are reported to be involved in homologous recombination, and depletion in HDAC 9 and 10 resulted in inhibition of homologous recombination [11].

5. HDACs and Cancer: Expression Pattern and Function

Altered acetylation level and mutation/or aberrant expression of various HDACs have been observed frequently in numerous human diseases including cancer, hence making them an important drug target [2]. Fraga et al. (2005) reported that change in genome-wide patterns of acetylation may lead to the initiation and progression of cancer by demonstrating that cancer cells undergo a loss of acetylation at lysine 16 of H4 [29]. HDACs have various histone and non-histone protein targets that not only regulate the chromatin activity, but also control apoptosis, cell cycle progression and differentiation. Association of HDACs with regulatory processes reflects their involvement in cancer phenotypes [30].

5.1. Class I HDACs

5.1.1. HDAC 1

HDAC 1 overexpression has been reported in Hodgkin's lymphoma (HL), gastric, ovarian, and prostate cancers [11,23]. Choi and co-workers (2001) have shown the overexpression of HDAC 1 in 60% cases compared with normal tissue [31]. This study was further validated by a recent study including 293 gastric cancer samples showing upregulation in expression of HDACs 1, 2, and 3 [32,33]. Elevated level of expression of HDAC 1, 2, and 3 was reported in pancreatic cancer involving 192 samples and this overexpression was responsible for dedifferentiation and enhanced proliferation of pancreatic cancer cell [34]. Overexpression of HDAC 1, 2, and 3 is associated with mortality rate in colorectal cancer. Expression of HDAC 2 has emerged as an independent prognostic marker in colorectal cancer [35]. Furthermore, overexpression of HDAC 1 is reported in hepatocellular carcinoma [36], lung cancer [37] and breast cancer [38]. Direct correlation between HDAC 1, 3 expression and estrogen and progesterone receptor expression have been reported by Krusche et al. [39].

HDAC 1 induces cell proliferation and inhibition of differentiation and apoptosis [23,38]. HDAC 1 and 3 knockdowns (KD) resulted in the inhibition of cell proliferation in Hela cells [40]. HDAC 1 KD has been shown to result in cell cycle arrest either at the G1 phase or at the G2/M transition phase, causing loss of mitotic cells, inhibition of cell growth, and an increase in the number of apoptotic cells in osteosarcoma and breast cancer cells. However, HDAC 2 KD showed no such effects in these cells [41]. HDAC1 might also be involved in multidrug resistance as they showed overexpression in a pattern in chemotherapeutically resistant neuroblastoma cells [42].

5.1.2. HDAC 2

Overexpression of HDAC2 reported in uterine, cervical, gastric, cutaneous T cell lymphoma (CTCL), HL, prostate and colorectal cancers [38]. Elevated expression of HDAC 2 along with HDAC 1 and 3 are associated with advance stage of disease and prognosis of gastric, colorectal, and prostate cancers [33–35].

Knockdown of HDAC2 in cervical cancer causes increased apoptosis and the differentiated phenotype of cells associated with increased $p21^{Cip1/WAF1}$ expression that was independent of p53 [43]. In breast carcinoma cells, HDAC 2 KD results into the increased DNA binding activity of tumor suppressor protein p53, which causes the inhibition of cell proliferation and induction of cellular senescence [44]. HDAC 2 KD also causes decreased viability, growth arrest, and increased apoptosis in colorectal and breast cancer cells [45].

5.1.3. HDAC 3

HDAC 3 overexpression has been reported in HL, ovarian and lung cancers, colon cancer, and chronic lymphocyte leukemia (CLL) [11,38,46]. An upregulated expression of HDAC1 along with HDAC3 was paradoxically related to disease-free survival in invasive breast cancer patients [24]. HDAC3 elevated expression together with HDAC 1 and 2 significantly causes poor prognosis in gastric, colon, and prostate cancers [33–35]. Decreased expression of HDAC 3 has been observed in liver cancer [45].

HDAC 3 KD in acute promyelocytic leukemia (APL) cells causes restoration of expression of a retinoic acid-dependent gene whose transcription repression was caused by promyelocytic leukemia retinoic acid receptor alpha (PML-RARα) [47]. While HDAC3 KD in colon cancer causes a decrease in the viability of cell by increasing the rate of apoptosis [45].

5.1.4. HDAC 8

Expression of HDAC 8 has been reported to increase in childhood neuroblastoma. HDAC KD shows reduction in proliferation of lung, colon, and cervical cancer. In childhood neuroblastoma cell HDAC 8 KD causes cell cycle arrest, reduction in cell proliferation [48,49]. HDAC 8 has also been reported in controlling telomerase activity [50].

5.2. Class IIA HDACs

5.2.1. HDAC4

A breast cancer sample showed overexpressed genotype of HDAC 4 [51]. However, lung and colon cancer analysis showed downregulated expression of HDAC 4 [11].

In APL, HDAC 4 was found to repress the expression of differentiation-associated genes by interacting with a leukemic fusion protein, PLZF-RARa [52]. HDAC 4 also regulates the activity of hypoxia inducing factor-1α (HIF-1α). HDAC4 has also been shown to help prostate cancer cells overcome hypoxic conditions by stabilizing HIF-1α. The binding of HDAC4 to HIF-1α generates a complex that regulates glycolysis and the cytotoxic stress of cell adaptation to hypoxic conditions [53]. HDAC4 KD in colon and glioblastoma cells causes an increased apoptosis rate and reduced growth rate [54].

5.2.2. HDAC 5

HDAC 5 overexpression has been reported in medulloblastoma [55] and colon cancer [51] while interestingly, the lung cancer sample showed a downregulated genotypic expression of HDAC5 [11]. HDAC 5 traverses from the nucleus to the cytosol upon interacting with transcription factor GATA-1 during differentiation of mouse erythroleukemia cells [56]. Knock down of HDAC 5 has been shown to cause reduced growth and viability of medulloblastoma cells [55].

5.2.3. HDAC 7

They are highly expressed in ALP, CLL, and colon cancer [46,51] and downregulated expression is reported in lung cancer samples [45,57]. HDAC 7 silencing in endothelial cells altered their morphology, their migration, and their capacity to form capillary tube-like structures in vitro but did not affect cell adhesion, proliferation, or apoptosis, suggesting that HDAC7 may represent a rational target for anti-angiogenesis in cancer [58].

5.2.4. HDAC 9

Elevated expression of HDAC 9 was reported in ALL and medulloblastoma [59,60] and in cervical cancer [31]. Silencing HDAC 9 results into inhibition of homologous recombination, sensitivity towards DNA damage and decreased viability and growth of medulloblastoma [45].

5.3. Class IIB HDACs

5.3.1. HDAC 6

A significantly higher expression of HDAC 6 was reported in oral squamous cell carcinoma, hepatocellular carcinoma, acute myeloid leukemia, CLL, breast cancer, CTCL and ovarian cancer, whereas its expression increased in the advanced stages of cancer compared to the early stages of cancer [5,61].

HDAC 6 overexpression causes increased migration of the fibroblast cell while the inhibition of HDAC 6 results in decreased fibroblast cell migration [62]. HDAC 6 targeted inhibition causes HSP 90 protein acetylation and disruption of its chaperone activity resulting in decreased viability of K562 leukemic cell [63]. HDAC4/6 has the potential to help prostate cancer cells overcome hypoxic conditions by stabilizing HIF-1 α [53]. HDAC 6 is also involved in metastasis, epithelial to mesenchymal transition in lung cancer cells by compromising TGF-β SMAD 3 pathway [64].

5.3.2. HDAC 10

Osada and colleague [57] described the potential role of HDAC 10 in cancer initiation and progression and reported the downregulated expression of HDAC 10 in non-small lung carcinoma cells and this is related with poor prognosis in lung cancer patients. Its role in gastric cancer and CLL is also reported [65].

HDAC 10 are shown to regulate the production of reactive oxygen species in gastric cancer cells [66]. HDAC 10 KD causes reduced vascular endothelial growth factor of receptor 1 and 2 (VEGF 1 and 2) and increased sensitivity towards DNA damage in cancer cells [67].

5.4. Class III HDACs

Sirtuins

Growing evidence supports the relation between cancer and sirtuins. As other HDACs they are also both tumor suppressors as well as pro-oncogenic in nature. SIRT 1 expression was shown to be upregulated in acute myeloid leukemia (AML), non-melanoma skin cancer and prostate cancer [68–70] while downregulated in colorectal cancer [51]. SIRT 2 expression decreased in glioma and gastric cancer [71]. However, a mutation in the catalytic domain of SIRT 2 has also been reported [72]. Expression pattern of SIRT 3 has been found to increase or decrease in different kinds of breast cancer tissues [73]. SIRT 6 expression was reported to decrease in liver cancer while increased expression pattern in CLL [46]. SIRT 7 shows an upregulated expression pattern in breast cancer [73].

SIRT 2 functions as a tumor suppressor protein and the mutation in its catalytic domain results in compromised cell cycle checkpoints leading to genomic instability and tumorigenesis [74]. In many cancerous cells, increased expression of SIRT 1 induces the p-glycoprotein expression responsible for chemotherapeutically resistant cancer cells whereas siRNA-mediated SIRT 1 KD causes a reversal of drug-resistant phenotype [75]. SIRT 3 functions both as a tumor suppressor and a tumor promoter protein. Higher expression of SIRT 3 was responsible for preventing bladder cancer cells from p53-mediated cell growth arrest [76]. SIRT 7 was shown to stabilize cancer cell phenotypes. SIRT 7 KD results in the tumorigenic potential of human cancer xenograft in mice [77].

5.5. Class IV HDACs

HDAC 11

The involvement of HDAC 11 in cancer is not well understood. However aberrant expression of HDAC 11 were reported in HL and Philadelphia-negative chronic myeloproliferative neoplasms (CMPN) [78].

siRNA-mediated HDAC 11, KD results in an increased apoptosis rate in HL, colon, prostate, breast, and ovarian cell lines [45,79]. Selective inhibition of HDAC 11 with histone deacetylase inhibitor (HDACi) reduces the chance of splenomegaly and other metabolic disorders reported in CMPN affected people [78].

6. Histone Deacetylase Inhibitors as an Anticancer Agent

The aberrant or altered expression of HDACs or their functions is frequently observed in a variety of cancer types and is the reason for targeting HDACs in cancer therapy. The availability of HDACi not only has accelerated our understanding of HDAC functions and its mechanism of actions but also presented a promising new class of compounds for cancer treatment. HDACi belong to a large and diverse family of both natural and synthetic compounds and can be categorized into four groups; i.e., hydroximic acid, benzamides, cyclic peptides, and aliphatic fatty acids [80]. Several natural or synthetic compounds are isolated and characterized for their potential as histone deacetylase inhibitors. The first significant compound identified as HDACi was *n*-butyrate, responsible for the accumulation of hyperacetylated histone inside the nucleus [81]. Subsequently, trichostatin A (TSA) and trapoxin A were found to be reversible and irreversible inhibitors of HDACs, respectively [11,82]. Schreiber et al. (1996) were first to discover and clone the human HDAC by using trapoxin A [80]. While developing these compounds as anticancer agents, parameters like their specificity, efficiency, pharmacokinetic and toxicological properties were analyzed [83]. Some HDACi, such as TSA, lycorine and zerumbone, are pan-HDAC inhibitors since they act on all isoform of zinc-dependent HDAC classes, while others are class specific.

HDCAs can reversibly modify the acetylation pattern of histone/non-histone protein resulted in abnormal gene expression without changing the DNA sequence. HDACi can overcome this problem and can resume the expression of tumor the suppressor genes responsible for apoptosis, cell cycle arrest, and the inhibition of angiogenesis and metastasis. Ungerstedt and co-workers [84] reported that cancerous cells are more sensitive than normal cells towards HDACi-induced apoptosis.

6.1. Natural HDACi

Altogether natural compounds provide pleiotropic and potent inhibitors of all hallmarks of cancer. Many of the HDACi discovered to date are of natural origin; for example in 1976, Tsuji et al. [85] isolated a naturally occurring HDACi, TSA from *Streptomyces hygroscopicus*. FK322, a cyclic peptide isolated from *Chromobacterium violaceum* selectively inhibits the activity of HDAC 1 and 2. TSA causes differentiation of cell and arrests the cell cycle of both normal and cancerous cells, resulting in the accumulation of acetylated histones [86]. Depudecin and trapoxin A and B are also the examples of naturally occurring HDACi extracted from a fungus. Marine organisms are also the source of natural HDACi, such as largazole and azumamides, and they are reported to be active even at nanomolar concentrations [11]. Other well-characterized naturally occurring HDACi, such as butein, kaempferol, protocatechuic aldehyde, sinapinic acid, resveratrol and zerumbone, are isolated from plant, fruits or vegetables (Table 2). Molecular modelling studies revealed the HDACi like activity of other dietary compounds; i.e., vitamin E, α-lipoic acid, and biotin [48]. For the first time, the clinical validation of natural HDACi was done by Riggs and colleague [81] in 1977. They analyzed the effect of butyrate on histone modificationin HeLa and Friend erythroleukemia cell lines [80]. Later in 1980, McKnight et al. [87] reported the effect of propionate on histone deacetylation in chick oviduct and showed it to have lesser activity than butyrate. Both these compounds were active at millimolar concentrations and synthesized by colonic bacteria. Valproic acid, a longer chain aliphatic fatty acid, also reported to have significant HDACi activity. Valproic acid inhibits HDACs activity by binding to its active site [87]. Detailed features of other natural histone deacetylase inhibitors and their sources are shown in Table 2.

Table 2. Examples of the natural compound with histone deacetylase inhibitory activity.

S.N	Class of Compounds	Name of the Compound	HDAC Target	Source (Species/Family)	Structure	Reference
1.	Phenolics	Aceroside VIII	HDAC6	*Betula platyphylla*		[87]
		Homobutein	Class I, II and IV	*Butea frondosa*		[88]
		Isoliquiritigenin	Class I, II and IV	*Glycyrrhiza glabra*		[89]
		Butein	Class I, II and IV	*Toxicodendron vernicifluum*		[88]
		Kaempferol	Class I, II and IV	*Aloe vera*		[89]
		Marein	Class I, II and IV	*Coreopsis maritima*		[88]
		Protocatechuic aldehyde	HDAC2	*Hordeum vulgare*		[23]

Table 2. *Cont.*

S.N	Class of Compounds	Name of the Compound	HDAC Target	Source (Species/Family)	Structure	Reference
		Psammaplin A	Class I	*Poecillastra* spp. and *Jaspis* spp.		[23]
		Sinapinic acid	Pan-HDAC	*Hydnophytum formicarum Jack*		[90]
		Resveratrol	Class I, II and IV	*Vitis vinifera*		[91]
2.	Polyketides	Depudecin	HDAC 1	*Alternaria brassicicola*		[92]
3.	Tetrapeptide	Apicidin	Class I HDAC	*Fusarium* spp.		[93]
		Azumamide E	Class I	*Mycale izuensis*		[94]

Table 2. *Cont.*

S.N	Class of Compounds	Name of the Compound	HDAC Target	Source (Species/Family)	Structure	Reference
		Chlamydocin	HDAC 1, 6	*Diheterospora chlamydosporia*		[95]
		Trapoxin A	Class I	*Helicoma ambiens* RF-1023		[96]
4.	Terpenoids	Zerumbone	Pan HDAC	*Zingiber zerumbet*		[23]
		β-Thujaplicin	HDAC 2	*Cupressaceae* spp.		[23]
		6-methoxy-2E,9E-humuladien-8-one	Pan HDAC	*Zingiber zerumbet*		[23]
5.	Alkaloid	Lycorine	Pan HDAC	*Amaryllidaceae*		[97]
6.	Fatty acid	9-Hydroxystearic acid	Class I	Lipid peroxidation product		[98]

Table 2. *Cont.*

S.N	Class of Compounds	Name of the Compound	HDAC Target	Source (Species/Family)	Structure	Reference
7.	Organosulphur compounds	Diallyl disulfide	Acetylation Level increased	*Allium sativum*		[99,100]
		(*S*)-allylmercaptocysteine		*Allium sativum*		[101]
8.	Hydroxamic acid	Trichostatin A	Class I and II	*Streptomyces hygroscopicus*		[2,11]
9.	Desipeptides	FK228	HDAC 1, 2	*Chromobacterium violaceum*		[11]
		Largazole	Class I	*Symploca* spp.		[99]

6.2. FDA-Approved and Under Clinical Trial HDACi

Aberrant expression of HDACs gene is reported in various cancer types. So, the scientists across the globe are searching for a therapeutic alternative, which not only can inhibit the increased activity of HDACs, but also reverse the malignant phenotype. The histone deacetylase inhibitors chiefly cause the gene to be in a hyperacetylated state, which in turn restarts the gene expression, and are also involved in chromatin stability, mitosis, and the DNA repair mechanism [23]. However, it has been reported that both normal and cancerous cells show accumulation of acetylated histone after treatment with HDACi, but healthy cells appear to be much less susceptible to apoptosis and growth inhibition than a cancerous cell. Four synthetic compounds, viz., vorinostat, romidepsin, belinostat, and panobinostat have been approved as HDACi for cancer treatment to date by the United States Food and Drug Administration (FDA). In addition, many other HDACi are under clinical trials in patients suffering from various types of cancer [101,102]. FDA-approved and other HDACi under clinical trials are presented in Table 3.

Vorinostat, a hydroximic acid-based drug, is also known as suberanilohydroxamic acid (SAHA) and is marketed with different names. Zolinza was the first FDA-approved vorinostat drug for cutaneous T cell lymphoma treatment (CTCL). It inhibits the HDACs except class III sirtuins and was developed by Merck & Co. (Kenilworth, NJ, USA). In phase II clinical trial study (NCT00958074) on 74 CTCL patients with a daily oral dose of vorinostat (400 mg), an objective response rate (ORR) of 30% was observed [11]. Vorinostat is also reported to be useful in other cancer types, such as brain metastasis, refractory colorectal, advanced solid tumors, melanoma, pancreatic, lung cancer and multiple myeloma [6]. A combinatorial therapy of vorinostat with temozolomide and radiotherapy is under clinical trial for the treatment of early stage of glioblastoma multiformae (NCT00731731).

Romidepsin, a cyclic tetrapeptide, was the second FDA-approved drug for treatment of CTCL in 2009 and in 2011, for treatment of peripheral T cell lymphoma (PTCL) with the response rate of 34% and 25%, respectively. However, romidepsin treatment was associated with side effects, such as nausea, vomiting, cardiac toxicity, and myelotoxicity [11,37]. Romidepsin has been evaluated for treatment of T-cell lymphoma either as a single agent (NCT00426764) or in combination with other drugs (NCT03141203) in 30 clinical trials. Romidepsin intake produced fatigue, nausea, vomiting, diarrhea, constipation, phlebitis, headache, and dyspnea as side effects [6]. Romidepsin either singly or in combination with paclitaxel exhibited elimination of both primary tumors and a metastatic lesion at multiple sites formed by the SUM149 IBC cell line in the Mary-X preclinical model [103].

In 2014, belinostat was the third drug approved by the FDA for PTCL treatment. It is a hydroxamate that inhibits the activity of class I and II HDACs. Clinical trial study (NCT00865969) on 120 PTCL patients showed an ORR of 26% [6]. Belinostat is now being investigated in more than 15 clinical trials for the treatment of CTCL (NCT00274651), multiple myeloma (NCT00431340), Burkitt lymphoma (NCT00303953), and solid tumors as in fallopian tube cancer (NCT00301756) [23].

Panobinostat was approved by the FDA in 2015 for the treatment of multiple myelomas [37]. It is a hydroxamate derivative causing the inhibition of class I, II, and IV HDACs. An ORR of 27% was reported for panobinostat. Diarrhoea and cardio-toxicity are side effects associated with Panobinostat. It has been used for treating other cancer types, such as CTCL (NCT00490776), AML (NCT01613976), Hodgkin's lymphoma (NCT00742027), MDS (NCT00594230), thyroid carcinoma (NCT01013597), and colorectal and prostate cancers (NCT00663832) in more than 50 clinical trials [23].

In contrast to the above mentioned clinical trials and studies reporting efficacy of HDACi in the treatment of various lymphomas, leukemia and myeloma, solid tumors have shown limited response against HDACi. The study conducted by Paller and colleagues [104] reported that HDACi VPA and vorinostat in combination with AMG 900, a pan-aurora kinase inhibitor, significantly enhanced cellular senescence, polyploidy, and apoptosis in prostate cancer cell lines (DU-145, LNCaP and PC3) as compared with a single agent treatment. Combination therapy with Janus kinase (JAK) inhibitor INCB018424 has been shown to improve the clinical efficacy of vorinostat in triple-negative breast cancer patients [105]. Similarly, combination therapies targeting HDACs and IκB kinase have shown potential against ovarian cancer [106].

229

Table 3. FDA approved and under clinical trials histone deacytylase inhibitors (HDACi).

S.N	Chemical Class	Name of the Compounds	HDAC Target	Cancer Specificity	Trial Stage	Structure of the Compound	Reference
1.	Hydroxamic acid	SAHA (Vorinostat)	Class I, II and IV	CTCL	FDA approved (2006)		[107]
		Belinostat	Class I, II and IV	PTCL	FDA approved (2014)		[108]
		Panobinostat	Class I, II and IV	MM	FDA approved in 2015		[109]
		Resminostat	Class I and II	Colorectal, HCC, HL	Phase II trial		[6]
		Givinostat	Class I and II	CLL, HL, MM	Phase II trial		[110]
		Pracinostat	Classes I, II and IV	AML	Phase II trial		[111]
		Abexinostat	Class I and II	CLL, HL, Non-HL, Solid tumors	Phase I trial		[45]
		Quisinostat	Class I and II	Solid tumor, CTCL	Phase I and II trial		[45]

Table 3. *Cont.*

S.N	Chemical Class	Name of the Compounds	HDAC Target	Cancer Specificity	Trial Stage	Structure of the Compound	Reference
		MPT0E028	HDAC 1, 2 and 6	Solid tumor, B-cell lymphoma	Phase I trial		[112]
		CHR 3996	Class I	Solid tumors	Phase I trial		[113]
		CUDC 101	Class I and II	Solid tumor	Phase I trial		[6]
		CUDC 907	Class I and II	MM; lymphoma; solid tumor	Phase I trial		[6]
		Entinostat	Class I	Solid tumors	Phase I and II trial		[113]
2.	Benzamides	Chidamide	HDAC 1, 2,3 and 10	Breast cancer	Phase II and III trial		[114]
		Ricolinostat	HDAC 6	MM, Lymphoma	Phase I and II trial		[115]

Table 3. *Cont.*

S.N	Chemical Class	Name of the Compounds	HDAC Target	Cancer Specificity	Trial Stage	Structure of the Compound	Reference
		Tacedinaline	Class I	Lung and pancreatic cancer, MM	Phase II and III trial		[6]
		Mocetinostat	Class I and IV	Solid malignancies	Phase I and II trial		[116]
3.	Cyclic peptides	Romidepsin	Class I	CTCL, PTCL	FDA approved in 2009		[6,117]
		Valproic acid	Class I and II	Solid and hematological tumors	Phase I and II trial		[118]
4.	Fatty acids	AR-42	Class I and IIb	AML	Phase I trial		[45]
		Phenyl butyrate	Class I and II	Solid and hematological tumors	Phase I and II trial		[118]
		Pivanex	Class I and II	NSCLC, Myeloma, CLL	Phase II trial		[113]

CTCL, cutaneous T cell lymphoma treatment; PTCL, peripheral T cell lymphoma; MM, multiple myeloma; HCC, hepatocellular Carcinoma; HL, Hodgkin lymphoma; CLL, chronic lymphocyte leukemia; AML, acute myeloid leukemia; NSCLC, non-small cell lung cancer.

7. Mechanisms of Action of HDACi

HDACi induces cell cycle arrest, differentiation, and apoptosis as well as inhibits angiogenesis [119]. The mechanism of the anticancer effect of HDACi depends upon the cancer type, individual, stage of cancer, dose, and some other factors [120]. The antiproliferative mechanisms of HDACi action are described below.

7.1. Cell Cycle Arrest

Various mechanisms are involved in HDACi-mediated cell cycle arrest. One of the most important mechanisms is the increased expression of the cyclin-dependent kinase (CDK) inhibitor gene CDKN1A (p21, WAF1/CIP1). An interesting fact is that the HDACi-mediated overexpression of p21 is independent of p53 [121,122]. The concentration-dependent cell cycle inhibitory effects of HDACi have been observed. At lower concentrations HDACi predominately induces G1 arrest while at higher concentrations induces both G1 and G2/M arrest [123]. p21 is mainly associated with G1 and G2/M arrest, inhibits the activity of CDKs (i.e., CDK 4/6), which regulates the progression of the G1 stage of cell cycle, CDK 2 responsible for G1/S transition and cdc2/CDK 1 causes G2/M transition. The p21 mutation abolishes the HDACi induced G1 arrest [124]. However, HDACi-mediated G1 arrest is also observed in a cell without p21. Hitomi et al. [125] reported that TSA causes G1 arrest in human colon p21 mutant cell by induction of p15 (INK4b), which subsequently causes inhibition of cyclin D-dependent kinases resulting in the absence of CDK 2. Protein p53 interacts with the p21 promoter by competing with HDAC1 and alters the expression of the p21 gene. HDAC1 is the transcriptional repressor of p21, which gets detached from the Sp1 (promoter-specific RNA polymerase II transcription factor) after HDACi treatment, resulting in increased p21 expression. Moreover, HDACi also causes an increase in the half-life of protein p53 thereby improving its interaction with p21 and increased levels of p21 inside the cell mediates cell cycle arrest and apoptosis [126]. HDACi treatment also compromises the CDK activity, which may account for the dephosphorylation of the retinoblastoma protein (Rb), which blocks the elongation factor, E2F function in the transcription of genes for G1 progression and G1/S transition [118].

7.2. Induction of Apoptosis in Transformed Cell

HDACi induces the rate of apoptosis in a transformed cell by regulating both pro-apoptotic and anti-apoptotic genes (Figure 3) and this involves the activation of both extrinsic and intrinsic apoptotic pathways. HDACi induced extrinsic pathway initiation involves the binding of death receptor such as Fas (Apo-1 or CD95), tumor necrosis factor (TNF) receptor-1 (TNFR-1), TNF-related apoptosis-inducing ligand (TRAIL) receptors (DR-4 and DR-5), DR-3 (Apo3) and DR-6 to their ligand FasL, TNF, TRAIL, and TL1A resulting into activation of caspase 8 and 10. In vitro and in vivo studies suggest that HDACi upregulates the expression of both death receptor and their ligand in transformed cells but no such effect is observed in normal cells [127]. Upregulated expression of Fas and FasL have been reported in the treatment of human neuroblastoma cells with m-carboxycinnamic acid bihydroxamide, nude mice xenograft of osteocarcinoma with FK228, acute promyelocytic leukemia model of a rat with valproic acid, and so on [128,129]. FK228 also induces the expression of TNF α in HL 60 and K562 cells. cFLIP, an inhibitor of the activity of the death receptor has been reported to be downregulated after HDACi treatment in cancer cells [127]. HDACi-mediated apoptosis also involves the activation of the intrinsic apoptotic pathway, which causes the release of inter mitochondrial membrane protein, such as cytochrome c, Smac, apoptosis-inducing factor (AIF), and the subsequent activation of caspase. HDACi activate the intrinsic apoptotic pathways by regulating the transcription of pro-apoptotic genes; i.e., Bid (BH3 interacting domain death agonist protein), Bad (Bcl-2 associated agonist of cell death protein), and Bim [130]. The mechanism of HDACi-mediated intrinsic pathway activation is not well understood, but it is suggested that HDACi causes leaking of mitochondrial intermembrane proteins, cytochrome c, AIF and Smac. The release of cytochrome c from mitochondria in turn causes activation of caspase-9 [131,132]. The intrinsic apoptotic pathway is regulated by changing the HDACi-mediated expression of factors. It can be concluded that HDACi upregulate the expression of proapoptotic genes and pathways (BAX, Apaf1 and BAK) and downregulate the expression of the antiapoptotic Bcl-2 family proteins, Bcl-2, Bcl-XL and Mcl-1 [133].

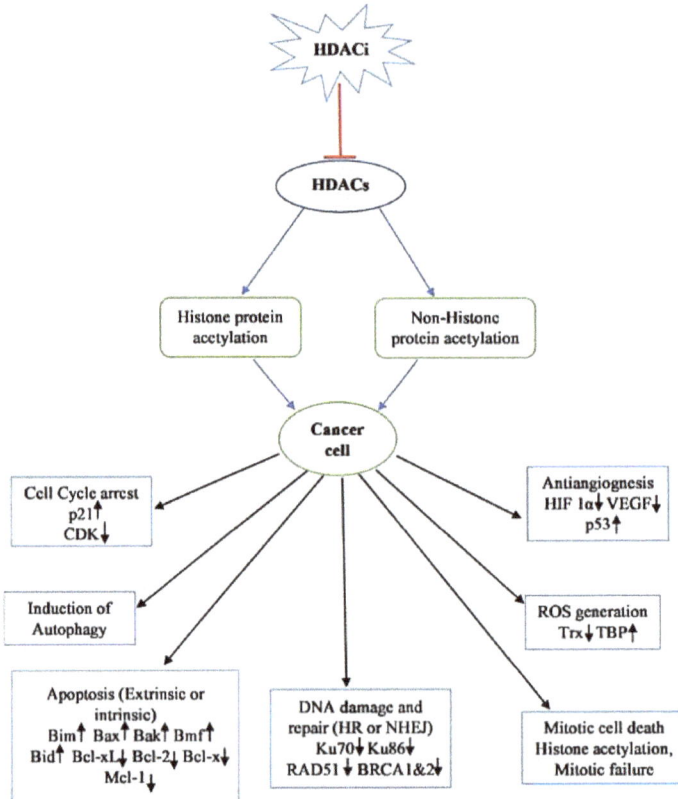

Figure 3. Multiple anti-tumor pathways such as, cell cycle arrest, induction of autophagy and apoptosis, DNA damage repair, ROS generation, angiogenesis inhibitor and mitotic cell death are activated by the action of HDACi in cancer cells. Arrows (↑ and ↓) indicates the increase and decrease, respectively, in the obtained variables. HIF, Hypoxia inducing factor; VEGF, Vascular endothelial growth factor; HR, homologous recombination; NHEJ, Non-homologous end joining; Trx, Thioredoxin; TBP, Thioredoxin binding protein.

7.3. Autophagic Cell Death

The role of HDACi in autophagy is not well understood. Recent findings suggest that autophagy serves as cell death mechanism, therefore, autophagy inhibitors or knockdown of autophagy-related gene decreases the anticancer effect of HDACi. When HeLa cell line having an Apaf-1 knockout or Bcl-XL overexpression was cultured with vorinostat or butyrate, it undergoes autophagic cell death by forming autophagosome inside cytoplasm [134]. Treatment of a colon carcinoma cell HCT116 with vorinostat resulted in the inhibition of cell growth as well as senescence type phenotype [135]. SAHA causes cell death in endometrial stromal sarcoma cell via autophagy [136]. In p53 mutant cancer cells, SAHA induces autophagy and cell death. HDACi-mediated autophagy involves several signaling pathways, one such pathway is the mechanistic target of the rapamycin (mTOR) pathway that is the main suppressor of autophagy via phosphorylation and the inactivation of the Unc51 like autophagy activating kinase 1 (ULK1) complex. SAHA inhibits the activity of mTOR and resumes the activity of ULK1, upstream component of autophagy pathway [137]. SAHA up-regulates the expression of autophagy-related protein by stimulating NF-κβ activity [138]. SAHA also induces autophagy via ROS production in leukemic and hepatocellular carcinoma cells. Romidepsin induces autophagy in HeLa cells [139]. SAHA inhibited the growth of glioblastoma cells xenograft in nude mice by inducing autophagy via downregulation of AKT-mTOR signaling [140]. In some cancer cells showing resistance towards apoptosis, HDACi can induce cell death via the induction of autophagy by bypassing the apoptosis. Hence, HDACi induced autophagy stimulation could be a promising anticancer strategy.

7.4. Inhibition of Angiogenesis

HDACi mediated inhibition of angiogenesis can interfere with the metastasis. HDAC inhibitors downregulate proangiogenic genes, such as the vascular endothelial growth factor gene (VEGF) and endothelial nitric oxide synthase gene [141]. The inhibition of the activity of hypoxia-inducible factor (HIF) by HDACi can block the angiogenesis. Hypoxia is a commonly occurring condition in tumor cells responsible for the overexpression of class I HDACs, except HDAC 8, which in turn causes activation of HIF 1α and promotes angiogenesis [142]. Several compounds viz., TSA, vorinostat, FK228, butyrate and LAQ824, have been reported to inhibit the angiogenesis process and thereby decrease the expression of proangiogenic (HIF 1α and VEGF) factors. Several mechanisms are responsible for the HDACi-mediated degradation of HIF 1α. These include the degradation of HIF 1α by acetylation at Lys532 leading to ubiquitination, class II HDACs associate with HIF 1α and cause siRNA-mediated degradation of HIF 1α [143,144]. HDACi also degrades HIF 1α through compromising its transactivation potential, and also reduces the sensitivity of cancerous cells towards the angiogenic signal generated by VEGF [145,146]. Vorinostat and TSA downregulate the expression of VEGF receptors. Valproic acid impedes angiogenesis by increasing the production of thrombospondin-1 and activin A, the antiangiogenic proteins [147]. Use of combination therapies with VEGF inhibitors finds support from the above reports.

7.5. ROS Generation

Oxidative stress has been implicated in cell death [148–151]. Experimental facts support the treatment of transformed cells with HDACi, such as TSA, vorinostat, butyrate or MS275, leading to the accumulation of reactive oxygen species (ROS) inside cells that subsequently induce cell death [152]. Ruelfi and co-workers [153] in 2001 reported that the quenching of ROS by N-acetylcysteine, a free radical scavenger decreases HDACi induced apoptosis, suggesting the role of HDACi in cell death. Thioredoxin (Trx), a hydrogen ion donor, is a ROS scavenger [154]. It is required in several redox reactions and is responsible for the activity of many protein, such as ribonucleotide reductase, which play an important role in the synthesis of DNA and the transcription factor. HDACi inhibits the activity of Trx by inducing the expression of Trx binding protein 2 (TBP2), which binds to it and inhibits its activity in cancer cells but not in normal cells [155]. Trx binds and inhibits the activity of ASK1. ASK1, an apoptosis signal regulating kinase, increases the rate of apoptosis by the activation of the SET1-JNK and MKK3/MKK6-p38 signaling pathways, and by elevating the expression of pro-apoptotic protein Bim. Therefore, higher expression of TBP2 by HDACi prevents the activity of Trx resulting in the increased expression of ASK1 and ultimately leading to apoptosis [156].

7.6. Mitotic Cell Death

HDACi treatment causes an abnormal acetylation pattern of histone protein in heterochromatin and centromere region. Newly synthesized chromatin contains acetylated histones and TSA treatment in transformed cells causes newly synthesized chromatin to remain acetylated, leading to the structural and functional disorder of centromere and pericentric heterochromatin [157], and this structural disturbance interferes with the phosphorylation of histone as well as disrupts the activity of mitotic spindle checkpoint proteins; i.e., BubR1, hBUB1, CENP-F, and CENP-E [123]. And this causes cell division arrest at the prometaphase stage followed by abnormal mitosis, such as the disaggregation and chromosomal loss leading to cell death either through apoptosis or mitotic cell death [2,124,158].

8. Potential Limitation and Side-Effects of HDACi

There are potential limitations to selective HDACi therapy. The effects of class I HDACi on DNA damage and repair pathways suggest that prolonged exposure to these agents could lead to unacceptable toxicities and secondary malignancies [159]. Class I HDACs may also play an oncogenic role depending on the context. Sontoro et al. [160] reported that in mouse tumor model, a single putative barrier to full transformation is surprisingly provided by HDAC 1 and HDAC2. Knock-down of HDAC 1 resulted in the both blockade of cellular differentiation and the increased genomic instability mediated by PML-RAR in hematopoietic progenitors. Either or both biological deregulations could be sufficient to cooperate with the tumor-promoting activities of oncoproteins, such as PML-RAR and Myc, and would provide a functional explanation for the observed increase in frequency of transformation to leukemia in HDAC1-deficient cells. Epigenetic changes are important for reprogramming somatic cells into pluripotent stem cells. Therefore, several inhibitors of epigenetic-modifying enzymes, including HDACi, are able to reprogram somatic cells into the pluripotent stem cells by modifying a chromatin structure and making it more permissive to transcription factors [119].

9. Conclusions

The present review summarizes the biological activities of HDAC. Further, emphasis has been given on the structural and functional features of the natural and synthetic inhibitors of HDAC as well as on their antitumor potential. HDACs are multisubstrate (histone and non-histone) enzyme involved in many biological processes; i.e., cell proliferation, differentiation, apoptosis, and senescence. According to scientific reports, histone deacetylase inhibitors have shown their efficacy as inhibitors of cancer initiation and progression. Generally, normal cells are resistant to HDACi, which selectively modulates gene expression in cancerous cells. Pan-HDAC inhibitors, such as vorinostat, belinostat, and panobinostat stimulate antitumor pathways, suggesting their therapeutic potential. FDA-approved HDACi are being used for the treatment of several types of cancers. Many HDACi are under clinical trial stages. HDACi show their anticancer action involving various mechanisms; i.e., cell cycle arrest, induction of apoptosis and autophagy in transformed cells, inhibition of angiogenesis, ROS as mediators of cell death, and mitotic cell death. Several natural HDACi are present in our diet: kaempferol (grapes, green tea, tomatoes, potatoes, and onions), resveratrol (grapes, red wine, blueberries and peanuts), sinapinic acid (wine and vinegar), diallyl disulfide (garlic) and zerumbone (ginger). Hence a better understanding of dietary HDACi regarding their target specificity and toxicity may underscore potential health benefits through nutritional intervention. Combination therapy might be another important direction to enhance the therapeutic efficacy of HDACi. Elucidation and validation of the detailed mechanistic aspects of HDACi action will provide a bright future for the use of HDACi as one of the important tools in the fight against cancer.

Author Contributions: A.K.S. and A.K.P. have equally contributed to the structure, preparation, and finalization of manuscript. A.K.S. conducted the literature search and prepared the first draft of the manuscript. A.K.P. and A.B. thoroughly reviewed the manuscript and made desired corrections in the final draft. All the authors have read and approved the final manuscript.

Acknowledgments: A.K.S. acknowledges the CSIR New Delhi for providing financial support in the form of Junior Research Fellowship. A.K.S. and A.K.P. also acknowledge the UGC-SAP and DST-FIST facilities of the Department of Biochemistry, University of Allahabad, Allahabad, India.

Conflicts of Interest: The authors declare no conflict of interest.

Nutrients **2018**, *10*, 731

References

1. Siegel, R.L.; Miller, K.D.; Jemal, A. Cancer Statistics, 2018. *CA Cancer J. Clin.* **2018**, *68*, 7–30. [CrossRef] [PubMed]
2. Kumar, S.; Ahmad, M.K.; Waseem, M.; Pandey, A.K. Drug Targets for Cancer Treatment: An Overview. *Med. Chem.* **2015**, *5*, 115–123. [CrossRef]
3. Sharma, U.K.; Sharma, A.K.; Pandey, A.K. Medicinal attributes of major phenylpropanoids present in cinnamon. *BMC Complement. Altern. Med.* **2016**, *16*, 156. [CrossRef] [PubMed]
4. Kumar, S.; Pandey, A.K. Oxidative stress-related microRNAs as diagnostic markers: A newer Insight in diagnostics. In *Oxidative Stress: Diagnostic Methods and Applications in Medical Science*; Maurya, P., Chandra, P., Eds.; Springer: Singapore, 2017; pp. 113–125.
5. Zahonero, B.B.; Parra, M. Histone deacetylases and cancer. *Mol. Oncol.* **2012**, *6*, 579–589. [CrossRef] [PubMed]
6. Mottamal, M.; Zheng, S.; Huang, T.L.; Wang, G. Histone Deacetylase Inhibitors in Clinical Studies as Templates for New Anticancer Agents. *Molecules* **2016**, *20*, 3898–3941. [CrossRef] [PubMed]
7. Allfrey, V.G.; Faulkner, R.; Mirsky, A.E. Acetylation and methylation of histones and their possible role in the regulation of Rna synthesis. *Proc. Natl. Acad. Sci. USA* **1964**, *51*, 786–794. [CrossRef] [PubMed]
8. Gershey, E.L.; Vidali, G.; Allfrey, V.G. Chemical studies of histone acetylation. The occurrence of epsilon-N-acetyllysine in the f2a1 histone. *J. Biol. Chem.* **1968**, *243*, 5018–5022. [PubMed]
9. Haberland, M.; Montgomery, R.L.; Olson, E.N. The many roles of histone deacetylases in development and physiology: implications for disease and therapy. *Nat. Rev. Genet.* **2009**, *10*, 32–42. [CrossRef] [PubMed]
10. Peng, L.; Seto, E. Deacetylation of Nonhistone Proteins by HDACs and the Implications in Cancer. In *Histone Deacetylases: The Biology and Clinical Implication*; Yao, T.P., Seto, E., Eds.; Handbook of Experimental Pharmacology; Springer: Berlin/Heidelberg, Germany, 2011; Volume 206, pp. 39–56. ISBN 978-3-642-21631-2.
11. Basset, S.A.; Barnett, M.P. The Role of Dietary Histone Deacetylases (HDACs) Inhibitors in Health and Disease. *Nutrients* **2014**, *6*, 4273–4301. [CrossRef] [PubMed]
12. Miller, P.E.; Snyder, D.C. Phytochemicals and cancer risk: A review of the epidemiological evidence. *Nutr. Clin. Pract.* **2012**, *27*, 599–612. [CrossRef] [PubMed]
13. Hou, I.C.; Amarnani, S.; Chong, M.T.; Bishayee, A. Green tea and the risk of genetic cancer: Epidemiological evidence. *World J. Gastroenterol.* **2013**, *19*, 3713–3722. [CrossRef] [PubMed]
14. Ivey, K.L.; Jensen, M.K.; Hodgson, J.M.; Eliassen, A.H.; Cassidy, A.; Rimm, E.B. Association of flavonoid-rich foods and flavonoids with risk of all-cause mortality. *Br. J. Nutr.* **2017**, *117*, 1470–1477. [CrossRef] [PubMed]
15. Kumar, S.; Pandey, A.K. Chemistry and biological activities of flavonoids: an overview. *Sci. World J.* **2013**, *2013*, 162750. [CrossRef] [PubMed]
16. Kim, H.J.; Bae, S.C. Histone deacetylase inhibitors: Molecular mechanisms of action and clinical trials as anti-cancer drugs. *Am. J. Transl. Res.* **2011**, *3*, 166–179. [PubMed]
17. Lawson, M.; Uciechowska, U.; Schemies, J.; Rumpf, T.; Jung, M.; Sippl, W. Inhibitors to understand molecular mechanisms of NAD$^+$-dependent deacetylases (sirtuins). *Biochim. Biophys. Acta* **2010**, *1799*, 726–739. [CrossRef] [PubMed]
18. Taunton, J.; Hassig, C.A.; Schreiber, S.L. A mammalian histone deacetylase related to the yeast transcriptional regulator Rpd3p. *Science* **1996**, *272*, 408–411. [CrossRef] [PubMed]
19. Yang, W.M.; Inouye, C.; Zeng, Y.; Bearss, D.; Seto, E. Transcriptional repression by YY1 is mediated by interaction with a mammalian homolog of the yeast global regulator RPD3. *Proc. Natl. Acad. Sci. USA* **1996**, *93*, 12845–12850. [CrossRef] [PubMed]
20. Yang, W.M.; Yao, Y.L.; Sun, J.M.; Davie, J.R.; Seto, E. Isolation and characterization of cDNAs corresponding to an additional member of the human histone deacetylase gene family. *J. Biol. Chem.* **1997**, *272*, 28001–28007. [CrossRef] [PubMed]
21. Grozinger, C.M.; Hassig, C.A.; Schreiber, S.L. Three proteins define a class of human histone deacetylases related to yeast Hda1p. *Proc. Natl. Acad. Sci. USA* **1999**, *96*, 4868–4873. [CrossRef] [PubMed]
22. Kao, H.Y.; Downes, M.; Ordentlich, P.; Evans, R.M. Isolation of a novel histone deacetylase reveals that class I and class II deacetylases promote SMRT-mediated repression. *Genes Dev.* **2000**, *14*, 55–66. [PubMed]
23. Losson, H.; Schnekenburger, M.; Dicato, M.; Diederich, M. Natural Compound Histone Deacetylase Inhibitors (HDACi): Synergy with Inflammatory Signalling Pathway Modulators and Clinical Applications in Cancer. *Molecules* **2016**, *21*, 1608. [CrossRef] [PubMed]

24. Lane, A.A.; Chabner, B.A. Histone deacetylase inhibitors in cancer therapy. *J. Clin. Oncol.* **2009**, *27*, 5459–5468. [CrossRef] [PubMed]

25. Minucci, S.; Pelicci, P.G. Histone deacetylase inhibitors and the promise of epigenetic (and more) treatments for cancer. *Nat. Rev. Cancer* **2006**, *6*, 38–51. [CrossRef] [PubMed]

26. Hubbert, C.; Guardiola, A.; Shao, R.; Kawaguchi, Y.; Ito, A.; Nixon, A.; Yoshida, M.; Wang, X.F.; Yao, T.P. HDAC6 is a microtubule associated deacetylase. *Nature* **2002**, *417*, 455–458. [CrossRef] [PubMed]

27. Seidel, C.; Schnekenburger, M.; Dicato, M.; Diederich, M. Histone deacetylase modulators provided by Mother Nature. *Genes Nutr.* **2012**, *7*, 357. [CrossRef] [PubMed]

28. Ropero, S.; Fraga, M.F.; Ballestar, E.; Hamelin, R.; Yamamoto, H.; Boix-Chornet, M.; Caballero, R.; Alaminos, M.; Setien, F.; Paz, M.F.; et al. A truncating mutation of HDAC2 in human cancers confers resistance to histone deacetylase inhibition. *Nat. Genet.* **2006**, *38*, 566–569. [CrossRef] [PubMed]

29. Fraga, M.F.; Ballestar, E.; Villar-Garea, A.; Boix-Chornet, M.; Espada, J.; Schotta, G.; Bonaldi, T.; Haydon, C.; Ropero, S.; Petrie, K.; et al. Loss of acetylation at Lys16 and trimethylation at Lys20 of histone H4 is a common hallmark of human cancer. *Nat. Genet.* **2005**, *37*, 391–400. [CrossRef] [PubMed]

30. Mai, A.; Massa, S.; Rotili, D.; Cerbara, I.; Valente, S.; Pezzi, R.; Simeoni, S.; Ragno, R. Histone deacetylation in epigenetics: An attractive target for anticancer therapy. *Med. Res. Rev.* **2005**, *25*, 261–309. [CrossRef] [PubMed]

31. Choi, J.H.; Kwon, H.J.; Yoon, B.I.; Kim, J.H.; Han, S.U.; Joo, H.J.; Kim, D.Y. Expression profile of histone deacetylase 1 in gastric cancer tissues. *Jpn. J. Cancer Res.* **2001**, *92*, 1300–1304. [CrossRef] [PubMed]

32. Witt, O.; Deubzer, H.E.; Milde, T.; Oehme, I. HDAC family: What are the cancer relevant targets? *Cancer Letters* **2009**, *277*, 8–21. [CrossRef] [PubMed]

33. Weichert, W.; Roske, V.A.; Gekeler, T.; Beckers, M.P.; Ebert, M.; Pross, M.; Dietel, C.; Denkert, C.; Rocken, C. Association of patterns of class I histone deacetylase expression with patient prognosis in gastric cancer: A retrospective analysis. *Lancet Oncol.* **2008**, *9*, 139–148. [CrossRef]

34. Weichert, W.; Roske, A.; Gekeler, V.; Beckers, T.; Stephan, C.; Jung, K.; Fritzsche, F.R.; Niesporek, S.; Denkert, C.; Dietel, M.; Kristiansen, G. Histone deacetylases 1, 2 and 3 are highly expressed in prostate cancer and HDAC2 expression is associated with shorter PSA relapse time after radical prostatectomy. *Br. J. Cancer* **2008**, *98*, 604–610. [CrossRef] [PubMed]

35. Weichert, W.; Roske, A.; Niesporek, S.; Noske, A.; Buckendahl, A.C.; Dietel, M.; Gekeler, V.; Boehm, M.; Beckers, T.; Denkert, C. Class I histone deacetylase expression has independent prognostic impact in human colorectal cancer: Specific role of class I histone deacetylases in vitro and in vivo. *Clin. Cancer Res.* **2008**, *14*, 1669–1677. [CrossRef] [PubMed]

36. Rikimaru, T.; Taketomi, A.; Yamashita, Y.; Shirabe, K.; Hamatsu, T.; Shimada, M.; Maehara, Y. Clinical significance of histone deacetylase 1 expression in patients with hepatocellular carcinoma. *Oncology* **2007**, *72*, 69–74. [CrossRef] [PubMed]

37. Sasaki, H.; Moriyama, S.; Nakashima, Y.; Kobayashi, Y.; Kiriyama, M.; Fukai, I.; Yamakawa, Y.; Fujii, Y. Histone deacetylase 1 mRNA expression in lung cancer. *Lung Cancer* **2004**, *46*, 171–178. [CrossRef] [PubMed]

38. Yoon, S.; Eom, G.H. HDAC and HDAC Inhibitor: From Cancer to Cardiovascular Diseases. *Chonnam Med. J.* **2016**, *52*, 1–11. [CrossRef] [PubMed]

39. Krusche, C.A.; Wulfing, P.; Kersting, C.; Vloet, A.; Bocker, W.; Kiesel, L.; Beier, H.M.; Alfer, J. Histone deacetylase-1 and -3 protein expression in human breast cancer: A tissue microarray analysis. *Breast Cancer Res. Treat.* **2005**, *90*, 15–23. [CrossRef] [PubMed]

40. Glaser, K.B.; Li, J.; Staver, M.J.; Wei, R.Q.; Albert, D.H.; Davidsen, S.K. Role of class I and class II histone deacetylases in carcinoma cells using siRNA. *Biochem. Biophys. Res. Commun.* **2003**, *310*, 529–536. [CrossRef] [PubMed]

41. Senese, S.; Zaragoza, K.; Minardi, S.; Muradore, I.; Ronzoni, A.S.; Passafaro, L.; Bernard, G.F.; Draetta, M.; Alcalay, C.; Seiser, S.; et al. Role for histone deacetylase 1 in human tumor cell proliferation. *Mol. Cell. Biol.* **2007**, *27*, 4784–4795. [CrossRef] [PubMed]

42. Keshelava, N.; Davicioni, E.; Wan, Z.; Ji, L.; Sposto, R.; Triche, T.J.; Reynolds, C.P. Histone deacetylase 1 gene expression and sensitization of multidrug-resistant neuroblastoma cell lines to cytotoxic agents by depsipeptide. *J. Natl. Cancer Inst.* **2007**, *99*, 1107–1119. [CrossRef] [PubMed]

43. Huang, B.H.; Laban, M.; Leung, C.H.; Lee, L.; Lee, C.K.; Salto-Tellez, M.; Raju, G.C.; Hooi, S.C. Inhibition of histone deacetylase 2 increases apoptosis and p21Cip1/WAF1 expression, independent of histone deacetylase 1. *Cell Death Differ.* **2005**, *12*, 395–404. [CrossRef] [PubMed]

44. Harms, K.L.; Chen, X. Histone deacetylase 2 modulates p53 transcriptional activities through regulation of p53-DNA binding activity. *Cancer Res.* **2007**, *67*, 3145–3152. [CrossRef] [PubMed]

45. West, A.C.; Johnstone, R.W. New and emerging HDAC inhibitors for cancer treatment. *J. Clin. Investig.* **2014**, *124*, 30–39. [CrossRef] [PubMed]

46. Wang, J.C.; Kafeel, M.I.; Avezbakiyev, B.; Chen, C.; Sun, Y.; Rathnasabapathy, C.; Kalavar, M.; He, Z.; Burton, J.; Lichter, S. Histone deacetylase in chronic lymphocytic leukemia. *Oncology* **2011**, *81*, 325–329. [CrossRef] [PubMed]

47. Atsumi, A.; Tomita, A.; Kiyoi, H.; Naoe, T. Histone deacetylase 3 (HDAC3) is recruited to target promoters by PML-RARa as a component of the N-CoR co-repressor complex to repress transcription in vivo. *Biochem. Biophys. Res. Commun.* **2006**, *345*, 1471–1480. [CrossRef] [PubMed]

48. Vannini, A.; Volpari, C.; Filocamo, G.; Casavola, E.C.; Brunetti, M.; Renzoni, D.; Chakravarty, P.; Paolini, C.; De Francesco, R.; Gallinari, P.; et al. Crystal structure of a eukaryotic zinc dependent histone deacetylase, human HDAC8, complexed with a hydroxamic acid inhibitor. *Proc. Natl. Acad. Sci. USA* **2004**, *101*, 15064–15069. [CrossRef] [PubMed]

49. Oehme, I.; Deubzer, H.E.; Wegener, D.; Pickert, D.; Linke, J.P.; Hero, B.; Kopp-Schneider, A.; Westermann, F.; Ulrich, S.M.; Von Deimling, A.; Fischer, M.; Witt, O. Histone deacetylase 8 in neuroblastoma tumorigenesis. *Clin. Cancer Res.* **2009**, *15*, 91–99. [CrossRef] [PubMed]

50. Lee, H.; Sengupta, N.; Villagra, A.; Rezai-Zadeh, N.; Seto, E. Histone deacetylase 8 safeguards the human ever-shorter telomeres 1B (hEST1B) protein from ubiquitin-mediated degradation. *Mol. Cell. Biol.* **2006**, *26*, 5259–5269. [CrossRef] [PubMed]

51. Ozdag, H.; Teschendorff, A.E.; Ahmed, A.A.; Hyland, S.J.; Blenkiron, C.; Bobrow, L.; Veerakumarasivam, A.; Burtt, G.; Subkhankulova, T.; Arends, M.J.; et al. Differential expression of selected histone modifier genes in human solid cancers. *BMC Genom.* **2006**, *7*, 90. [CrossRef] [PubMed]

52. Chauchereau, A.; Mathieu, M.; de Saintignon, J.; Ferreira, R.; Pritchard, L.L.; Mishal, Z.; Dejean, A.; Harel-Bellan, A. HDAC4 mediates transcriptional repression by the acute promyelocytic leukaemiaassociated protein PLZF. *Oncogene* **2004**, *23*, 8777–8784. [CrossRef] [PubMed]

53. Geng, H.; Harvey, C.T.; Pittsenbarger, J.; Liu, Q.; Beer, T.M.; Xue, C.; Qian, D.Z. HDAC4 protein regulates HIF1alpha protein lysine acetylation and cancer cell response to hypoxia. *J. Biol. Chem.* **2011**, *286*, 38095–38102. [CrossRef] [PubMed]

54. Wilson, A.J.; Byun, D.S.; Nasser, S.; Murray, L.B.; Ayyanar, K.; Arango, D.; Figueroa, M.; Melnick, A.; Kao, G.D.; Augenlicht, L.H.; et al. HDAC4 promotes growth of colon cancer cells via repression of p21. *Mol. Biol. Cell.* **2008**, *19*, 4062–4075. [CrossRef] [PubMed]

55. Milde, T.; Oehme, I.; Korshunov, A.; Kopp-Schneider, A.; Remke, M.; Northcott, P.; Deubzer, H.E.; Lodrini, M.; Taylor, M.D.; von Deimling, A.; et al. HDAC5 and HDAC9 in medulloblastoma: Novel markers for risk stratification and role in tumor cell growth. *Clin. Cancer Res.* **2010**, *16*, 3240–3252. [CrossRef] [PubMed]

56. Watamoto, K.; Towatari, M.; Ozawa, Y.; Miyata, Y.; Okamoto, M.; Abe, A.; Naoe, T.; Saito, H. Altered interaction of HDAC5 with GATA-1 during MEL cell differentiation. *Oncogene* **2003**, *22*, 9176–9184. [CrossRef] [PubMed]

57. Osada, H.; Tatematsu, Y.; Saito, H.; Yatabe, Y.; Mitsudomi, T.; Takahashi, T. Reduced expression of class II histone deacetylase genes is associated with poor prognosis in lung cancer patients. *Int. J. Cancer* **2004**, *112*, 26–32. [CrossRef] [PubMed]

58. Mottet, D.; Bellahcene, A.; Pirotte, S.; Waltregny, D.; Deroanne, C.; Lamour, V.; Lidereau, R.; Castronovo, V. Histone deacetylase 7 silencing alters endothelial cell migration, a key step in angiogenesis. *Circ. Res.* **2007**, *101*, 1237–1246. [CrossRef] [PubMed]

59. Kotian, S.; Liyanarachchi, S.; Zelent, A.; Parvin, J.D. Histone deacetylases 9 and 10 are required for homologous recombination. *J. Biol. Chem.* **2011**, *286*, 7722–7726. [CrossRef] [PubMed]

60. Moreno, D.A.; Scrideli, C.A.; Cortez, M.A.; de Paula Queiroz, R.; Valera, E.T.; da Silva Silveira, V.; Yunes, J.A.; Brandalise, S.R.; Tone, L.G. Differential expression of HDAC3, HDAC7 and HDAC9 is associated with prognosis and survival in childhood acute lymphoblastic leukaemia. *Br. J. Haematol.* **2010**, *150*, 665–673. [CrossRef] [PubMed]

61. Seidel, C.; Schnekenburger, M.; Dicato, M.; Diederich, M. Histone deacetylase 6 in health and disease. *Epigenomics* **2015**, *7*, 103–118. [CrossRef] [PubMed]

62. Sakuma, T.; Uzawa, K.; Onda, T.; Shiiba, M.; Yokoe, H.; Shibahara, T.; Tanzawa, H. Aberrant expression of histone deacetylase 6 in oral squamous cell carcinoma. *Int. J. Oncol.* **2006**, *29*, 117–124. [CrossRef] [PubMed]

63. Haggarty, S.J.; Koeller, K.M.; Wong, J.C.; Grozinger, C.M.; Schreiber, S.L. Domain-selective small-molecule inhibitor of histone deacetylase 6 (HDAC6)-mediated tubulin deacetylation. *Proc. Natl. Acad. Sci. USA* **2003**, *100*, 4389–4394. [CrossRef] [PubMed]

64. Bali, P.; Pranpat, M.; Bradner, J.; Balasis, M.; Fiskus, W.; Guo, F.; Rocha, K.; Kumaraswamy, S.; Boyapalle, S.; Atadja, P.; et al. Inhibition of histone deacetylase 6 acetylates and disrupts the chaperone function of heat shock protein 90: A novel basis for antileukemia activity of histone deacetylase inhibitors. *J. Biol. Chem.* **2005**, *280*, 26729–26734. [CrossRef] [PubMed]

65. Shan, B.; Yao, T.P.; Nguyen, H.T.; Zhuo, Y.; Levy, D.R.; Klingsberg, R.C.; Palmer, M.L.; Holder, K.N.; Lasky, J.A. Requirement of HDAC6 for TGF-β 1-induced epithelial-mesenchymal transition. *J. Biol. Chem.* **2008**, *283*, 21065–21073. [CrossRef] [PubMed]

66. Lee, J.H.; Jeong, E.G.; Choi, M.C.; Kim, S.H.; Park, J.H.; Song, S.H.; Park, J.; Bang, Y.J.; Kim, T.Y. Inhibition of histone deacetylase 10 induces thioredoxin-interacting protein and causes accumulation of reactive oxygen species in SNU-620 human gastric cancer cells. *Mol. Cell.* **2010**, *30*, 107–112. [CrossRef] [PubMed]

67. Johnson, E.K.; Wilgus, A.T. Vascular endothelial growth factor and angiogenesis in the regulation of cutaneous wound repair. *Adv. Wound Care (New Rochelle)*, **2014**, *3*, 647–661. [CrossRef] [PubMed]

68. Park, J.H.; Kim, S.H.; Choi, M.C.; Lee, J.; Oh, D.Y.; Im, S.A.; Bang, Y.J.; Kim, T.Y. Class II histone deacetylases play pivotal roles in heat shock protein 90-mediated proteasomal degradation of vascular endothelial growth factor receptors. *Biochem. Biophys. Res. Commun.* **2008**, *368*, 318–322. [CrossRef] [PubMed]

69. Bradbury, C.A.; Khanim, F.L.; Hayden, R.; Bunce, C.M.; White, D.A.; Drayson, M.T.; Craddock, C.; Turner, B.M. Histone deacetylases in acute myeloid leukaemia show a distinctive pattern of expression that changes selectively in response to deacetylase inhibitors. *Leukemia* **2005**, *19*, 1751–1759. [CrossRef] [PubMed]

70. Hida, Y.; Kubo, Y.; Murao, K.; Arase, S. Strong expression of a longevity-related protein, SIRT1, in Bowen's disease. *Arch. Dermatol. Res.* **2007**, *299*, 103–106. [CrossRef] [PubMed]

71. Huffman, D.M.; Grizzle, W.E.; Bamman, M.M.; Kim, J.S.; Eltoum, I.A.; Elgavish, A.; Nagy, T.R. SIRT1 is significantly elevated in mouse and human prostate cancer. *Cancer Res.* **2007**, *67*, 6612–6618. [CrossRef] [PubMed]

72. Hiratsuka, M.; Inoue, T.; Toda, T.; Kimura, N.; Shirayoshi, Y.; Kamitani, H.; Watanabe, T.; Ohama, E.; Tahimic, C.G.; Kurimasa, A.; et al. Proteomics-based identification of differentially expressed genes in human gliomas: Down-regulation of SIRT2 gene. *Biochem. Biophys. Res. Commun.* **2003**, *309*, 558–566. [CrossRef] [PubMed]

73. Lennerz, V.; Fatho, M.; Gentilini, C.; Frye, R.A.; Lifke, A.; Ferel, D.; Wolfel, C.; Huber, C.; Wolfel, T. The response of autologous T cells to a human melanoma is dominated by mutated neoantigens. *Proc. Natl. Acad. Sci. USA* **2005**, *102*, 16013–16018. [CrossRef] [PubMed]

74. Ashraf, N.; Zino, S.; Macintyre, A.; Kingsmore, D.; Payne, A.P.; George, W.D.; Shiels, P.G. Altered sirtuin expression is associated with node-positive breast cancer. *Br. J. Cancer* **2006**, *95*, 1056–1061. [CrossRef] [PubMed]

75. Dryden, S.C.; Nahhas, F.A.; Nowak, J.E.; Goustin, A.S.; Tainsky, M.A. Role for human SIRT2 NAD-dependent class II histone deacetylases in a Sin3-independent repression pathway. *Genes Dev.* **2003**, *14*, 45–54.

76. Chu, F.; Chou, P.M.; Zheng, X.; Mirkin, B.L.; Rebbaa, A. Control of multidrug resistance gene mdr1 and cancer resistance to chemotherapy by the longevity gene sirt1. *Cancer Res.* **2005**, *65*, 10183–10187. [CrossRef] [PubMed]

77. Yang, H.; Yang, T.; Baur, J.A.; Perez, E.; Matsui, T.; Carmona, J.J.; Lamming, D.W.; Souza-Pinto, N.C.; Bohr, V.A.; Rosenzweig, A.; et al. Nutrient-sensitive mitochondrial NAD⁺ levels dictate cell survival. *Cell* **2007**, *130*, 1095–1107. [CrossRef] [PubMed]

78. Bell, E.L.; Emerling, B.M.; Ricoult, S.J.; Guarente, L. SirT3 suppresses hypoxia inducible factor 1alpha and tumor growth by inhibiting mitochondrial ROS production. *Oncogene* **2011**, *30*, 2986–2996. [CrossRef] [PubMed]

79. Skov, V.; Larsen, T.S.; Thomassen, M.; Riley, C.H.; Jensen, M.K.; Bjerrum, O.W.; Kruse, T.A.; Hasselbalch, H.C. Increased gene expression of histone deacetylases in patients with Philadelphia-negative chronic myeloproliferative neoplasms. *Leuk. Lymphoma* **2012**, *53*, 123–129. [CrossRef] [PubMed]

80. Gao, L.; Cueto, M.A.; Asselbergs, F.; Atadja, P. Cloning and functional characterization of HDAC11, a novel member of the human histone deacetylase family. *J. Biol. Chem.* **2002**, *277*, 25748–25755. [CrossRef] [PubMed]

81. Riggs, M.G.; Whittaker, R.G.; Neumann, J.R.; Ingram, V.M. *n*-Butyrate causes histone modification in HeLa and Friend erythroleukaemia cells. *Nature* **1977**, *268*, 462–464. [CrossRef] [PubMed]

82. Kijima, M.; Yoshida, M.; Sugita, K.; Horinouchi, S.; Beppu, T. Trapoxin, an antitumor cyclic tetrapeptide, is an irreversible inhibitor of mammalian histone deacetylase. *J. Biol. Chem.* **1993**, *268*, 22429–22435. [PubMed]

83. Li, Y.; Seto, E. HDACs and HDAC Inhibitors in Cancer Development and Therapy. *Cold Spring Harb. Perspect. Med.* **2016**, *6*, 10. [CrossRef] [PubMed]

84. Ungerstedt, J.S.; Sowa, Y.; Xu, W.S.; Shao, Y.; Dokmanovic, M.; Perez, G.; Ngo, L.; Holmgren, A.; Jiang, X.; Marks, P.A. Role of thioredoxin in the response of normal and transformed cells to histone deacetylase inhibitors. *Proc. Natl. Acad. Sci. USA* **2005**, *102*, 673–678. [CrossRef] [PubMed]

85. Tsuji, N.; Kobayashi, M.; Nagashima, K.; Wakisaka, Y.; Koizumi, K. A new antifungal antibiotic, trichostatin. *J. Antibiot.* **1976**, *29*, 1–6. [CrossRef] [PubMed]

86. Yoshida, M.; Kijima, M.; Akita, M.; Beppu, T. Potent and specific inhibition of mammalian histone deacetylase both in vivo and in vitro by trichostatin A. *J. Biol. Chem.* **1990**, *265*, 17174–17179. [PubMed]

87. Mcknight, G.S.; Hanger, L.; Palmiter, R.D. Butyrate and related inhibitors of histone deacetylation block the induction of egg white genes by steroid harmones. *Cell* **1980**, *22*, 469–477. [CrossRef]

88. Orlikova, B.; Schnekenburger, M.; Zloh, M.; Golais, F.; Diederich, M.; Tasdemir, D. Natural chalcones as dual inhibitors of HDACs and NF-κB. *Oncol. Rep.* **2012**, *28*, 797–805. [CrossRef] [PubMed]

89. Berger, A.; Venturelli, S.; Kallnischkies, M.; Bocker, A.; Busch, C.; Weiland, T.; Noor, S.; Leischner, C.; Weiss, T.S.; Lauer, U.M.; et al. Kaempferol, a new nutrition-derived pan-inhibitor of human histone deacetylases. *J. Nutr. Biochem.* **2013**, *24*, 977–985. [CrossRef] [PubMed]

90. Senawong, T.; Misuna, S.; Khaopha, S.; Nuchadomrong, S.; Sawatsitang, P.; Phaosiri, C.; Surapaitoon, A.; Sripa, B. Histone deacetylase (HDAC) inhibitory and antiproliferative activities of phenolic-rich extracts derived from the rhizome of Hydnophytum formicarum Jack.: Sinapinic acid acts as HDAC inhibitor. *BMC Complement. Altern. Med.* **2013**, *13*, 232. [CrossRef] [PubMed]

91. Venturelli, S.; Berger, A.; Bocker, A.; Busch, C.; Weiland, T.; Noor, S.; Leischner, C.; Schleicher, S.; Mayer, M.; Weiss, T.S.; et al. Resveratrol as a pan-HDAC inhibitor alters the acetylation status of histone [corrected] proteins in human-derived hepatoblastoma cells. *PLoS ONE* **2013**, *8*, 73097. [CrossRef]

92. Ryu, H.W.; Lee, D.H.; Shin, D.H.; Kim, S.H.; Kwon, S.H. Aeroside VIII is a natural selective HDAC6 inhibitor that synergistically enhances the anticancer activity of HDAC inhibitor in HT29 cells. *Planta Med.* **2015**, *81*, 222–227. [CrossRef] [PubMed]

93. Jones, P.; Altamura, S.; Chakravarty, P.K.; Cecchetti, O.; de Francesco, R.; Gallinari, P.; Ingenito, R.; Meinke, P.T.; Petrocchi, A.; Rowley, M.; et al. A series of novel, potent, and selective histone deacetylase inhibitors. *Bioorg. Med. Chem. Lett.* **2006**, *16*, 5948–5952. [CrossRef] [PubMed]

94. Maulucci, N.; Chini, M.G.; Micco, S.D.; Izzo, I.; Cafaro, E.; Russo, A.; Gallinari, P.; Paolini, C.; Nardi, M.C.; Casapullo, A.; et al. Molecular Insights into Azumamide E Histone Deacetylases Inhibitory Activity. *J. Am. Chem. Soc.* **2007**, *129*, 3007–3012. [CrossRef] [PubMed]

95. De Schepper, S.; Bruwiere, H.; Verhulst, T.; Steller, U.; Andries, L.; Wouters, W.; Janicot, M.; Arts, J.; vanHeusden, J. Inhibition of histone deacetylases by chlamydocin induces apoptosis and proteasome-mediated degradation of survivin. *J. Pharmacol. Exp. Ther.* **2003**, *304*, 881–888. [CrossRef] [PubMed]

96. Itazaki, H.; Nagashima, K.; Sugita, K.; Yoshida, H.; Kawamura, Y.; Yasuda, Y.; Matsumoto, K.; Ishii, K.; Uotani, N.; Nakai, H.; et al. Isolation and structural elucidation of new cyclotetrapeptides, trapoxins A and B, having detransformation activities as antitumor agents. *J. Antibiot.* **1990**, *43*, 1524–1532. [CrossRef] [PubMed]

97. Li, L.; Dai, H.J.; Ye, M.; Wang, S.L.; Xiao, X.J.; Zheng, J.; Chen, H.Y.; Luo, Y.H.; Liu, J. Lycorine induces cell-cycle arrest in the G0/G1 phase in K562 cells via HDAC inhibition. *Cancer Cell Int.* **2012**, *12*, 49. [CrossRef] [PubMed]

98. Parolin, C.; Calonghi, N.; Presta, E.; Boga, C.; Caruana, P.; Naldi, M.; Andrisano, V.; Masotti, L.; Sartor, G. Mechanism and stereoselectivity of HDAC I inhibition by (R)-9-hydroxystearic acid in colon cancer. *Biochim. Biophys. Acta* **2012**, *1821*, 1334–1340. [CrossRef] [PubMed]

99. Ghosh, A.K.; Kulkarni, S. Enantioselective total synthesis of (+)-largazole, a potent inhibitor of histone deacetylase. *Org. Lett.* **2008**, *10*, 3907–3909. [CrossRef] [PubMed]

100. Druesne, N.; Pagniez, A.; Mayeur, C.; Thomas, M.; Cherbuy, C.; Duee, P.H.; Martel, P.; Chaumontet, C. Diallyl disulfide (DADS) increases histone acetylation and p21(waf1/cip1) expression in human colon tumor cell lines. *Carcinogenesis* **2004**, *25*, 1227–1236. [CrossRef] [PubMed]

101. Lea, M.A.; Rasheed, M.; Randolph, V.M.; Khan, F.; Shareef, A.; desBordes, C. Induction of histone acetylation and inhibition of growth of mouse erythroleukemia cells by S-allylmercaptocysteine. *Nutr. Cancer* **2002**, *43*, 90–102. [CrossRef] [PubMed]

102. Ververis, K.; Hiong, A.; Karagiannis, T.C.; Licciardi, P.V. Histone deacetylase inhibitors (HDACIs): Multitargeted anticancer agents. *Biologics* **2013**, *7*, 47–60. [CrossRef] [PubMed]

103. Robertson, F.M.; Chu, K.; Boley, K.M.; Ye, Z.; Liu, H.; Wright, M.C.; Moraes, R.; Zhang, X.; Green, T.L.; Barsky, S.H.; et al. The class I HDAC inhibitor romidepsin targets inflammatory breast cancer tumor emboli and synergizes with paclitaxel to inhibit metastasis. *J. Exp. Ther. Oncol.* **2013**, *10*, 219–233. [PubMed]

104. Paller, C.J.; Wissing, M.D.; Mendonca, J.; Sharma, A.; Kim, E.; Kim, H.S.; Kortenhorst, M.S.Q.; Gerber, S.; Rosen, M.; Shaikh, F.; et al. Combining the pan-aurora kinase inhibitor AMG 900 with histone deacetylase inhibitors enhances antitumor activity in prostate cancer. *Cancer Med.* **2014**, *3*, 1322–1335. [CrossRef] [PubMed]

105. Ferrarelli, L.K. HDAC inhibitors in solid tumors and blood cancers. *Sci. Signal.* **2016**, *9*, ec216. [CrossRef]

106. Vancurova, I.; Uddin, M.M.; Zou, Y.; Vancura, A. Combination Therapies Targeting HDAC and IKK in Solid Tumors. *Trends Pharmacol. Sci.* **2018**, *39*, 295–306. [CrossRef] [PubMed]

107. Marks, P.A.; Breslow, R. Dimethyl sulfoxide to vorinostat: Development of this histone deacetylase inhibitor as an anticancer drug. *Nat. Biotechnol.* **2007**, *25*, 84–90. [CrossRef] [PubMed]

108. Giaccone, G.; Rajan, A.; Berman, A.; Kelly, R.J.; Szabo, E.; Lopez-Chavez, A.; Trepel, J.; Lee, M.J.; Cao, L.; Espinoza-Delgado, I.; et al. Phase II study of belinostat in patients with recurrent or refractory advanced thymic epithelial tumors. *J. Clin. Oncol.* **2011**, *29*, 2052–2059. [CrossRef] [PubMed]

109. Duvic, M.; Dummer, R.; Becker, J.C.; Poulalhon, N.; Ortiz Romero, P.; Grazia Bernengo, M.; Lebbé, C.; Assaf, C.; Squier, M.; Williams, D.; et al. Panobinostat activity in both bexarotene- exposed and -naive patients with refractory cutaneous T-cell lymphoma: Results of a phase II trial. *Eur. J. Cancer* **2013**, *49*, 386–394. [CrossRef] [PubMed]

110. Rambaldi, A.; Dummer, R.; Becker, J.C.; Poulalhon, N.; Ortiz, R.P.; Grazia, B.M.; Lebbe, C.; Assaf, C.; Squier, M.; Williams, D.; et al. A pilot study of the Histone-Deacetylase inhibitor Givinostat in patients with JAK2V617F positive chronic myeloproliferative neoplasms. *Br. J. Haematol.* **2010**, *150*, 446–455. [CrossRef] [PubMed]

111. Razak, A.R.; Hotte, S.J.; Siu, L.L.; Chen, E.X.; Hirte, H.W.; Powers, J.; Walsh, W.; Stayner, L.A.; Laughlin, A.; Novotny-Diermayr, V.; et al. Phase I clinical, pharmacokinetic and pharmacodynamic study of SB939, an oral histone deacetylase (HDAC) inhibitor, in patients with advanced solid tumours. *Br. J. Cancer* **2011**, *104*, 756–762. [CrossRef] [PubMed]

112. Pili, R.; Salumbides, B.; Zhao, M.; Altiok, S.; Qian, D.; Zwiebel, J.; Carducci, M.A.; Rudek, M.A. Phase I study of the histone deacetylase inhibitor entinostat in combination with 13-cis retinoic acid in patients with solid tumours. *Br. J. Cancer* **2012**, *106*, 77–84. [CrossRef] [PubMed]

113. Banerji, U.; van Doorn, L.; Papadatos-Pastos, D.; Kristeleit, R.; Debnam, P.; Tall, M.; Stewart, A.; Raynaud, F.; Garrett, M.D.; Toal, M.; et al. A phase I pharmacokinetic and pharmacodynamics study of CHR-3996, an oral class I selective histone deacetylase inhibitor in refractory solid tumors. *Clin. Cancer Res.* **2012**, *18*, 2687–2694. [CrossRef] [PubMed]

114. Dong, M.; Ning, Z.Q.; Xing, P.Y.; Xu, J.L.; Cao, H.X.; Dou, G.F.; Meng, Z.Y.; Shi, Y.K.; Lu, X.P.; Feng, F.Y. Phase I study of chidamide (CS055/HBI-8000), a new histone deacetylase inhibitor, in patients with advanced solid tumors and lymphomas. *Cancer Chemother. Pharmacol.* **2012**, *69*, 1413–1422. [CrossRef] [PubMed]

115. Eckschlager, T.; Plch, J.; Stiborova, M.; Hrabeta, J. Histone Deacetylase Inhibitors as Anticancer Drugs. *Int. J. Mol. Sci.* **2017**, *18*, 1414. [CrossRef] [PubMed]

116. Younes, A.; Oki, Y.; Bociek, R.G.; Kuruvilla, J.; Fanale, M.; Neelapu, S.; Copeland, A.; Buglio, D.; Galal, A.; Besterman, J.; et al. Mocetinostat for relapsed classical Hodgkin's lymphoma: An open-label, single-arm, phase 2 trial. *Lancet Oncol.* **2011**, *12*, 1222–1228. [CrossRef]

117. Coiffier, B.; Pro, B.; Prince, H.M.; Foss, F.; Sokol, L.; Greenwood, M.; Caballero, D.; Borchmann, P.; Morschhauser, F.; Wilhelm, M.; et al. Results from a pivotal, open-label, phase II study of romidepsin in relapsed or refractory peripheral T-cell lymphoma after prior systemic therapy. *J. Clin. Oncol.* **2012**, *30*, 631–636. [CrossRef] [PubMed]

118. Bolden, J.E.; Peart, M.J.; Johnstone, R.W. Anticancer activities of histone deacetylase inhibitors. *Nat. Rev. Drug Discov.* **2006**, *5*, 769–784. [CrossRef] [PubMed]

119. Bao, L.; Diao, H.; Dong, N.; Xu, S.; Wang, B.; Mo, Q.; Yu, H.; Wang, X.; Chen, C. Histone deacetylase inhibitor induces cell apoptosis and cycle arrest in lung cancer cell via mitochondrial injury and p53 up-acetylation. *Cell Biol. Toxicol.* **2016**, *32*, 469–482. [CrossRef] [PubMed]

120. Kretsovali, A.; Hadjimichael, C.; Charmpilas, N. Histone deacetylase inhibitors in cell pluripotency, differentiation, and reprogramming. *Stem Cells Int.* **2012**, *2012*, 184154. [CrossRef] [PubMed]

121. Vrana, J.A.; Decker, R.H.; Johnson, C.R.; Wang, Z.; Jarvis, W.D.; Richon, V.M.; Ehinger, M.; Fisher, P.B.; Grant, S. Induction of apoptosis in U937 human leukemia cells by suberoylanilide hydroxamic acid (SAHA) proceeds through pathways that are regulated by Bcl-2/Bcl-XL, c-Jun, and p21CIP1, but independent of p53. *Oncogene* **1999**, *18*, 7016–7025. [CrossRef] [PubMed]

122. Richon, V.M.; Sandhoff, T.W.; Rifkind, R.A.; Marks, P.A. Histone deacetylase inhibitor selectively induces p21WAF1 expression and gene-associated histone acetylation. *Proc. Natl. Acad. Sci. USA* **2000**, *97*, 10014–10019. [CrossRef] [PubMed]

123. Xu, W.S.; Parmigiani, R.B.; Marks, P.A. Histone deacetylase inhibitors: molecular mechanisms of action. *Oncogene* **2007**, *26*, 5541–5552. [CrossRef] [PubMed]

124. Singh, A.K.; Kumar, R.; Pandey, A.K. Hepatocellular carcinoma: Causes, mechanism of progression and biomarkers. *Curr. Chem. Genom. Transl. Med.* **2018**, Accepted-in press.

125. Hitomi, T.; Matsuzaki, Y.; Yokota, T.; Takaoka, Y.; Sakai, T. p15 (INK4b) in HDAC inhibitor-induced growth arrest. *FEBS Lett* **2003**, *554*, 347–350. [CrossRef]

126. Suzuki, T.; Yokozaki, H.; Kuniyasu, H.; Hayashi, K.; Naka, K.; Ono, S.; Ishikawa, T.; Tahara, E.; Yasui, W. Effect of trichostatin A on cell growth and expression of cell cycle- and apoptosis-related molecules in humangastric and oral carcinoma cell lines. *Int. J. Cancer* **2000**, *88*, 992–997. [CrossRef]

127. Nakata, S.; Yoshida, T.; Horinaka, M.; Shiraishi, T.; Wakada, M.; Sakai, T. Histone deacetylase inhibitors upregulate death receptor 5/TRAIL-R2 and sensitize apoptosis induced by TRAIL/APO2-L in human malignant tumor cells. *Oncogene* **2004**, *23*, 6261–6271. [CrossRef] [PubMed]

128. Glick, R.D.; Swendeman, S.L.; Coffey, D.C.; Rifkind, R.A.; Marks, P.A.; Richon, V.M.; Michael, P.; La-Quaglia, M.P. Hybrid polar histone deacetylase inhibitor induces apoptosis and CD95/ CD95 ligand expression in human neuroblastoma. *Cancer Res.* **1999**, *59*, 4392–4399. [PubMed]

129. Insinga, A.; Monestiroli, S.; Ronzoni, S.; Gelmetti, V.; Marchesi, F.; Viale, A.; Altucci, L.; Nervi, C.; Minucci, S.; Pelicci, P.G. Inhibitors of histone deacetylases induce tumor-selective apoptosis through activation of the death receptor pathway. *Nat. Med.* **2005**, *11*, 71–76. [CrossRef] [PubMed]

130. Zhao, Y.; Tan, J.; Zhuang, L.; Jiang, X.; Liu, E.T.; Yu, Q. Inhibitors of histone deacetylases target the Rb-E2F1 pathway for apoptosis induction through activation of proapoptotic protein Bim. *Proc. Natl. Acad. Sci. USA* **2005**, *102*, 16090–16095. [CrossRef] [PubMed]

131. Ruefli, A.A.; Bernhard, D.; Tainton, K.M.; Kofler, R.; Smyth, M.J.; Johnstone, R.W. Suberoylanilide hydroxamic acid (SAHA) overcomes multidrug resistance and induces cell death in P-glycoprotein-expressing cells. *Int. J. Cancer* **2002**, *99*, 292–298. [CrossRef] [PubMed]

132. Sharma, A.K.; Kumar, S.; Chashoo, G.; Saxena, A.K.; Pandey, A.K. Cell cycle inhibitory activity of Piper longum against A549 cell line and its protective effect against metal-induced toxicity in rats. *Ind. J. Biochem. Biophys.* **2014**, *51*, 358–364.

133. Rosato, R.R.; Maggio, S.C.; Almenara, J.A.; Payne, S.G.; Atadja, P.; Spiegel, S.; Dent, P.; Grant, S. The histone deacetylase inhibitor LAQ824 induces human leukemia cell death through a process involving XIAP down-regulation, oxidative injury, and the acid sphingomyelinase-dependent generation of ceramide. *Mol. Pharmacol.* **2006**, *69*, 216–225. [CrossRef] [PubMed]

134. Shao, Y.; Gao, Z.; Marks, P.A.; Jiang, X. Apoptotic and autophagic cell death induced by histone deacetylase inhibitors. *Proc. Natl. Acad. Sci. USA* **2004**, *101*, 18030–18035. [CrossRef] [PubMed]

135. Zhang, J.; Ng, S.; Wang, J.; Zhou, J.; Tan, S.H.; Yang, N.; Lin, Q.; Xia, D.; Shen, H.M. Histone deacetylase inhibitors induce autophagy through FOXO1-dependent pathways. *Autophagy* **2015**, *11*, 629–642. [CrossRef] [PubMed]

136. Hrzenjak, A.; Kremser, M.L.; Strohmeier, B.; Moinfar, F.; Zatloukal, K.; Denk, H. SAHA induces caspase-independent, autophagic cell death of endometrial stromal sarcoma cells by influencing the mTOR pathway. *J. Pathol.* **2008**, *216*, 495–504. [CrossRef] [PubMed]

137. Liu, Y.L.; Yang, P.M.; Shun, C.T.; Wu, M.S.; Weng, J.R.; Chen, C.C. Autophagy potentiates the anti-cancer effects of the histone deacetylase inhibitors in hepatocellular carcinoma. *Autophagy* **2010**, *6*, 1057–1065. [CrossRef] [PubMed]

138. Shulak, L.; Beljanski, V.; Chiang, C.; Dutta, M.; Van Grevenynghe, J.; Belgnaoui, S.M.; Nguyen, L.; Di Lenardo, T.; Semmes, O.J.; Lin, R.; et al. Histone deacetylase inhibitors potentiate vesicular stomatitis virus oncolysis in prostate cancer cells by modulating NF-κB-dependent autophagy. *J. Virol.* **2014**, *88*, 2927–2940. [CrossRef] [PubMed]

139. Oh, M.; Choi, I.K.; Kwon, H.J. Inhibition of histone deacetylase1 induces autophagy. *Biochem. Biophys. Res. Commun.* **2008**, *369*, 1179–1183. [CrossRef] [PubMed]

140. Chiao, M.T.; Cheng, W.Y.; Yang, Y.C.; Shen, C.C.; Ko, J.L. Suberoylanilide hydroxamic acid (SAHA) causes tumor growth slowdown and triggers autophagy in glioblastoma stem cells. *Autophagy* **2013**, *9*, 1509–1526. [CrossRef] [PubMed]

141. Zupkovitz, G.; Tischler, J.; Posch, M.; Sadzak, I.; Ramsauer, K.; Egger, G.; Grausenburger, R.; Schweifer, N.; Chiocca, S.; Decker, T.; et al. Negative and positive regulation of gene expression by mouse histone deacetylase 1. *Mol. Cell Biol.* **2006**, *26*, 7913–7928. [CrossRef] [PubMed]

142. Liang, D.; Kong, X.; Sang, N. Effects of histone deacetylase inhibitors on HIF-1. *Cell Cycle* **2006**, *5*, 2430–2435. [CrossRef] [PubMed]

143. Jeong, J.W.; Bae, M.K.; Ahn, M.Y.; Kim, S.H.; Sohn, T.K.; Bae, M.H.; Yoo, M.A.; Song, E.J.; Lee, K.J.; Kim, K.W. Regulation and destabilization of HIF-1alpha by ARD1-mediated acetylation. *Cell* **2002**, *111*, 709–720. [CrossRef]

144. Qian, D.Z.; Kachhap, S.K.; Collis, S.J.; Verheul, H.M.; Carducci, M.A.; Atadja, P.; Pili, R. Class II histone deacetylases arenassociated with VHL-independent regulation of hypoxiainducible factor 1{alpha}. *Cancer Res.* **2006**, *66*, 8814–8821. [CrossRef] [PubMed]

145. Fath, D.M.; Kong, X.; Liang, D.; Lin, Z.; Chou, A.; Jiang, Y.; Fang, J.; Caro, J.; Sang, N. Histone deacetylase inhibitors repress the transactivation potential of hypoxia-inducible factors independently of direct acetylation of HIF-alpha. *J. Biol. Chem.* **2006**, *281*, 13612–13619. [CrossRef] [PubMed]

146. Deroanne, C.F.; Bonjean, K.; Servotte, S.; Devy, L.; Colige, A.; Clausse, N.; Blacher, S.; Verdin, E.; Foidart, J.M.; Nusgens, B.V.; et al. Histone deacetylases inhibitors as anti-angiogenic agents altering vascular endothelial growth factor signaling. *Oncogene* **2002**, *21*, 427–436. [CrossRef] [PubMed]

147. Cinatl, J.; Kotchetkov, R.; Blaheta, R.; Driever, P.H.; Vogel, J.U.; Cinatl, J. Induction of differentiation and suppression of malignant phenotype of human neuroblastoma BE(2)-C cells by valproic acid: Enhancement by combination with interferon α. *Int. J. Oncol.* **2002**, *20*, 97–106. [CrossRef] [PubMed]

148. Sharma, U.K.; Kumar, R.; Gupta, A.; Ganguly, R.; Pandey, A.K. Renoprotective effect of cinnamaldehyde in food color induced toxicity. *3 Biotech* **2018**, *8*, 212. [CrossRef] [PubMed]

149. Sharma, U.K.; Sharma, A.K.; Gupta, A.; Kumar, R.; Pandey, A.; Pandey, A.K. Pharmacological activities of cinnamaldehyde and eugenol: antioxidant, cytotoxic and anti-leishmanial studies. *Cell. Mol. Biol. (Noisy-le-grand)* **2017**, *63*, 73–78. [CrossRef] [PubMed]

150. Kumar, S.; Pandey, S.; Pandey, A.K. In vitro antibacterial, antioxidant, cytotoxic activities of Parthenium hysterophorus and characterization of extracts by LC MS analysis. *BioMed Res. Int.* **2014**, *2014*, 495154. [CrossRef] [PubMed]

151. Sharma, A.K.; Sharma, U.K.; Pandey, A.K. Protective effect of *Bauhinia variegata* leaf extracts against oxidative damage, cell proliferation and bacterial growth. *Proc. Natl. Acad. Sci. India, Sect. B Biol. Sci.* **2017**, *87*, 47–51. [CrossRef]

152. Rosato, R.R.; Almenara, J.A.; Grant, S. The histone deacetylase inhibitor MS-275 promotes differentiation or apoptosis in human leukemia cells through a process regulated by generation of reactive oxygen species and induction of p21CIP1/WAF1 1. *Cancer Res.* **2003**, *63*, 3637–3645. [PubMed]

153. Ruefli, A.A.; Ausserlechner, M.J.; Bernhard, D.; Sutton, V.R.; Tainton, K.M.; Kofler, R.; Smyth, M.J.; Johnstone, R.W. The histone deacetylase inhibitor and chemotherapeutic agent suberoylanilide hydroximic acid (SAHA) induces a cell-death pathway characterized by cleavage of Bid and production of reactive oxygen species. *Proc. Natl. Acad. Sci. USA* **2001**, *98*, 10833–10838. [CrossRef] [PubMed]

154. Kumar, S.; Pandey, A.K. Free radicals: Health implications and their mitigation by herbals. *Br. J. Med. Med. Res.* **2015**, *7*, 438–457. [CrossRef]

155. Xu, W.; Ngo, L.; Perez, G.; Dokmanovic, M.; Marks, P.A. Intrinsic apoptotic and thioredoxin pathways in human prostate cancer cell response to histone deacetylase inhibitor. *Proc. Natl. Acad. Sci. USA* **2006**, *103*, 15540–15545. [CrossRef] [PubMed]

156. Saitoh, M.; Nishitoh, H.; Fujii, M.; Takeda, K.; Tobiume, K.; Sawada, Y.; Kawabata, M.; Miyazono, K.; Ichijo, H. Mammalian thioredoxin is a direct inhibitor of apoptosis signal-regulating kinase (ASK) 1. *EMBO J.* **1998**, *17*, 2596–2606. [CrossRef] [PubMed]

157. Cimini, D.; Mattiuzzo, M.; Torosantucci, L.; Degrassi, F. Histone hyperacetylation in mitosis prevents sister chromatid separation and produces chromosome segregation defects. *Mol. Biol. Cell* **2003**, *14*, 3821–3833. [CrossRef] [PubMed]

158. Kumar, S.; Chashoo, G.; Saxena, A.K.; Pandey, A.K. *Parthenium hysterophorus*: A Probable Source of Anticancer, Antioxidant and Anti-HIV Agents. *BioMed Res. Int.* **2013**, *2013*, 810734. [CrossRef] [PubMed]

159. Khabele, D. The Therapeutic Potential of Class I Selective Histone Deacetylase Inhibitors in Ovarian Cancer. *Front. Oncol.* **2014**, *4*, 111. [CrossRef] [PubMed]

160. Santoro, F.; Botrugno, O.A.; Dal, Z.R.; Pallavicini, I.; Matthews, G.M.; Cluse, L.; Barozzi, I.; Senese, S.; Fornasari, L.; Moretti, S.; et al. dual role for Hdac1: oncosuppressor in tumorigenesis, oncogene in tumor maintenance. *Blood* **2013**, 3459–3468. [CrossRef] [PubMed]

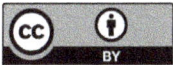

nutrients

MDPI

Review

Cancer Prevention and Therapy with Polyphenols: Sphingolipid-Mediated Mechanisms

Michele Dei Cas and Riccardo Ghidoni *

Department of Health Sciences, University of Milan, 20142 Milan, Italy; michele.deicas@unimi.it
* Correspondence: riccardo.ghidoni@unimi.it, Tel.: +39-025-032-3250

Received: 30 May 2018; Accepted: 19 July 2018; Published: 21 July 2018

Abstract: Polyphenols, chemically characterized by a polyhydroxylated phenolic structure, are well known for their widespread pharmacological properties: anti-inflammatory, antibiotic, antiseptic, antitumor, antiallergic, cardioprotective and others. Their distribution in food products is also extensive especially in plant foods such as vegetables, cereals, legumes, fruits, nuts and certain beverages. The latest scientific literature outlines a resilient interconnection between cancer modulation and dietary polyphenols by sphingolipid-mediated mechanisms, usually correlated with a modification of their metabolism. We aim to extensively survey this relationship to show how it could be advantageous in cancer treatment or prevention by nutrients. From this analysis it emerges that a combination of classical chemotherapy with nutrients and especially with polyphenols dietary sources may improve efficacy and decreases negative side effects of the antineoplastic drug. In this multifaceted scenario, sphingolipids play a pivotal role as bioactive molecules, emerging as the mediators of cell proliferation in cancer and modulator of chemotherapeutics.

Keywords: sphingolipids; ceramide; flavonoids; resveratrol; genistein; curcumin; nutrients; nutraceuticals; chemotherapeutics

---

1. Polyphenols

1.1. Polyphenols: Chemical Classification

Polyphenols are one of the biggest class of phytochemicals (more than 8000 compounds) chemically characterized by common polyhydroxylated phenolic structures. Polyphenols are easily found in many plant-based products [1].

They can be divided into two main classes: flavonoids and non-flavonoids (Table 1). Flavonoids generally contain two phenolic rings (A and B rings) connected by a carbon chain or, more commonly, by an O-ring (C ring) which is similar to a phenylbenzopyrane structure. Based on the respective position of the B and C rings, functional groups and the presence of unsaturation in the C ring, they have been separated into subclasses: flavones, isoflavones, flavanones, flavonols, anthocyanidins, chalcones and flavanols, containing catechins and tannins. Hydroxylation and conjugation patterns characterize individual compounds in each subclass. In nature polyphenols (flavanols are an exception) exist as glycosides or other conjugates. Polyphenols can polymerize into large molecules, such as tannins, which are able to bind and precipitate proteins. The most important subclasses of tannins are proanthocyanidins, derived tannins and hydrolyzable tannins. Proanthocyanidins consist of monomeric units of flavans which are linked through carbon-carbon and ether linkages. They also may contain gallates. Relevant proanthocyanidins are procyanidins ([epi]catechin polymers), prodelephinidins ([epi]gallocatechin polymers) and propelargonidins ([epi]afzelechin). There is a second class of tannins which is comprised of tannins formed primarily beneath aerobic conditions during the manipulation of plants and subsequent processing into foods such as oolong and black teas, red wines and coffee. Important members of this subclass are theaflavins and thearubigins, easily found in tea. The last subclass of tannins comprises hydrolyzable tannins namely esters of gallic acid (gallotannins) or ellagic acid (ellagitannins) with a non-aromatic polyol [2].

Table 1. Polyphenols classes and examples of more relevant compounds.

Flavonoid Polyphenols	
Flavones	apigenin, chrysin, diosmin, luteolin, baicalein
Isoflavones	daidzein, daidzin, genistein
Flavanones	hesperetin, narigenin
Flavonols	kaempferol, quercetin, rutine, myricetin, morin
Anthocyanidins	cyanidin, dephinidin, malvidin, pelargonidin, peonidin
Chalcones	butein, curcumin, xanthohumol
Flavanols	catechins, tannins
Non-Flavonoid Polyphenols	
Benzoic acids	vanillic acid, gallic acid, syringic acid
Cinnamic acids	caffeic acid, chlorogenic acid, CAPE, tannic acid
Stilbenes	resveratrol, piceatannol, isorhapontigenin, oxyresveratrol

Non-flavonoid polyphenols are divided into three main classes: phenolic acids (benzoic acid derivatives and cinnamic acid derivatives), stilbenoids and other polyphenols. Phenolic acids can be further divided, depending on the number of carbons, into two subclasses: benzoic acid derivatives (7 atoms of carbon) and cinnamic acid derivatives (9 atoms of carbon). In fruits and vegetables they are in a free-form whereas in grains and seeds they are in a conjugated form, that could be hydrolyzed by acid, alkaline or enzyme catalysis [1]. Stilbenoids class includes basic stilbenes, bibenzyls or dihydrostilbenes, bis(bibenzyls), phenanthrenes, 9,10-dihydrophenanthrenes and related compounds derived from the phenylpropanoid pathway. Stilbenes are structurally identified by a 1,2-diphenylethylene nucleus. They exist as both monomers and complex oligomers. The common monomeric skeleton consists of two aromatic rings linked by an ethylene bridge, commonly in *trans* configuration. The oligomers are formed by stilbene units (resveratrol-oxyresveratrol, resveratrol-piceatannol, resveratrol-isorhapontigenin, oxyresveratrol-isorhapontigenin and piceatannol-isorhapontigenin) linked by either C-C or C-O-C bonds [3]. Figure 1 shows the chemical structures of polyphenols considered in this review article.

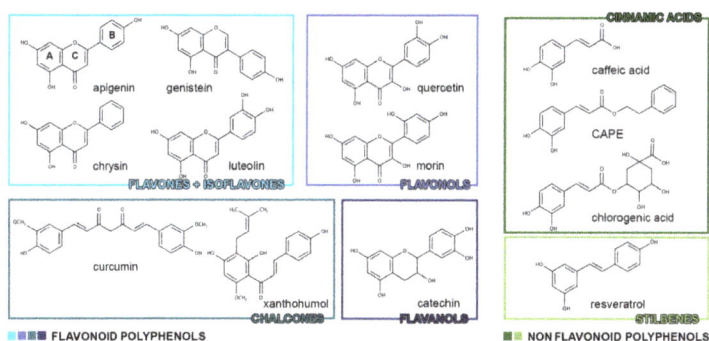

Figure 1. Chemical structures of polyphenols that are connected with a sphingolipid-based mechanism for cancer prevention and treatment.

1.2. Distribution of Polyphenols in Food

Many plants and herbs consumed by humans are known to contain relevant amounts of polyphenols, which have been demonstrated to have many beneficial effects such as anti-inflammatory, antibiotic, antiseptic, antitumor, antiallergic, cardioprotective and others. They are ubiquitous in plant foods such as vegetables, cereals, legumes, fruits, nuts and beverage such as wine, cider, beer, tea, cocoa.

Their levels are mainly influenced by genetic factors, environmental conditions, variety, cultivars, processing and storage [4]. Specifically, the greatest dietary sources of flavonoids are tea (*Camellia sinensis*), onions (*Allium cepa*), apples (*Malus domestica*), citrus fruits (*Citrus* spp.), berries (blackberry *Rubus ulmifolius*, blueberry *Vaccinium* spp., elderberry *Sambucus* spp., raspberry *Rubus* spp., strawberry *Fragaria* × *ananassa*), legumes (*Fabaceae* spp.) and red wine (*Vitis vinifera*). Human flavonoid intake was estimated in the USA to be approximately 170 mg/day and in Netherlands 23 mg/day (both expressed as aglycones) using the content of only five flavonoids (quercetin, kaempferol, myricetin, luteolin and apigenin). Consequently, the effective intake may be much higher [5]. The dietary consumption of polyphenols consists principally of 80% flavanols, 8% for flavonols, 6% for flavanones, 5% for anthocyanidins, and less than 1% for isoflavones and flavones [6]. The major dietary sources of stilbenes are grapes and red wine (*Vitis vinifera*). Within this family resveratrol (Res) derivatives predominate, with several patterns of oligomerization and glycosylation [3]. For benzoic acid derivatives, the dietary sources were especially açaí oil (obtained from the fruit of *Euterpe oleracea*) [7], wine and vinegar [8]. For cinnamic acid compounds the food distribution was abundantly widespread: cereal grains, rice (*Oryza sativa*), wheat bran, coffee (*Coffea Arabica*), sweet potato (*Ipomoea batatas*), artichoke (*Cynara cardunculus*), cinnamon (*Cinnamomum cassia*), citrus fruits (*Citrus* spp.), grape (*Vitis vinifera*), tea (*Camellia sinensis*), cocoa (*Theobroma cacao*), spinach (*Spinacia oleracea*), celery (*Apium graveolens*), brassicas vegetables (*Brassicaceae* spp.), peanuts (*Arachis hypogaea*), basil (*Ocimum basilicum*) and garlic (*Allium sativum*) [9].

1.3. Bioavailability, Absorption and Metabolism of Polyphenols

The absorption and metabolism of polyphenols are consequent to: their chemical structure, the degree of glycosylation/acylation, the molecular size, the degree of polymerization and solubility [10]. Polyphenolic compounds can be distinguished into extractable and non-extractable according to their molecular weight and solubility: extractable polyphenols have a low-medium molecular mass and can be extracted using different solvents, whereas non-extractable remain insoluble due to their high molecular weight or complex phenols structures. Non-extractable polyphenols were highly recovered in feces, confirming the lack of absorption/digestion [11]. Concerning their metabolism, aglycones and simple monomeric polyphenols can be absorbed through the intestinal mucosa. On the other hand, glycosides cannot be absorbed because mammals lack in the proper β-glycosidases. However, some glycosides can be partially absorbed by the intervention of an enzyme present in the gastrointestinal microbiota [12]. Polyphenols undergo liver-mediated metabolism: methylation and/or conjugation with glucuronic acid or sulfate. Metabolites were secreted in the urine or in the bile, according to their lipophilic nature. In bile, some of them can be deconjugated and reabsorbed for many times (enterohepatic cycle) [13]. The level of absorbed polyphenols in the body and consequently their potential physiologic effects are still not clear [11,14].

2. Sphingolipids

2.1. Sphingolipid Classification

Sphingolipids are a complex family of amino alcohols compounds sharing a common structure: a sphingoid base backbone that is synthesized *de novo* from serine and acyl-CoA [15]. Sphingolipids can be divided into several different classes: sphingoid bases, ceramides, phosphosphingolipids, phosphonosphingolipids, neutral glycosphingolipids, acidic glycosphingolipids, including gangliosides, basic glycosphingolipids, amphoteric glycosphingolipids, arsenosphingolipids and others. The major sphingoid base of mammals is commonly referred to as sphingosine (Sph), that is (2S,3R,4E)-2-aminooctadec-4-ene-1,3-diol. Sphingoid bases found in nature could diverge in alkyl chain length and branching, the number and positions of unsaturation, the presence of additional hydroxyl groups and other features. These differences are mostly related to their specific role as for example by skin phytoceramides enriched in hydroxylation. Thus, interaction with nearby molecules strengthens the permeability barrier of the skin. In addition, a large number of fungi and sponges produces compounds with structural similarity to sphingoid bases some of which (such as myriocin and the fumonisins) are potent inhibitors of the enzymes of sphingolipid metabolism. In mammals sphingolipids are mainly represented by sphingomyelins (SM) which are formed by a polar head of phosphocholine and a core of ceramide (Cer). The latter is formed by a sphingosine amide-linked to fatty acids, mostly saturated or monounsaturated, bearing from 14 to 26 carbon atoms [16]. The major sphingolipid in insects is Cer-phosphoethanolamines whereas fungi have phytoCer-phosphoinositols and mannose-containing head groups [17]. SM is a dominant structural molecule, not only in plasma membrane but also in ER-to-Golgi vesicles as well as in membrane buddings (endocytosis and exocytosis). A high ratio of SM over cell lipids is present in blood cells, platelets and in the eye lens, which exhibits a peculiar increase of dihydro-sphingomyelin [18]. Cer is the central core of another important class named glycosphingolipids, in which Cer links one or more uncharged sugars such as glucose, galactose and fucose or modified sugars such as N-acetylglucosamine and N-acetylgalactosamine. Gangliosides are particular glycosphingolipids showing N-acetyl or N-glycolyl neuraminic acid as glycol-residues. Finally, there are basic glycosphingolipids and amphoteric glycosphingolipids. Water-living organism replace the phosphate polar group with either phosphono-group or arsenic acid. Sphingolipids can be linked to proteins, such as the inositol-phospho-Cers that are used by fungi to anchor membrane proteins and ω-hydroxyCers and ω-glucosylCers that are attached to surface proteins in human epidermal cells [17].

2.2. Sphingolipid Metabolism

Sphingolipids are synthesized in eukaryotic cells in the endoplasmic reticulum (ER) through a multiple step process whose rate is limited by serine palmitoyltransferase (SPT), an enzyme that catalyzes the initial condensation of serine with palmitic acid, forming 3-keto-sphinganine (3-KDS) [19]. Hereditary sensory and autonomic neuropathy type 1 has been recently associated with SPT mutations that enhance the affinity of the enzyme for alanine, instead of serine, thus forming neurotoxic deoxysphingolipids [20]. Reduction of 3-KDS by 3-KDS reductase (KDSR) releases dihydrosphingosine (or sphinganine, DHSph), which can be differentially acylated to form dihydroceramide (DHCer). Acylation is catalyzed by six different Cer synthases (CerS) [21] each using specific acyl chains, typically with saturated or mono-unsaturated fatty acids with 14 to 26 carbons. Cers are then formed by dehydrogenation *via* DHCer desaturase (DHCD). The enzymes involved in the Cer biosynthesis are included in the ER while in the Golgi occurs: (1) the synthesis of SM; (2) the synthesis of glycosphingolipids; and (3) the unusual phosphorylation of Cer, by Cer kinase (CerK), to Cer-1-phosphate (Cer-1P). Cer can be translocated from ER to Golgi by vesicular transport or anchored to a protein transporter (CERT). The transport *via* CERT was demonstrated to be specific for SM synthesis whereas vesicular trafficking for glycosphingolipids synthesis [22,23].

SM is synthesized through the transfer of the phosphocholine head group of phosphatidylcholine to Cer by two enzymes: SM synthase 1 (SMS1) and 2 (SMS2). SMS1 is responsible for the *de novo* synthesis of SM whereas SMS2 probably resynthesizes SM from Cer generated by the catabolism of SM [22]. The whole production of glycosphingolipids starts from two direct derivatives of Cer, galactosylceramide (GalCer) and glucosylceramides (GlcCer). From the latter it is produced lactosylceramide (LacCer), that is the precursor of the neolacto-, lacto-, globo-, asialoganglio- and ganglio- series of glycosphingolipids [23]. Sphingolipids have a rapid turnover and their levels are constantly in change between synthesis and degradation. They are degraded in lysosomes by glycosidases or acid sphingomyelinases (aSMase) which remove the head groups to form Cers. Deacylation of Cer by ceramidases (CDase) is the only pathway known to generate Sph, that can be recycled back to Cer. Sph could also be phosphorylated by Sph kinases (SphK1 and SphK2) forming Sph-1-phosphate (Sph-1P). Sph-1P could either be dephosphorylated by phosphatases (SPPase1 and SPPase2) or degraded by Sph-1P lyase (SPL) to ethanolamine-1-phosphate and *trans*-hexadecenal. Sphingomyelinase (SMase) cleaves SM to Cer and phosphatidylcholine by a reversible reaction.

Five types of SMase have been described and classified on their cation dependence and pH optima of action. The more relevant are Mg-dependent neutral sphingomyelinase (nSMase) and lysosomal aSMase [24]. An overview of sphingolipids metabolism and chemical structure of the principal ones is shown in Figure 2.

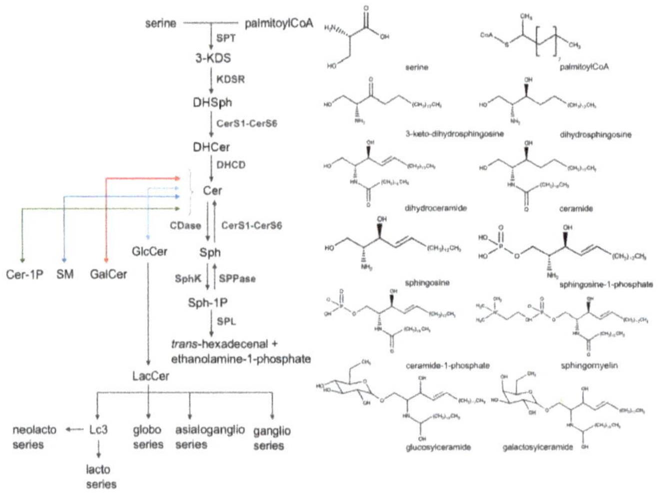

Figure 2. Sphingolipids metabolism and their chemical structures. Lc3: GlcNAcβ1-3Galβ1-4Glcβ-Cer for others see the abbreviation list.

2.3. Sphingolipids Modulation of Cellular Functions

The structural diversity of sphingolipids reflects a correspondent diversification in pathophysiological functions: regulation of apoptosis [25], proliferation, differentiation, autophagy [26], invasiveness, modification of signaling cascade and mediation of inflammatory responses by cytokines [27,28].

Cer promotes cell-type specific apoptosis by (1) activating both protein kinases such as protein kinase C (PKC), protein phosphatases 1-2 and proteases, including caspases and cathepsin D; (2) formation of pores in the mitochondrial membrane; and (3) modulation of pro-apoptotic Bcl-2-family proteins [29,30]. Also, Sph *via* PKC upholds apoptosis [31].

In contrast to Cer, that is predominantly pro-apoptotic, Sph-1P is mainly an anti-apoptotic messenger by stimulating G-protein-coupled receptors activating RAS, RAC, phosphatidylinositide 3-kinases (PI3K), protein kinase B (AKT), phospholipase C (PLC) and Rho kinase. The regulation of a signaling cascade mediated by Sph-1P includes modulation in mitogenesis, cell migration, cytoskeletal rearrangement and angiogenesis. Sphingolipids could also be correlated with pro-inflammatory cytokines through different mechanisms [31,32]. Sph-1P stimulate inflammation by either upregulation of cyclooxygenase 2 (COX-2) with overproduction of prostaglandin E_2 and activation of nuclear factor kappa-light-chain-enhancer of activated B cells (NF-κB). In the same way, Cer-1P through activation of cytosolic phospholipases A2 (cPLA2) enhances the production of pro-inflammatory arachidonic acid [33].

2.4. Sphingolipids and Cancer

Sphingolipids have emerged as mediators of cell proliferation in cancer and as potential chemotherapeutics (Table 2). In general, Cer regulates anti-cancer cellular fate whereas Sph-1P is pro-oncogenic and pro-metastatic.

Table 2. Roles of sphingolipids in cancer.

Sphingolipids	Biological Target	Effect in Cancer	References
Cer	PKC, I2PP2A, cathepsin D, caspases, telomerase	Apoptosis, growth arrest, senescence	[23,26–31,34–37]
Cer-1P	cPLA$_2$	Release of arachidonic acid and activation of inflammatory cascade	[31,33,37]
DAG (from SM)	PKC	Cellular proliferation	[38,39]
Sph-1P	NFKB, COX-2, ERK	Malignant transformation, anti-apoptosis, angiogenesis, survival, metastatization	[31–33,40]

Cer normally mediates antiproliferative responses such as cell growth inhibition, apoptosis induction, senescence modulation, ER stress response and autophagy. Interestingly, recent studies [34,35] suggest that *de novo*-generated Cers present an ambivalent role in the promotion/suppression of tumors reliant to their fatty acid chain lengths, subcellular localization and direct downstream targets. In a study [36] on head and neck squamous cell carcinoma (HNSCC) decreased levels of C18 Cer are correlated with lymphovascular invasion and nodal metastasis. Conversely, overexpression of CerS1 and increased levels of *de novo* synthesized C16 Cer show a reduction of tumoral cell growth by inhibition of telomerase activity. Overexpression of *de novo* synthesized C16 Cer was associated with tumor proliferation whereas downregulation of *de novo* synthesized C16 Cer induce ER stress and apoptosis of HSNCC cells by activating the ATF6/CHOP pathway. Furthermore, elevated levels of C16 Cer, CerS2 and CerS6 were associated with breast cancer. Moreover, the interaction of Cer with cathepsin D, PKC, I2PP2A, caspases and telomerase leads to apoptosis, growth suppression and senescence.

Cer-1P has been shown to induce the release of arachidonic acid in cancer cells leading to an inflammatory condition [37].

SM contributes to release diacylglycerol from phosphatidylcholine, a well-known activator of PKC, thus promoting cellular proliferation. GlcCer indeed leads to drug resistance.

Sph-1P induces anti-apoptosis processes engaging with Sph-1P receptors 1–5 (S1PR1–5). In addition, elevated levels of Sph-1P have been observed in different cancer and tumor tissues [38,39].

The SphK1 expression has been found to be upregulated in a number of solid tumors. High levels of SphK1 has been correlated with poor survival of patients who suffer from glioblastoma, gastric and breast cancers. In accordance, anticancer regimens have been shown to down-regulate SphK1 activity in various cancer cell and animal models. This enzyme-increased transcription is proposed to be responsible for chemo- and radio-resistance of cancer cells and to favor the progression of hormone-refractory state. As an example, it was proved a direct correlation of SphK1 activity and expression with prostate tumor grade as well as with the clinical outcome after prostatectomy [40].

3. Focus on Cancer: Dietary Polyphenols and Sphingolipids

3.1. Apigenin

Apigenin (4′,5,7-trihydroxyflavone) is a flavone found in fruits, vegetables and other plants. It counteracts inflammation, oxidative stress and development of cancer [41]. Major apigenin-containing food sources include thyme (*Thymus vulgaris*), cherries (*Prunus avium*), tea (*Camellia sinensis*), olives (*Olea europaea*), broccoli (*Brassica oleracea*), celery (*Apium graveolens*), and legumes (*Fabaceae* spp.). The most abundant sources are the leafy herb parsley (*Petroselinum cripspum*) and dried flowers of chamomile (*Matricaria chamomilla*) [42]. Although a few contradictory reports [43,44], apigenin exerts anti-tumoral effect influencing mitochondria activity, gene expression and partially through targeting of the JAK/STAT pathway [45].

Moussavi et al. [46] investigated the effect of apigenin as a dietary component in colon cancer by testing its relationship with cell death, mediated alternately by Cer and reactive oxygen species (ROS).

Apigenin was reported to elevate Cer levels and apoptosis in colon cancer cells (HCT116) in a concentration- and time-dependent manner but independently on the *de novo* synthesis pathway (Figure 3A).

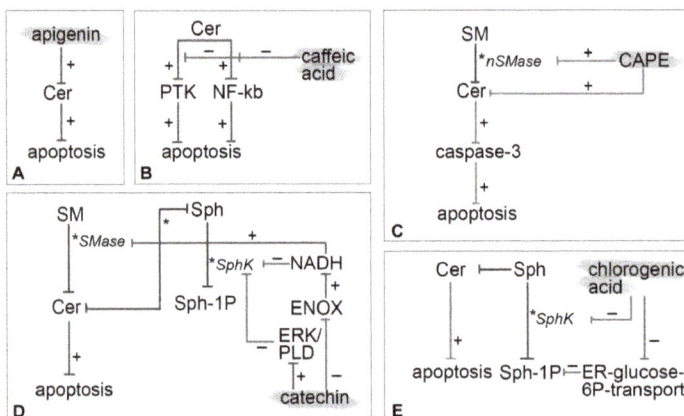

Figure 3. Mechanism of modulation on sphingolipids by apigenin (**A**), caffeic acid (**B**), CAPE (**C**), catechin (**D**) and chlorogenic acid (**E**). It is depicted with an asterisk (*) enzymatic pathway, with plus (+) red-regulated pathway and with minus (−) down-regulation ones. PTK: protein tyrosine kinase.

3.2. Caffeic Acid

Caffeic acid (3,4-dihydroxycinnamic acid) is a widespread hydroxycinnamic acid, naturally found in many plant species as a secondary metabolite of the shikimate pathway. It displays the classical framework of phenylpropanoids (C6-C3) with a 3,4-dihydroxylated aromatic ring connected to a carboxylic acid moiety by a *trans*-ethylene ether. It is the most abundant hydroxycinnamic acid and the diet sources are argan oil (*Argania spinosa*), oats (*Avena nuda*), wheat (*Triticum* spp.), rice (*Oryza sativa*), olive oil (*Olea europaea*), narrow-leaved purple coneflower (*Echinacea angustifolia*), and berries (blackberry *Rubus ulmifolius*, blueberry *Vaccinium* spp., elderberry *Sambucus* spp., raspberry *Rubus* spp., strawberry *Fragaria* × *ananassa*). Other dietary sources include potatoes (*Solanum tuberosum*), carrots (*Daucus carota*), artichokes (*Cynara cardunculus*) and obviously coffee (*Coffea arabica*) [47,48]. The average phenolic acids intake in humans is in the order of 210 mg/day within a broad range, depending on nutritional habits. Caffeic acid has been reported to account for up to 90% of total phenolic acids intake [49]. The wide spectrum of biological effects induced by caffeic acid includes: enzyme activity inhibition (5- and 12-lipoxygenases, glutathione S-transferase, xanthine oxidase), antitumor activity, anti-inflammatory properties, modulation of cellular response to ROS and inhibition of HIV replication [50–52].

Nardini et al. [50] reported that caffeic acid significantly inhibits Cer-induced activation of NF-κB in human monocytic U937 cells, with consequent suppression of acute inflammation, septic shock, HIV replication, acute phase response, viral replication, radiation damage, atherogenesis and possibly some neoplastic degeneration. The NF-κB inhibition mechanisms may be different: countering the changes of the intracellular redox status induced by Cer, inhibition of 5 and 12 lipoxygenases activities or PKC and PKA activity arrest. Additionally, some data indicate that caffeic acid inhibits protein tyrosine kinase activity [53,54]. This ability may be the mechanism liable for the inhibition of Cer-induced apoptotic response rather than its antioxidant properties. This hypothesis was also in agreement with the observation that no tested antioxidants inhibit DNA fragmentation and therefore apoptosis. The action of caffeic acid is two-faced: it shows pro-apoptotic effects at high concentrations (>200 μM) and antiapoptotic ones at lower levels explaining a conflicted range of activities [50]. At low concentrations, close to those expected *in vivo*, it mediates a double inhibition mechanism on Cer-induced NF-κB activation and Cer-induced apoptosis by protein tyrosine kinase. Under this perspective, caffeic acid could not be used as a coadjuvant to chemotherapy in low concentrations since it reduces Cer-mediated apoptosis (Figure 3B).

3.3. CAPE

Caffeic acid phenethyl ester (CAPE) or 2-phenylethyl (2E)-3-(3,4-dihydroxyphenyl)acrylate is a natural bioactive compound. It occurs in many plants and the main human source is propolis. Propolis is a resinous substance made by honeybees mixing saliva, beeswax and exudate collected from botanical sources. CAPE is a cinnamic acid polyphenol characterized by a hydroxyl catechol ring. It has different biological activities on infections, oxidative stress, inflammation, cancer, diabetes, neurodegeneration and anxiety [55].

Tseng et al. [56] demonstrated that CAPE-induced apoptosis involves nSMase activation and accumulation of Cer in C6 glioma cells. CAPE modulates two parallel signaling pathways both leading to activation of caspase 3 as an ultimate effector of apoptosis. On one hand CAPE increases nSMase activity triggering the activation of ERK/NGFR/NGF/JNK pathway and on the other hand it causes an accumulation of Cer which initiates the p38 MAPK/p53/BAX signaling path. In addition to the apoptotic potential of CAPE in cancer cells a coherent manipulation of Cer levels may improve the efficacy of chemotherapy agents (Figure 3C).

3.4. Catechin

The catechin family presents two benzene rings and a 3-OH-dihydropyran heterocycle with two chiral centers on C2 and C3. Thus, it has four diastereoisomers: two in *trans* configuration called catechin and two in *cis* configuration called epicatechin. In plants they are usually conjugated with gallic acid.

Epigallocatechin-3-gallate (EGCG) is the most potent catechin with antioxidant properties and it is mainly present in green tea together with its related compounds epicatechin [57]. High concentrations of catechin can be found in fresh tea leaves (*Camellia sinensis*), red wine, broad beans (*Vicia faba*), black grapes, apricots (*Prunus armeniaca*) and strawberries (*Fragaria* × *ananassa*) nevertheless epicatechin could be found in high concentrations in apples (*Malus domestica*), blackberries, broad beans (*Vicia faba*), cherries (*Prunus cerasus*), black grapes, pears (*Pyrus* spp.), raspberries (*Rubus* spp.), and chocolate (*Theobroma cacao*). Catechins showed *in vitro* protection against degenerative diseases and a strong inverse relationship between the intake of catechins and risk of mortality by cardiovascular heart diseases [58]. It has been reported that catechins have antimicrobic activity (gram-positive more than gram-negative) and inhibit carcinogenesis of the skin, lung, esophagus, stomach, liver, small intestine, colon, bladder, prostate, and mammary glands. EGCG has been described to have many potential targets for action against carcinogens and among them also sphingolipids [58].

Brizuela et al. [40] reported, for the first time, that green tea polyphenols (EGCG and polyphenon E, PPE) inhibit SphK1 activity, *via* a novel ERK/PLD-dependent mechanism in prostate cancer cells (C4-2B hormone-responsive and PC-3 hormone-refractory). The treatment with ECGC and PPE in both PC-3 and C4-2B cell lineages showed a remarkable inhibition of cell growth by altering the sphingolipid balance correlated with SphK1 inhibition and increment of pro-apoptotic Cer. The mechanisms underlying SphK1 inhibition by green tea extract are dependent on the down-regulation of the ERK1/2 and consequently with PLD/PA signaling pathway [40,59]. *In vivo* studies, confirmed the data obtained *in vitro*, suggesting that animals with SphK1 overexpressing PC-3 cells implanted in a subcutaneous district develop larger tumors and resistance to green tea due to disruption of sphingolipid equilibrium. In conjunction, EGCG and PPE diet is also associated with a significant metastasis reduction in the orthotopic PC-3 model. Preventive approaches [60,61] using catechins have been shown to inhibit other cancers as the colon one. Hence, a combination of green tea polyphenols and chemotherapeutic agents or radiation therapy would be promising.

Another mechanism of Cer-mediated apoptosis proposed by Wu et al. [62] involves ENOX2 (tNOX) inhibition by EGCG. Inhibition of the ENOX family commonly results in an accumulation of cytosolic NADH at the inner leaflet of the plasma membrane. Regarding sphingolipid metabolism, NADH modulates SphK inhibition and SMase stimulation. The disruption of sphingolipid rheostat, which is clearly connected with apoptosis, occurs when Sph-1P levels increase and Cer levels decrease (Figure 3D).

3.5. Chlorogenic Acid

Chlorogenic acid, a non-flavonoid polyphenol, is a quinic acid conjugate of caffeic acid found in high levels in coffee beans (*Coffea arabica*). An average coffee drinker tends to consume 0.5–1 g of chlorogenic acids daily. It could be found also in apples (*Malus domestica*), pears (*Pyrus* spp.), eggplants (*Solanum melongena*), tomatoes (*Solanum lycopersicum*), blueberries (*Vaccinium myrtillus*), strawberries (*Fragaria* × *ananassa*), bamboo (Bambuseae spp.) and potatoes (*Solanum tuberosum*) [63,64]. It has various biological activities such as anti-inflammatory, anti-diabetic, anti-tumorigenic, antioxidative, anti-gout and anti-obesity.

Lee et al. [65] demonstrated that the inhibition of Hypoxia-Inducible factor-1α (HIF-1α) by chlorogenic acid involves the SphK-1 pathway under hypoxia in the DU145 human prostate cancer cell line. Hypoxia is a common condition in solid tumors enhancing its rough development. HIF-1α is a transcription factor that regulates cancer progression such as angiogenesis, metastasis, anti-apoptosis, cell proliferations whereby it imparts resistance to chemotherapy. SphK-1 regulates and stabilizes HIF-1α through the AKT/GSK-3 leading to his accumulation. It was shown that under hypoxia, chlorogenic acid significantly decreases HIF-1α and SphK-1 activity. Besides, it prevents phosphorylation of AKT and GSK-3β which are involved in stabilization of HIF-1α by SphK. In summary, chlorogenic acid decreased cancer cell growth by (1) inhibition of SphK-1 and reduction of HIF-1α; (2) decrement of phosphorylation of HIF-1α stabilizing agent; (3) decrease of VEGF (vascular endothelial growth factor) and angiogenesis.

Additionally, according to Belkaid et al. [66], chlorogenic acid possesses anticancer properties in highly invasive U-87 glioblastoma cells. The competitive inhibition of ER-glucose-6-phosphate transport was shown causing a consequent downregulation of Sph-1P-induced cell migration and a hindrance to Sph-1P-induced ERK phosphorylation. Sph-1P is present at high levels in brain tissue acting as a potent mitogen for glioblastoma multiform cells, triggering intracellular signaling by MAPK pathway and causing the release of intracellular calcium pools (Figure 3E).

3.6. Chrysin

Chrysin is a naturally occurring flavone found in human diet products such as *Passiflora caerulea*, *Passiflora incarnate* infuse, *Oroxylum indicum* and mushroom, *Pleurotus ostreatus* [67]. Traditional Chinese medicine uses the seed of *Oroxylum indicum* in the treatment of cough, acute or chronic bronchitis, pharyngitis, pertussis and other respiratory disorders. Other parts of this small tree such as leaves, flowers and immature boiled fruits are commonly used in the daily diet in Thailand and Laos. Baicalein, oroxylin A and chrysin which can be isolated from its bark play an important role in cancer, as well as viral and bacterial infections [68]. Chrysin has been shown to have a broad range of pharmacological effects such as anti-oxidation, anti-viral, anti-inflammatory properties and anti-cancer properties on breast cancer cells.

Hong et al. [69] evaluated the effects of chrysin treatment on human estrogen receptor (ER)-negative breast cancer cells (MDA-MB-231). This study provides mechanistic evidence that chrysin treatment inhibits the cancer cell growth with a direct or indirect increased expression of PPARα mRNA. PPARs activation can result in intracellular accumulation of Cer, which mediates downstream effects such as apoptosis. Besides, Cer accumulation is assumed to be dependent on a modulation of arachidonic acid (Figure 4A) [70].

3.7. Curcumin

Curcumin is one of the main substances found in the rhizome of turmeric (*Curcuma longa*) and other *Curcuma* spp. Commercially available curcumin contains about 77% in curcuminoids that include pure curcumin, demethoxycurcumin and bis-demethoxycurcumin. [71].

Curcumin inhibits cell proliferation and stimulates apoptosis by affecting various key targets in signal transduction pathways, including Akt, cyclooxygenase, NF-kB, c-myc, Bcl-2, c-Jun N-terminal kinase (JNK), and epithelial growth factor (EGF) receptor (Figure 4B).

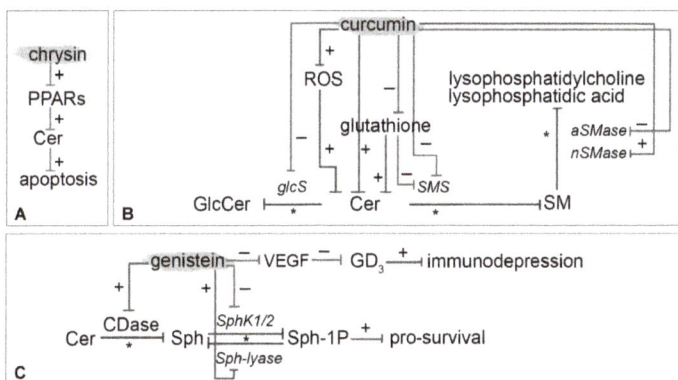

Figure 4. Mechanism of modulation on sphingolipids by chrysin (**A**), curcumin (**B**) and genistein (**C**). It is depicted with an asterisk (*) enzymatic pathway, with plus (+) red-regulated pathway and with minus (−) down-regulation ones.

Cheng et al. [72] demonstrated that curcumin inhibits cell growth and induces apoptosis in colon cancer cells (Caco-2 cells) affecting aSMase activity. It reduces the hydrolytic capacity of the enzyme associated with a slight increase of cellular SM. No modification of alkaline, nSMase and phospholipase D was found after curcumin treatment. Reduction of aSMase activity was not due to a direct inhibitory effect of curcumin on the enzyme, but rather to an inhibition of the enzyme biosynthesis. The up-mentioned action is particularly evident in specific cell type: stronger in monolayer Caco-2 cells than in polarised ones. The role of aSMase in cancer is still debated and there is evidence suggesting that this enzyme activity may affect phospholipase A_2 and thus the formation of lysophosphatidylcholine and lysophosphatidic acid which are required for colon cancer metastasis [73,74].

In contrast, Moussavi et al. [75] found that curcumin significantly increased the Cer levels in colon cancer HCT 116 cells without detectable changes of aSMase and nSMase. Cer generation by curcumin occurred through *de novo* synthesis since cell death could be reversed by myriocin, an inhibitor of serine palmitoyltransferase. Colon cancer cell apoptosis by curcumin was strongly related with JNK activation mediated principally by ROS generation and to a minor extent *via* a parallel Cer-associated pathway.

Another study on anti-colorectal cancer effects by curcumin was conducted by Chen et al. [76]. They showed that co-administration of curcumin and perifosine, an orally bioactive alkylphospholipid, increases colorectal cancer cell apoptosis by modulating multiple signaling pathways such as inactivation of Akt and NF-κβ, activation of c-Jun, downregulation of Bcl-2 and cyclin D1 and increment in intracellular levels of both ROS and Cer. Furthermore, they suggested that ROS/Cer production after co-administration of curcumin and perifosine and ER stress response were independent of Akt inhibition and Bcl-2/cyclin D1 downregulation.

Yu et al. [77] showed that curcumin-induced cell growth inhibition and apoptosis in melanoma cell lines (WM-115 and B16) could be facilitated by PDMP (DL-threo-1-phenyl-2-decanoylamino-3-morpholino-1-propanol). PDMP is a well-known inhibitor of sphingolipid biosynthesis especially directed to the formation of GlcCer, thus resulting in an accumulation of its endogenous precursor. Combination of PDMP and curcumin may be used as a new therapeutic intervention against melanoma. Curcumin induces an early increase of Cer (12 h), that melanoma cells could remove, after long-term (24 h), by glycosylation. Upon incubation on PDMP, Cer levels remain elevated causing further cell death and apoptosis. In addition, exogenous cell-permeable C6-Cer sensitizes melanoma cell lines to curcumin-induced apoptosis.

The curcumin effect was investigated in clinical trials of patients with multiforme glioblastoma, ideally as a second line therapy after failure of radiation and temozolomide [78]. The optimal method should be setting curcumin in combination with an established cytotoxic chemotherapy agent such as carmustine or lomustine. A progression of this aggressive brain cancer is related to a decrease in Cer levels: curcumin has been shown to enhance Cer production influencing CerS activity.

According to Thayyullathil et al. [79], curcumin has been shown to be a pro-autophagic drug in malignant gliomas. Malignant glioma cells are likely responding to therapy better *via* autophagy than apoptosis but, for apoptosis-resistant glioblastoma patients, a pro-autophagic drug could be extremely advantageous. Curcumin induces autophagy by Par-4 (prostate apoptosis response-4) upregulation and Cer generation *via* ROS-dependent mechanism. Cer generation was correlated to the nSMase pathway in U87MG malignant glioma cells since GW4869, an inhibitor of nSMase, significantly blocked curcumin-induced Cer generation and autophagy.

Hilchie et al. [80] determined the mechanism by which curcumin induces cytotoxicity in prostate cancer cells (PC3). This treatment caused time- and dose-dependent apoptosis and depletion of cellular reduced glutathione, Cer accumulation, activation of p38, JNK and release of different caspases and cytochrome c. The authors conclude that apoptosis in prostate cancer is due principally to Cer accumulation causing mitochondrial membrane integrity damage, a consequent release of cytochrome c and apoptosis-inducing factor. By contrast, clinical trials have confirmed that curcumin is poorly absorbed in the gastrointestinal tract owing to the efficient efflux of monoglutathionyl curcumin conjugates from intestinal epithelial cells into the lumen. Achieving a useful plasma concentration to trigger apoptosis is the major obstacle to the clinical application of curcumin-based therapy. Combination of curcumin and piperine or more stable analogs of curcumin may overcome these pharmacokinetics problems.

Kizhakkayil et al. [81] investigated more deeply the glutathione decline as a mechanism by which curcumin acts on human leukemic cells. A decrease of intracellular glutathione regulates caspase-dependent inhibition of SMS activity and Cer generation, and thus apoptosis. Curcumin-induced Cer generation and apoptosis were inhibited by extracellular supplementation of glutathione, N-acetylcysteine and caspase inhibitor z-VAD-fmk, supporting these findings. In particular, an important role in Cer generation was found to be related to the regulation of the SMS cycle and not to the *de novo* pathway.

Scharstuhl et al. [82] revealed that curcumin induces apoptosis by the formation of channels in the outer mitochondrial membranes and the release of apoptosis-inducing factors. The formation of channels was correlated to the combined action of Cers, VDAC and BAX and not to caspases pathways. Nevertheless, inhibition of the *de novo* synthesis and inhibition of SMase did not significantly block curcumin-induced apoptosis, indicating that Cers are partially involved.

Shakor et al. [83] examined curcumin-induced apoptosis in human leukemia HL60 cells and their HL60/VCR multidrug-resistant counterparts. The molecular mechanism of curcumin action consists in a biphasic Cer accumulation in the cells firstly by rapid activation of nSMase2 and then by inhibition of SMS, accompanied in the drug-resistant cells by glucosylceramide synthase (GlcS, the enzyme involved in GlcCer synthesis from Cer) inhibition. The intracellular increase of Cer modulates the transcription of apoptosis-regulating genes, such as BAX, Bcl-2 and caspase-3. The glycosylation of Cer, *via* GlcS, is recognized as a chemoresistance strategy and enhanced by several tumors. On the other side, the down-regulation of this Golgi enzyme seems to be related to P-gp inhibition. P-gp, an ATP consuming flippase, translocates GlcCer. P-gp antagonists (cyclosporine A or tamoxifen) impair Cer clearance and enhance its cytotoxicity. Moreover, molecular modeling studies confirmed that curcumin binds to P-gp in its substrate binding site possibly competing with GlcCer binding. Finally, apoptosis is associated with Cer increase, glutathione depletion and ROS generation after curcumin treatments.

Another study by Shakor et al. [84] indicated a complex crosstalk among Bcl-2, Bcl-xL, caspases and glutathione during curcumin-induced apoptosis. This point to the superior role of caspase-8 activity, Bcl-xL down-regulation and glutathione depletion in the pro-apoptotic cascade leading to nSMase activation and hence generation of Cer. The signaling cascade controlling Cer-mediated apoptosis in curcumin-treated cells was: caspase-8 activation, Bcl-xL degradation, glutathione depletion, nSMase activation and Cer accumulation. Caspase-3 activation and Bcl-2 degradation, both regulated by glutathione levels and reciprocally interconnected, are also co-involved in SMase initiation. SMS degradation was indeed regulated only by caspase-3 activation.

Yang et al. [85] analyzed the impact of the SphK1 inhibitor on Cer production, particularly as a potential curcumin chemo-sensitizer in ovarian cancer cells (CaOV3). Inhibition of SphK1, by pharmacological tools as SKI-II (2-(p-Hydroxyanilino)-4-(p-chlorophenyl)thiazole) or by RNA interference, dramatically enhanced curcumin-induced apoptosis and growth inhibition in ovarian cancer cells *via* Cer production and p38 activation and Akt inhibition.

A further supplement to curcumin treatment (Qui et al. [86]) was the addition of exogenous cell-permeable short-chain, C6-Cer. It sensitizes melanoma cells (B16 and WM-115) to curcumin-mediated apoptosis due to the augment of the mitochondrial apoptosis pathway, especially through (1) the cleavage of caspases 3 and 9 and (2) the downregulation of anti-apoptosis protein Bcl-xL and X-IAP.

3.8. Genistein

Genistein is essentially present in soy-derived products and the soybeans contain the compound in ranges from 5.6 to 276 mg/100 g. In addition to genistein soy foods contain another major isoflavone, daidzein. Daidzein differs from genistein by the lack of the hydroxyl group on position 5. Both isoflavones may exist in their aglycone or glycoside forms. The most common glycoside forms of genistein and daidzein are O-β-D-glucoside derivatives. Due to soy consume the average dietary isoflavone intake in Asian countries is in the range of 25–50 mg/day, whereas in Western countries, the intake is approximately 2 mg/day. In lower concentrations genistein and daidzein are also present in legumes. The genus *Lupinus* (commonly known as lupin) represents a typical example of the legume that is now widely cultivated for its seeds, which possess a nutritional value similar to soybean. Other important legumes are broad beans (*Vicia faba*) and chickpeas (*Cicer arietinum*), but the flavones can be detected also in fruit, nuts, and vegetables where their content can vary considerably, ranging being from 0.03 to 0.2 mg/100 g [87].

This soybean isoflavone exerts many cellular effects, namely apoptosis activation, and protein-tyrosine kinase activity and angiogenesis inhibition (Figure 4C). It is important to note that genistein affects in a dose-dependent manner, both positively and negatively tumorigenesis.

Engel et al. [88] reported the influence of phytoestrogens, such as genistein, on the metabolome of breast cancer cells. They compare either MCF-7, positive for ERα and ERβ, and MCF-12A, a non-tumorigenic epithelial breast cell line. Three sphingolipids were analyzed: Sph, DHSph and ethanolamine-phosphate. These metabolites were elevated in MCF-7 under control conditions and genistein treatment normalizes their levels. Whereas their amounts, in MCF-12A, were not affected. By contrast, DHSph was not normalized by genistein treatment in MCF-7 to gain the level of MCF-12A under control conditions. Western blotting-coupled immunofluorescence experiments revealed a significant, concentration-dependent, decrease in the amount of SphK1 and SphK2 enzyme in MCF-7 after genistein exposure. In MCF-12A phytoestrogen exposure revealed boosted SphK1 amounts and undetectable expression of SphK2. These findings suggested that SphK1 is expressed in cancerous as well as non-tumorigenic cells while Sphk2 is overexpressed in cancer line. SPL expression was also investigated. MCF-7 has a weaker expression than MCF-12A but after exposure with genistein, the SPL amount increases dramatically. Exposure to phytoestrogens in higher concentrations (10 μM of genistein) resulted in (1) decreased tumor progression *via* sphingolipids pathway and (2) enhanced the reaction of SPL causing a higher conversion of Sph-1P to phosphoethanolamine.

Lucki et al. [89] showed that nanomolar concentrations of genistein induces aCDase transcription in MCF-7 breast cancer cells *via* ERK1/2 dependent mechanism.

The proliferative properties of genistein are supposed to be related to its ability to stimulate estrogenic pathways by binding ERα and GPR30. GPR30 is a transmembrane G-protein-coupled receptor that binds most ER ligands triggering estrogenic signaling and proliferation. aCDase is a lipid hydrolase, that degrades Cer to Sph and a free fatty acid, thus playing a key role in cellular homeostasis regulation by controlling the Cer/Sph/Sph-1P balance within the cell. Activation of this pathway promotes: (1) histone acetylation; (2) recruitment of the phospho-estrogen receptor α; and (3) translocation of Sp1 transcription factor to the aCDase promoter. This activation culminated in an increased enzymatic activity, which results in increased Sph-1P production. Nanomolar concentrations of genistein stimulates the growth of ER-positive breast cancer cells by modulating expression of aCDase. Such modulation produces two synergic but different events: (1) an increment of Sph-1P levels, which activates proliferative pathways by binding to cell surface receptors and (2) the modulation of cyclin B2 expression, driving mitotic progression and cell growth.

Another study by Engel et al. [90] showed that high doses of genistein promote the growth of bone cancer cells. They explored the co-administration of genistein and calcitriol in order to inhibit immature osteosarcoma cells MG-63. The malignant proliferation induced by 100 µM genistein could be normalized to control levels after simultaneous exposure to 10 nM calcitriol. This synergistic effect may be consistent with (1) an overexpression of ERβ, (2) a reduction of extracellular acidification and respiration rates and (3) an increased ethanolamine production by the overexpression of SPL.

The use of genistein as an anti-cancer compound is usually limited because a relatively high concentration is necessary. Ji et al. [91] counteracted this limitation by adding exogenous cell-permeable short-chain Cers to enhance genistein activity. In this study, melanoma cell line (B16, WM451, MeWo) were sensitized to genistein by increasing cellular level of Cers, both exogenously and endogenously. In B16 melanoma cells, genistein caused only a moderate increase of intracellular Cers, which are poorly related to significant cell apoptosis. Co-administration of PDMP, a Cer glycosylation inhibitor, or SKI-II facilitated Cers accumulation and significantly enhanced genistein-induced melanoma cell apoptosis. Moreover, adding to genistein some exogenous cell-permeable short-chain Cers (C2, C4 and C6) lead to a major anti-melanoma effect by increasing cytotoxicity and apoptosis (especially C6). This mechanism could be explained by the JNK activation of and Akt inhibition.

Tiper et al. [92] showed that VEGF and ganglioside GD3 production by ovarian cancers suppress NKT- mediated anti-tumor response. The growth of cancer and the development of metastases strongly depend on the divert of the immune system response. Previous reports [93,94] showed that the ganglioside GD3 and VEGF levels in ovarian cancer ascites (OV-CAR-3 and SK-OV-3) are much higher than in ascites associated with other solid tumors. They proposed that VEGF and ganglioside GD3 synthesis pathway might be linked, working in tandem to suppress immune responses. The data proposed suggest that VEGF could modulate ganglioside GD3 expression confirming that ovarian cancer associated GD3 is responsible for suppressing CD1d-mediated NKT cell activation. This malignant overproduction of immunodepressive ganglioside could be reduced after 72 h of genistein treatment.

Phenoxodiol is a sterically modified version of genistein, with a higher bioavailability, a lower rate of metabolism and increased antitumor potency. According to Gamble et al. [95] phenoxodiol may be an effective anticancer drug, targeting the proliferation of the tumor cells and the angiogenic and inflammatory stimulation of the vasculature. These findings involve different enzymatic pathways, one of them concerning sphingolipids. It inhibited SphK which has been recently correlated with endothelial cell activation [96], angiogenesis and oncogenesis [97]. Hence, the inhibitory effect of phenoxodiol on pro-survival signals, mediated by SphK and Sph-1P, might contribute to arrest mitosis, to reduce angiogenesis and to promote apoptosis [95].

3.9. Luteolin

Luteolin (3′,4′,5,7-tetrahydroxyflavone) is a naturally occurring flavone, another subtype of flavonoid, found in food sources such as broccoli (*Brassica oleracea*), green chili (*Capsicum* spp.), onion leaf (*Allium unifolium*), French bean (*Phaseolus vulgaris*), carrot (*Daucus carota*), white radish (*Raphanus sativus var. longipinnatus*) and in infusion of clover blossom (*Trifolium pratense*) [67].

On a broad range of malignancies, luteolin displays different effects such as inhibition of cell proliferation, angiogenesis, metastasis, induction of apoptosis and sensitization to chemotherapy. Nevertheless, the molecular mechanisms of luteolin still remain unclear.

Hadi et al. [98] conducted an important study aimed to demonstrate a connection between luteolin and apoptosis in colon cancer cells. First, luteolin elevated Cer levels, followed by the apoptotic death of colon cancer cells, but not in differentiated enterocytes. Second, luteolin impaired the vesicle-mediated transport of Cer from ER to Golgi. The consequent dysregulation of sphingolipids equilibrium consisted of Cer elevation and significant reduction of both SM and glycosphingolipids. This effect may be correlated with the inhibition of AKT phosphorylation which emerges as a key mechanism affecting this vesicles route. Third, luteolin inhibited the production of Sph-1P by a SphK2 hindrance. Moreover, luteolin was proven to unbalance the sphingolipid rheostat by bending it to apoptosis in colon cancer cells (Figure 5A).

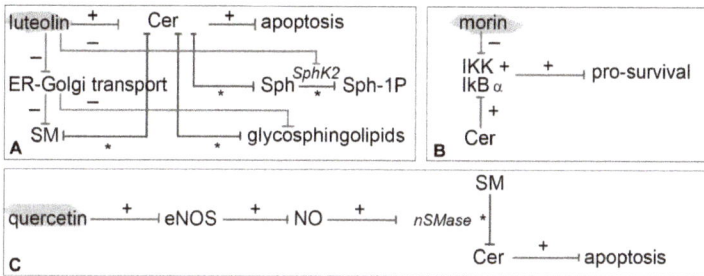

Figure 5. Mechanism of modulation on sphingolipids by luteolin (**A**), morin (**B**) and quercetin (**C**). It is depicted with an asterisk (*) enzymatic pathway, with plus (+) red-regulated pathway and with minus (−) down-regulation ones.

3.10. Morin

Morin (3,5,7,2′,4′-pentahydroxyflavone) is a flavonoid polyphenol of the class of flavonols. It is a yellow pigment that could be isolated from non-edible Osage orange (*Maclura pomifera*) and old fustic (*Maclura tinctoria*). Morin is also present in dietary infusions of white mulberry leaves (*Morus alba*), in figs (*Ficus carica*), almond (*Prunus dulcis*), guava (*Psidium guajava*) and wine [99]. Morin is a flavonol that exhibits antiproliferative, antitumor, and anti-inflammatory effects through a mechanism that is not well understood.

Manna et al. [100] proposed that morin mediates its effects by modulating NF-κB in the control of cell survival, proliferation, and tumorigenesis. NF-κB is a heterodimeric protein complex of members of the Rel protein family. NF-κB morin-mediated transcription can be promoted by a wide variety of inflammatory stimuli, including Cer (Figure 5B).

3.11. Quercetin

Quercetin is a naturally occurring flavonol found in high concentrations in red onions (*Allium cepa*), citrus fruits (*Citrus* spp.), apples (*Malus domestica*), red wine, and sour cherry seeds (*Prunus cerasus*) [67].

A study done by Ferrer et al. [101] showed that intravenous administration of quercetin prevented the metastatic growth of highly malignant B16 melanoma F10 cells, by enhancing NO release from the vascular endothelium through an increment of eNOS expression. The rise of NO promotes a tumor cytotoxicity and an activation of nSMase, thus increasing Cer and apoptosis.

Torres et al. [102] reported that the derivative of quercetin THDF (5,7,3'-trihydroxy-3,4'-dimethoxyflavone) inhibits cell proliferation and induces apoptosis in human leukemia cells (HL-60 and U937) by a disruption of tubulin polymerization and an activation of aSMase-dependent generation of Cer correlated with cell death (Figure 5C).

3.12. Resveratrol

Res (3,5,4'-trihydroxy-trans-stilbene) is a natural stilbene found in several plants including blueberries (*Vaccinium* sect. *Cyanococcus*), mulberries (*Morus* spp.), cranberries (*Vaccinium* subgenus *Oxycoccus*), peanuts (*Arachis hypogaea*), grapes (*Vitis* spp.), rhubarb (*Rheum* spp.) and wine. It has been reported to have anti-cancer, anti-inflammatory, anti-cardiovascular disease and blood-sugar lowering properties [103,104]. It has been classified as phytoalexin for being synthesized in spermatophytes in response to injury, UV irradiation and fungal attack. It exists in both *trans*, the more frequent, and *cis* isomeric forms. In plants, Res is generally found in glycosylated forms, known as 3-*O*-β-D-glucosides, and called piceids. Other natural Res analogs contain pterostilbene and piceatannol [105]. Anticancer properties of Res are quite complex and composed of different mechanisms. It can affect the processes underlying all stages of carcinogenesis, angiogenesis and metastasis. Its activity against cancer appears to be closely associated with: mutational activation of Ras, deregulation of myc, overexpression of AP-1, amplification of cell cycle regulator cyclins D/E and Cdks 2/4, mutation of Fas and Bax, deletion of p53, disruption of DNA-damage response regulators Chk1/2 and ATM/ATR, overexpression of survival kinase AKT1, mutation of cell cycle inhibitors and translocation of anti-apoptotic Bcl-2 [106]. Here we focus on the several Res anticancer properties triggered by modulation of sphingolipid metabolism (Figure 6C).

Signorelli et al. [107] demonstrated a strict correlation between sphingolipid metabolism, Res and autophagy in gastric cancer cells (HCGC-27). Res inhibits DHCD and subsequently induces an imbalanced accumulation of DHCers *versus* Cers thus promoting autophagy rather than apoptosis.

Shin et al. [108] established that Res leads to the accumulation of endogenous Cers and significantly increases DHCers especially DHCer-C24:0 (containing lignoceric acid) in SNU-1 gastric cancer cells and HT-29 colon adenocarcinoma cells. The accumulation of DHCer with different fatty acid chain lengths (C24:0 > C16:0 > C24:1 > C22:0) was powerfully associated with Res- induced cell cytotoxicity although the inhibition of DHCD was not found to be a critical mechanism. The effect of Res was drastically increased by dimethylsphingosine (a non-specific SphK inhibitor) and retinamide (4-HPR, a non-specific DHCD inhibitor) but not by GT-11 (a specific DHCD inhibitor). The Res cytotoxic effect is cell-specific: SNU-1 and HT-29 are highly sensitive in contrast with SNU-668.

According to Lin et al. [109], Res and Cer could be used in sequence or in combination for chemoprevention and cancer treatment due to their similarities in transduction pathways to induce apoptosis in human ovarian cancer OVCAR-3 cells. Cer and Res uses an endocytic- and activated ERK1/2 dependent pathway to induces apoptosis in human ovarian cancer cells. Additionally, exposure to these compounds induces expression and nuclear accumulation of COX-2 without affecting COX-1, Ser-15 phosphorylation of p53 and accumulation of BcL-xS. By contrast, only Cer utilizes both p38 kinase-dependent pathway and ERK 1/2-dependent pathway whereas Res only the latter one. However, the relationship of COX-2 protein on cancer is not easy to establish: some studies reported an expression of COX-2 in cells associated with tumor cell growth, metastasis, enhanced cellular adhesion and inhibition of apoptosis [110] whereas others suggested a pro-apoptotic activity [111].

Lim et al. [112] showed that Res and its dimers (ampelopsin A and balanocarpol) could perturb SphK 1-mediated signaling in MCF-7 breast cancer cells. Ampelopsin A and balanocarpol are dimers of Res formed by the fusion of *cis*- and *trans*-isomers and they could be extracted and isolated from plants in the Dipterocarpaceae family. In this family *Hopea dryobalanoides* and *Hopea odorata* supply a very limited food products. In this study, Res was found to be a competitive inhibitor of SphK1 and balanocarpol is about twice as potent as Res on kinase inhibition because of its binding to two catalytic sites simultaneously. The mechanism of down-regulation of SphK1 expression might involve changes in its protein turnover by ubiquitin-proteasomal or modification in lysosomal-cathepsin B proteolysis or alterations in gene promoter activity.

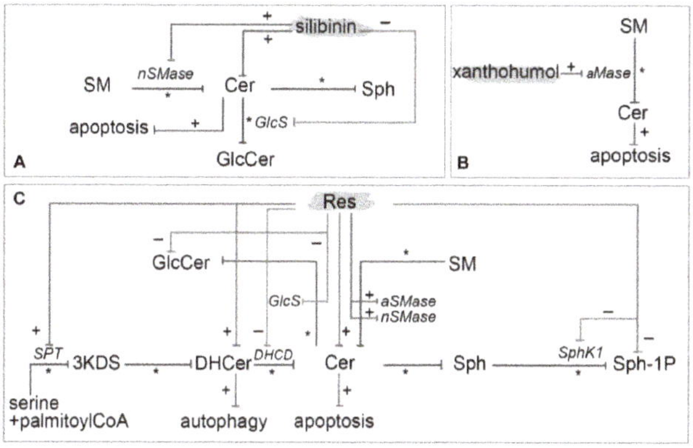

Figure 6. Mechanism of modulation on sphingolipids by silibinin (**A**), xanthohumol (**B**) and Res (**C**). It is depicted with an asterisk (*) enzymatic pathway, with plus (+) red-regulated pathway and with minus (−) down-regulation ones.

In agreement with Lim et al. [112], Tiang et al. [113] proposed Res to be an apoptotic agent in the myelogenous leukemia cell line K562 by modulation of SphK1 and translocation of the enzyme from the membrane to the cytosol. The kinase activity is clearly repressed granting a restoration of sphingolipid balance. Sph-1P level decreases whereas Cer level increases.

Cakir et al. [114] showed that Res induces apoptosis through a concurrent increase of *de novo* Cer and decrease of anti-apoptotic Sph-1P and GlcCer. Not only, targeting Cer metabolism increased chemosensitivity to Res in acute myeloid leukemia cells.

Kartal's study [115] was also focused on the relationship between the sphingolipid pathway, Res and human K562 chronic myeloid leukemia cells. A synergistic anti-proliferative effect was observed with Res in combination with: (1) Cer-C8, a cell-permeable analog of natural Cer inducing *de novo* generation; (2) PDMP, an inhibitor of GlcS; and (3) PF-543, a SphK1 inhibitor. Moreover, they showed that Res triggers apoptosis through raising expression of longevity assurance genes (LASS2, LASS4, LASS5, LASS6) correlated with down-regulation of GlcS and SphK 1.

Chow et al. [116] reported an abnormal accumulation of Cer *via* activation of SPT resulting in an ER dilation/expansion and thus ER stress. ER stress is, indeed, firmly associated with cell apoptosis by mechanisms involving direct activation of ER-associate caspases (3, 9 and 12) and CHOP, a common downstream pro-apoptotic molecule of unfolded protein response.

Wang et al. [117] described two divergent mechanisms of Res in melanoma B16 cells. They showed an inhibition of B16 cell growth *via* induction of mitochondrial apoptosis and contemporary inducing protective autophagy through Cer accumulation and AKT/mTOR pathway inhibition. Interruption of the autophagy program leads to an improvement of the efficacy of Res cytotoxicity and apoptosis. It was the first study revealing that Res-induced accumulation of Cer conferred protection of B16 cells against apoptosis inducing protective autophagy.

Another mechanism was proposed according to Mizutani et al. [118]. Inhibition in K562 (a human leukemia cell line) and HTC116 (a human colon cancer cell line) by Res was correlated to up-regulation of Cer and aSMase expression and down-regulation of Sph-1P. This study suggested a possible relationship between Res-induced cell growth inhibition and the sphingolipid metabolism modulation.

As previously mentioned, catechin and Res synergically inhibit SphK1 activity, *via* a novel ERK/PLD-dependent mechanism in prostate cancer cells (C4-2B hormone-responsive and PC-3 hormone- refractory) acting as a possible anti-cancer effector [40].

According to Scarlatti et al. [119] activation of the *de novo* Cer synthesis by Res is the mechanism underlying its growth inhibitory effect on the metastatic, drug-resistant and highly invasive breast cancer cell line MDA-MB-231. This accumulation derives from both *de novo* Cer synthesis and SM hydrolysis by activation respectively of SPT and nSMase.

Another work by Scarlatti et al. [120] presented that pretreatment with Res enhances tumor cell killing and inhibits the clonogenic survival in resistant irradiated-DU145 prostate cancer cells, synergistically affecting the cellular response to ionizing radiation. This event was mediated by an increase in cellular *de novo* Cer levels.

Dolfini et al. [121] demonstrated that targeting Cer signaling with Res might offer a potential strategy to prevent the growth of hormone-independent breast cancer. Res exerts a severe inhibitory effect on the growth of MDA-MB-231 both *in vitro* and *in vivo*. It affects the aggregation properties of MDA-MB-231 cells into multicellular tumor spheroids in association with induction of *de novo* synthesis of Cer.

Minutolo et al. [122] showed that a synthesized derivative of Res [5-(6-hydroxynaphthalen-2-yl)benzene-1,3-diol] is more effective in triggering apoptosis, coupled with the induction of endogenous Cer in human cancer cells MDA-MB-231. Since the Res biological activity in cancer cells is limited by its photosensitivity and metabolic instability, the authors replaced the 3,5-hydroxy groups with more stable methoxy groups, thus obtaining a compound with increased anti-proliferative activity. Moreover, the stabilization of the stilbene double bond of Res by a naphthalene ring increases the molecular rigidity. This dramatically improves the biological activity *via* Cer-mediated pro-apoptotic mechanism coupled to cleavage of PARP.

3.13. Silibinin

Silibinin is the most active and major component (60–70%) of silymarin, a standardized extract from the seeds of the milk thistle seeds (*Silybum marianum*). Other flavonolignans consist in silibinin, isosilibinin, silychristin, isosilychristin and silydianin. Silibinin is a mixture of two diastereomers, silybin A and silybin B, in approximately equimolar ratio [123].

It has been used in the prevention and treatment of viral hepatitis, cirrhosis caused by alcohol abuse and liver damage caused by medications or industrial toxins, in traditional and modern medicine. Silibinin effects are due to free radical trapping, prevention of lipid peroxidation, an increment of proapoptotic protein (Bax, p53), a decrement of anti-apoptotic proteins (Bcl-2 and Bcl-xL) and anti-cancer activity.

Boojara et al. [124] investigated the effects of four silibinin derivatives that is silybin A, silybin B, 3-*O*-galloyl-silybin A and 3-*O*-galloyl-silybin B on cell viability, caspase assessment, total Cer levels and Cer-metabolizing enzyme in Hep G2 hepatocarcinoma cell line. Exposure to silibinin isomers and gallate derivatives in human liver carcinoma cells resulted in increased Cer levels. Gallate derivatives had a stronger ability in Cer elevation in comparison with silybin A and B. The activity of aCDase, the enzyme involved in the catabolism of Cer to Sph, was markedly inhibited by silybin B, 3-*O*-galloyl-silybin A and 3-*O*-galloyl-silybin B. The activity of nSMase was increased by treatment with silybin A, silybin B and 3-*O*-galloyl-silybin A whereas the activity of GlcS was inhibited by silibin A, silibin B and 3-*O*-galloyl-silybin B (Figure 6A).

3.14. Xanthohumol

Xanthohumol (3'-[3,3-dimethyl allyl]-2',4',4-trihydroxy-6'-methoxychalcone) is the principal prenylated chalcone of the female inflorescences of the hop plant (*Humulus lupulus*). It is the main ingredient of beer and together with prenylflavonoids it is used to add bitterness and flavor.

The naturally occurring chalcones are heat-degraded during the brewing process therefore relatively high levels are due to a second addition of hops to the boiling wort.

Xanthohumol has been shown to elicit anti-inflammatory, antiangiogenic, anticancer, antibacterial, antifungal, antimalarial and antiviral effects. It favorably influences also sleep disorders and menopausal symptoms in women, acting as estrogen by its metabolites isoxanthohumol and 8-prenylnaringenin. According to Xuan et al. [125] xanthohumol stimulates aSMase in dendritic cells, derived from mouse bone marrow, leading to Cer formation and caspase activation. The sequence of events postulated was: (1) translocation of aSMase onto cell surface; (2) formation of Cer; (3) autocatalysis of caspase 8; (4) activation of caspase 3; and (5) DNA fragmentation and proteolysis of intracellular proteins (Figure 6B).

4. Conclusions

Cancer treatment and cancer prevention are a constant challenge for clinicians and the whole scientific community. Nutrients on their own appear to offer a good strategy in prevention more than in cancer therapy. However, chemotherapy has gradually transitioned from monotherapy to multidrug therapy. It is believed that a combination of classical chemotherapy with nutrients and especially with polyphenols dietary sources may improve efficacy and decreases negative side effects of the antineoplastic drug. In this multifaceted scenario, sphingolipids play a pivotal role as bioactive molecules, controlling several aspects of cancer from cell growth and proliferation to anti-cancer therapeutics. Further research on the crosstalk between polyphenols and sphingolipids could lead to better understand their reciprocal roles and to develop new therapeutic strategies against cancer.

Funding: This research received no external funding.

Acknowledgments: M.D.C. is supported by the PhD program in Molecular and Translational Medicine of the University of Milan, Italy.

Conflicts of Interest: The authors declare no conflict of interest.

Abbreviations

3-KDS	3-keto dihydrosphingosine
4-HPR	retinamide
aCDase	acid ceramidase
AIF	apoptosis inducing factor
AKT	protein kinase B
AP-1	activator protein 1
aSMase	lysosomal acidic sphingomyelinase
ATF6	activating transcription factor-6
ATM	ataxia-telangiectasia mutated kinase
ATR	serine/threonine-protein kinase ATR or ataxia telangiectasia and Rad3-related protein
BAX	apoptosis regulator BAX
BAX	apoptosis regulator BAX
Bcl-2	B-cell lymphoma 2
Bcl-xL	B-cell lymphoma-extra large
Bcl-xS	B-cell lymphoma-xS
BCR/ABL	Philadelphia chromosome
c-FOS	cellular DNA-binding proteins encoded by the c-fos genes
CAPE	caffeic acid phenethyl ester
CDase	ceramidase
Cdc25C	gene for M-phase inducer phosphatase 3
Cdk1	cyclin-dependent kinase 1
Cer	ceramide
CERT	ceramide transfer protein

Cer-1P	ceramide-1-phosphate
CerK	ceramide kinase
CerS	ceramide synthases
CERT	ceramide transfer protein
cGMP	cyclic guanosine monophosphate
Chk1/2	checkpoint kinase $\frac{1}{2}$
CHOP	C/EBP homology protein
CHOP	transcription factor CCAAT-enhancer-binding protein homologous protein
COX	cyclooxygenase
COX-2	cyclooxygenase 2
cPLA2	cytosolic phospholipases A2
CREB	cAMP response element-binding protein
DHCD	dihydroceramide desaturase
DHCer	dihydroceramides
DHSph	dihydrosphingosine or sphinganine
EGCG	epigallocatechin-3-gallate
EGF	epithelial growth factor
ELISA	enzyme-linked immunosorbent assay
ENOX	Ecto-NOX disulfide-thiol exchanger
ENSA	electrophoretic mobility shift assay
ER	estrogen receptor
ER	endoplasmic reticulum
ERK	extracellular signal regulated kinase
FACS	fluorescence activated cell sorted
Fas	first apoptosis signal receptor
FITC	fluorescein isothiocyanate
GalCer	galactosylceramide
GC/MS	gas chromatography tandem mass spectrometry
GD3	ganglioside GD3 or disialosyllactosylceramide
GlcCer	glucosylceramide
GlcS	glucosylceramide synthase
GPR30	G protein-coupled receptor for estrogen
GSK-3	glycogen synthase kinase 3
GT-11	*N*-[(1*R*,2*S*)-2-hydroxy-1-hydroxymethyl-2-(2-tridecyl-1-cyclopropenyl)ethyl]octanamide
GW4869	*N*,*N'*-Bis[4-(4,5-dihydro-1*H*-imidazol-2-yl)phenyl]-3,3'-p-phenylene-bis-acrylamide
HIF-1α	hypoxia-inducible factor-1α
HNSCC	head and neck squamous cell carcimona
HPLC	high performance liquid chromatography
HPTLC	high performance thin layer chromatography
I2PP2A	protein phosphatase 2A inhibitor 2
IKK	IκBα kinase
IκBα	inhibitory subunit of NF-κB
JAK	janus kinase
JNK	c-Jun N-terminal kinase
KDSR	3-ketodihydrosphingosine reductase
LacCer	lactosylcercamide
LASS	longevity assurance genes
Lc3	GlcNAcβ1-3Galβ1-4Glcβ-Cer
LPS	lipopolysaccharides
MAPK	mitogen activated protein kinase
MPM-2	mitotic protein monoclonal 2
mTOR	mammalian target of rapamycin
MTT	3-(4,5-dimethylthiazol-2-yl)-2,5-diphenyltetrazolium bromide
NADH	reduced form of Nicotinamide adenine dinucleotide
NF-κB	nuclear factor kappa-light-chain-enhancer of activated B cells

NGF	nerve growth factor
NGFR	nerve growth factor receptor
nSMase	neutral sphingomyelinase Mg-dependent
P-gp	permeability glycoprotein
p38 MAPK	p38 mitogen activated protein kinase
p53	tumor protein p53
p75NTR	low-affinity nerve growth factor receptor or p75 neurotrophin receptor
PA	phosphatidic acid
Par-4	prostate apoptosis response 4
PARP	poly (ADP-ribose) polymerase
PDMP	DL-threo-1-phenyl-2-decanoylamino-3-morpholino-1-propanol
PI3K	phosphatidylinositide 3-kinases
PKC/PKA	protein kinase C/protein kinase A
PLC	phospholipase C
PLD	phospholipase D
PPAR	peroxisome proliferator-activated receptors
PPE	polyphenon E
Res	resveratrol
ROS	reactive oxygen species
S1PR1-5	sphingosine-1-phosphate receptors 1–5
SEAP	secreted embryonic alkaline phosphatase
SKI-II	2-(p-Hydroxyanilino)-4-(p-chlorophenyl)thiazole
SM	sphingomyelin
SMase	sphingomyelinase
SMS1/2	sphingomyelin synthase 1/2
Sph	sphingosine
Sph-1P	sphingosine-1-phosphate
SphK1/2	sphingosine kinase 1/2
SPL	sphingosine-1-phosphate lyase
SPPase1/2	sphingosine-1-phosphate phosphatases 1/2
SPT	serinepalmitoyl transferase
STAT	signal transducer and activator of transcription protein
THDF	5,7,3′-trihydroxy-3,4′-dimethoxyflavone
THDF	5,7,3′-trihydroxy-3,4′-dimethoxyflavone
TLC	thin layer chromatography
TLC	thin layer chromatography
TNF	tumor necrosis factor alpha
VDAC	voltage-dependent anion-selective channel
VEGF	vascular endothelial growth factor
XM462	Octanoic acid (1S,2S)-(2-hydroxy-1-hydroxymethyl-3-tridecylsulfanyl-propyl)-amide

References

1. Tsao, R. Chemistry and biochemistry of dietary polyphenols. *Nutrients* **2010**, *2*, 1231–1246. [CrossRef] [PubMed]
2. Beecher, G.R. Overview of dietary flavonoids: Nomenclature, occurrence and intake. *J. Nutr.* **2003**, *133*, 3244S–3246S. [CrossRef] [PubMed]
3. Rivière, C.; Pawlus, A.D.; Mérillon, J.-M. Natural stilbenoids: Distribution in the plant kingdom and chemotaxonomic interest in Vitaceae. *Nat. Prod. Rep.* **2012**, *29*, 1317–1333. [CrossRef] [PubMed]
4. Husain, N.; Gupta, S. A critical study on chemistry and distribution of phenolic compounds in plants, and their role in human health. *IOSR J. Environ. Sci. Toxicol. Food Technol.* **2015**, *1*, 57–60.
5. Cook, N. Flavonoids—Chemistry, metabolism, cardioprotective effects, and dietary sources. *J. Eur. Ceram. Soc.* **1996**, *7*, 66–76. [CrossRef]

6. Kim, K.; Vance, T.M.; Chun, O.K. Estimated intake and major food sources of flavonoids among US adults: Changes between 1999–2002 and 2007–2010 in NHANES. *Eur. J. Nutr.* **2016**, *55*, 833–843. [CrossRef] [PubMed]

7. Frankel, E.N. Chemistry of extra virgin olive oil: Adulteration, oxidative stability, and antioxidants. *J. Agric. Food Chem.* **2010**, *58*, 5991–6006. [CrossRef] [PubMed]

8. Gálvez, M.C.; Barroso, C.G.; Pérez-Bustamante, J.A. Analysis of polyphenolic compounds of different vinegar samples. *Z. Lebensm. Unters. Forsch.* **1994**, *199*, 29–31. [CrossRef]

9. Adisakwattana, S. Cinnamic acid and its derivatives: Mechanisms for prevention and management of diabetes and its complications. *Nutrients* **2017**, *9*, 163. [CrossRef] [PubMed]

10. D'Archivio, M.; Filesi, C.; Varì, R.; Scazzocchio, B.; Masella, R. Bioavailability of the polyphenols: Status and controversies. *Int. J. Mol. Sci.* **2010**, *11*, 1321–1342. [CrossRef] [PubMed]

11. Bravo, L. Polyphenols: Chemistry, dietary sources, metabolism, and nutritional significance. *Nutr. Rev.* **2009**, *56*, 317–333. [CrossRef]

12. Scalbert, A.; Morand, C.; Manach, C.; Rémésy, C. Absorption and metabolism of polyphenols in the gut and impact on health. *Biomed. Pharmacother.* **2002**, *56*, 276–282. [CrossRef]

13. Lewandowska, U.; Szewczyk, K.; Hrabec, E.; Janecka, A.; Gorlach, S. Overview of metabolism and bioavailability enhancement of polyphenols. *J. Agric. Food Chem.* **2013**, *61*, 12183–12199. [CrossRef] [PubMed]

14. Manach, C.; Scalbert, A.; Morand, C.; Remesy, C.; Jimenez, L. Polyphenols—Food sources and bioavailability. *Am. J. Clin. Nutr.* **2004**, *79*, 727–747. [CrossRef] [PubMed]

15. Chen, Y.; Liu, Y.; Sullards, M.C.; Merrill, A.H. An introduction to sphingolipid metabolism and analysis by new technologies. *NeuroMol. Med.* **2010**, *12*, 306–319. [CrossRef] [PubMed]

16. Zheng, W.; Kollmeyer, J.; Symolon, H.; Momin, A.; Munter, E.; Wang, E.; Kelly, S.; Allegood, J.C.; Liu, Y.; Peng, Q.; et al. Ceramides and other bioactive sphingolipid backbones in health and disease: Lipidomic analysis, metabolism and roles in membrane structure, dynamics, signaling and autophagy. *Biochim. Biophys. Acta Biomembr.* **2006**, *1758*, 1864–1884. [CrossRef] [PubMed]

17. Fahy, E.; Subramaniam, S.; Brown, H.A.; Glass, C.K.; Merrill, A.H.; Murphy, R.C.; Raetz, C.R.H.; Russell, D.W.; Seyama, Y.; Shaw, W.; et al. A comprehensive classification system for lipids. *J. Lipid Res.* **2005**, *46*, 839–862. [CrossRef] [PubMed]

18. Slotte, J.P. Biological functions of sphingomyelins. *Prog. Lipid Res.* **2013**, *52*, 424–437. [CrossRef] [PubMed]

19. Gault, C.R.; Obeid, L.M.; Hannun, Y.A. An overview of sphingolipid metabolism: From synthesis to breakdown. *Adv. Exp. Med. Biol.* **2010**, *688*, 1–23. [CrossRef] [PubMed]

20. Murphy, S.M.; Ernst, D.; Wei, Y.; Laurà, M.; Liu, Y.T.; Polke, J.; Blake, J.; Winer, J.; Houlden, H.; Hornemann, T.; Reilly, M.M. Hereditary sensory and autonomic neuropathy type 1 (HSANI) caused by a novel mutation in SPTLC2. *Neurology* **2013**, *80*, 2106–2111. [CrossRef] [PubMed]

21. Park, W.J.; Park, J.W. The effect of altered sphingolipid acyl chain length on various disease models. *Biol. Chem.* **2015**, *396*, 693–705. [CrossRef] [PubMed]

22. Aguilera-Romero, A.; Gehin, C.; Riezman, H. Sphingolipid homeostasis in the web of metabolic routes. *Biochim. Biophys. Acta Mol. Cell Biol. Lipids* **2014**, *1841*, 647–656. [CrossRef] [PubMed]

23. Yamaji, T.; Hanada, K. Sphingolipid metabolism and interorganellar transport: Localization of sphingolipid enzymes and lipid transfer proteins. *Traffic* **2015**, *16*, 101–122. [CrossRef] [PubMed]

24. MacEyka, M.; Spiegel, S. Sphingolipid metabolites in inflammatory disease. *Nature* **2014**, *510*, 58–67. [CrossRef] [PubMed]

25. Patwardhan, G.A.; Beverly, L.J.; Siskind, L.J. Sphingolipids and mitochondrial apoptosis. *J. Bioenerg. Biomembr.* **2016**, *48*, 153–168. [CrossRef] [PubMed]

26. Young, M.M.; Kester, M.; Wang, H.-G. Sphingolipids: Regulators of crosstalk between apoptosis and autophagy. *J. Lipid Res.* **2013**, *54*, 5–19. [CrossRef] [PubMed]

27. Nakamura, H.; Murayama, T. The role of sphingolipids in arachidonic acid metabolism. *J. Pharmacol. Sci.* **2014**, *124*, 307–312. [CrossRef] [PubMed]

28. Ghidoni, R.; Caretti, A.; Signorelli, P. Role of sphingolipids in the pathobiology of lung inflammation. *Mediat. Inflamm.* **2015**, *2015*, 487508. [CrossRef] [PubMed]

29. Lahiri, S.; Futerman, A.H. The metabolism and function of sphingolipids and glycosphingolipids. *Cell. Mol. Life Sci.* **2007**, *64*, 2270–2284. [CrossRef] [PubMed]

30. Hannun, Y.A.; Obeid, L.M. The ceramide-centric universe of lipid-mediated cell regulation: Stress encounters of the lipid kind. *J. Biol. Chem.* **2002**, *277*, 25847–25850. [CrossRef] [PubMed]

31. Hannun, Y.A.; Obeid, L.M. Principles of bioactive lipid signalling: Lessons from sphingolipids. *Nat. Rev. Mol. Cell Biol.* **2008**, *9*, 139–150. [CrossRef] [PubMed]

32. Taha, T.A.; Hannun, Y.A.; Obeid, L.M. Sphingosine kinase: Biochemical and cellular regulation and role in disease. *J. Biochem. Mol. Biol.* **2006**, *39*, 113–131. [CrossRef] [PubMed]

33. Cowart, L.A. Sphingolipids: Players in the pathology of metabolic disease. *Trends Endocrinol. Metab.* **2009**, *20*, 34–42. [CrossRef] [PubMed]

34. Sridevi, P.; Alexander, H.; Laviad, E.L.; Min, J.; Mesika, A.; Hannink, M.; Futerman, A.H.; Alexander, S. Stress-induced ER to Golgi translocation of ceramide synthase 1 is dependent on proteasomal processing. *Exp. Cell Res.* **2010**, *316*, 78–91. [CrossRef] [PubMed]

35. Siskind, L.J.; Mullen, T.D.; Rosales, K.R.; Clarke, C.J.; Hernandez-Corbacho, M.J.; Edinger, A.L.; Obeid, L.M. The BCL-2 protein BAK is required for long-chain ceramide generation during apoptosis. *J. Biol. Chem.* **2010**, *285*, 11818–11826. [CrossRef] [PubMed]

36. Karahatay, S.; Thomas, K.; Koybasi, S.; Senkal, C.E.; ElOjeimy, S.; Liu, X.; Bielawski, J.; Day, T.A.; Gillespie, M.B.; Sinha, D.; et al. Clinical relevance of ceramide metabolism in the pathogenesis of human head and neck squamous cell carcinoma (HNSCC): Attenuation of C18-ceramide in HNSCC tumors correlates with lymphovascular invasion and nodal metastasis. *Cancer Lett.* **2007**, *256*, 101–111. [CrossRef] [PubMed]

37. Pettus, B.J.; Bielawska, A.; Subramanian, P.; Wijesinghe, D.S.; Maceyka, M.; Leslie, C.C.; Evans, J.H.; Freiberg, J.; Roddy, P.; Hannun, Y.A.; et al. Ceramide 1-phosphate is a direct activator of cytosolic phospholipase A2. *J. Biol. Chem.* **2004**, *279*, 11320–11326. [CrossRef] [PubMed]

38. Ponnusamy, S.; Meyers-Needham, M.; Senkal, C.E.; Saddoughi, S.A.; Sentelle, D.; Selvam, S.P.; Salas, A.; Ogretmen, B. Sphingolipids and cancer: Ceramide and sphingosine-1-phosphate in the regulation of cell death and drug resistance. *Future Oncol.* **2010**, *6*, 1603–1624. [CrossRef] [PubMed]

39. Saddoughi, S.A.; Song, P.; Ogretmen, B. Roles of bioactive sphingolipids in cancer biology and therapeutics. *Subcell. Biochem.* **2008**, *49*, 413–440. [CrossRef] [PubMed]

40. Brizuela, L.; Dayon, A.; Doumerc, N.; Ader, I.; Golzio, M.; Izard, J.C.; Hara, Y.; Malavaud, B.; Cuvillier, O. The sphingosine kinase-1 survival pathway is a molecular target for the tumor-suppressive tea and wine polyphenols in prostate cancer. *FASEB J.* **2010**, *24*, 3882–3894. [CrossRef] [PubMed]

41. Zbidah, M.; Lupescu, A.; Jilani, K.; Fajol, A.; Michael, D.; Qadri, S.M.; Lang, F. Apigenin-induced suicidal erythrocyte death. *J. Agric. Food Chem.* **2012**, *60*, 533–538. [CrossRef] [PubMed]

42. Lefort, É.C.; Blay, J. Apigenin and its impact on gastrointestinal cancers. *Mol. Nutr. Food Res.* **2013**, *57*, 126–144. [CrossRef] [PubMed]

43. Choi, A.Y.; Choi, J.H.; Lee, J.Y.; Yoon, K.S.; Choe, W.; Ha, J.; Yeo, E.J.; Kang, I. Apigenin protects HT22 murine hippocampal neuronal cells against endoplasmic reticulum stress-induced apoptosis. *Neurochem. Int.* **2010**, *57*, 143–152. [CrossRef] [PubMed]

44. Balez, R.; Steiner, N.; Engel, M.; Muñoz, S.S.; Lum, J.S.; Wu, Y.; Wang, D.; Vallotton, P.; Sachdev, P.; O'Connor, M.; et al. Neuroprotective effects of apigenin against inflammation, neuronal excitability and apoptosis in an induced pluripotent stem cell model of Alzheimer's disease. *Sci. Rep.* **2016**, *6*, 1–16. [CrossRef] [PubMed]

45. Zbidah, M.; Lupescu, A.; Shaik, N.; Lang, F. Gossypol-induced suicidal erythrocyte death. *Toxicology* **2012**, *302*, 101–105. [CrossRef] [PubMed]

46. Moussavi, M. Insight into the Mechanisms by Which Apigenin, Curcumin and Sulfasalazine Induce Apoptosis in Colon Cancer Cells. Master's Thesis, University of British Columbia, Vancouver, BC, Canada, 2003.

47. Stojković, D.; Petrović, J.; Soković, M.; Glamočlija, J.; Kukić-Marković, J.; Petrović, S. In situ antioxidant and antimicrobial activities of naturally occurring caffeic acid, p-coumaric acid and rutin, using food systems. *J. Sci. Food Agric.* **2013**, *93*, 3205–3208. [CrossRef] [PubMed]

48. Silva, T.; Oliveira, C.; Borges, F. Caffeic acid derivatives, analogs and applications: A patent review (2009–2013). *Expert Opin. Ther. Pat.* **2014**, *24*, 1257–1270. [CrossRef] [PubMed]

49. El-Seedi, H.R.; El-Said, A.M.A.; Khalifa, S.A.M.; Göransson, U.; Bohlin, L.; Borg-Karlson, A.K.; Verpoorte, R. Biosynthesis, natural sources, dietary intake, pharmacokinetic properties, and biological activities of hydroxycinnamic acids. *J. Agric. Food Chem.* **2012**, *60*, 10877–10895. [CrossRef] [PubMed]

50. Nardini, M.; Leonardi, F.; Scaccini, C.; Virgili, F. Modulation of ceramide-induced NF-κB binding activity and apoptotic response by caffeic acid in U937 cells: Comparison with other antioxidants. *Free Radic. Biol. Med.* **2001**, *30*, 722–733. [CrossRef]

51. Hagiwara, A.; Kokubo, Y.; Takesada, Y.; Tanaka, H.; Tamano, S.; Hirose, M.; Shirai, T.; Ito, N. Inhibitory effects of phenolic compounds on development of naturally occurring preneoplastic hepatocytic foci in long-term feeding studies using male F344 rats. *Teratog. Carcinog. Mutagen.* **1996**, *16*, 317–325. [CrossRef]

52. Tanaka, T.; Kojima, T.; Kawamori, T.; Wang, A.; Suzui, M.; Okamoto, K.; Mori, H. Inhibition of 4-nitroquinoline-1-oxide-induced rat tongue carcinogenesis by the naturally occurring plant phenolics caffeic, ellagic, chlorogenic and ferulic acids. *Carcinogenesis* **1993**, *14*, 1321–1325. [CrossRef] [PubMed]

53. Nardini, M.; Scaccini, C.; Packer, L.; Virgili, F. In vitro inhibition of the activity of phosphorylase kinase, protein kinase C and protein kinase A by caffeic acid and a procyanidin-rich pine bark (Pinus marittima) extract. *Biochim. Biophys. Acta Gen. Subj.* **2000**, *1474*, 219–225. [CrossRef]

54. Kang, N.J.; Lee, K.W.; Shin, B.J.; Jung, S.K.; Hwang, M.K.; Bode, A.M.; Heo, Y.S.; Lee, H.J.; Dong, Z. Caffeic acid, a phenolic phytochemical in coffee, directly inhibits Fyn kinase activity and UVB-induced COX-2 expression. *Carcinogenesis* **2009**, *30*, 321–330. [CrossRef] [PubMed]

55. Murtaza, G.; Karim, S.; Akram, M.R.; Khan, S.A.; Azhar, S.; Mumtaz, A.; Bin Asad, M.H.H. Caffeic acid phenethyl ester and therapeutic potentials. *Biomed. Res. Int.* **2014**, *2014*, 145342. [CrossRef] [PubMed]

56. Tseng, T.H.; Shen, C.H.; Huang, W.S.; Chen, C.N.; Liang, W.H.; Lin, T.H.; Kuo, H.C. Activation of neutral-sphingomyelinase, MAPKs, and p75 NTR-mediating caffeic acid phenethyl ester-induced apoptosis in C6 glioma cells. *J. Biomed. Sci.* **2014**, *21*, 61. [CrossRef] [PubMed]

57. Wang, R.; Zhou, W.; Jiang, X. Reaction kinetics of degradation and epimerization of epigallocatechin gallate (EGCG) in aqueous system over a wide temperature range. *J. Agric. Food Chem.* **2008**, *56*, 2694–2701. [CrossRef] [PubMed]

58. Gadkari, P.V.; Balaraman, M. Catechins: Sources, extraction and encapsulation: A review. *Food Bioprod. Process.* **2015**, *93*, 122–138. [CrossRef]

59. Singh, B.N.; Shankar, S.; Srivastava, R.K. Green tea catechin, epigallocatechin-3-gallate (EGCG): Mechanisms, perspectives and clinical applications. *Biochem. Pharmacol.* **2011**, *82*, 1807–1821. [CrossRef] [PubMed]

60. Ju, J.; Hong, J.; Zhou, J.N.; Pan, Z.; Bose, M.; Liao, J.; Yang, G.Y.; Liu, Y.Y.; Hou, Z.; Lin, Y.; et al. Inhibition of intestinal tumorigenesis in Apcmin/+ mice by (−)-epigallocatechin-3-gallate, the major catechin in green tea. *Cancer Res.* **2005**, *65*, 10623–10631. [CrossRef] [PubMed]

61. Xiao, H.; Hao, X.; Simi, B.; Ju, J.; Jiang, H.; Reddy, B.S.; Yang, C.S. Green tea polyphenols inhibit colorectal aberrant crypt foci (ACF) formation and prevent oncogenic changes in dysplastic ACF in azoxymethane-treated F344 rats. *Carcinogenesis* **2008**, *29*, 113–119. [CrossRef] [PubMed]

62. Wu, L.Y.; De Luca, T.; Watanabe, T.; Morré, D.M.; Morré, D.J. Metabolite modulation of HeLa cell response to ENOX2 inhibitors EGCG and phenoxodiol. *Biochim. Biophys. Acta Gen. Subj.* **2011**, *1810*, 784–789. [CrossRef] [PubMed]

63. Clifford, M.N. Chlorogenic acids and other cinnamates—Nature, occurrence, dietary burden, absorption and metabolism. *J. Sci. Food Agric.* **2000**, *80*, 1033–1043. [CrossRef]

64. Olthof, M.R.; Hollman, P.C.H.; Katan, M.B. Human nutrition and metabolism chlorogenic acid and caffeic acid are absorbed in humans. *J. Nutr.* **2001**, *131*, 66–71. [CrossRef] [PubMed]

65. Lee, M.S.; Lee, S.O.; Kim, K.R.; Lee, H.J. Sphingosine kinase-1 involves the inhibitory action of HIF-1α by chlorogenic acid in hypoxic DU145 cells. *Int. J. Mol. Sci.* **2017**, *18*, 325. [CrossRef] [PubMed]

66. Belkaid, A.; Currie, J.C.; Desgagnés, J.; Annabi, B. The chemopreventive properties of chlorogenic acid reveal a potential new role for the microsomal glucose-6-phosphate translocase in brain tumor progression. *Cancer Cell Int.* **2006**, *6*, 7. [CrossRef] [PubMed]

67. Basu, A.; Das, A.S.; Majumder, M.; Mukhopadhyay, R. Antiatherogenic roles of dietary flavonoids chrysin, quercetin, and luteolin. *J. Cardiovasc. Pharmacol.* **2016**, *68*, 89–96. [CrossRef] [PubMed]

68. Yan, R.Y.; Cao, Y.Y.; Chen, C.Y.; Dai, H.Q.; Yu, S.X.; Wei, J.L.; Li, H.; Yang, B. Antioxidant flavonoids from the seed of Oroxylum indicum. *Fitoterapia* **2011**, *82*, 841–848. [CrossRef] [PubMed]

69. Samokhvalov, V.; Zlobine, I.; Jamieson, K.L.; Jurasz, P.; Chen, C.; Lee, K.S.S.; Hammock, B.D.; Seubert, J.M. PPARδ signaling mediates the cytotoxicity of DHA in H9c2 cells. *Toxicol. Lett.* **2015**, *232*, 10–20. [CrossRef] [PubMed]

70. Hull, M.A.; Gardner, S.H.; Hawcroft, G. Activity of the non-steroidal anti-inflammatory drug indomethacin against colorectal cancer. *Cancer Treat. Rev.* **2003**, *29*, 309–320. [CrossRef]

71. Lestari, M.L.A.D.; Indrayanto, G. *Curcumin. Profiles of Drug Substances, Excipients and Related Methodology*; Elsevier: New York, NY, USA, 2013; Volume 39, pp. 113–204, ISBN 9780128001738.

72. Cheng, Y.; Kozubek, A.; Ohlsson, L.; Sternby, B.; Duan, R.D. Curcumin decreases acid sphingomyelinase activity in colon cancer caco-2 cells. *Planta Med.* **2007**, *73*, 725–730. [CrossRef] [PubMed]

73. Koumanov, K.S.; Quinn, P.J.; Béréziat, G.; Wolf, C.; Bereziat, G. Cholesterol relieves the inhibitory effect of sphingomyelin on type II secretory phospholipase A2. *Biochem. J.* **1998**, *336*, 625–630. [CrossRef] [PubMed]

74. Shida, D.; Kitayama, J.; Yamaguchi, H.; Okaji, Y.; Tsuno, N.H.; Watanabe, T.; Takuwa, Y.; Nagawa, H. Lysophosphatidic acid (LPA) enhances the metastatic potential of human colon carcinoma DLD1 cells through LPA1. *Cancer Res.* **2003**, *63*, 1706–1711. [PubMed]

75. Moussavi, M.; Assi, K.; Gómez-Muñoz, A.; Salh, B. Curcumin mediates ceramide generation via the *de novo* pathway in colon cancer cells. *Carcinogenesis* **2006**, *27*, 1636–1644. [CrossRef] [PubMed]

76. Chen, M.B.; Wu, X.Y.; Tao, G.Q.; Liu, C.Y.; Chen, J.; Wang, L.Q.; Lu, P.H. Perifosine sensitizes curcumin-induced anti-colorectal cancer effects by targeting multiple signaling pathways both in vivo and in vitro. *Int. J. Cancer* **2012**, *131*, 2487–2498. [CrossRef] [PubMed]

77. Yu, T.; Li, J.; Qiu, Y.; Sun, H. 1-Phenyl-2-decanoylamino-3-morpholino-1-propanol (PDMP) facilitates curcumin-induced melanoma cell apoptosis by enhancing ceramide accumulation, JNK activation, and inhibiting PI3K/AKT activation. *Mol. Cell. Biochem.* **2012**, *361*, 47–54. [CrossRef] [PubMed]

78. Sordillo, L.A.; Sordillo, P.P.; Helson, L. Curcumin for the treatment of glioblastoma. *Anticancer Res.* **2015**, *35*, 6373–6378. [PubMed]

79. Thayyullathil, F.; Rahman, A.; Pallichankandy, S.; Patel, M.; Galadari, S. ROS-dependent prostate apoptosis response-4 (Par-4) up-regulation and ceramide generation are the prime signaling events associated with curcumin-induced autophagic cell death in human malignant glioma. *FEBS Open Bio.* **2014**, *4*, 763–776. [CrossRef] [PubMed]

80. Hilchie, A.L.; Furlong, S.J.; Sutton, K.; Richardson, A.; Robichaud, M.R.J.; Giacomantonio, C.A.; Ridgway, N.D.; Hoskin, D.W. Curcumin-induced apoptosis in PC3 prostate carcinoma cells is caspase-independent and involves cellular ceramide accumulation and damage to mitochondria. *Nutr. Cancer* **2010**, *62*, 379–389. [CrossRef] [PubMed]

81. Kizhakkayil, J.; Thayyullathil, F.; Chathoth, S.; Hago, A.; Patel, M.; Galadari, S. Glutathione regulates caspase-dependent ceramide production and curcumin-induced apoptosis in human leukemic cells. *Free Radic. Biol. Med.* **2012**, *52*, 1854–1864. [CrossRef] [PubMed]

82. Scharstuhl, A.; Mutsaers, H.A.M.; Pennings, S.W.C.; Russel, F.G.M.; Wagener, F.A.D.T.G. Involvement of VDAC, Bax and ceramides in the efflux of AIF from mitochondria during curcumin-induced apoptosis. *PLoS ONE* **2009**, *4*, e6688. [CrossRef] [PubMed]

83. Abdel Shakor, A.B.; Atia, M.; Ismail, I.A.; Alshehri, A.; El-Refaey, H.; Kwiatkowska, K.; Sobota, A. Curcumin induces apoptosis of multidrug-resistant human leukemia HL60 cells by complex pathways leading to ceramide accumulation. *Biochim. Biophys. Acta Mol. Cell Biol. Lipids* **2014**, *1841*, 1672–1682. [CrossRef] [PubMed]

84. Abdel Shakor, A.B.; Atia, M.; Alshehri, A.S.; Sobota, A.; Kwiatkowska, K. Ceramide generation during curcumin-induced apoptosis is controlled by crosstalk among Bcl-2, Bcl-xL, caspases and glutathione. *Cell Signal.* **2015**, *27*, 2220–2230. [CrossRef] [PubMed]

85. Yang, Y.L.; Ji, C.; Cheng, L.; He, L.; Lu, C.C.; Wang, R.; Bi, Z.G. Sphingosine kinase-1 inhibition sensitizes curcumin-induced growth inhibition and apoptosis in ovarian cancer cells. *Cancer Sci.* **2012**, *103*, 1538–1545. [CrossRef] [PubMed]

86. Qiu, Y.; Yu, T.; Wang, W.; Pan, K.; Shi, D.; Sun, H. Curcumin-induced melanoma cell death is associated with mitochondrial permeability transition pore (mPTP) opening. *Biochem. Biophys. Res. Commun.* **2014**, *448*, 15–21. [CrossRef] [PubMed]

87. Spagnuolo, C.; Russo, G.L.; Orhan, I.E.; Habtemariam, S.; Daglia, M.; Sureda, A.; Nabavi, S.F.; Devi, K.P.; Loizzo, M.R.; Tundis, R.; et al. Genistein and cancer: Current status, challenges, and future directions. *Adv. Nutr. Int. Rev. J.* **2015**, *6*, 408–419. [CrossRef] [PubMed]

88. Engel, N.; Lisec, J.; Piechulla, B.; Nebe, B. Metabolic Profiling reveals sphingosine-1-phosphate kinase 2 and lyase as key targets of (phyto-) estrogen action in the breast cancer cell line MCF-7 and not in MCF-12A. *PLoS ONE* **2012**, *7*, e47833. [CrossRef] [PubMed]

89. Lucki, N.C.; Sewer, M.B. Genistein stimulates MCF-7 breast cancer cell growth by inducing acid ceramidase (ASAH1) gene expression. *J. Biol. Chem.* **2011**, *286*, 19399–19409. [CrossRef] [PubMed]

90. Engel, N.; Adamus, A.; Schauer, N.; Kühn, J.; Nebe, B.; Seitz, G.; Kraft, K. Synergistic action of genistein and calcitriol in immature osteosarcoma MG-63 cells by SGPL1 up-regulation. *PLoS ONE* **2017**, *12*, e0169742. [CrossRef] [PubMed]

91. Ji, C.; Yang, Y.L.; He, L.; Gu, B.; Xia, J.P.; Sun, W.L.; Su, Z.L.; Chen, B.; Bi, Z.G. Increasing ceramides sensitizes genistein-induced melanoma cell apoptosis and growth inhibition. *Biochem. Biophys. Res. Commun.* **2012**, *421*, 462–467. [CrossRef] [PubMed]

92. Tiper, I.V.; Temkin, S.M.; Spiegel, S.; Goldblum, S.E.; Giuntoli, R.L.; Oelke, M.; Schneck, J.P.; Webb, T.J. VEGF potentiates GD3-mediated immunosuppression by human ovarian cancer cells. *Clin. Cancer Res.* **2016**, *22*, 4249–4258. [CrossRef] [PubMed]

93. Zebrowski, B.K.; Liu, W.; Ramirez, K.; Akagi, Y.; Mills, G.B.; Ellis, L.M. Markedly elevated levels of vascular endothelial growth factor in malignant ascites. *Ann. Surg. Oncol.* **1999**, *6*, 373–378. [CrossRef] [PubMed]

94. Bamias, A.; Koutsoukou, V.; Terpos, E.; Tsiatas, M.L.; Liakos, C.; Tsitsilonis, O.; Rodolakis, A.; Voulgaris, Z.; Vlahos, G.; Papageorgiou, T.; et al. Correlation of NK T-like CD3+CD56+ cells and CD4+CD25+(hi) regulatory T cells with VEGF and TNFα in ascites from advanced ovarian cancer: Association with platinum resistance and prognosis in patients receiving first-line, platinum-based chemotherapy. *Gynecol. Oncol.* **2008**, *108*, 421–427. [CrossRef] [PubMed]

95. Gamble, J.R.; Xia, P.; Hahn, C.N.; Drew, J.J.; Drogemuller, C.J.; Brown, D.; Vadas, M.A. Phenoxodiol, an experimental anticancer drug, shows potent antiangiogenic properties in addition to its antitumour effects. *Int. J. Cancer* **2006**, *118*, 2412–2420. [CrossRef] [PubMed]

96. Limaye, V.; Li, X.; Hahn, C.; Xia, P.; Berndt, M.C.; Vadas, M.A.; Gamble, J.R. Sphingosine kinase-1 enhances endothelial cell survival through a PECAM-1-dependent activation of PI-3K/Akt and regulation of Bcl-2 family members. *Blood* **2005**, *105*, 3169–3177. [CrossRef] [PubMed]

97. Plano, D.; Amin, S.; Sharma, A.K. Importance of sphingosine kinase (SphK) as a target in developing cancer therapeutics and recent developments in the synthesis of novel SphK inhibitors. *J. Med. Chem.* **2014**, *57*, 5509–5524. [CrossRef] [PubMed]

98. Hadi, L.A.; Di Vito, C.; Marfia, G.; Ferraretto, A.; Tringali, C.; Viani, P.; Riboni, L. Sphingosine kinase 2 and ceramide transport as key targets of the natural flavonoid luteolin to induce apoptosis in colon cancer cells. *PLoS ONE* **2015**, *10*, e0143384. [CrossRef]

99. Madankumar, P.; Naveenkumar, P.; Devaraj, H.; Niranjalidevaraj, S. Morin, a dietary flavonoid, exhibits anti-fibrotic effect and induces apoptosis of activated hepatic stellate cells by suppressing canonical NF-κB signaling. *Biochimie* **2015**, *110*, 107–118. [CrossRef] [PubMed]

100. Manna, S.K.; Aggarwal, R.S.; Sethi, G.; Aggarwal, B.B.; Ramesh, G.T. Morin (3,5,7,2′,4′-pentahydroxyflavone) abolishes nuclear factor-κB activation induced by various carcinogens and inflammatory stimuli, leading to suppression of nuclear factor-κB—Regulated gene expression and up-regulation of apoptosis. *Clin. Cancer Res.* **2007**, *13*, 2290–2297. [CrossRef] [PubMed]

101. Ferrer, P.; Asensi, M.; Priego, S.; Benlloch, M.; Mena, S.; Ortega, A.; Obrador, E.; Esteve, J.M.; Estrela, J.M. Nitric oxide mediates natural polyphenol-induced Bcl-2 down-regulation and activation of cell death in metastatic B16 melanoma. *J. Biol. Chem.* **2007**, *282*, 2880–2890. [CrossRef] [PubMed]

102. Torres, F.; Quintana, J.; Estévez, F. 5,7,3′-Trihydroxy-3,4′-Dimethoxyflavone Inhibits the Tubulin Polymerization and Activates the Sphingomyelin Pathway. *Mol. Carcinog.* **2011**, *50*, 113–122. [CrossRef] [PubMed]

103. Lee, P.S.; Chiou, Y.S.; Ho, C.T.; Pan, M.H. Chemoprevention by resveratrol and pterostilbene: Targeting on epigenetic regulation. *BioFactors* **2018**, *44*, 26–35. [CrossRef] [PubMed]

104. Zulueta, A.; Caretti, A.; Signorelli, P.; Ghidoni, R. Resveratrol: A potential challenger against gastric cancer. *World J. Gastroenterol.* **2015**, *21*, 10636–10643. [CrossRef] [PubMed]

105. Xianfeng, H.; Zhu, H.-L. Resveratrol and Its Analogues: Promising Antitumor Agents. *Anticancer. Agents Med. Chem.* **2011**, *11*, 479–490. [CrossRef]

106. Signorelli, P.; Ghidoni, R. Resveratrol as an anticancer nutrient: Molecular basis, open questions and promises. *J. Nutr. Biochem.* **2005**, *16*, 449–466. [CrossRef] [PubMed]

107. Signorelli, P.; Munoz-Olaya, J.M.; Gagliostro, V.; Casas, J.; Ghidoni, R.; Fabriàs, G. Dihydroceramide intracellular increase in response to resveratrol treatment mediates autophagy in gastric cancer cells. *Cancer Lett.* **2009**, *282*, 238–243. [CrossRef] [PubMed]

108. Shin, K.-O.; Park, N.-Y.; Seo, C.-H.; Hong, S.-P.; Oh, K.-W.; Hong, J.-T.; Han, S.-K.; Lee, Y.-M. Inhibition of sphingolipid metabolism enhances resveratrol chemotherapy in human gastric cancer cells. *Biomol. Ther.* **2012**, *20*, 470–476. [CrossRef] [PubMed]

109. Lin, H.Y.; Delmas, D.; Vang, O.; Hsieh, T.C.; Lin, S.; Cheng, G.Y.; Chiang, H.L.; Chen, C.E.; Tang, H.Y.; Crawford, D.R.; et al. Mechanisms of ceramide-induced COX-2-dependent apoptosis in human ovarian cancer OVCAR-3 cells partially overlapped with resveratrol. *J. Cell. Biochem.* **2013**, *114*, 1940–1954. [CrossRef] [PubMed]

110. Dixon, D. A Dysregulated post-transcriptional control of COX-2 gene expression in cancer. *Curr. Pharm. Des.* **2004**, *10*, 635–646. [CrossRef] [PubMed]

111. Zahner, G.; Wolf, G.; Ayoub, M.; Reinking, R.; Panzer, U.; Shankland, S.J.; Stahl, R.A. Cyclooxygenase-2 overexpression inhibits platelet-derived growth factor- induced mesangial cell proliferation through induction of the tumor suppressor gene p53 and the cyclin-dependent kinase inhibitors p21waf-1/cip-1 and p27kip-1. *J. Biol. Chem.* **2002**, *277*, 9763–9771. [CrossRef] [PubMed]

112. Lim, K.G.; Gray, A.I.; Pyne, S.; Pyne, N.J. Resveratrol dimers are novel sphingosine kinase 1 inhibitors and affect sphingosine kinase 1 expression and cancer cell growth and survival. *Br. J. Pharmacol.* **2012**, *166*, 1605–1616. [CrossRef] [PubMed]

113. Tian, H.; Yu, Z. Resveratrol induces apoptosis of leukemia cell line K562 by modulation of sphingosine kinase-1 pathway. *Int. J. Clin. Exp. Pathol.* **2015**, *8*, 2755–2762. [PubMed]

114. Cakir, Z.; Saydam, G.; Sahin, F.; Baran, Y. The roles of bioactive sphingolipids in resveratrol-induced apoptosis in HL60 acute myeloid leukemia cells. *J. Cancer Res. Clin. Oncol.* **2011**, *137*, 279–286. [CrossRef] [PubMed]

115. Kartal, M.; Saydam, G.; Sahin, F.; Baran, Y. Resveratrol triggers apoptosis through regulating ceramide metabolizing genes in human K562 chronic myeloid leukemia cells. *Nutr. Cancer* **2011**, *63*, 637–644. [CrossRef] [PubMed]

116. Chow, S.E.; Kao, C.H.; Liu, Y.T.A.; Cheng, M.L.; Yang, Y.W.; Huang, Y.K.; Hsu, C.C.; Wang, J.S. Resveratrol induced ER expansion and ER caspase-mediated apoptosis in human nasopharyngeal carcinoma cells. *Apoptosis* **2014**, *19*, 527–541. [CrossRef] [PubMed]

117. Wang, M.; Yu, T.; Zhu, C.; Sun, H.; Qiu, Y.; Zhu, X.; Li, J. Resveratrol triggers protective autophagy through the ceramide/Akt/mTOR pathway in melanoma B16 cells. *Nutr. Cancer* **2014**, *66*, 435–440. [CrossRef] [PubMed]

118. Mizutani, N.; Omori, Y.; Kawamoto, Y.; Sobue, S.; Ichihara, M.; Suzuki, M.; Kyogashima, M.; Nakamura, M.; Tamiya-Koizumi, K.; Nozawa, Y.; et al. Resveratrol-induced transcriptional up-regulation of ASMase (SMPD1) of human leukemia and cancer cells. *Biochem. Biophys. Res. Commun.* **2016**, *470*, 851–856. [CrossRef] [PubMed]

119. Scarlatti, F.; Sala, G.; Somenzi, G.; Signorelli, P.; Sacchi, N.; Ghidoni, R. Resveratrol induces growth inhibition and apoptosis in metastatic breast cancer cells via *de novo* ceramide signaling. *FASEB J.* **2003**, *17*, 2339–2341. [CrossRef] [PubMed]

120. Scarlatti, F.; Sala, G.; Ricci, C.; Maioli, C.; Milani, F.; Minella, M.; Botturi, M.; Ghidoni, R. Resveratrol sensitization of DU145 prostate cancer cells to ionizing radiation is associated to ceramide increase. *Cancer Lett.* **2007**, *253*, 124–130. [CrossRef] [PubMed]

121. Dolfini, E.; Roncoroni, L.; Dogliotti, E.; Sala, G.; Erba, E.; Sacchi, N.; Ghidoni, R. Resveratrol impairs the formation of MDA-MB-231 multicellular tumor spheroids concomitant with ceramide accumulation. *Cancer Lett.* **2007**, *249*, 143–147. [CrossRef] [PubMed]

122. Minutolo, F.; Sala, G.; Bagnacani, A.; Bertini, S.; Carboni, I.; Placanica, G.; Prota, G.; Rapposelli, S.; Sacchi, N.; Macchia, M.; et al. Synthesis of a resveratrol analogue with high ceramide-mediated proapoptotic activity on human breast cancer cells. *J. Med. Chem.* **2005**, *48*, 6783–6786. [CrossRef] [PubMed]

123. Davis-Searles, P.R.; Nakanishi, Y.; Kim, N.C.; Graf, T.N.; Oberlies, N.H.; Wani, M.C.; Wall, M.E.; Agarwal, R.; Kroll, D.J. Milk thistle and prostate cancer: Differential effects of pure flavonolignans from Silybum marianum on antiproliferative end points in human prostate carcinoma cells. *Cancer Res.* **2005**, *65*, 4448–4457. [CrossRef] [PubMed]

124. Boojar, M.M.A.; Hassanipour, M.; Mehr, S.E.; Boojar, M.M.A.; Dehpour, A.R. New aspects of silibinin stereoisomers and their 3-o-galloyl derivatives on cytotoxicity and ceramide metabolism in hep G2hepatocarcinoma cell line. *Iran. J. Pharm. Res.* **2016**, *15*, 421–433.

125. Xuan, N.T.; Shumilina, E.; Gulbins, E.; Gu, S.; Götz, F.; Lang, F. Triggering of dendritic cell apoptosis by xanthohumol. *Mol. Nutr. Food Res.* **2010**, *54*. [CrossRef] [PubMed]

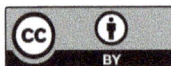

MDPI

St. Alban-Anlage 66

4052 Basel

Switzerland

Tel. +41 61 683 77 34

Fax +41 61 302 89 18

www.mdpi.com

Nutrients Editorial Office

E-mail: nutrients@mdpi.com

www.mdpi.com/journal/nutrients